A MIDWIFE'S HANDBOOK

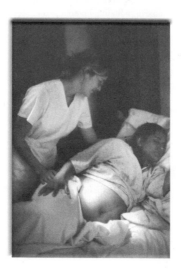

CONSTANCE SINCLAIR, CNM, MSN

Staff Nurse-Midwife
Kaiser Permanente Medical Center
Santa Rosa, California

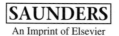

SAUNDERS

An Imprint of Elsevier

SAUNDERS

An Imprint of Elsevier

11830 Westline Industrial Drive
St. Louis, Missouri 63146

A MIDWIFE'S HANDBOOK   0-7216-8168-9
Copyright © 2004, Elsevier (USA). All rights reserved.

Notice

Library of Congress Cataloging in Publication Data

Sinclair, Constance
    A midwife's handbook/Constance Sinclair.
      p. cm.
    Includes bibliographical references and index.
    ISBN 0-7216-8168-9 (alk. paper)
    I. Midwifery—Handbooks, manuals, etc. I. Title.
RG950.S565 2004
618.2—dc21   2003050553

Executive Editor: Michael S. Ledbetter
Developmental Editor: Amanda Sunderman Politte
Publishing Services Manager: Deborah L. Vogel
Project Manager: Kelley Barbarick, Ann E. Rogers, Jodi M. Willard
Designer: Teresa Breckwoldt
Cover Art: Daphne Waldo

Printed in the United States of America.

Last digit is the print number: 9   8   7   6   5   4   3   2   1

Dedication

My family and I recently visited Sutter's Mill in Coloma, California, where gold was discovered. The ranger briefly mentioned a nearby site where Indian women had ground acorns. We walked over to the huge boulder and read that the Maidu Indians had lived in the little valley for 12,000 years before 1864. On the boulder were a dozen or more indentations—actually inches-deep from centuries of use. I was deeply moved as I imagined all the women who had gathered in that place to work together. The mothers would surely have shared birth stories with babies alongside and children playing at the base of the rock; older women would have shared their knowledge; the healers—the midwives—would have taught their craft. I could nearly hear their conversations, their singing, their laughter. It is to these women—all of those who came before us—that I wish to dedicate this book.

My maternal grandmother, Jeannie Robb Howard, emigrated from Scotland when she was 21. She bore undiagnosed twins—my mother and her sister—in 1930, the depth of the depression. She was the quintessential "Grandma" with her brogue, her knitting, her shortbread, and the way she attended with rapt interest as she listened. I dedicate this book to her with love.

My paternal grandmother, Margaret "Madge" Spears Sinclair, was Canadian. She and my grandfather homesteaded in Southern Saskatchewan, where she bore her four youngest children on a stark prairie with neighbor women to help her. As the preacher's wife, she was a midwife to women in the community. She died the year I was born. I dedicate this book to her, wishing I had known her.

I have been blessed with two daughters. I hope that they will find a profession that offers them as much gratification as midwifery has given me. I dedicate this book to Hannah and Olivia. They have taught me the one thing I could never have imagined from all my study and experience of midwifery: the breathtaking dimensions of a mother's love.

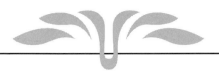

Primary Reviewers

Gina Jensen-Hill, CNM, MSN
CommuniCare Health Centers
Davis, California

Carolyn B. Moes, RN, MSN, CNM
Clinical Research Coordinator/Nurse Clinician
Department of Obstetrics and Gynecology
University Hospitals of Cleveland
Clinical Instructor
Department of Reproductive Biology
School of Medicine
Case Western Reserve University
Cleveland, Ohio

Cynthia N. Opderbeck, CNM, MSN
Obstetrics/Gynecology
Fort Defiance Indian Hospital
Fort Defiance, Arizona

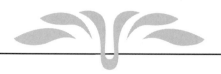

Reviewers

Patricia Burkhardt, CNM, DrPH
Program Director, Midwifery Program
New York University
New York, New York

Lee Clay, CNM, MS
Staff Midwife
Morristown Memorial Hospital
Morristown, New Jersey

Virginia Crandall, MSN, CNM, ACCE
Nurse Practitioner, Women's Health Care
Indian River County Health Department
Indian River County, Florida

H. Frances Cushenberry, MSN, CNM, JD, EDD(c)
Program Director, Nurse-Midwifery Education Program
College of Allied Health
Charles R. Drew University of Medicine and Science
Los Angeles, California

Carol Howe, CNM, DNSc, FACNM
Director, Nurse-Midwifery
Oregon Health & Science University
Portland, Oregon

Lauren P. Hunter, RN, PhD, CNM
Director, Graduate Nurse-Midwifery Education
School of Nursing
College of Health and Human Services
San Diego State University
San Diego, California

Kathleen Utter King, CNM, MS
Senior Associate
University of Rochester
School of Nursing
Rochester, New York

Gloria M. Mondor, MS, CNM, RN
Senior Teaching Specialist
School of Nursing
University of Minnesota
Minneapolis, Minnesota

Donna Scheideberg, CNM, PhD
Adjunct Faculty
Clarke College
Department of Nursing;
Nurse-Midwife
Medical Associates
Dubuque, Iowa

Marilyn L. Stewart
University of Utah
College of Nursing
Salt Lake City, Utah

Preface

This handbook is written for midwifery students and for experienced midwives. Its scope is broad, including most areas of midwifery practice. A list format is often used, words and phrases within the text are set in **boldface** type, and a management icon 🄜 indicates the management sections. This makes the book useful as a tool to scan and quickly determine the completeness of an evaluation or a plan. Its organization, cross-referencing, and indexing are meant to make it easily accessible for use. It includes visit and examination formats for the student. It provides an update for the experienced midwife, as well as reviewing conditions that may arise infrequently in clinical practice. In many practices, midwives work closely with physician specialists, often managing the uncomplicated aspects of the patient's care while the physician manages the complications. A basic overview of medical and gynecologic complications and their treatment is included here to give the midwife a more comprehensive understanding of the woman's health, needs, and medical management. In other cases, a patient may be referred for physician care. This handbook provides the anticipatory guidance needed when the woman asks about her condition and its treatment. I offer this handbook in the hopes that it will be as interesting and useful to others as it has been for me to research.

Many complementary measures are included in this text. I am not a specialist in any of the complementary areas but wish, as do many midwives, to become more knowledgeable about these arts and sciences. I offer a brief overview of several healing arts in Chapter 11 and include complementary suggestions for a number of conditions throughout the book. Charts are included to help the practitioner learn relevant Chinese acupressure points and reflexology zones. The reader is encouraged to read the section regarding the safety of herbal remedies and to determine his or her own comfort level with herbal practice. This handbook offers a first step in developing a familiarity with herbal remedies by listing those herbs recommended by three or more herbalists. In some cases where authors did not duplicate their suggestions, I refer the reader to an herbalist who has suggestions for a particular condition. Inclusion of herbal suggestions in this text does not imply that I have used these remedies nor is it an endorsement of their use. Finally, the art of homeopathy offers remedies for many of the conditions described. Choosing the right remedy, however, requires a lengthy holistic evaluation of the woman. In the interest of space, I could not list all of the criteria that should be considered for every homeopathic prescription. Instead, I list homeopathic authors who include a discussion of that malady and its remedies for the interested reader. The complementary sections were fascinating to write and I hope they are of value to the reader.

Acknowledgments

At the beginning of our midwifery program at the University of Pennsylvania, we were encouraged to keep a notebook of all those things that could not be kept in our brain—a "peripheral brain." I kept a few notes, but my classmate Elizabeth Parr, CNM, showed me her impressive peripheral brain well into the program and inspired me to compile a more complete reference during integration. Rebecca Morris, CNM, my former integration student, looked at my peripheral brain and encouraged me to publish it. James Campisano, Chief of Obstetrics, and Carol Thomason, Director of Midwifery at Kaiser Medical Center, Santa Rosa, allowed me to take the time that I needed to complete the book. Carol also lent me her own peripheral brain for inspiration. Leeni Balogh, Kaiser librarian, patiently and generously obtained multiple articles for me and assisted immeasurably in the research for the book. Richard Klekman, Brad Golditch, and Austin Kooba, Kaiser obstetricians, provided literature, insight, information, and encouragement. Elizabeth Smith, CNM, an integration student at the time, offered ideas and resources. David Walker, acupuncturist, gave me encouragement, information, and resources regarding the Chinese medicine complementary measures in this text. The section on doulas was inspired by Humm Berryessa, a doula with whom I am privileged to work. Humm combines commitment, knowledge, insight, and wisdom and has taught me the potential of the doula role. I am delighted that the front of the book is graced with a photograph by Daphne Waldo. Besides creating beautiful images, Daphne is a joy to work with. Thank you to Rebecca McLeod and especially to Carmen Rodriguez, and her beautiful little daughter, Kaylee, who graciously participated in the photo shoot, as well as to other Kaiser colleagues, who let us photograph them at work.

It's a scary thing to write about midwifery. Words are often inadequate to the task of describing a profession that is so grounded in intuition, experience, and touch. Moreover, there are as many ways to be a good midwife as there are labors to attend. As I have slowly brought this project to its fruition, once again I must express my deep regard for all the folks at Saunders/Mosby, who invested wholeheartedly in this work long before it was finished. To the most patient of midwives, Michael Ledbetter, my editor, I express my deepest appreciation. Always encouraging and positive, Michael could not have been more supportive or more flexible. I am so grateful for his guidance and his belief in me.

Other Mosby/Saunders personnel participated in the editing process: Victoria Bruno began this project with me in Philadelphia and was always supportive and helpful. Amanda Politte has patiently kept track of countless charts, boxes, figures, chapters, reviews, illustrations, and permissions. Kelley Barbarick began the book production process with skill and friendly, encouraging concern. Ann Rogers and Jodi Willard assumed the book production when it was at full throttle. Their commitment to this project was truly as if they had been there from the beginning, and they have made valuable additions to the book. The illustrator, Will Horton, added immeasurably to this book with his illustrations. Carolyn Jarvis and Pat Thomas were kind enough to allow me to borrow the beautiful illustration for Leopold's maneuvers and others from their Saunders text, *Physical Examination and Health Assessment.*

Two personal friends, whose knowledge and practice of midwifery I deeply respect, participated directly in the making of this book. Gina Jensen-Hill, CNM, and Cynthia Opderbeck, CNM, offered to review the manuscript. Neither of them realized the extent of the task for which they had volunteered. Cynthia made time around her work, her family, her gardens, and her lamb farm to make suggestions, especially for the intrapartum chapter. Gina persevered faithfully through the entire manuscript. She made excellent suggestions and was supportive and interested in the final outcome. I so appreciate the help by both provided. Several other midwives blindly reviewed parts of the manuscript. One of these, Carolyn Moes, was particularly generous in her efforts. She reviewed the entire manuscript. She enclosed references and even articles that she thought might be useful. She wrote notes of encouragement in the margins. She invested great effort trusting a midwife she did not know to take her comments and integrate them into a worthy end product. I am deeply moved by her giving spirit and am appreciative of her input. All of these individuals gave their best to help me make this book the best that it could be, and I am deeply grateful.

Finally—and especially—I could not have completed this project without the support of my husband, Steve Cordis. Besides providing technical support (ah! the computer age), he has never complained about the time I was investing or about never seeing me in daylight hours without a book chapter in my hands.

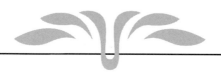

Contents

Chapter 4 **The Puerperium,** 224

Chapter 5 **The Newborn,** 248

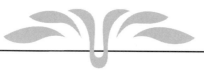

Chapter 1

Normal Pregnancy

• PRECONCEPTION VISIT FORMAT

The preconception visit includes assessment, education, and health-promoting interventions. Take the opportunity to provide this information and care to all women who might become pregnant, because women who experience unintended pregnancies are likely to have at least as many risk factors for complications as women who plan to become pregnant.

Assessment

- **Family history:** Including history of congenital disorders (especially phenylketonuria, neural tube defects, or chromosomal disorders)
- **Medical/surgical history:** Including childhood diseases, hepatitis, vaccination status, risk factors for diabetes (early glucose control, which is critical in preventing anomalies), and tuberculosis exposure
- **Gynecologic history:** Whether the woman has been attempting pregnancy and for how long, human immunodeficiency virus (HIV) risk behaviors and testing results, type of contraception (if any) used, presence of infection or other condition such as an abnormal Pap smear result, and risk factors for breast cancer
- **Obstetric history:** Complications in previous pregnancy that present risk factors for subsequent pregnancies
- **Teratogenic risks: Medication use,** including use of over-the-counter (OTC) drugs; **substance abuse,** including cigarette smoking; and **occupational hazards**
- **Lifestyle history: Exercise** patterns, **nutritional assessment** including use of supplements, pica, vegetarianism, eating disorders, adequacy of financial resources, and special dietary considerations such as phenylketonuria or lactose intolerance
- **Dental health:** Date of last dental visit, whether woman has untreated dental problems
- **Social history:** Quality of primary relationship and support system, domestic or sexual **abuse,** adequacy of **housing and financial**

resources including health insurance, any **relevant cultural practices,** and presence of **cats** in home
- **Partner's family history:** Including congenital disorders, **HIV** status and risk behaviors, and **environmental hazards** that may affect sperm health
- **Sexual practices: Frequency and timing** of intercourse, **positions and practices** (use of any oils, creams, or other substances), whether both partners are **monogamous**
- **Physical examination** for normalcy of all systems, screening for gynecologic **infections,** a **Pap** smear, and a **CBC;** offer an **HIV** test

Education and Health Promotion Interventions

- Arrange **genetic counseling** for the woman at risk because of genetic predisposition or teratogenic exposure. Offer **cystic fibrosis screening.**[2]
- Because **medical conditions** such as diabetes or hypertension should be closely controlled before pregnancy, refer the client to her primary care provider for management of these conditions. Baseline studies may be required. Counsel regarding the impact of any condition on pregnancy, her health, and that of her planned fetus. Counsel regarding the **safety of any medication.** Facilitate the prescribing of alternatives to potentially teratogenic medications.
- Treat ongoing infections or **gynecologic conditions** before pregnancy. Discuss high-risk behaviors. Offer **HIV** testing. Refer the HIV-positive woman for treatment and counseling regarding the risks of sexual activity to an HIV-negative partner, risks to the fetus, and current interventions available to minimize risk.
- Offer **immunization** for rubella, varicella, hepatitis B, and tetanus to the nonimmune woman when pregnancy can be delayed for 3 months after a live viral immunization.[87]
- Advise the woman that the breast changes of pregnancy and lactation may delay detection of breast lumps. Increased density renders mammograms less reliable. Offer a **mammogram** before pregnancy.
- Review **risks for pregnancy complications** associated with the obstetric history and suggest appropriate interventions.
- Counsel regarding **lifestyle risk factors** such as poor nutritional status, overweight or underweight, exercise pattern, cigarette smoking, and alcohol intake, which decrease fertility and increase the risk for pregnancy complications. Refer for support if necessary (e.g., for assistance with substance abuse). Discuss **fetal vulnerability during organogenesis** and the need for optimal lifestyle during the preconception and conception periods.
- Counsel regarding **sexual practices** and fertility: menstrual cycle and fertility, eliminating the use of lubricants, ideal sexual positioning and frequency.

- Counsel regarding **nutritional needs** during the childbearing years. Advise regarding excesses (such as oversupplementation of fat-soluble vitamins). Refer for nutritional counseling if needs are complex. Suggest **supplementation** for specific deficiencies. Most women benefit from supplementation with calcium. Women with no family history of neural tube defects should **supplement folic acid** with 400 μg daily for 6 to 8 weeks before conception. If a family history of neural tube defects is present, 4 mg is suggested.[9]
- Counsel regarding the importance of gestational dating in pregnancy management, the need for **keeping accurate menstrual records,** and the importance of an **early first prenatal visit.**
- Teach the cat owner about **toxoplasmosis** risks and safety measures (see p. 373).
- Suggest obtaining necessary **dental care** before conception.
- **Refer for counseling or social service** support as advisable for signs of, for example, domestic abuse, mental health problems, or financial needs.
- Counsel regarding **ideal pregnancy spacing.** Eighteen months after a live birth, maternal nutritional stores are replenished, and postpartum stress is resolved. Conception at this time reduces adverse perinatal outcomes.[112]
- Integrate **cultural** practices, beliefs, and concerns into all counseling.

• ANTEPARTUM VISIT FORMAT

Initial Antepartum Visit Format

Some of the following functions are performed by nursing support staff in some practices. Physician referral and consultation are individualized for each practice and according to each state's requirements.

Interview/History

1. Make **introductions** and review agenda.
2. Determine **whether pregnancy is desired,** and if not, whether the woman wants information regarding termination or adoption. The woman desiring termination requires menstrual and gynecologic histories and uterine sizing.
3. Perform **social assessment,** including support network, housing, food, domestic abuse, safety, whether a social services referral is indicated, cultural traditions, or concerns.
4. Provide **written information** regarding practice arrangements.
5. Take family, medical/ surgical/gynecologic, and menstrual **histories.**
6. Take **obstetric history:** year and place of each delivery, number of weeks gestation, type of delivery, perineal injury for vaginal delivery, indication and type of incision for cesarean delivery, anesthesia, sex and weight of infant and whether alive now, and any complications.

Present Pregnancy History

1. **Establish estimated date of confinement (EDC).**
   a. Determine the **last normal menstrual period (LNMP)** and the certainty of the date. Use Naegele's rule to determine the EDC: add 7 days to the first day of the last known menstrual period and count back 3 months.
   b. Determine the date of positive **pregnancy test** result and whether serum or urine was used. Does the test confirm the EDC?
   c. Note the date on which **quickening** was noted and whether there is ongoing fetal movement. Does the quickening date confirm the EDC?
   d. What **contraceptive** was used most recently, and when was use discontinued?
2. Determine the woman's health status since becoming pregnant. Ask the following questions:
   a. Has the woman been seen by any **health care provider** (including alternative) since becoming pregnant?
   b. Has she had a fever, rash, or any type of **infection?**
   c. Has she been involved in any **accidents?**
   d. Has she taken any prescribed or OTC **medications?** Does she have a history of **substance abuse** (including cigarettes)?
   e. Has she had an **x-ray** examination?
   f. Have **supplements** (including vitamins), tinctures, herbs, homeopathy, or other complementary remedies been used?
   g. Has the woman consumed raw meat or been exposed to hazardous materials (potential **teratogenic** events)?
   h. Has she experienced **vaginal bleeding** or signs of **vaginal infection:** lesions, itching, burning, or discharge? Does she or her partner have a history of genital **herpes?**
   i. Has she experienced signs of **urinary tract infection (UTI):** burning or frequency?
   j. Has she experienced urinary incontinence? (Twenty-one percent of women report urinary incontinence after spontaneous vaginal delivery; 34% after instrumental vaginal delivery.)[74a]
   k. Has she experienced fecal incontinence? (From 5.5% to 22% of women report fecal incontinence after vaginal delivery.)[43a,74a]
   l. What was her **weight** before pregnancy? What are her dietary habits? Is she having cravings?
   m. Has she experienced **gastrointestinal (GI) symptoms:** nausea, vomiting, heartburn, constipation, or hemorrhoids?
   n. Has she experienced **central nervous system (CNS) symptoms:** headaches, fatigue, dizziness, syncope, or visual problems?
   o. Has she had back or abdominal pain?
   p. Has she had **leg** cramps? Are varicosities present?
   q. What changes has she observed in her **breasts?**
   r. Has she experienced **shortness of breath?**
   s. Has she had **edema,** especially of hands and face?

    t. How is she **sleeping?** Is she **exercising?**
    u. Are there **cats** in the home?
    v. What other **concerns** does the woman have?
3. Determine whether **genetic screening** should be performed. Indications for genetic screening include maternal age >35 years; maternal history of three or more first-trimester spontaneous abortions (SABs); stillbirth; use of medications or street drugs since last menses; or in either parent or his or her family a history of any of the following: thalassemia, neural tube defects, Down syndrome, Tay-Sachs disease, muscular dystrophy, hemophilia, sickle cell anemia, cystic fibrosis, Huntington's chorea, mental retardation (etiology?), or any inherited genetic or chromosomal disorder.

Physical Examination

The woman's weight and urine measurement of glucose and protein levels are obtained. Give the woman drapes and have her undress completely. Perform a physical examination, including the following.

TAKE THE BLOOD PRESSURE. If the woman is anxious, or if the BP is high, it may alternately be taken at the end of the physical examination.

BREASTS. Inspect with hands on waist, at sides, over head, leaning over. Palpate axillary nodes, breasts (including the tail of Spence), and nipples (express). Teach breast self-examination. Note skin and breast changes of pregnancy including hyperpigmentation of nipples and areolae, prominent veins, mammary souffle, and tenderness and nodularity of breast tissue.

ABDOMEN. Inspect for contour, symmetry, hernias, distention, abnormal pulsations, scars, linea nigra, and striae. Auscultate for bowel sounds in all quadrants. Percuss the abdominal area, noting the bladder, liver, spleen (tenth rib with deep inspiration), and gastric air. Palpate each quadrant lightly then deeply over the liver, spleen, kidneys, and aorta. Note any rigidity, guarding, tenderness, or masses.

After 12 weeks, measure fundal height and auscultate fetal heart tones (FHTs), noting location. After 20 weeks, determine fetal position by using Leopold's maneuvers to locate FHTs. At 20 weeks, listen for FHTs with fetoscope to confirm dating. Note the condition of the uterus—whether tender, soft, irritable, or contracting. Observe for fetal movement. At 34 or more weeks, if a nonvertex position is noted, this must be addressed (see p. 157). At term, estimate fetal weight.

LEOPOLD'S MANEUVERS. Assessment of the fetal variety, presentation, position, and lie is conducted after the fundal height is measured (a contraction may be stimulated by the maneuvers, altering fundal height). The woman's bladder should be empty for accuracy and comfort. See Figure 1-1.
First maneuver: Determine the contents of the fundus.

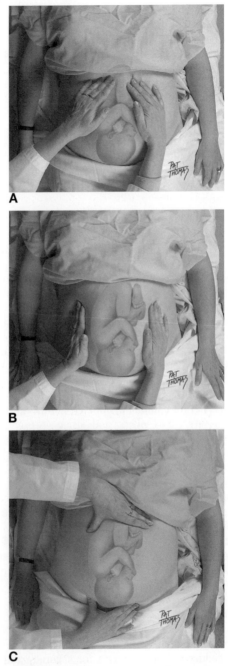

Figure 1-1 • Leopold's maneuvers. **A,** First maneuver; **B,** second maneuver; **C,** third
maneuver (or Pawlik's maneuver). *Continued*

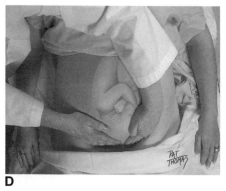

D

Figure 1-1 • cont'd **D,** fourth maneuver. (From Jarvis C: *Physical examination and health assessment,* ed 3, Philadelphia, 2000, WB Saunders.)

Second maneuver: Palpate the sides of the uterus to locate the small parts and the back. Determine the lie of the fetus and the orientation in relation to the maternal pelvis.

Third maneuver (Pawlik's maneuver): With the woman's knees slightly bent, grasp the lower portion of the abdomen between thumb and middle finger to determine the presenting part.

Fourth maneuver: With the woman's knees still bent, press the fingers of both hands on the lower abdomen, pointing toward the pelvis. Press centrally, attempting to move your fingers in front of the presenting part. If you can, the presenting part is unengaged. If the head is presenting, and if it is engaged, your fingers will meet a hard round object on one or both sides. If the object is on both sides, then you are palpating the occiput and the chin, and the head is entering the pelvis in an unflexed (military) position. If you feel the round object on one side only—the same side as the fetal back—you are palpating the occiput of a deflexed head, and the infant is entering the pelvis in a face presentation. If you feel the round object on the opposite side from the back, then you are palpating the forehead of a well-flexed head entering the pelvis in an occiput presentation. Presenting part, position, and engagement are thus determined.

PELVIC EXAMINATION. This examination is conducted with the woman's bladder empty for comfort and accuracy. The woman positions herself on the examination table with her legs in stirrups.

1. **External examination:** Palpate Bartholin's glands, the urethra, and Skene's glands; note any discharge. Note any scarring of the perineum or other genitalia. Note any hemorrhoids. Observe for **Chadwick's sign** of pregnancy (discoloration of vulva and vaginal walls).

2. **Speculum examination:**
   a. **Vagina:** Note color (Chadwick's sign?), inflammation, vaginal secretions (quantity, color, character, consistency, and odor)

and any lesions. The **pH** of the secretions is determined using narrow-range pH paper. A pH >4.5 suggests bacterial vaginosis or Trichomonas infection (see pp. 474 and 480). A wet mount is used to diagnose suspected vaginal infection (see p. 579).

b. **Cervix:** Note location, size, and shape; any scarring, polyps, inflammation, or secretions; whether dilated; presence of Nabothian cysts or other lesions; discharge (color, quantity, character, consistency, odor); friability; and ectropion. Box 1-1 describes variations that may be seen on the cervical examination.

3. Bimanual examination: The second and third fingers of the examiner's prominent hand are lubricated and placed into the vagina. The examiner's other hand rests on the woman's lower abdomen.

a. **Cervix:** Note size, consistency, position, dilation, effacement, mobility, and any tenderness. Observe for **Goodell's sign** of pregnancy (softened consistency of the cervix).

b. **Vagina:** Note the integrity of the anterior and posterior vaginal walls, as well as the presence of cysts, nodules, or masses. Have the woman demonstrate her vaginal tone and teach the **Kegel exercise.**

c. **Uterus:** Note size, consistency, mobility, shape, position, and any tenderness. Is the uterus levo-rotated or dextro-rotated? Observe for **Piskacek's sign** of pregnancy (slight enlargement of one cornu at the implantation site) and **Hegar's sign** of pregnancy (compressible neck of the uterus).

d. **Adnexa:** Are ovaries palpable? If so, note size, shape, and any tenderness. Are any masses present?

e. **Rectovaginal examination:** Using the dominant hand, the examiner places the second finger in the vagina and the third finger in

---

• *Box 1-1* / **Variations in Cervical Examination Findings** •

- **Cancer:** Small hardened granular area that bleeds at the slightest touch. Surrounding tissue may be normal OR may show chronic cervicitis.
- **Nabothian cysts:** White or opaque blebs.
- **Ectropion or eversion:** Rolling of endocervix out toward ectocervix.
- **Erosion:** Red, granular zone where superficial epithelium has been lost; friable.
- **Acute cervicitis:** Red, swollen; WBCs observed on the wet mount; profuse, purulent discharge.
- **Chronic cervicitis:** Endocervix thickened, white purulent discharge, erythema around the os; must be differentiated from neoplasm.
- **Polyps:** Hyperplasia of endocervical epithelium appearing as red, fragile, spongy fingerlike masses.
- **Herpes:** Vesicles, ulcers, surrounded by inflammation and edema.
- **Leukoplakia:** White or gray irregular angular plaques, slightly raised from surface. May be neoplastic.

the rectum. A rectovaginal examination is indicated annually for women ≥40 years or if bimanual findings are uncertain.[48] Do findings confirm above findings? Note masses, sphincter tone, polyps, nodules, strictures, and rectovaginal musculature. Obtain stool sample and test stool for occult blood for women ≥ 40 years.

PELVIMETRY. Pelvimetry can be postponed until the third trimester when vaginal walls are more distensible. Assess the pelvic outlet, noting its suitability for vaginal birth. See Figure 1-2. The gynecoid measurements noted in the following list indicate those considered large enough to pass the average-sized fetus:

1. Note width of the **pubic arch** in fingerbreadths (FBs). *Gynecoid: 2 to 3 FBs*
2. Note curvature and direction of the **sidewalls.** *Gynecoid: straight sidewalls*
3. Locate and assess the shape and encroachment of the **ischial spine.** *Gynecoid: flat spines*
4. Estimate the **interspinous diameter.** *Gynecoid: 10 cm*
5. Note the shape and direction of the **sacrum** and the dimensions of the posterior pelvis. *Gynecoid: concave sacrum parallel to symphysis pubis*
6. Note whether the **coccyx** is mobile, fixed, or encroaching into pelvis. *Gynecoid: mobile*
7. Locate the **sacrospinous ligament,** measure the width in FBs. *Gynecoid: 2 to 3 FBs*
8. Note the shape of the **sacrospinous arch.** *Gynecoid: rounded*
9. Assess the **opposite side of the pelvis** for similarity.
10. Estimate the length of the diameter from the suprapubic arch to the sacral promontory—the **diagonal conjugate**—or state the measurement as being greater than the measurement of one's hand (e.g., >12 cm). *Gynecoid: >12 cm*
11. Measure the diameter between the ischial tuberosities by pressing the knuckles on one's fisted hand against them externally. Estimate this **biischial diameter** (also called the *bituberous* or *intertuberous diameter*) or note a measurement greater than the measurement of one's hand, such as >8 cm. *Gynecoid: ≥8 cm*
12. Record findings, describing pelvis according to its shape and size. See Figure 1-3 for descriptions of the pelvic types.

Conclusion of Visit

1. **Discuss findings.** Answer **questions.** Review **danger signs and symptoms** and how to call in an emergency.
2. Schedule **next prenatal visit.** Prescribe prenatal **vitamins.** Make **referrals.** Order ultrasound examination and laboratory tests: Pap smear, gonorrhea (GC) and chlamydia (CT) cultures, blood type, Rhesus factor, antibody screening, VDRL (alternatively, serologic

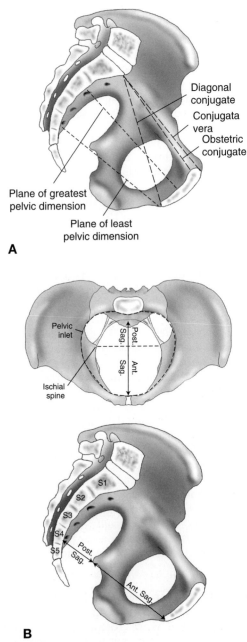

Figure 1-2 • Planes of the pelvis and their diameters. **A,** The inlet of the pelvis. **B,** The midplane of the pelvis. (From Walsh LV: *Midwifery: community-based care during the child-bearing year*, Philadelphia, 2001, WB Saunders.)

Continued

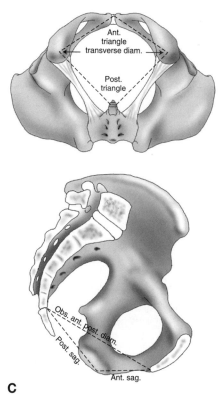

C

Figure 1-2 • cont'd **C,** The outlet of the pelvis. (From Walsh LV: *Midwifery: community-based care during the childbearing year,* Philadelphia, 2001, WB Saunders.)

test for syphilis [STS] or rapid plasmin reagin [RPR]), hepatitis B antigen, rubella titer, CBC, urinalysis (UA). Order time-appropriate laboratory tests (e.g., triple screening at 16 weeks). Offer HIV testing. Order a TSH for women with symptoms or a personal or family history of thyroid disease.[3] Additionally, in some practices the following tests will be ordered: sickle cell prep, hemoglobin electrophoresis, PPD (unless known to be positive), varicella titer, urine culture, cervical cultures for *Mycoplasma hominis* and bacterial vaginosis.

3. Document the visit and findings in the client's chart.

Return Antepartum Visit Format

1. Review client's chart.
2. Determine weight and obtain urine sample for determination of protein and glucose.
3. Interval history: Ask client about quickening date and fetal movement, vaginal bleeding, abdominal pain, urinary difficulties, and

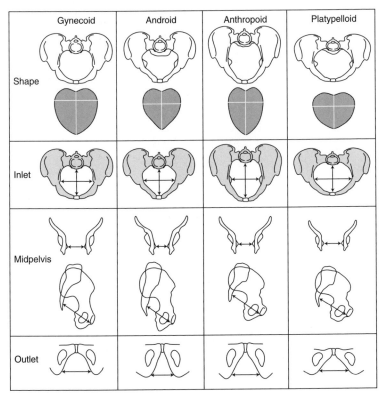

	Gynecoid	Android	Anthropoid	Platypelloid
Shape				
Inlet				
Midpelvis				
Outlet				

Figure 1-3 • Common pelvic types and their planes. (From Walsh LV: *Midwifery: community-based care during the childbearing year*, Philadelphia, 2001, WB Saunders.)

edema. After 20 weeks, ask about signs and symptoms of preeclampsia including headaches, visual disturbances, epigastric pain, and edema.

4. Take blood pressure.
5. Review test results.
6. Measure fundal height. Note concordance with dates.
7. After 20 weeks, perform Leopold's maneuvers to facilitate auscultation of FHTs. The nonvertex presentation is otherwise clinically significant only after 34 weeks.
8. Auscultate FHTs, noting location. Auscultation with fetoscope confirms 20-week dating.
9. Teach client about danger signs, comfort measures for common discomforts, signs and symptoms of labor.
10. Laboratory tests: At 16 to 18 weeks, offer maternal serum alpha-fetoprotein (MSAFP) test or triple screening. At 24 to 28 weeks, schedule 50-g glucose tolerance screening test and repeat hema-

tocrit (Hct) and hemoglobin (Hb). Perform antibody screening for the Rh-negative woman, and if the result is negative, offer her RhoGAM. At 32 to 34 weeks, repeat GC and CT. An RPR may be repeated. A vaginal/rectal GBS culture is performed. In the anemic woman, Hct and Hb may be repeated at 32 and/or 36 weeks.

11. Fetal surveillance: At 41 weeks, schedule postdate testing for fetal well-being every 3 to 4 days until delivery (NST, AFI, or BPP) (see p. 75).
12. Review the management plan with the client, addressing concerns. Schedule tests and the return visit.
13. Document the visit and findings in the client's chart.

Prenatal Visit Frequency

1. **ACOG recommends** prenatal visits every 4 weeks up to 28 to 32 weeks' gestation, every 2 weeks until 36 weeks, and every week thereafter until delivery.
2. A **reduced-frequency visit schedule** includes one visit in each of the following intervals: weeks 6 to 8, weeks 14 to 16, weeks 24 to 28, week 32, week 36, week 38, then weekly until delivery.[108]

• DIAGNOSIS OF PREGNANCY

Differential Diagnoses:

Pregnancy is diagnosed by evaluating the following signs:

Presumptive Signs of Pregnancy	Probable Signs of Pregnancy	Positive Signs of Pregnancy
Cessation of menses	Enlarged abdomen	Fetal movement perceived by the examiner
Breast pain and tingling	Ballottement	FHTs present
Fatigue	Change in uterine shape, size, consistency	Fetus visible on x-ray or ultrasound examination[36]
Breast enlargement	Palpable outline of fetus	
Chadwick's sign (see p. 7)	Softening of the cervix	
Skin pigmentation changes, including breasts, linea nigra	Braxton Hicks contractions	
Nausea and/or vomiting	Positive human chorionic gonadotropin (hCG) test result (home urine pregnancy test kits 99% correct when performed accurately within a few days of missed menses)[110]	
Increased urinary frequency		
Development of Montgomery's tubercles		
Perception of fetal movement		
The woman's belief that she is pregnant		

Irregular menses may be due to lactation, menopause, menarche, starvation, chronic disease, excessive exercise, or stress. Breast and skin changes may be caused by oral contraceptive use, use of certain tranquilizers, or tumors. Palmer erythema of the first trimester should be differentiated from hepatitis. An enlarged uterus may be due to subserous fibroids or adenomyosis. The positive HCG test result may have been contaminated or run too early or too late. HCG is secreted by bronchogenic carcinoma, and the hCG concentration may be elevated in a woman with systemic lupus erythematosus. Menopause causes elevation of the luteinizing hormone (LH) level, which can cause a false-positive result. Cervical ripening may be a side effect of oral contraceptives. Phenothiazines can cause amenorrhea, breast changes, and false-positive pregnancy test results. Spurious pregnancy and pseudocyesis present with pregnancy symptoms.[36]

• DANGER SIGNS AND SYMPTOMS DURING PREGNANCY

Reportable Warning Signs[36]

Signs of Possible Preterm Labor or Preterm Premature Rupture of the Membranes (PPROM):

- Contractions ≥ 4 times/hr (may be perceived as abdominal pain, tightening, backache, menstrual cramping, or vaginal pressure)
- Change in vaginal secretions (thick, thin, mucoid, any color)
- Vaginal bleeding
- Fluid coming from the vagina

Signs of an Illness with the Potential for Dehydration:

- Persistent vomiting
- Generalized, flu-like aching
- Chills or fever

Signs of Urinary Tract Infection (UTI):

- Dysuria, urgency, increased frequency

Signs of Preeclampsia:

- Severe or continuous headache, unrelieved by acetaminophen, or varying in character from usual headaches
- Visual problems (blurring or scotoma)
- Epigastric or right upper abdominal pain
- New or sudden increase in swelling of extremities or face
- Rapid weight gain

Nonreassuring Sign of Fetal Well-Being:

- Change in intensity or frequency of fetal movement

• FETAL GROWTH AND DEVELOPMENT

Women often enjoy learning about the current development of their fetuses. Such information may also enhance prenatal bonding in the adolescent or other women. See Table 1-1 for fetal size and developmental information.

• PSYCHOLOGICAL TASKS OF THE PREGNANT COUPLE

The parental role is developed anew for each child during the pregnancy.[15] The woman's development is affected by her relationship with her mother and with the baby's father. Some authors have described the

Table 1-1 / Fetal Size and Characteristics

Age (wk from LNMP)	CR Length (mm)*	Foot Length (mm)	Fetal Weight (g)†	Main External Characteristics
Previable Fetuses				
11	50	7	8	Eyes closing or closed. Head more rounded. External genitalia still not distinguished as male or female. Intestines in umbilical cord.
12	61	9	14	Intestine in abdomen. Early fingernail development.
14	87	14	45	Sex distinguishable externally. Well-defined neck.
16	120	20	110	Head erect. Lower limbs well developed.
18	140	27	200	Ears stand out from head.
20	160	33	320	Vernix caseosa present. Early toenail development.
22	190	39	460	Head and body hair (lanugo) visible.
Viable Fetuses‡				
24	210	45	630	Skin wrinkled and red.
26	230	50	820	Fingernails present. Lean body.
28	250	55	1000	Eyes partially open. Eyelashes present.
30	270	59	1300	Eyes open. Good head of hair. Skin slightly wrinkled.
32	280	63	1700	Toenails present. Body filling out. Testes descending.
34	300	68	2100	Fingernails reach fingertips. Skin pink and smooth.
38	340	79	2900	Body usually plump. Lanugo hairs almost absent. Toenails reach toe tips. Flexed limbs; firm grasp.
40	360	83	3400	Prominent chest; breasts protrude. Testes in scrotum or palpable in inguinal canals. Fingernails extend beyond fingertips.

Modified from Moore K, Persaud TVN: *The developing human: clinically oriented embryology*, ed 7, Philadelphia, 2003, Saunders.

*These measurements are averages and so may not apply to specific cases; dimensional variations increase with age.

†These weights refer to fetuses that have been fixed for about 2 wk in 10% formalin. Fresh specimens usually weigh about 5% less.

‡There is no sharp limit of development, age, or weight at which a fetus automatically becomes viable or beyond which survival is ensured, but experience has shown that it is rare for a baby to survive whose weight is <500 g or whose fertilization age is <22 wk. The term *abortion* refers to all pregnancies that terminate before the period of viability.

father as "grappling for relevance": struggling with the reality of pregnancy, being recognized as a parent—especially by the pregnant woman—and forming his concept of the father role. Box 1-2 describes the tasks of the parents in each of the trimesters.

Maternal attachment to the fetus has been described as having five dimensions: differentiation of self from fetus, interaction with the fetus, attributing characteristics to the fetus, giving of self, and role taking.

• Box 1-2 / Psychological Tasks of Pregnancy •

First Trimester	Second Trimester	Third Trimester
MOTHER		
Resolution of ambivalence. Observes pregnancy changes, accepts fetus as real, becomes introverted, self-image changes, may be moody. May fear sex or be too uncomfortable for sexual activity.	Feels good but less satisfied with body changes as pregnancy progresses. May enjoy sex or may avoid it. Preoccupied with development of maternal identity. Explores and may move toward relationship with own mother.	Trying on new roles. Vulnerable, wants nurturance. Anxious for pregnancy to end yet fearful. Has dreams, fantasies about baby. Begins preparation for labor and delivery. Makes plans for postpartum period. Needs social acceptance and support. Less confident. Sex may become less comfortable; usually wants to be held.
FATHER		
Accepting the reality of pregnancy, pride and/or guilt. Resolving ambivalence. May experience couvade. May feel need to protect, control; focuses on provider role.	Networks with other men to hear their experiences; is developing father identity. May experience anxiety, irritability. Men have varied reactions to the physical changes in their partners and may be more or less interested in sexual contact.	Getting prepared for labor and delivery. May have anxiety regarding partner's body. Becomes introspective; explores relationship with own father while developing his image of "father." Role as "provider" important.

Data from Malnory ME: Development of the pregnant couple, *J Obstet Gynecol Neonatal Nurs* 25:525-532, 1996.

Attachment increases as the pregnancy advances. Maternal-fetal attachment may affect the competence of mothering during infancy.[13] Attachment behaviors include talking about the fetus as an individual, talking to the fetus in response to fetal movement, calling the fetus by a name, noting differences in movements, reading about fetal and child development, health promotion behaviors, and preparing the home. Attachment may be threatened by factors such as lack of support from the father and the pregnant woman's mother.[15]

Interventions to Facilitate Accomplishment of These Tasks

Confirm the reality of the fetus by listening to FHTs with the parents and encouraging the father to attend ultrasound examinations. Monitor the mother's relationship with the father, including him in prenatal care, supporting his involvement, and assisting as mother and father assume their parenting roles.[15] Affirm the normalcy of ambivalence during the first trimester for both parents. Let them share their stories as their parent-identities start to form. Point out changes related to pregnancy. Share information regarding the development of the fetus (see Table 1-1). Normalize dreams and fantasies. Help the father understand "couvade" as his taking part in the pregnancy. Offer anticipatory guidance regarding changes he can expect in the woman and what he can do to support her. Discuss safety and comfort measures in relation to sexual activity. In the second and third trimesters, help the mother become aware of fetal movement. Reinforce her interactions with the baby, and educate the couple about fetal capabilities. Explore the couple's feelings about the woman's changing body. Support their efforts to learn about birth and early parenting. Encourage communication between the partners regarding their fears and imaginings. Observe for maternal-fetus and maternal-infant attachment behaviors. Throughout the pregnancy, explore and remain sensitive to cultural differences that influence the couple's perceptions and concerns.[71]

• PREGNANCY IN ADOLESCENCE

The pregnant adolescent faces many risks. Like all adolescents, she is at increased risk for substance abuse, sexually transmitted infections (STIs) including HIV, violence, abuse, depression, suicide, and accidental trauma.[8] Adolescents more often experience the following complications of pregnancy: anemia, intrauterine growth restriction (IUGR), preterm birth, preeclampsia, gestational diabetes mellitus (GDM), and increased perinatal mortality.[82] The pelvis continues to grow through late adolescence, and young teens have an increased risk for cephalopelvic disproportion.[75] Meanwhile, barriers to health care for these women include uninsured or underinsured status, limited availability of appropriate services, out-of-pocket co-payments, transportation, lack of culturally appropriate care, and confidentiality issues. Teens more often have poor prepregnancy nutritional status, poor diets during pregnancy, and body image concerns that put them at nutritional risk during pregnancy.[54] Infants of adolescents may weigh less because the maternal need for nutrients (because of skeletal immaturity) competes with the nutritional needs of the fetus.[90]

Pregnancy may complicate the emotional growth of the adolescent, making her achievement of the developmental tasks of adolescence and the completion of her education more difficult. Family structure and living arrangements and the relationship with the baby's father have been found to significantly affect her ability to attach. In the first trimester the woman receiving emotional support from the father of the baby shows more differentiation of the baby from herself and more role-taking behavior. In the second trimester, a good relationship with the father of the baby increases interaction with the fetus, attribution of characteristics to the fetus, and giving of herself. After delivery, support from either the infant's father or her own mother affects the adolescent mother's ability to attach to the newborn.[15]

Psychosocial Tasks of Adolescence as Related to Pregnancy[38]

Early Adolescence: 11 to 15 Years

During early adolescence, a girl has just moved from concrete to abstract operations and is learning to conceptualize. In turmoil from hormonal influences and physical changes, the young adolescent girl may try to exert control by lashing out at her parents. She is preoccupied with her appearance as her body changes. Because of this concern with self, a fetus may seem abstract or unreal, and a girl in this stage of adolescence may deny and hide pregnancy. She may conform to advice only to avoid punishment or obtain favors. Pregnancy may interrupt and prevent identity formation. The relationship with the father of the baby is often casual, and a girl of this age usually looks to same-sex friends for support. She needs parental or adult support to emotionally parent and to provide for the child.

Middle Adolescence: 14 to 18 Years

The young woman in middle adolescence is developing her identity as a sexual being, and pregnancy changes may be unwelcome. She is thinking about long-term plans and developing her self-image as an adult. At this age, female teens want loving relationships with male counterparts, but male teens are focused more on the sexual aspect of relationships. Women in this stage of adolescence are able to modify behaviors for the well-being of the coming baby but need parental or adult support to provide for a child.

Late Adolescence: 17 to 20 Years

In late adolescence the young woman assumes the identity formed in middle adolescence and begins to cope with adult challenges. She may advance her education to assume a professional role. She is usually capable of abstract thinking and adult decision-making processes and is able to curb activities in consideration of consequences for the fetus. A woman of this age is comfortable with her adult body and is able to accept the changes of pregnancy. Women in late adolescence are able to parent independently and may have clear career goals.

Interventions to Facilitate and Support Achievement of Psychosocial Tasks

Observe maternal-fetus and maternal-infant attachment behaviors. During pregnancy assist the adolescent to focus on the fetus and her development as a mother. Monitor the relationship with the father of the baby, including him in prenatal care, supporting his involvement, and assisting as both mother and father assume their parenting roles.[15] Encourage resolution of family conflicts if possible to allow provision of support to the new parents.[38]

• FUNDAL HEIGHT MEASUREMENT

Fundal height is measured from the symphysis pubis to the uterine fundus in centimeters. Consistency of method is essential. Between 18 and 30 wk, the number of centimeters coincides with the fundal height in centimeters. A variance of 2 to 3 cm indicates inappropriate fetal growth.[36] See Figure 1-4 for normal fundal height parameters during pregnancy.

• ULTRASOUND EXAMINATION FOR GESTATIONAL DATING

Although there is a theoretic risk for tissue damage associated with ultrasound examination at high intensities from the effects of heat and cavitation, no biologic effects have been confirmed in mammals in the ranges of frequency used in humans.[36] Ultrasound is used to determine gestational age by measuring different fetal structures. See Table 1-2 regarding structures measured and the accuracy of these measurements.

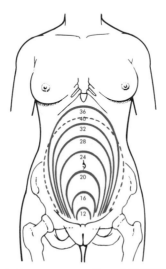

Figure 1-4 • Fundal height during pregnancy. (From Seidel HM et al: *Mosby's guide to physical examination,* ed 5, St Louis, 2003, Mosby.)

Table 1-2 / Ultrasonic Gestational Age Estimation and Accuracy

Fetal Structures Measured	Gestational Age at Testing	Accuracy
Gestational sac diameter	Performed from 4.5-5.5 wk	Accuracy ± 5 days
Embryonic crown-rump length	Performed at 6-12 wk	Accuracy ± 3 days
Biparietal diameter (BPD), femur length,	Performed from 15-22 wk	Accuracy ± 10 days
or cerebellar transverse diameter	Performed at 22 or more wk	Accuracy ± 14-20 days

Data from Burrow GN, Ferris TF: *Medical complications during pregnancy*, ed 4, Philadelphia, 1995, WB Saunders.

• WEIGHT GAIN DURING PREGNANCY

The average weight gain during pregnancy is 12.5 kg (27.5 lb). Of this, 9 kg is made up of the fetus, placenta, amniotic fluid, uterine hypertrophy, increased maternal blood volume, breast enlargement, and maternal intracellular and extracellular volume. The remainder of weight gain is composed of increased maternal fat stores.[36]

Variables affecting weight gain include age, parity, income, maternal education, race, and ethnic background. Weight gain and nutritional needs are influenced by prepregnancy weight, energy expenditure, preparation for lactation, and multiple gestation. Normal outcomes occur among women within a wide range of weight gain. Women who gain little weight have a greater risk of having preterm or small-for-gestational-age (SGA) babies (see pp. 74 or 150). Women who gain a large amount of weight have a higher risk of having a large-for-gestational-age (LGA) baby (see p. 98). Excessive weight gain during pregnancy also contributes to long-term maternal obesity, increasing the woman's risks for cardiovascular disease and diabetes in later life.[90]

In 1990, the National Academy of Science through the Institute of Medicine recommended weight gain according to the body mass index (see p. 574): 28 to 40 lb for underweight women, 15 to 35 lb for normal-weight women, and 15 to 25 lb for overweight women. Women who are underweight at the beginning of pregnancy are at risk for delivery of low-birthweight (LBW) and premature babies. Underweight women and women at risk of having LBW babies should gain 5 lb during the first trimester and slightly more than 1 lb/wk during the last two trimesters. For normal-weight women, the rate of gain should be 2 to 4 lb during the first trimester and 1 lb/wk for the remainder of pregnancy. Women who are overweight at the beginning of pregnancy do not necessarily have nutrient stores, depending on the quality of their diet.[111] Overweight women should gain 2 lb during the first trimester and then slightly <1 lb/wk for the last 2 trimesters.[90]

The weight gain of early pregnancy is attributable to maternal tissue deposition and expanded blood volume. Early pregnancy weight gain of

< 4.3 kg by 24 weeks' gestation is associated with a significantly greater risk of having an SGA baby, regardless of whether the total weight gain for the pregnancy is adequate (relative risk = 1.88).[94] Late second- and third-trimester gains have more to do with the fetus, amniotic fluid, and placenta. Inadequate late gain is associated with preterm delivery regardless of whether the total weight gain for the pregnancy is adequate.[54,99] Women who have gained only 10 lb by mid-pregnancy and women who gain <2 lb or >6$\frac{1}{2}$ lb/mo should be referred for nutritional counseling.[63]

The infant's weight and proportions at birth may have a long-term effect on the infant's health, contributing to future hypertension, obesity, glucose intolerance, and cardiovascular disease.[99] Adequate nutrition during pregnancy results in offspring with improved muscle mass, greater height, increased capacity for work, and improved intellectual performance at ages 10 to 20 years.[90]

Receiving information from the health care provider is associated with normal weight gain during pregnancy, and an active role in nutrition counseling is a critical component of prenatal care.[30] Pregnancy adds 200 to 300 kcal/d to nonpregnant requirements.[111] Kolasa and Weismiller[63] suggest an increase of 100 kcal/d for the adult woman of normal weight during the first trimester, increasing to 300 kcal/d for the remainder of the pregnancy.

• GENETIC TESTING

Formal genetic testing is offered to women ≥35 years of age (at delivery), when the risk of the procedure to the fetus equals the risk that they will have an infant affected with a genetic syndrome (see Table 1-3). Genetic screening is also offered when the woman, a member of her family, another child, the father of the baby, or a member of his family has a history of thalassemia (persons of Italian, Greek, Mediterranean, or Asian descent), neural tube defects, Down syndrome, Tay-Sachs disease (persons of Jewish descent), muscular dystrophy, hemophilia,

Table 1-3 / Genetic Procedures: Success, Accuracy, and Fetal Loss Rates*

Procedure	Time Performed	Successful Procedures (%)	Accuracy (%)	Fetal Loss (%)
Midtrimester amniocentesis	16-19 wk	99	99.4	0.05%-0.033%
Early amniocentesis	11-15 wk	94	99.4	2.98%
Chorionic villous sampling (CVS)	10-12 wk	97.7-99.7	97.5	1%

Data from Cunningham FG et al: *Williams obstetrics*, ed 20, Stamford, Conn, 1997, Appleton and Lange.
*Fetal loss rate will vary with each agency.

sickle cell disease, cystic fibrosis, Huntington's chorea, mental retardation, fragile X syndrome, cleft lip or palate, or another inherited genetic or chromosomal disorder. More than three first-trimester SABs, a stillbirth, or possible teratogenic exposure since the last menses are also indications for referral for genetic testing.[36]

Genetic screening specific for cystic fibrosis should be offered to women planning to conceive or those seeking prenatal care and may be ordered by the nurse-midwife.[3]

Amniocentesis

Early Amniocentesis

Early amniocentesis is performed between 11 and 15 weeks' gestation to obtain fetal cells to culture for cytogenic studies and enzyme and DNA analysis. The procedure involves cleansing of the skin, introduction of a 20- to 22-gauge needle into the amniotic sac under ultrasonic guidance, and withdrawal of amniotic fluid. In multiple pregnancy, dye is injected after the first withdrawal to ensure that a sample is obtained from each fetus. The Rh-negative mother is given RhoGAM after the procedure. The procedure was still termed investigational by the Centers for Disease Control and Prevention (CDC) in 1995 because of its loss rate—up to 2.5 times greater than that associated with midtrimester procedures.[36] A 1996 study showed that women who had an early amniocentesis (rather than mid-trimester) were more likely to have postprocedure amniotic fluid leakage (2.9% vs. 0.2%), postprocedure vaginal bleeding (1.9% vs. 0.2%), and fetal loss within 30 days (2.2% vs. 0.2%). The rates of stillbirth, preterm delivery, IUGR, and neonatal death were equal.[20] The Canadian Early and Mid-trimester Amniocentesis Trial Group[23] duplicated these findings, with a 2.98% greater pregnancy loss rate and a greater incidence of talipes equinovarus (1.3% vs. 0.1%) in the first-trimester group.

Mid-trimester Amniocentesis

Performed at 16 to 19 weeks, the procedure for mid-trimester amniocentesis is the same as for early amniocentesis. The Rh-negative mother is given RhoGAM after the procedure. Complications include maternal or fetal trauma, infection, SAB, preterm labor, placental perforation, fetomaternal hemorrhage (which may cause isoimmunization), and placental hemorrhage.[36] Leakage of amniotic fluid after second-trimester amniocentesis resulted in PROM in 1.2% (seven women) in one study of 603 second-trimester amniocentesis procedures. In all seven cases, leakage stopped with strict bedrest and expectant management.[47]

Chorionic Villus Sampling

In chorionic villus sampling (CVS), another prenatal genetic testing procedure, chorionic villus material is withdrawn from the center of the chorion, either transcervically or transabdominally, and analyzed.

Advantages over amniocentesis include rapid results and early diagnosis, allowing easier and safer termination of pregnancy, when it is chosen, because of an abnormal result.

Disadvantages include the identification of many abnormal fetuses that would have been spontaneously aborted without the testing. Maternal cell contamination can invalidate the test results. In 1991 and 1992, fetal limb reduction defects were noted after CVS procedures, but the occurrence rate varies greatly among researchers.[79] The estimated risk of limb reduction defects is 1:3000.[36]

Finally, placental mosaicism is present in 1.3% of CVS samples. Mosaicism describes an individual who has two different cell lines derived from the same zygote. Mosaicism may be present in some tissues and not others. Its manifestation depends on when the cell line developed during embryogenesis. If a normal cell line develops, as well as one with a chromosomal abnormality, the fetus may come to term and be viable; it may even lose the abnormal cell line.[79] The finding of mosaicism is equivocal: the majority of fetuses will have no abnormalities, but the IUGR and perinatal loss rates are increased (16.7% vs. 2.7%).[36]

CVS is a relatively safe alternative to amniocentesis, which may be considered between 10 and 12 weeks' gestation. It is not recommended before 10 weeks. Genetic counseling is required before the procedure.[36]

Ultrasonographic Markers of Down Syndrome

Ultrasonographic indicators of Down syndrome include increased nuchal thickness (nuchal translucency [NT]), shortened humerus length, hyperechogenic bowel, and hypoplastic fifth digit. These markers may be used as an initial screening device, or they may be calculated with maternal age to estimate the risk for Down syndrome for the woman who declines amniocentesis.[11] NT is caused by a cystic hygroma (a rapidly growing cyst of lymphatic origin) or nuchal edema; the latter is strongly associated with fetal aneuploidies, especially Down syndrome. NT in the late first-trimester fetus is a marker for structural abnormalities, foremost cardiac defects, but also abdominal wall defects, diaphragmatic hernias, skeletal dysplasia, and others. NT is also associated with high rate of fetal death. In the general population, the detection rate of Down syndrome by means of NT alone is between 60% and 80% for a 5% screen-positive rate. (The biochemical markers have a 60% to 65% detection rate for Down syndrome with a 5% screen-positive rate.[68])

• MATERNAL SERUM ALPHA-FETOPROTEIN

Alpha-fetoprotein (AFP) is a major serum protein produced mainly in the fetal liver, present in fetal blood and in small amounts in the amniotic fluid through fetal urinary excretion. A small amount crosses the placenta and is detectable in the maternal serum where it is called *maternal serum alpha-fetoprotein (MSAFP)*. When the fetus has open spina bifida, anencephaly, or an abdominal wall defect, the AFP level is elevated, and this is detectable in maternal serum. With a Down syndrome fetus, the AFP level is reduced. In some states, this screening test is combined with the hCG (level higher than usual during the second trimester) for Down syndrome; and unconjugated estriol (uE3; lower than usual in Down syndrome pregnancies).[37] Combined testing is called triple screening.

Conditions Detected

Together, these screening tests detect 97% of fetuses with anencephaly, 80% of fetuses with open spina bifida, and 85% of fetuses with abdominal wall defects (gastroschisis and omphalocele). Maternal age and the serum markers are used to calculate the risk for Down syndrome, and when this value is >1:250, it is expressed as positive. The rate of detection varies with maternal age (at 20 years, the detection rate is 40%; at 25 years, 44%; at 30 years, 52%; at 35 years, 71%; at 40 years, 90%; and at 45 years, 99%). Sixty percent of fetuses with trisomy 18 are identified. For every 16 women who receive a positive report for trisomy 18, one will actually have a fetus with trisomy 18.[37]

Maternal Serum Alpha-Fetoprotein

Reference ranges for serum MSAFP levels at 13 to 16 weeks' gestation are set by regional laboratories for their own population and are expressed as multiples of the mean (MoM). Most laboratories identify 3 to 5 standard deviations above the mean as the positive cutoff point. Should the level be abnormal, a second serum test is done. If this test confirms the abnormal test result, amniocentesis and ultrasound examination are offered.[92] The interval from the time that blood is drawn for determination of the MSAFP level until the results of a follow-up amniocentesis are received is 12 to 28 days. Early testing preserves as many choices as possible for the woman.[37]

Interpretation of false positive MSAFP results:

- **False high positive MSAFP screen:** Occurs because of normal variation, underestimation of gestational age, multiple gestation, renal abnormalities, fetal demise, and fetomaternal hemorrhage. An otherwise unexplained elevated MSAFP is associated with increased rates of fetal demise, preterm labor, and LBW.[37] Preeclampsia is also seen more frequently among these women. The mechanism is probably poor placentation, and fetal surveillance is indicated in the third trimester for these women.[25]
- **False low positive MSAFP screen:** Occurs because of normal variation, overestimation of fetal age, and other chromosomal syndromes such as triploidy and Turner's syndrome.[37]

Aneuploidy Screening

Two other markers have been combined with the MSAFP level to increase the test's accuracy in identifying fetuses with Down syndrome and other aneuploidies: hCG and the uE3 levels. Down syndrome is evidenced by low MSAFP and uE3 levels and a high hCG. This test identifies 65% of all fetuses with Down syndrome, with a false-positive rate of 5%. When all the levels are low, trisomy 18 is the diagnosis.[25]

• COMMON DISCOMFORTS OF PREGNANCY AND THEIR REMEDIES

Backache

Forty-eight to ninety percent of women experience back pain at some time during their pregnancies. Obesity, a history of back problems, and greater parity increase the likelihood of back pain during pregnancy.[86]

Perkins et al[86] state that two major types of lower back pain occur during pregnancy: lumbar pain (LP) and posterior pelvic pain (PPP). LP occurs in the lumbar spine with or without radiation into the leg; is like the back pain experienced by nonpregnant women; and is aggravated by prolonged postures. Some of the pain of LP may not be related to the pregnancy. PPP is experienced as a deep pain distal and lateral to the L5/S1 vertebrae, bilateral or unilateral, over the sacroiliac joint and the posterior superior iliac spine, possibly radiating to the posterior thigh or knee. Four times as prevalent during pregnancy and usually triggered by the pregnancy, PPP is aggravated by prolonged postures, asymmetric loading of the pelvis, flexion of the upper body and lifting with twisting, climbing stairs, turning at night, and walking. It may be experienced with symphysis pubis pain. Pain may persist long after such activities have ceased.

A test to determine which pain the woman is experiencing is called the **posterior pelvic pain provocation test.** The woman lies supine. The hip on the affected side is flexed 90 degrees. The examiner stabilizes the opposite iliac crest and applies vertical pressure into the bent hip. If the woman's pain is reproduced, she has PPP. PPP tends to resolve more quickly after pregnancy, though the severity of pain generally predicts the length of time required for resolution, regardless of whether the pain was LP or PPP. Some women experience chronic back pain after pregnancy.[86]

The cause of back pain is probably multifactorial. Back pain increases early in pregnancy and levels off during week 24 (except for women with preexisting back pain who experience increasing discomfort until delivery).[65] Relaxin levels, the increase in weight, and the degree of anterior tilt of the pelvis do not correlate with back pain. Pain occurring only at night that is unrelated to position changes may be due to hypervolemia and pressure on the inferior vena cava in the supine position.[86]

ⓜ Management

1. **R/O preterm labor** and **urinary tract disease.**[86]
2. **Provide the following comfort suggestions and advice: Avoid the supine position** if back pain occurs at night. Maintain good **posture** and wear a **supportive bra. Avoid excessive bending, walking** without resting, and **lifting.** Use good **body mechanics:** lift with the legs, not the back; distribute weight equally when carrying weight; and avoid bending while rotating the spine. In the last trimester, eliminate, or at least share, heavy lifting. **Sleep** on a firm mattress with pillows. Support the top leg and the abdomen with pillows for sleep. To arise from bed, roll to the side with hips and knees bent and use arms to push up. **Exercise** may offer relief, including prenatal exercise class, yoga, swimming, and relaxation exercises, squatting down with back to a wall, "tailor sits" (sit on ground with soles of feet together; press knees toward floor), and the "knee chest twist" (while lying on floor with arms out to the sides, bend knees to straight above hips, and keeping knees together, touch the floor on one side and then the other). Use **seats** that support the spine with back cushions. Perform activities in a **neutral spine position.** Lying with feet supported on a stool, sitting backwards in a chair leaning forward on the chair back, and stretching with the hands in the small of the back are all **restful positions** for the back. Brief periods of rest are helpful. **Heat** and **ice** applications may bring relief. For severe cases, a pregnancy **girdle** may provide relief. Wear low-heeled supportive **shoes.**[86] Changing the height of shoes may help.[106]
   a. **For the woman with LP:** When prolonged standing cannot be avoided, weight shifting from foot to foot or using a small stool will reduce tension in the back. Recalcitrant LP pain may be reduced, for a small number of women, by use of maternity supports.[86]
   b. **For the woman with PPP:** Avoid unsymmetrical loading of the pelvis and jarring exercises. Use of sacral belts and sacral support in chairs may provide relief. The woman's return to normal activities after delivery should be gradual.[86]

   Fuchs[43] suggests the following **massage** technique for lower back pain. Have the woman lie on her left side on an examination or massage table with the edge of the table just behind her. Her lower arm is under a pillow; her upper arm is over her head in alignment with her body. Standing behind her with one of your feet placed about 18 inches behind the other, both feet parallel to the woman's back pointing toward her feet, place the web between your left thumb and first finger over the woman's upper iliac crest and lean forward, using your body weight as you shift from the back to the forward foot. Hold for 15 to 30 seconds, and release slowly. Reverse your body so that your feet are parallel to the woman's back, pointing toward her head. Put your hands on either side of the lower ribcage, and lift the ribcage upward in the same manner, using your body weight as you shift to the foot nearer the head. Place your forearms together, parallel, and place them between the patients' iliac crest and lower ribcage, then stretch outward, stretching the woman's muscles. Finally, stand above her head, grasp her upper arm and pull, stretching the muscles of the entire body length. Hold 15 to 30 seconds, and release slowly. Repeat on the other side.

Maintenance of a good body weight after pregnancy will minimize subsequent back problems.[105]

3. **Indications for consultation or referral** include lower back pain that fails to improve with rest, fails to respond to conservative management, or is unaffected by movement or position change. Make an appropriate referral if you suspect GI or cardiovascular disease, or for the woman with neurologic signs such as sensory, motor, or reflex changes, or bowel or bladder dysfunction that may indicate a herniated disk.[86]

4. **Complementary measures:**
   a. **Acupuncture, chiropractic care, osteopathy, physical therapy, Bowen therapy** (Australian body work), **massage,** and **shiatsu** may be useful. **Yoga** and **back-strengthening exercises** are useful for maintaining back health.[21,61,101,102,105]
   b. **Homeopathy:** Experts suggest a number of remedies.[34,52,91,96,105]
   c. **Nutritional suggestions: Calcium,** 1500 mg, and **magnesium,** 750 mg, daily may reduce muscle spasms.[105]
   d. **Reflexology:** The spinal zones of the feet, located along the inner edges of the feet, may be worked. Laxity of the symphysis pubis may be treated by stimulation of the pituitary zone.[104] **See charts and information on reflexology, p. 567.**

Carpal Tunnel Syndrome

Compression of the median and ulnar nerves as a result of changing posture, edema, or repetitive motion may cause burning, tingling, pain and/or numbness in the central portion of the hand, the thumb, first two fingers, and the medial aspect of the ring finger. One or both hands may be affected. Symptoms may worsen with use of the hands or at night.[64] **Tinel's sign** is elicited by tapping the median nerve at the wrist (tap centrally on crease between ligaments on inner aspect of wrist). With carpal tunnel syndrome (CTS), the tapping sends a shock-like tingling into the hand. **Phalen's maneuver** is positive for CTS if the woman feels burning and a reproduction of the pain after flexing her wrist down 90 degrees for 1 minute.[60]

ⓜ Management

1. **Provide the following comfort suggestions and advice: Discontinue repetitive motions.** Maintaining good **posture** with shoulders back and wearing a supportive bra, as described in the

section on upper backache, may help. Lying down and **elevating the arms** may help. **Relaxation exercises** focused on the muscles surrounding the joints where the nerve enters the spine—that is, along the upper back, chest, and shoulder—may be useful.

Stabilization of the wrist in a neutral position with a **splint** and restricting its use and range of motion may relieve the discomfort. The splint is used primarily at night but may be used during the day if it does not interfere with daily activities or if the condition is severe.

Massage techniques that may be helpful for CTS include squeezing each finger with the hand; kneading the palm, alternating pressure with the two thumbs; and holding the carpal trigger point, which is located on the back of the wrist.[43]

2. **Indication for referral:** If the comfort measures do not provide relief, make a referral to an orthopedist. Corticosteroid injections into the joint may give some women temporary relief. Surgery is a last resort to release the carpel tunnel and would not be done during pregnancy. Nonsteroidal analgesics are not effective in managing this discomfort.[64]

3. **Complementary measures:**
   a. **Osteopathic** treatment of the wrist and forearm helps to drain the joints and improves mobility of the wrist.[31] **Chiropractic** treatment may help.[83]
   b. Some **homeopathy** experts suggest homeopathic remedies for CTS.[105]
   c. **Nutritional suggestions:** Some carpal tunnel problems are attributed to vitamin B_6 and magnesium deficiencies and improve with supplementation.[83,105]
   d. **Chinese medicine:** Using **acupressure,** work the Kidney meridian of the leg. Apply pressure to Pericardium 6 for 7 to 10 seconds 3 times.[61] **Acupuncture**[21] and **shiatsu** may be useful. **See charts and information on Chinese medicine, p. 559.**

Constipation

Hardening of stool may occur as a result of a progesterone-mediated decreased peristalsis rate, displacement of the bowel by the growing uterus, or iron supplementation. A decrease in the woman's normal activity level may be additive.

Ⓜ Management

1. **Provide the following suggestions and advice for alleviation: Exercise,** adequate **rest,** and decreased **stress** may be helpful. **Dietary measures** include consumption of whole grains, fibrous fruits and vegetables, dried fruits (especially prunes and figs), and other fruits and juices to add bulk and fiber to the diet. The woman should drink eight glasses of noncaffeinated liquid a day. **Avoid lax-**

atives unless suggested by the health care provider.[12] Establish a **regular bowel habit.** Hot or cold liquids may stimulate peristalsis and a bowel movement on arising in the morning. Wait until the urge to have a bowel movement is present and then sit down and try to have a bowel movement in an unhurried manner. Do not delay having a bowel movement when the urge is present. While sitting on the toilet, elevate feet on a stool.

2. **Medical interventions** include changing the **brand of iron supplement**[63] and suggesting the use of **natural bulk laxatives** (Metamucil or Citrucel)—natural food products made of psyllium—that draw water into the bowel to soften the stool. Colace is a safe **stool softener** to be used only when natural measures have failed.[12]

3. **Complementary measures:**
   a. **Homeopathy** experts suggest remedies for constipation.[83,91,96,105]
   b. **Chinese medicine: Acupuncture** has been used with success in treating the woman with constipation.[21] **Shiatsu** massage of the Stomach meridian or **acupressure** of Stomach 36 (application of pressure 3 times for 7 to 10 seconds) may help.[61] **See charts and information on Chinese medicine, p. 559.**
   c. **Nutritional suggestions:** Tarr[101] advocates eating **vitamin B–rich** foods. Koehler[62] suggests **limiting consumption of muscle meats** to 2 to 3 times weekly. Gladstar[46] suggests adding **carob powder** to blenderized drinks or cereals or mixing it into foods.
   d. **Reflexology:** Stimulation of the intestinal zone, located in the arch of the foot, may relieve constipation. Massage is done in a clockwise motion with the thumbs.[103] **See charts and information on reflexology, p. 567.**
   e. **Herbs: Psyllium** seeds, 1 to 2 tsp, soaked in water, act as a mucilaginous bulk laxative and soften stool.* Decoctions of **dandelion** have a laxative effect.[49,62,69,97] **See information on herbs, p 563.**

Dyspareunia

Discomfort during intercourse may occur during pregnancy as a result of fatigue, pelvic vasocongestion, decreased vaginal lubrication, subluxation of the pubic symphysis and sacroiliac joints, a retroverted uterus in early weeks, weight of the partner on the enlarged uterus in later months, deep engagement of the fetal presenting part, stress incontinence, backache, vaginal infection, UTI, hemorrhoids, or vulvar varicosities. Psychological barriers may be present because of anxiety about infertility, repeated miscarriages, fetal handicap, or neonatal death. The woman experiencing an uncomplicated pregnancy may also have concerns regarding her body image, the changes in the relationship, and myths about the safety of intercourse during pregnancy.[88]

---

*References 32, 46, 49, 69, 81, 95, 101, 105.

ⓜ Management

1. **R/O preexisting dyspareunia** (see p. 466).
2. **Provide the following comfort suggestions and advice: Reassure** the woman and her partner that sexual activity is safe during normal pregnancy. **Alternative positions** may offer comfort as the abdomen grows or may prevent discomfort with deep thrusting. **Ice** may be applied to the perineum for vascular engorgement. **Alternate means** of sexual gratification may be discussed.

Dyspnea of Pregnancy

The enlarging pregnant uterus encroaches on the diaphragm, increasing diaphragmatic pressure and decreasing functional residual capacity. Progesterone acts on the respiratory center to increase the threshold for oxygen.[50] Increased tidal volume drives the P_{CO_2} down,[36] resulting in dyspnea among 60% to 70% of pregnant women. Dyspnea of pregnancy is not associated with decreased capacity or decreased oxygen uptake.[22]

ⓜ Management

1. **Indications for consultation include** cyanosis, pain, abnormal lung or heart sounds, deterioration of other vital signs, decreased pulse oximetry readings, and fever or cough.
2. **Provide the following comfort suggestions and advice:** Offer **reassurance** that shortness of breath often occurs during pregnancy for the reasons noted above. The following measures may be helpful: **Get fresh air. Breathe slowly** and deliberately. **Stand up** and stretch, taking deep breaths. Breathe with **arms stretching over head. Good posture** allows fullest lung expansion. **Elevate the head of the bed** to decrease lung compression during the night. Avoid lying flat on the back. Use relaxation exercises. Get onto hands and knees to decrease pressure of uterus on other organs.[62]
3. **Complementary measures:**
   a. **Chinese medicine: Shiatsu** treatment of the Lung 1 point and Pericardium 6 may relieve some of the breathlessness of pregnancy.[61] **See charts and information on Chinese medicine, p. 559.**

Edema of the Lower Extremities

Physiologic edema worsens as pregnancy advances, because venous return is impaired by the weight of the growing uterus.

ⓜ Management

1. **Exclude preeclampsia** (see p. 85), **varicosities** (see p. 45), and **thrombophlebitis** and consult or refer appropriately.
2. **Provide the following comfort suggestions and advice: Avoid restrictive clothing** that impairs venous return. **Vary position often.** Minimize long periods of standing or walking. **Elevate legs** at inter-

vals during the day. Do not sit with a weight in the lap further imped-ing circulation. Rest **lying in the left lateral position** to maximize drainage of the blood vessels in the legs. Get **exercise.**[12]

Fuchs[43] suggests the following **massage:** With the woman in the semi-Fowler position, use warmed lotion or oil and long, moderately firm, upward strokes to massage the leg from knee upward toward groin. Have the woman bend her knee, then massage from ankle upward toward knee, kneading the calf muscle. Stroke the sole of the foot with alternating thumbs, from heel toward toes while the fingers are massag-ing the upper foot. With the thumbs, make circles around the balls of the foot. Continue down the entire foot. Rub the heel with the palm. Stroke the foot with thumbs from toes toward ankle. Avoid acupressure points in the ankle that may stimulate labor (see p. 560). Wring each toe from base to tip using thumb and index finger. Again, using long strokes, stroke from foot to knee to groin. Repeat on the other leg.

3. **Complementary measures:**
   a. **Osteopathic treatment** may release restrictions at the joint and facilitate resolution of edema secondary to gravity.[31]
   b. **Chinese medicine: Acupuncture** may be used in the treatment of edema during pregnancy,[21] as may **shiatsu.** Using **acupressure,** work applied to the Kidney meridian, Kidney 7, Stomach 36, Bladder 23, and Kidney 3 to treat edema.[61] **See charts and infor-mation on Chinese medicine, p. 559.**
   c. **Reflexology:** Regular stimulation of the lymphatic system zone, kidneys, liver, and GI tract will relieve edema.[104] **See charts and information on reflexology, p. 567.**
   d. **Herbs: Dandelion** tea is a diuretic.[32,46,49,101] **Parsley** (¼ oz fresh parsley/d[32]) increases renal function; it is also a uterine stimulant and is contraindicated for women with GI disease but is safe if **eaten in moderation.* See information on herbs, p. 563.**

Fatigue

Fatigue often occurs until 12 to 14 weeks' gestation because of an increased basal metabolic rate. The third trimester also brings fatigue as the growing fetus becomes heavier.

m *Management*

1. **Exclude anemia** (see p. 352) or, if diagnosed, prescribe iron supple-mentation. Exclude depression and/or anxiety (consider social ser-vice referral if present). Exclude inadequate nutrition, referring as appropriate to social services for resources and/or dietician for infor-mational needs.

---

*References 32, 49, 56, 62, 69, 101.

2. **Provide the following comfort suggestions and advice: Provide reassurance** that the experience of fatigue in the first trimester is normal and should improve at 12 to 14 weeks. **Regular exercise, good posture, well-balanced meals,** and **naps** are preferable to drinking coffee. Advise the woman to **rest** and avoid assuming extra responsibilities now.

3. **Complementary measures** (see section on insomnia if woman has difficulty sleeping):
   a. **Chinese medicine: Shiatsu** may be useful in the treatment of fatigue during pregnancy.[61] **See information on Chinese medicine, p. 559.**
   b. **Nutritional suggestions:** Evaluate the diet for adequacy of **B vitamins.**[46,62,101] Tarr[101] suggests increasing **protein** in the diet.

Gas Discomfort

Increased intestinal gas may occur more frequently during pregnancy because of slowed motility and the tendency for constipation.

ⓜ Management

1. **Exclude preterm labor** (see p. 150), **UTI** (see p. 389), and **round ligament discomfort** (see p. 43).

2. **Provide the following suggestions and advice for comfort alleviation:** Get adequate **exercise.** Use measures to **prevent constipation** (see p. 28). **Dietary interventions** include eating four to five small meals a day. Chew food well. Eat four or more fresh fruits and vegetables a day. Cook vegetables by quick steaming rather than by prolonged boiling. Avoid gas-forming foods. To reduce gas-forming compounds in legumes, place the beans in water and boil for 1 minute; pour the water off and begin again with fresh water.[12] The **knee-chest** position, squatting, or abdominal massage in the direction of the colon may ease the discomfort from unexpelled gas. Avoid combining proteins and carbohydrates at the same meal. Eat fruit by itself for better digestion.[105]

3. **Medical interventions:** Simethicone decreases surface tension of gas bubbles. Although its efficacy has not been demonstrated in studies, this drug is apparently not absorbed from the GI tract and so is safe for use during pregnancy and lactation.[19] Maalox Maximum Strength and Mylanta Gas Relief are two products that contain simethicone.

4. **Complementary measures:**
   a. Some **homeopathy** experts recommend homeopathic remedies for gas discomfort.[83,105]
   b. **Nutritional suggestions:** Koehler[62] states that gas is usually formed by undesirable bacteria in the intestinal tract, which **yogurt or kefir** will keep at bay.
   c. **Herbs: Dill** eases flatulence.[32,56,69,83] **Papaya** tablets taken with meals relieve gas by increasing secretion of stomach

acids.[49,83,85,101] **Ginger** may relieve gas (see p. 40 regarding safety in pregnancy).[32,49,56,69,83] **Peppermint** reduces colic discomfort.[49,56,69,81] **See information on herbs, p. 563.**

Headache

Headaches unrelated to any pathologic process and of unknown etiology may begin during pregnancy.[36] See p. 380 regarding evaluation of headaches.

m Management

1. **Exclude pathologic processes** such as sinusitis, seasonal allergies, ocular strain, migraines, or other pathology as the cause of headaches (see p. 380). After 20 weeks' gestation, R/O **preeclampsia** (see p. 85).[36]
2. **Provide the following comfort suggestions and advice:** Get adequate **rest** and **fresh air. Yoga** may relieve headaches. Drink enough **fluids.** Eat **small frequent meals.**[12] **Relax** in a quiet place. Use relaxation techniques. Place a **cool or warm wet washcloth** on the forehead and the back of the neck. An **ice pack** may be used on the head while the hands and feet are placed in warm water. Soothing music, a hot bath with Epsom salts, and slow deep breathing may help.

   Massage of the neck, shoulders, face, and scalp may also help. Fuchs[43]suggests the following series of pressure points in a facial massage for relief of a sinus headache. Using a stool if necessary, stand behind the woman's head as she reclines. Beginning centrally above the eyebrows with the thumbs pointing at each other, pull outward until you reach the temple, where you lighten the pressure. Begin again, about an inch above the first position, repeating until the entire forehead has been pressed in three to four strips. Repeat the sequence 3 times. Massage the entire nose, alternating fingers, from the top to tip. Above the inner canthus where the upper aspect of the nose and the ocular orbit join, using an index finger on each side, simultaneously press toward the forehead in a lifting motion for 5 seconds, then release. Repeat 3 times. Move outward bilaterally along the orbit and press downward with the index fingers, every inch or so, until you have completed a total of four pressure points and have covered the orbits equally. With thumbs, press on either side of the nostrils, 1 cm from the end of the nose (tender with sinus involvement). Press firmly for 5 seconds, release slowly, and stroke toward the ear. Repeat 3 times. Repeat if the woman is extremely congested.

   For neck and shoulder tension that often accompanies headaches, Fuchs recommends standing behind and to one side of the seated woman. With one hand, push the right shoulder down to the right, and with the other hand over the head and holding the occiput, push the head to the left. Place the palms over the scapulae and squeeze the trapezius muscle. Apply pressure to any tight areas using thumb or knuckles.[43]

3. **Medical interventions: Acetaminophen (Tylenol)** may be taken for relief of headaches.
4. **Complementary measures:**
   a. **Chiropractic, biofeedback, massage,** and **magnet** therapy may all be helpful for relief of vascular headaches.[83]
   b. **Homeopathy** experts suggest remedies.[35,91,96,105]
   c. **Chinese medicine: Acupuncture** may be used with success in the treatment of headaches,[21,83] as may **shiatsu.**[61] An **acupressure** point for headaches called *In Do* is located between the eyebrows.[83] Pressing on the two Bladder 10 points is suggested, releasing when the pain stops.[105] **See charts and information on Chinese medicine, p. 559.**

Heartburn (Pyrosis)

Heartburn, a burning sensation in the esophagus, may be caused by the relaxing effect of progesterone on the cardiac sphincter of the stomach, decreased GI motility, displacement of the stomach up and to the right, decreased esophageal peristalsis,[36] increased intragastric pressure, or decreased intraesophageal pressure. During pregnancy, 30% to 50% of women experience heartburn.[72]

ⓜ Management

1. **Provide the following comfort suggestions and advice:**
   a. **Mealtimes** should be relaxed and tension-free, and the woman should focus on eating slowly and chewing thoroughly. Eat several small meals a day. Avoid causative foods (coffee, alcohol, chocolate, fats [depress motility of the stomach and secretion of gastric juices], and spicy foods). Avoid very cold foods or liquids with meals because this inhibits the secretion of gastric juices. Eating a pat of butter before starting a meal may help. Eat more raw foods. During meals, drink only a glass of water containing 1 Tblsp of raw apple cider vinegar. Avoid eating or lying down for 3 hours before bedtime. Avoid carbonated beverages, processed foods, and sugars. Once heartburn occurs, **yogurt** or **raw almonds** chewed slowly may give relief.[109]
   b. Use good **posture.** Do the **"flying exercise":** sitting tailor style, raise and lower your arms quickly, joining the backs of your hands over your head. Wear **loose-fitting clothing. Avoid cigarettes.**[109] If heartburn occurs at night, **sleep** with an extra pillow or place bricks under the head of the bed. Side-lying may help.
2. **Medical interventions:**
   a. **Antacids** may be used, although they decrease iron absorption. Maalox and Gelusil are acceptable antacids.[106] Tums and other calcium carbonate products provide calcium and temporary relief of heartburn but may cause severe rebound heartburn. Milk of Magnesia (magnesium) causes diarrhea and is contraindicated in

women with kidney stones. Chronic use may result in magnesium toxicity. Amphojel (aluminum) may cause constipation and interfere with calcium absorption. Simethicone is often combined with other ingredients in antacids, such as Mylanta II and Maalox Plus. It decreases the surface tension of gas bubbles. Although its efficacy has not been demonstrated in studies, this drug is apparently not absorbed from the GI tract and so is safe for use during pregnancy and lactation.[19]

b. **Antisecretory antihistamines** inhibit gastric acid secretions. Examples are Pepcid AC, Tagamet, Zantac, and Axid Pulvules. Tagamet (cimetidine) is classified as Food and Drug Administration (FDA) category B (no evidence of teratogenesis or impaired fertility), because it has been associated with benign testicular tumors when given in massive doses to rats and because studies regarding antiandrogenic effects on male fetuses have had conflicting results. Zantac (ranitidine) and Pepcid AC (famotidine) are also FDA category B drugs. Axid Pulvules (nizatidine) is a category C drug because of its association with an increased rate of SAB in animal studies.[19]

3. **Complementary measures:**

   a. **Osteopathic treatment** may relieve heartburn by producing relaxation of the diaphragm and increased mobility of the ribcage and thoracic spine.[31]

   b. **Homeopathy** experts suggest remedies.[34,83,91,96,105]

   c. **Chinese medicine: Acupuncture** has been successful in the treatment of heartburn,[21] as has **shiatsu.** Using **acupressure,** work the Stomach meridian; apply pressure to Stomach 36 and Pericardium 6. The Bladder meridian and Conception Vessel 22 may be worked by the woman herself.[61] **See charts and information on Chinese medicine, p. 559.**

   d. **Reflexology:** Stimulation of the zones for the esophagus, stomach, and intestines along with sedation (prolonged pressure) of the solar plexus and diaphragm may bring relief.[104] **See charts and information on reflexology, p. 567.**

   e. **Herbs:** Fresh **papaya,** papaya leaf tea (1 tsp plant/1 cup water boiled for 10 minutes, tid[80]) or papaya enzyme capsules may prevent heartburn when chewed with a meal.* **Marshmallow root,**[12,32,46,49] **catnip,**[12,56,69] and **ginger**† are suggested for relief of heartburn. See p. 40 regarding the safety of ginger in pregnancy. **Peppermint** tea aids digestion by an antispasmodic action and by improving bile-acid flow. One tsp may be steeped in 1 cup

---

*References 12, 46, 49, 62, 80, 83, 85, 101, 109.
†References 12, 49, 56, 69, 83, 85, 97.

of water for 20 minutes, or 5 gtt tincture may be added to $\frac{1}{4}$ cup water; may repeat prn.[*] **See information on herbs, p. 563.**

Hemorrhoids

Varicosities of the rectum, or hemorrhoids, worsen during pregnancy as a result of the progesterone-mediated relaxation of venous walls, the weight of the uterus, pelvic venous congestion, and the added strain of constipation.[111]

ⓜ Management

1. **Provide the following comfort suggestions and advice:** To minimize hemorrhoid formation, **prevent constipation** by increasing fiber and drinking lots of water. Rest in the **left lateral position,** which promotes drainage of the blood vessels below the uterus. Elevate the foot of the bed. As for any varicosity, **avoid standing or sitting for long periods.** Use proper lifting techniques to **avoid straining.** Perform **Kegel exercises.** When using the **toilet,** do not sit or strain for long periods and place a stool under the feet. **Exercise** daily. Warm **sitz** baths may be taken 4 to 6 times/d for 15 to 20 minutes, followed by 1 minute in cold water (repeat cycle 2 to 3 times). Cornstarch or baking soda in the sitz water will decrease itching, or the cornstarch can be used as powder after the bath. Apply cold **witch hazel** compresses or **ice. Avoid inflated "donut" pillows,** which compromise circulatory drainage.[12] **Avoid spicy foods** that may irritate hemorrhoids.
2. **Medical interventions:** Preparation H and other topical or anti-inflammatory analgesics may be suggested.[106]
3. **Complementary measures:**
   a. **Homeopathy** experts suggest remedies for hemorrhoids.[91,96,105,109] **See p. 566 regarding homeopathy.**
   b. **Chinese medicine: Acupuncture, shiatsu,** or **acupressure** treatments may improve hemorrhoids.[21,61] **See p. 559 regarding Chinese medicine.**
   c. **Nutritional suggestions:** Try taking **vitamin B$_6$,** 25 mg, with each meal.[101] A diet high in vitamin B may be helpful.[62] **Vitamin C** is suggested by many herbalists.[46,62,83,101] **Vitamin E** is suggested by Koehler[62] and Weed.[109] **Bioflavonoids** are said to strengthen capillaries.[46,83] Raw **garlic** and **onions** are considered powerful stimulants of circulation that improve elasticity of vessels.[64,97,109] **Okra, buckwheat, oats, wheat germ,** and **dark green leafy vegetables** strengthen the circulatory system as a whole.[109]
   d. **Reflexology:** Stimulation of the lymphatic system and intestinal zones and sustained pressure (having the effect of "sedation") applied to the rectal zone will bring relief from hemorrhoids, ease discomfort and constipation, and may reduce swelling.[83,104] **See charts and information on reflexology, p. 567.**

---

[*]References 32, 46, 49, 56, 62, 69, 81.

e. **Herbs: Comfrey** may be used in a compress for hemorrhoids.[69,97,109] However, it is contraindicated during pregnancy because of its hepatotoxic effects, except in small doses for limited periods of external use only.[85] **Horse chestnut** may be taken internally to strengthen the venous walls[56,69,81] and may also be used as a compress.[81] **Plantain leaves** may provide relief (4 oz herb to $\frac{1}{2}$ gallon of water steeped 8 hours, used as sitz bath), or plantain ointment may be used.[56,83,109] **Pilewort** is specific for hemorrhoids. An astringent that tones blood vessels, it may be made into an ointment (5 g/100 mL ointment[85]) or a suppository (0.1 to 1 g herb/suppository[85]), or it may be taken internally.[56,69,81] **Nettle leaf tea** (1 cup/d) is high in vitamin C and bioflavonoids and increases the elasticity of the vessels.[46,97,109]

One peeled clove of **garlic,** wrapped in one layer of gauze and oiled, can be inserted into the rectum overnight to minimize swelling; or a garlic-infused oil may be applied locally.[12,101,105,109] **Grated raw potato** may also be used as a suppository.[97,101,109] **See information on herbs, p. 563.**

Insomnia

Emotional concerns, fetal movement, or other discomforts may keep the pregnant woman awake at night.

Ⓜ Management

1. **Provide the following comfort suggestions and advice: Exercise** daily. **Avoid caffeine. Decrease fluid intake before bedtime. Avoid large meals** within 2 hours of bedtime. **Sleep regular hours.** Choose **nonstimulating activities before bedtime.** Take a warm bath or have a warm drink, particularly warm milk, before bed. Decrease the noise and lights in the environment. Get a massage. Have plenty of pillows for comfort. Use **relaxation techniques.** Take **naps.** These new habits will be useful in the early weeks of parenting as well.
2. **Complementary measures:**
   a. **Homeopathy** experts suggest remedies for insomnia.*
   b. **Chinese medicine: Acupuncture** may be used in the treatment of insomnia,[21] as may **shiatsu.**[61] An **acupressure** point for insomnia is on the back of the head, at the hairline on either side of the spine (Bladder 10).[83] Alternately, someone can apply 10 to 15 lb of pressure with the heel of one hand to the sacrum for 2 to 3 minutes at bedtime to bring on relaxation and sleep (Bladder 31 and 32).[101] **See charts and information on Chinese medicine, p. 559.**
   c. **Nutritional suggestions:** Balch and Balch[12] suggest that **vitamin B** deficiencies can cause insomnia. Tarr[101] suggests that a **calcium/**

---

*References 34, 35, 52, 83, 91, 96, 105.

magnesium supplement taken at bedtime may promote sleep. Consumption of **oats** may help sleep.[32,49,83]

d. **Herbs: Valerian root** may be taken for sleep.[56,81,105] NOTE: Valerian root acts as sedative.[12,56,69,80,85] Dosage is 10 to 25 gtt tincture, bid to tid,[80] or 1 cup of tea (1 tsp herb/150 mL water) up to several cups/d.[85] Prolonged use and large doses, which may lead to addiction, are to be avoided.[56,80] **Skullcap** tea[32,62,83,97,105] or **catnip** tea at bedtime is suggested.[49,62,101] **See information on herbs, p. 563.**

Leg Cramps

Leg cramps may be due to a diet low in calcium or the use of a new exercise. The pressure of the uterus impairs circulation to the lower extremities and may place pressure on nerves coursing through the obturator foramen.

Management

1. **Supplement calcium and magnesium.**[111]
2. **Provide the following comfort suggestions and advice:** Minimize cramps by **exercising,** using good **posture,** and **elevating the legs** periodically during the day. At night, do stretching **exercises** without pointing the toes before bed. Take a **warm bath** at bedtime (Epsom salts may be used), and **keep the legs warm** while sleeping. **Elevate** the legs while sleeping, and change their position frequently. The **push-away exercise** may help: Stand facing a wall one arm's length away. Lean forward, holding oneself with the hands, and hold the position for 10 seconds, keeping heels on floor and body in a straight line. Push away from wall, returning to standing position. Repeat 4 times, bid.[106] **Once a cramp is present,** flex feet with toes pointing upward, and apply heat.[12] **Massage** the leg toward the heart.[105]
3. **Complementary measures:**
   a. Some **homeopathy** experts suggest remedies for leg cramps.[105]
   b. **Chinese medicine:** An **acupressure** treatment for leg cramps involves pressure to the Stomach, Gallbladder, and Bladder meridians. Pressure to Bladder 57 while dorsiflexing the foot will relieve the cramp in the moment, and the woman can be taught to do this herself.[61] **See charts and information on Chinese medicine, p. 559.**
   c. **Herbs: Cramp bark** is indicated for muscle cramps.[56,69,74] **See information on herbs, p. 563.**

Leukorrhea

A heavier than usual white vaginal discharge, caused in part by increased cervical gland mucoid production, may occur during pregnancy. In addition, the amount of glycogen being converted by *Lactobacillus acidophilus* in vaginal epithelial cells increases, and the acidic secretions protect against infection during pregnancy.[36]

m *Management*

1. **Rule out vaginal infection and rupture of membranes.**
2. **Offer reassurance** that increased secretions are normal during pregnancy as a result of hormonal changes. **Provide the following comfort suggestions and advice:** Wearing **cotton underwear** and taking the necessary **hygienic measures** will provide comfort. **Avoid use of commercial products** including feminine hygiene products, douching, bubble baths, and scented toilet paper or sanitary products. Use a mild laundry detergent.[12]
3. **Complementary measures:**
   a. Some herbal experts suggest various **herbs** for leukorrhea.[12,49,74,80,95]
   b. Some **homeopathy** experts suggest remedies.[96]
   c. **Chinese medicine: Shiatsu** may relieve the leukorrhea, with work focusing on the Kidney meridian.[61] **See charts and information on Chinese medicine, p. 559.**
   d. **Nutritional suggestions:** Balch and Balch[12] suggest supplementing essential fatty acids, as directed by the manufacturer, for the antifungal properties; taking *L. acidophilus*, two capsules tid to promote normal flora; vitamin B complex, 100 mg tid; vitamin B, 50 mg tid (because vitamin B deficiency is associated with leukorrhea); and vitamin C with bioflavonoids qd to boost natural immunity.

Nausea and Vomiting

The pattern of nausea and vomiting (N&V) among 160 pregnant women were described in a study carried out in 2000. Although the mean beginning of N&V was at 8.2 weeks, 76% of the women reported nausea from the week of conception that lasted a mean of 34 days (range, 1 to 114 days). Severity peaked at 11 weeks. Fifty percent reported resolution by 14 weeks, but not until 22 weeks had nausea resolved in 90%. Nausea of pregnancy occurs all day long, and nausea scores were comparable to those induced by chemotherapy. N&V were more likely to occur in women with less education; women with low to middle income; women employed part-time; and women who also experienced N&V when taking medications (including OTC drugs), during illness, when under stress, during menses, or while traveling.[66]

N&V have been associated with positive pregnancy outcome—a decreased risk of SAB, preterm birth, IUGR, and perinatal death. Low energy intake stimulates placental growth in early pregnancy, and N&V may be a mechanism that favors placental growth.[58] Low blood sugar, gastric overloading, slowed peristalsis, an enlarged uterus, hormonal factors (especially hCG), dietary habits, and emotional factors have also been implicated.[111]

ⓜ Management

1. For N&V that persists after the first trimester, rule out **emotional problems, hydatidiform mole (see p. 81),** and **hyperemesis gravidarum (see p. 83).**

2. **Provide the following suggestions and advice for alleviation and comfort:** For **morning nausea,** eat dry, unsalted crackers (such as graham crackers) before arising. **Get out of bed slowly** and smoothly. A **light protein snack** at bedtime may decrease nausea through the night. **Dietary measures** include eating small frequent meals. Easily digested energy foods such as carbohydrates are often more easily tolerated. **Always carry food.** Avoid dehydration. **Take** vitamins, iron, and other **supplements after meals.** Eat a **high-protein** diet. **Avoid** strong **odors, spicy foods,** and **fatty foods.** Take **liquids between meals. Dry foods and carbonated drinks** may be better tolerated. Try eating **salty and tart** foods in combination (such as lemonade with potato chips) and sucking on **hard candies.** Spending time outside in the **fresh air** and/or **reducing mobility** may relieve symptoms. To explore the possible **emotional component** of nausea, Susan Weed[109] suggests that the pregnant woman who finds no relief from her nausea consider the following questions: What is it that I can't accept? What is it that I can't stomach? What wants clearing out?

   Eat foods rich in **vitamin B** (brewers' yeast, wheat germ, kale, blackstrap molasses).[12,46,62,106] In one randomized, double-blind, placebo-controlled study, 25 mg of vitamin B_6 was given to pregnant women tid. The severely affected women showed a significant reduction of symptoms.[93] Another randomized, double-blind, placebo-controlled study showed that taking 30 mg of vitamin B_6 qd significantly reduced N&V.[107]

   Ginger (soda, tea, ginger snaps, or chewing crystallized ginger pieces) is suggested by many authors (tea: $1/4$-inch slice of ginger boiled in 1 cup of water for 15 minutes).* Kolasa and Weismiller[63] suggest use of ginger in tea, soda, or tablets (250 mg qid for 4 to 5 days). Ginger root has been found to reduce N&V in randomized, double-blind, placebo-controlled trials.[42,78] Edelman and Logan[40] note that ginger has been found to be effective in one randomized, double-blind, crossover trial but that no studies have addressed the safety of ginger in pregnancy. They also note that the FDA does not regulate ginger products. Chez[26] writes that the question of its safety is based on results of in vitro studies with large doses. The German Commission E states that ginger is contraindicated during pregnancy but does not provide data or references; however, pharmacopoeias of China, Britain, Austria, Belgium, Switzerland, India, Japan, the

---

*References 12, 32, 46, 63, 83, 103, 105.

Netherlands, and the United States cite no harmful effects, and many cultures use ginger widely in foods.[26] Ginger is recommended by many herbalists.* However, *The PDR for Herbal Medicines*[85] states that ginger is an emetic and is contraindicated for treatment of nausea in pregnancy. Ody[81] states that ginger powder (1 g in capsules qd) or 2 to 5 gtt tincture (up to 1 mL/d) may be taken but should be used with caution in early pregnancy and the stated dose should not be exceeded.

3. **Medical interventions:** No **drugs** are FDA approved for the treatment of N&V in pregnancy. Antiemetics or antihistamines may be prescribed, but their associated risks should be weighed against the risks of prolonged starvation and dehydration.[40] **Doxylamine and pyridoxine** in combination (provided by one half of a 25-mg tablet of Unisom—a sleep aid—and 25 mg of vitamin B_6 qd or bid—the components of Bendectin) may be recommended, since they have been extensively studied, determined not to be related to birth defects, and determined to be safe for use in pregnancy by the FDA in 1999. Doxylamine is an antihistamine and, like all antihistamines, is discontinued if preterm labor occurs because of an increased incidence of retrolental fibroplasia in premature infants delivered within 2 weeks of intrauterine exposure. Hydroxyzine is used in combination with metoclopramide **(Vistaril)** or used in combination with pyridoxine instead of doxylamine. **Dramamine** (oral dimenhydrinate) is used extensively in Canada, but not in the United States. When given IV near term, it may have oxytocic effects.[16] **Compazine** (prochlorperazine) (25 mg q12h PR or 5 to 10 mg given IM, IV, or PO q6-8h prn) may be given for relief of N&V; however, it may be additive with other CNS depressants and may cause dystonia, dyskinesia, pseudoparkinsonism, and neuroleptic malignant syndrome.[40] **Droperidol** (a butyrophenone derivative), a dopamine antagonist, is potent against N&V and hyperemesis gravidarum but may cause extrapyramidal effects.[16] **Phenergan** (promethazine) (12.5 to 25 mg PO, PR, or IV q4h) is an antihistamine and an antiemetic with sedative properties. It potentiates other CNS depressants or anticonvulsants. Phenergan is used with caution in persons with glaucoma.[40] Selective serotonin receptor antagonists (dolasetron **[Anzemet]**, granisetron **[Kytril]**, and ondansetron **[Zofran]**) have not been studied extensively but do not appear to be teratogenic.[16]

4. **Complementary measures:**
   a. **Homeopathy** experts suggest remedies for N&V.†
   b. **Hypnosis** has been reported to be useful, although it has not been studied.[78]

---

*References 32, 46, 49, 62, 69, 84, 97, 101, 109.
†References 34, 52, 83, 91, 96, 105, 109.

c. **Chinese medicine:** The Nei-Kuan **acupressure** point (Pericardium 6) diminishes nausea for many women. A wristband available OTC as a seasickness aid may be worn to stimulate this point by acupressure. Alternatively, Stomach 36, as well as the entire Bladder meridian, may be worked.[61,105] **Acupuncture** may be helpful.[21,61,63,78,101] **See charts and information on Chinese medicine, p. 559.**

d. **Reflexology:** Stimulation of the solar plexus may provide relief from N&V. **See charts and information on reflexology, p. 567.**

e. **Nutritional suggestions:** One herbalist noted that once the woman has had vomiting and/or diarrhea long enough to cause dehydration and electrolyte imbalance, the nausea will not stop. She composed the following formula based on Ringer's lactate solution: $\frac{1}{3}$ cup lemon juice, $\frac{1}{4}$ tsp salt, 11-grains calcium tablet crushed, with enough water added to make a quart and sweetened to taste. Sweetened Pedialyte and electrolyte drinks also work.[41]

   A broth made with barley and/or oats is suggested by many herbalists.[45,46,49] After it is cooked, it should be strained and may be flavored with tamari or soup seasoning. It should be consumed in small sips. **Yogurt or kefir** (may be flavored with cinnamon) are easy to tolerate.[45,46] One teaspoon of **apple cider vinegar** in 8 oz of warm water, taken first thing in the morning, has been found to aid digestion and ease GI upset.[62,101,109]

f. **Herbs: Red raspberry** tea (1 oz leaves/2 cups water for tea[80] or 1 mL tincture[74]) sipped all day may help.* It may be combined with peppermint tea.[80] It may be taken as capsules (1 to 2) of freeze-dried leaf or in tincture form (1 mL): qd to bid for first 6 months of gestation; during seventh month, bid to tid; during remainder of pregnancy, 1 to 2 cups/d, and continued for 4 to 6 weeks postpartum.[74] **Peppermint** tea is an antispasmodic that is used to treat stomach discomfort and is useful for relief of nausea in pregnancy.† **Black horehound** tea flavored with honey is a sedative useful for nervous dyspepsia.[32,55,81] **Catnip** tea relieves indigestion and smooth-muscle spasms.[12,49,62,101] **Meadowsweet** is used to treat GI upset.[49,55,97] **Peach leaf** tea,[32,62,84,109] **spearmint** tea,[62,97,101,109] **lemon balm** tea,[32,62,81,97] and **basil** tea[62,81,84] are also suggested by herbalists. Remedies may be effective only briefly and may need to be rotated. **See information on herbs, p. 563.**

Ptyalism

Excessive salivation occurs as a result of excess acidity in the mouth, or it may be stimulated by the intake of starch. It often occurs in a cyclic fashion with nausea.[36] This discomfort appears to occur more com-

---

*References 12, 49, 62, 74, 84, 85, 97, 101, 109.
†References 12, 32, 45, 49, 56, 62, 69, 81, 97, 101, 109.

monly than recognized. In a Wisconsin clinic, 17% of 850 women reported excessive salivation, though previous reports indicated that <1% of women report ptyalism. These women reported that the onset was in the first trimester. Forty percent reported interference with swallowing, 30% indicated that taste was adversely affected, 30% stated that it interfered with sleep, and 27% said that it affected speech.[59]

ⓜ Management

1. **Provide the following comfort suggestions and advice:** Suck on **hard candies. Decreasing starch intake** may provide some relief. **Dairy products** may worsen ptyalism, and **fruit** may be tolerated best.[59]
2. **Complementary measures:** The **homeopathic** remedy **ipeca-cuanha** is suggested for ptyalism.* **See information on homeopathy, p. 566.**

Round Ligament Discomfort

Round ligament discomfort occurs with the stretching and hypertrophy of these ligaments as the uterus grows. Often, the discomfort will worsen with parity as uterine and abdominal tone diminish, placing more strain on the ligaments.

ⓜ Management

1. **R/O** pathologic conditions, including **UTI, preterm labor, and GI** or other abdominal organ complications.
2. **Provide the following comfort suggestions and advice:** The application of moist heat, as in a warm bath or shower, may provide relief. **In bed,** use pillows under the uterus and between the knees. Lying in bed toward the affected side and getting up by pushing up with the arms prevents straining these ligaments further. A **pelvic girdle** may be necessary. **Exercise:** Flex the knees onto the abdomen or bend forward to relieve pain.[12] Andrews and O'Neill[10] found that pelvic rocking reduced the intensity, the frequency, and, to a lesser degree, the duration of round ligament discomfort. They taught women to stand, wearing low heels or none, supporting themselves with one hand on a chair, and raise the affected leg vertically from the pelvis, 1.5 to 2 inches off the ground for 6 seconds, creating a unilateral pelvic tilt. Begin on the affected side for 10 repetitions; repeat with the other leg.
3. **Medical interventions: Acetaminophen** may be taken for persistent discomfort.
4. **Complementary measures: Osteopathic** manipulation of the tissues around the inguinal canal may reduce round ligament pain.[31]

---

*References 52, 83, 91, 96, 105, 109.

Sciatica

During pregnancy the fetus may be positioned in such a way that the sciatic nerve is compressed. Women experience this discomfort as sharp pain in the center of the hip, as a shooting pain down the leg, and sometimes as a sense that the leg is going to give out when pressure is placed on it while taking a step.

ⓜ Management

1. **Provide the following comfort suggestions and advice:** Fuchs[43] suggests using a **pressure point** to relieve sciatic pain. With the woman lying on her side, using oil, massage the entire upper gluteal muscle with the fist. Then find the piriformis trigger point, located in the center of the buttock (if it were divided into quadrants). To be certain the location is correct, note tenderness in the point. Press gently on this area with the thumb, making small circles, 3 times, then slowly release. Repeat the procedure with slightly firmer pressure; repeat a third time with still firmer pressure. Knead the area again. Have the woman turn and massage the other side.

   To encourage a fetus to move to a new position, the woman can stand behind a sofa. Someone stands behind her for safety. She lies on the back of the sofa along the headrest area. If the sciatica is on the left, the woman places her right leg up along the back of the sofa as she reclines to her left, with her left arm and a small pillow under her head. Her left leg is bent with the foot on the floor. Her abdomen is resting with pressure along the left side to encourage movement of the fetus to the right.[43]

   Moist **heat** applied to the low back and buttocks is soothing. **Back-strengthening exercises** and **proper body mechanics** may be used to prevent future episodes. Being overweight contributes to sciatica, and the **return to an appropriate body weight** after pregnancy is encouraged.[105] **Ice** packs, possibly alternating with application of wet heat but ending with cold, may relieve the pain.[83]

2. **Complementary measures:**
   a. **Acupuncture, chiropractic** care, **Bowen therapeutic technique** (Australian body work), and physical therapy may all be helpful with sciatica.[21,105] **Osteopathic** care may also be successful.[31,105] Some **homeopathy** experts also suggest remedies for sciatica.[105]
   b. **Nutritional suggestions:** Calcium, 1500 mg/d, and magnesium, 750 mg/d, given orally may help relieve related muscle cramps.[105]
   c. **Reflexology:** Stimulate the reflexology point for the sciatic nerve.[83] **See charts and information on reflexology, p. 567.**

Urinary Frequency

In early pregnancy, the enlarging uterus with its softened isthmus puts pressure on the bladder. Late in pregnancy, as the fetal presenting part engages, pressure is again applied on the bladder. Nocturia may occur in part because the woman is in a recumbent position and there is less pressure on the inferior vena cava, improving blood flow to the kidneys and increasing the glomerular filtration rate.

Management

1. **Exclude UTI.**
2. Offer **reassurance** that urinary frequency occurs during pregnancy for the reasons noted above. **Provide the following comfort suggestions and advice:** Increasing fluids during the day and **drinking less before bedtime,** as well as **limiting caffeine,** may ameliorate symptoms.[12]
3. **Complementary measures: Shiatsu** treatment of the Kidney meridian may relieve frequency.[61] **See information on Chinese medicine, p. 559.**

Varicosities

Varicosities may occur in the labia or the legs. Hemorrhoids are one form of varicosity, and the tendency to varicosities is partially familial. During pregnancy, progesterone relaxes venous walls, and the venous return from the lower extremities is compromised by the growing uterus, so the venous system is under increased pressure and varicosities may flourish. Excess weight, heavy lifting, and constipation may also play a part in the formation of varicosities.[12] Varicosities predispose the woman to thrombus formation. After delivery, the varicosities will improve, though with the next pregnancy, they will return and may worsen.[36]

Management

1. **Provide the following comfort suggestions and advice:** Wear **maternity support hose** or ace wraps applied in the morning after the legs have been elevated. **Avoid constrictive clothing. Avoid crossing the legs.** When possible, sit with legs raised rather than standing. Engage in mild **exercise** such as walking. **Avoid long periods of standing.** Spend time lying in the **left lateral position,** which removes the weight of the uterus from the inferior vena cava, improving return to the heart from the legs. Several times a day, lie on the floor with legs elevated against the wall, and if vulvar varicosities are present, elevate the hips as well. For the woman with **vulvar varicosities: wear a** foam rubber **pad** held in place with a maternity belt or two sanitary napkins on a sanitary belt **for support. Ice packs** decrease swelling.
2. **Teach** the woman the **signs and symptoms of deep vein thrombosis** and to **avoid injury to the varicosities** that may cause thrombus formation.[36]

3. During delivery, **avoid laceration** to a vulvar varicosity that may result in hemorrhage. **Progressive ambulation** should occur soon after delivery.[36]

4. **Complementary measures:**
   a. **Homeopathy:** Some experts suggest homeopathic remedies for varicosities.[83,91,96] **See information on homeopathy, p. 566.**
   b. **Chinese medicine: Acupuncture** and **shiatsu** have been used with success in the treatment of varicosities.[21,61] **See information on Chinese medicine, p. 559.**
   c. **Nutritional suggestions: Vitamin C** is suggested by many herbalists.[46,62,83,101] **Vitamin E** is also suggested.[62,109] **Bioflavonoids** are said to strengthen capillaries.[46,83] Raw **garlic** and **onions** are considered powerful stimulants of circulation that improve elasticity of vessels.[46,97,109] **Okra, buckwheat, oats, wheat germ,** and **dark green leafy vegetables** are believed to strengthen the circulatory system as a whole.[109]
   d. **Herbs: Comfrey** can be used in a compress for varicosities.[69,97,109] Comfrey is contraindicated during pregnancy because of its hepatotoxic effects except in small doses for limited periods of external use only.[85] **Horse chestnut** may be taken internally to strengthen the venous walls[56,69,81] and may also be used in a compress.[81] **Nettle leaf** tea (1 cup/d) is high in vitamin C and bioflavonoids and increases the elasticity of the vessels.[46,97,109] **See information on herbs, p. 563.**

• SAFETY ISSUES DURING PREGNANCY

Automobile Safety

Physical trauma complicates 1 in every 12 pregnancies. Motor vehicle accidents are the most significant cause of fetal deaths from trauma. All pregnant women should be reminded to wear their seatbelts. The lap belt should be worn across the iliac crest and suprapubic bone. The shoulder harness should be worn between the breasts. Airbags do not appear to increase fetal or maternal injuries, and it is not recommended that they be disabled during pregnancy.[7]

Oral and Dental Care

Timing of dental care before and during pregnancy is important. Ideally, women should seek preventative and restorative care before conception to remove a potential source of infection. During the first trimester, only emergency care should be given. One or two dental x-ray exposures, if necessary for dental work during pregnancy, are considered "not contraindicated."[57]

Pregnancy affects the teeth and gums by causing increased carbohydrate needs, increasing the risk for dental caries. **Pregnancy gingivi-**

tis—in which gums become swollen, vascular, tender, and bleed easily—is caused by maternal hormones. Occasionally, local irritation and poor dental hygiene result in a benign lesion of the gums called **pregnancy tumor.** The tumor may resolve spontaneously after pregnancy, or a dentist may remove the tumor and the local irritant that caused it. The woman who experiences hyperemesis gravidarum may have **acid erosion of the teeth** caused by gastric acid contact, appearing as cupped-out erosions behind the anterior teeth.[57]

Proper oral hygiene minimizes permanent damage to teeth during pregnancy. Holder et al[57] state that topical fluoride treatments are not contraindicated during pregnancy, although systemic fluoride is controversial. Mouthwashes that contain more than 10% alcohol should not be used because of alcohol's effects of the fetus.

Exercise

Exercise is associated with a number of benefits during pregnancy. Exercise may lead to a lower incidence of preterm delivery.[14,53] Women who exercise during pregnancy require less intervention in labor, have substantially fewer cesarean births, and may have shorter stages of labor.[27] For women who have a body mass index (see p. 574) above 33, exercise may reduce the risk of GDM.[39] Exercise improves the spirits, and exercise with a peer group may provide emotional support from other pregnant women. Previously inactive women or those with pregnancy complications should be evaluated before they gradually begin an exercise program.[4]

The FHR usually rises during exercise; however, after strenuous exercise in 15% to 16% of pregnant women, fetal bradycardia is observed. This bradycardia has not been associated with increased morbidity or mortality.[73]

Exercise has different effects on pregnant and nonpregnant women. Exercise requires more work for the pregnant woman. Increasing fetal weight, laxity of the joints, postural changes, fatigue, and increased cardiovascular workload may decrease the physical abilities of the pregnant woman. The hyperinsulinemia of pregnancy may decrease the body fat–reduction effects of exercise. Although the usual heart rate guidelines are not applicable for the pregnant woman, better guidelines are not known. Thus maternal perception of exertion together with heart rate parameters are still suggested as guidelines for exercise.[73]

The occurrence of SAB, FHR abnormalities, PIH, congenital anomalies, IUGR, placental abruption, and fetal demise are not increased with exercise.[28,70] Prenatal exercise does not increase the frequency of preterm delivery.[14,51] The hyperthermia associated with exercise has not been shown to be teratogenic. Women who exercise until delivery produce babies who are 300 to 500 g lighter with lower body fat, but not growth restricted in weight or body structures. No studies have been conducted to determine whether there are long-term developmental effects from this decreased body fat.[73]

Precautions and Suggestions for Planning Exercise

Women who were previously physically inactive and those who have any of the following complications should be evaluated before they begin an exercise program.

Contraindications to Exercise:

IUGR[36]	Lung disease[4]
Preeclampsia[36]	PPROM[4]
Severe heart disease[36]	Preterm labor in present or
Multiple gestation[36]	previous pregnancies[4]
Incompetent cervix or cerclage[4]	Placenta previa after 26 weeks[4]
Persistent second- or	
third-trimester bleeding[4]	

Relative Contraindications to Exercise[4]:

Severe anemia	Being extremely underweight
Chronic bronchitis	Poorly controlled hyperthyroidism
Extreme morbid obesity	Seizure disorder
Heavy smoking	Diabetes type 1
Unevaluated maternal arrhythmia	Hypertension

The following are guidelines for planning safe exercise during pregnancy:

1. **Thirty minutes or more of moderate exercise** almost every day is appropriate for the pregnant woman.[4]
2. **Avoid the supine position** and **prolonged motionless standing.**[4]
3. The **appropriate level** of exertion is guided by maternal perception of exertion and the age-predicted heart rate target.[73]
4. **Avoid exercises in which falling or abdominal trauma is a risk. Avoid scuba diving. Exercise at altitude above 6000 ft** may cause altitude sickness.[4] **Avoid balance-requiring exercises. Non–weight-bearing exercise** is better tolerated than weight-bearing exercise.
5. **Discontinue exercise if any of the following occur[4]:**

Amniotic fluid leakage	Dyspnea before exertion
Calf pain or swelling	Headache
Chest pain	Muscle weakness
Decreased fetal movement	Preterm labor
Dizziness	Vaginal bleeding

6. Provide the body with **adequate hydration, calories, and nutrition.**

Pica

Pica is the ingestion of non-nutritive substances such as ice (pagophagia), starch (amylophagia), clay (geophagia), burnt matches, hair, and any other nonfood substance. The condition is seen more often among women of lower economic status, black women, those in rural areas, and those with a family history of pica. Both the toxicity of the item being consumed and the displacement of healthy nutrients are considered in treating this client. Congenital lead poisoning has affected fetuses of women who eat wall plaster; maternal fecal impaction may occur with ingestion of clay; fetal hemolytic anemia may occur when the woman is eating mothballs or toilet fresheners; maternal parotid enlargement and GI obstruction may occur with ingestion of excessive laundry starch; and parasitic infections may result from the consumption of clay or dirt.[111] Pica may or may not be associated with iron deficiency anemia.[36]

Teratogens

Effects of Teratogens

Before 15 days' gestation, there is no differentiation of fetal tissue, and, when exposed to a teratogen, the fetus either experiences no effect or an SAB occurs. After 8 weeks, teratogens usually affect the fetus by causing IUGR or functional disturbances. Figure 1-5 shows the timing of embryologic development of different body systems and when those systems are most vulnerable to teratogenic exposure.

The embryonic period (2 to 8 weeks' gestation) is the most critical period during which to avoid teratogens because of the organogenesis that occurs at this time. Fewer drugs have an effect during the second half of pregnancy. Some drugs' effects are not seen for years (e.g., DES daughters; see p. 482). Maternal absorption and metabolism of the drug, protein binding and storage, molecular size, electrical charge, and lipid solubility affect passage of the drug across the placenta.[36] It is advisable to prescribe the lowest possible dose to achieve the desired effect during pregnancy. Possible effects on the fetus and the infant include structural malformations; neonatal effects such as neonatal intoxication or neonatal withdrawal; intrauterine fetal death; altered fetal growth; and neurobehavioral toxicity that includes long-term CNS defects that result in delayed behavioral maturation, impaired problem-solving, and impaired learning.[1]

CAFFEINE USE. Caffeine is a CNS stimulant. It increases the heart rate and may contribute to supraventricular tachycardia and sleeplessness.[98] Caffeine is contained in foods that supply nonnutritive calories, thus suppressing appetite. Withdrawal symptoms may include headache, restlessness, and irritability.[89] Table 1-4 lists the caffeine content of some foods.

Caffeine crosses the placenta, and fetal tachycardia is observed after consumption of large doses by the mother.[106] The half-life of caffeine is increased twofold to threefold during pregnancy.[22] Caffeine intake has been associated, in a dose-related manner, with SAB in some studies,[29] but the association between anomalies and caffeine intake has not been consistently replicated. Caffeine consumption of >300 mg/d has been inconsistently related to LBW.[22] Caffeine has been shown to increase the frequency, although not the incidence, of fetal breathing move-

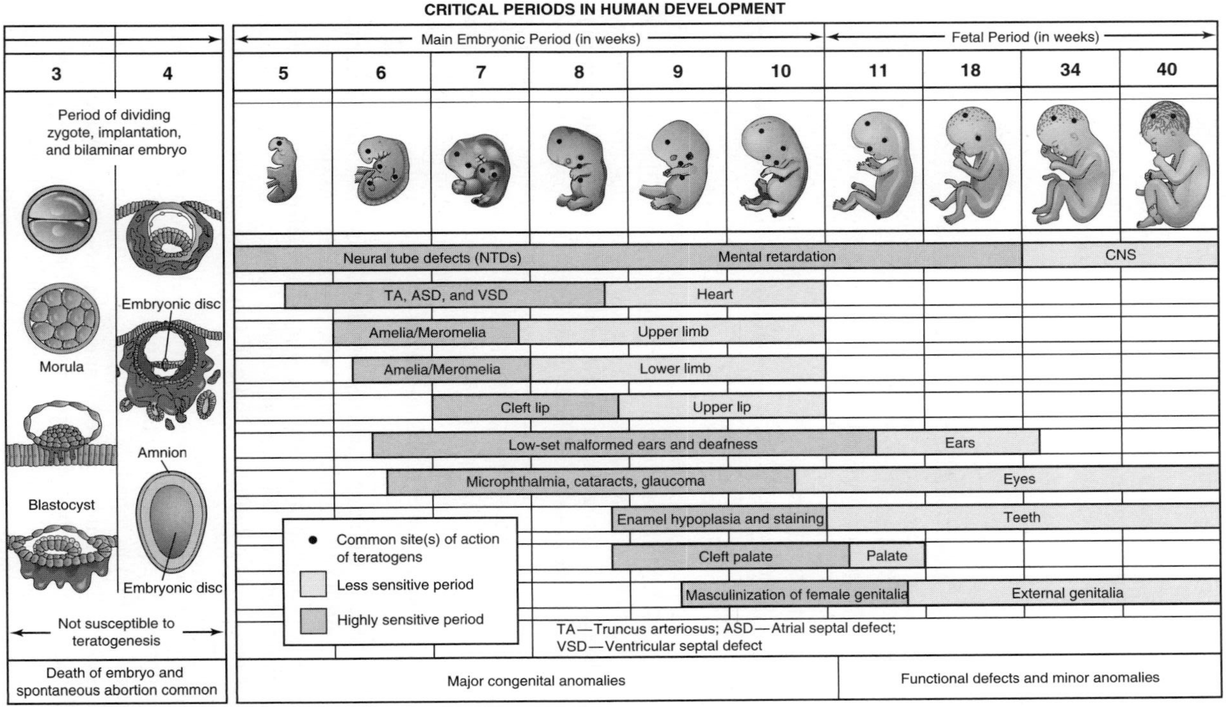

Figure 1-5 • Timing of systems development in the human embryo. Areas indicated by dark color denote periods of high sensitivity to teratogens; light colors indicate periods of lesser sensitivity. (From Moore K, Persaud TVN: *The developing human: clinically oriented embryology*, ed 7, Philadelphia, 2003, Saunders.)

Table 1-4 / Caffeine Content of Various Foods and Beverages

Food/Beverage	Caffeine Content (mg)
150 mL brewed coffee	115
150 mL boiled coffee	90
150 mL instant coffee	60
150 mL tea made with loose tea or teabag	39
150 mL herbal tea	0
150 mL soft drink (cola)	15
150 mL cocoa	4
1 g chocolate bar	0.3
Some medications	50-100/tablet

Data from Cnattinguis S et al: Caffeine intake and the risk of first-trimester spontaneous abortion, *Engl J Med* 343(25):1839-1845, 2000.

ments.[33] When caffeine was administered IV to sheep, it decreased uterine blood flow by 5% to 10%.[36] Rarely, withdrawal symptoms are seen in the neonate.[22] In 1980, the FDA advised pregnant women to limit their intake of caffeine.[36] Burrow and Ferris[22] suggest that 150 mg of caffeine/d in the first trimester would be a prudent limit, particularly in women with a history of habitual SAB.

HAIR TREATMENTS. Hair dye and permanents are safe.[5]

NUTRASWEET (ASPARTAME) USE. The major metabolite of aspartame is phenylalanine, concentrated in the fetus by the placenta. The only known risk of NutraSweet use during pregnancy is in the presence of maternal phenylketonuria (PKU), in which sustained high blood levels of phenylalanine are associated with mental retardation in the fetus. NutraSweet has never been shown to harm unborn children. The pregnant woman would have to consume one diet drink every 8 minutes for 24 hours to exceed the level of phenylalanine that can be safely metabolized by the healthy individual.[111]

PAINT EXPOSURE. Paint is not a proven teratogen, but minimal exposure is wise.[44]

RADIATION EXPOSURE. Recommendations for safe limits of radiation exposure have varied over the years and among experts. Radiation is cumulative and mutagenic, and the DNA of some individuals is more vulnerable to radiation than that of others. If the individual is affected, the exposure increases the person's risk of leukemia, and certain other indicator diseases including asthma, eczema, urticaria, pneumonia, dysentery, and rheumatic fever.[17]

The recommended occupational limit for the 40 weeks of pregnancy is estimated to be 500 mrad. Therapeutic abortion is recommended when exposure exceeds 10,000 mrad. Doses between 1000 and 3000 mrad may increase the risk of childhood malignancy.[79] In the setting of major maternal trauma, weighing the risks and benefits, Coleman et al [30a] state that >2500 mrad (a routine trauma x-ray examination series) presents very little risk for the fetus. An 18-exposure full-mouth series of dental x-ray films exposes the fetus to 0.001 mrad or less.[57] Exposure is 1 mrad for a chest x-ray film and 221 mrad for an abdominal film.[79] A computed axial tomography scan exposes the fetus to approximately 3.5 rad.[7] The gestational timing of exposure (with 8 to 15 weeks being the most susceptible[36]) and the maternal body part irradiated (distance is protective) are factors in the assessment of risk.[17]

Travel

The second trimester is recommended for travel because of the increased risk of SAB during the first trimester and the risks of preterm labor, hypertension, or other complications that would require medical care during the third trimester. Airlines have regulations regarding travel during pregnancy and should be consulted regarding their policies. Most allow domestic travel until 36 weeks' gestation. Relative contraindications to air travel include severe anemia, a history of thromboembolic disease, and placental problems. International travel may be considered relatively contraindicated in the following circumstances: history of SAB, incompetent cervix, ectopic pregnancy, preterm labor or PPROM, history of placentation abnormalities, threatened abortion, history of preeclampsia, diabetes, hypertension, multiple gestation, infertility, thromboembolic disease, severe anemia, heart disease, chronic medical problems, as well as the primigravida <15 years or >35 years. Areas that are problematic include those of high altitudes, areas where food-borne or insect-borne diseases are endemic, areas where live-virus vaccines are required, and areas where malaria is endemic.[24]

Safety Suggestions for Travel

1. Information and **immunizations** required for international travel are available at local public health facilities.
2. Travel with a **companion.**
3. Make sure **health insurance** is valid overseas.
4. Identify **medical facilities** at the destination for management of complications, and delivery if needed.
5. Arrange to receive **prenatal care** during the visit if necessary.
6. Know whether **blood** is screened for hepatitis and HIV at the destination, and know one's blood type.
7. Use appropriate **automobile safety** measures (see p. 46).
8. **When flying,** maintain hydration, use seatbelt correctly and continuously, wear support stockings, move the legs regularly, and ambulate q30min during the flight.[24]

9. **Seek medical attention for** the **danger signs** of pregnancy (see p. 14). Carry a copy of the pregnancy medical record.
10. Learn about the **safety of food and beverages** at the destination. Eat well-cooked foods and pasteurized dairy products. Avoid pre-prepared salads.
11. Should traveler's **diarrhea** occur, keep hydrated.[24]

Work

Physically demanding work is associated with preterm birth (odds ratio [OR] 1.22), IUGR (OR 1.37), and hypertension or preeclampsia (OR 1.60). Prolonged standing is significantly associated with preterm birth (OR 1.26), as are shift and night work (OR 1.24) and a high cumulative fatigue score (OR 1.63). Long work hours are not associated with preterm birth.[77] Heavy lifting has been linked to SAB and preterm labor, as well as varicosities of the lower extremities.[67]

Other factors that may be hazardous to the working pregnant woman include radiation (discussed previously), magnetic fields, travel (see p. 52), vibrations, impacts, noise, heat, stress, and infections. Vibration may alter circulation in the pelvis, may affect spinal reflexes, and in later pregnancy, may cause back or abdominal discomfort. High noise levels have been associated with preterm delivery or delivery of LBW infants in some studies, and a noisy setting may diminish fetal hearing. Stress increases the risk of preterm labor and LBW infants. Work in bacteriology or virology laboratories is associated with high maternal serum viral levels and an increased incidence of perinatal deaths. No risk factors are associated with use of computer visual display units.[67] Occupational exposure to substances is discussed in the following section.

Occupational Substance Exposures

Approximately 5% of the some 60,000 chemicals used in industry have actually been tested for their effects on reproduction.[67] Occupational exposure to substances such as dry cleaning chemicals, paint, rubber, semi-conductor manufacturing materials, and glycol ethers used among fabrication workers increases the risk of SAB, and other effects are uncertain.[44] Chemicals in the following groups are known to cause malformations: solvents, anesthetic gases, cytostatica, halogenated hydrocarbons, and heavy metals.[67]

• COMPLEMENTARY MEASURES FOR GENERAL WELL-BEING AND BIRTH PREPARATION

Some herbs are suggested to be taken daily for the final weeks of gestation to tone the uterus, promote timely and efficient labor, and prevent postpartum hemorrhage (PPH):

1. **Blue cohosh** (From 36 weeks on, 1 capsule, 1 cup tea, or 1 tsp tincture/cup liquid tid[80]).[12,69,74,80,101]
2. **Red raspberry** (1 cup tea/d last 2 months of pregnancy[81]).*
3. **Squawvine** (1 cup tea/d[81]).† **See information on herbs, p. 563.**

• REFERENCES

1. American Academy of Pediatrics (AAP) Committee on Drugs: Use of psychoactive medication during pregnancy and possible effects on the fetus and newborn, *Pediatrics* 105:880-887, 2000.
2. American College of Nurse-Midwives (ACNM): Guidelines for providers: cystic fibrosis genetic screening, *Quickening* 33(1):23, 2002.
3. ACNM: Society releases position paper on hypothyroidism, *Quickening* 30(5):20, 1999.
4. American College of Obstetricians and Gynecologists (ACOG): *Exercise during pregnancy and the postpartum period,* ACOG Committee Opinion No. 267, Washington, DC, 2002, ACOG.
5. ACOG: Will this hurt my fetus? *ACOG Woman's Health* Jan 1999, accessed at *http://www.acog.com/from_home/publications/womans_ health/wh12-15-7.htm.*
6. Reference deleted in galleys.
7. ACOG: *Obstetric aspects of trauma management,* ACOG Educational Bulletin No. 249, Washington, DC, 1998, ACOG.
8. ACOG: Now is the time to help adolescent girls avoid lifelong health problems report OB/GYNs, *ACOG News Release* Dec 9, 1997, accessed at *http://www.acog.com/from_ home/publications/press_releases/nr12-9-97.htm.*
9. ACOG: *Preconceptional care,* ACOG Technical Bulletin No. 205, Washington, DC, 1995, ACOG.
10. Andrews CM, O'Neill LM: Use of pelvic tilt exercise for ligament pain relief, *J Nurse Midwifery* 39:370-374, 1994.
11. Bahado-Singh R et al: An alternative for women initially declining genetic amniocentesis: individual Down syndrome odds on the basis of maternal age and multiple ultrasonographic markers, *Am J Obstet Gynecol* 179:514-519, 1998.
12. Balch JF, Balch PA: *Prescription for nutritional healing,* ed 2, Garden City Park, NY, 1997, Avery Publishing Group.
13. Beck CT: Available instruments for research on prenatal attachment and adaptation to pregnancy, *MCN Am J Matern Child Nurs* 24:25-32, 1999.
14. Berkowitz GS et al: Physical activity and the risk of preterm labor, *J Reprod Med* 28: 581-588, 1983.
15. Bloom KC: Perceived relationship with the father of the baby and maternal attachment in adolescents, *J Obstet Gynecol Neonatal Nurs* 27:420-430, 1998.
16. Briggs GG: Nausea and vomiting of pregnancy. In drugs, pregnancy, and lactation, *OBGYN News* 36(15):8, 2001.
17. Bross IDJ, Natarajan N: Cumulative genetic damage in children exposed to preconception and intrauterine radiation, *Invest Radiol* 15(1):52-64, 1980.
18. Brucker MC: Management of the third stage of labor: an evidence-based approach, *J Midwifery Womens Health* 46:381-392, 2001.
19. Brucker MC, Faucher MA: Pharmacologic management of common gastrointestinal health problems in women, *J Nurse Midwifery* 42:145-162, 1997.
20. Brumfield CG et al: Pregnancy outcome following genetic amniocentesis at 11-14 weeks versus 16-19 weeks' gestation, *Obstet Gynecol* 88:114-118, 1996.

---

*References 18, 49, 56, 69, 81, 83, 100.
†References 12, 49, 56, 69, 81, 83.

21. Budd S: Acupuncture. In Tiran D, Mack S, editors: *Complementary therapies for pregnancy and childbirth*, ed 2, Edinburgh, 2000, Baillière Tindall.

22. Burrow GN, Ferris TF: *Medical complications during pregnancy*, ed 4, Philadelphia, 1995, WB Saunders.

23. The Canadian Early and Mid-trimester Amniocentesis Trial (CEMAT) Group: Randomized trial to assess safety and fetal outcome of early and midtrimester amniocentesis, *Lancet* 351:242-247, 1998.

24. Centers for Disease Control and Prevention (CDC): *Pregnancy, breast-feeding and travel*, July 2000. Available at: *http://www.cdc.gov/travel/pregnant.htm*.

25. Chescheir NC, Hansen WF: New in perinatology, *Pediatr Rev* 20:57-63, 1999.

26. Chez RA: Herbal remedies in pregnancy, *Contemp Ob Gyn* 46:112, 2001 (letter).

27. Clapp JF: The course of labor after endurance exercise during pregnancy, *Am J Obstet Gynecol* 163:1799-1805, 1990.

28. Clapp JF: The effects of maternal exercise on early pregnancy outcome, *Am J Obstet Gynecol* 161:1453-1457, 1989.

29. Cnattinguis S et al: Caffeine intake and the risk of first-trimester spontaneous abortion, *N Engl J Med* 343:1839-1845, 2000.

30. Cogswell ME et al: Medically advised, mother's personal target, and actual weight gain during pregnancy, *Obstet Gynecol* 94:616-622, 1999.

30a. Coleman MT, Trianfo VA, Rund DA: Nonobstetric emergencies in pregnancy: trauma and surgical conditions, *Am J Obstet Gynecol* 177:497-502, 1997.

31. Conway PL: Osteopathy during pregnancy. In Tiran D, Mack S, editors: *Complementary therapies for pregnancy and childbirth*, ed 2, Edinburgh, 2000, Baillière Tindall.

32. Crawford AM: *Herbal remedies for women*, Rocklin, Calif, 1997, Prima.

33. Creasy RK, Resnick R: *Maternal-fetal medicine: principles and practice*, Philadelphia, 1994, WB Saunders.

34. Cummings B, Tiran D: Homeopathy for pregnancy and childbirth. In Tiran D, Mack S, editors: *Complementary therapies for pregnancy and childbirth*, ed 2, Edinburgh, 2000, Baillière Tindall.

35. Cummings S, Ullman D: *Everybody's guide to homeopathic medicines*, New York, 1997, Jeremy P. Tarcher/Putnam.

36. Cunningham FG et al: *Williams obstetrics*, ed 20, Stamford, Conn, 1997, Appleton and Lange.

37. Department of Health Services Genetic Disease Branch: *California Expanded Alpha-Fetoprotein Screening Program prenatal care provider handbook*, Berkeley, Calif, 1995, Author.

38. Drake P: Addressing developmental needs of pregnant adolescents, *J Obstet Gynecol Neonatal Nurs* 256:518-524, 1996.

39. Dye TD et al: Physical activity, obesity, and diabetes in pregnancy, *Am J Epidemiol* 146:961-965, 1997.

40. Edelman A, Logan JR: *Pregnancy, hyperemesis gravidarum*, last updated Aug 24, 2001, accessed at *http://www.emedicine.com/emerg/topic479.htm*.

41. Feral C: Natural remedies, *Midwifery Today* 26:35-38, 1993.

42. Fischer-Rasmussen W et al: Ginger treatment of hyperemesis gravidarum, *Eur J Obstet Gynecol Biol* 38:19-24, 1990.

43. Fuchs D: *Massage for common discomforts of pregnancy for use in clinical practice*, American College of Nurse-Midwives Annual Convention, San Francisco, May 1998 (handout from workshop: Prenatal Massage).

43a. Fynes M et al: Effect of second vaginal delivery on anorectal physiology and faecal incontinence: a prospective study, *Lancet* 354:983-986, 1999.

44. Gabbe SG, Niebyl JR, Simpson JL: *Obstetrics: normal & problem pregnancies*, ed 3, New York, 1996, Churchill Livingstone.

45. Gardner J: *Healing yourself*, ed 7 revised, Trumansburg, NY, 1982, The Crossing Press.

46. Gladstar R: *Herbal healing for women*, New York, 1993, Simon & Schuster.

47. Gold RB et al: Conservative management of second trimester post-amniocentesis fluid leakage, *Obstet Gynecol* 74:745-747, 1989.

48. Gordon JD et al: *Obstetrics gynecology & infertility*, Glen Cove, NY, 1998, Scrub Hill Press.

49. Griffith HW: *Healing herbs: the essential guide*, Tucson, Ariz, 2000, Fisher Books.

50. Hacker NF, Moore JG: Essentials of obstetrics and gynecology, ed 3, Philadelphia, 1998, WB Saunders.

51. Hale RW, Milne L: The elite athlete and exercise in pregnancy, *Semin Perinatol* 20: 277-284, 1996.

52. Hanafin MJ: *An introduction to homeopathy*, American College of Nurse-Midwives Annual Convention, San Francisco, May 1998 (lecture handout and notes).

53. Hatch M et al: Maternal leisure-time exercise and timely delivery, *Am J Public Health* 88:1528-1533, 1998.

54. Hediger ML et al: Patterns of weight gain in adolescent pregnancy: effects on birth weight and preterm delivery, *Obstet Gynecol* 74:6-12, 1989.

55. Hoffmann D: *The complete illustrated holistic herbal*, Boston, 1996, Element Books Limited.

56. Hoffmann D: *The holistic herbal*, Findhorn, Scotland, 1985, The Findhorn Press.

57. Holder R et al: Preventative dentistry during pregnancy, *Nurse Pract* 24:21-24, 1999.

58. Huxley RR: Nausea and vomiting in early pregnancy: its role in placental development, *Obstet Gynecol* 95:779-782, 2000.

59. Jancin B: Accelerated salivation common in pregnancy, *OBGYN News* Aug 1, 2001, p 10.

60. Jarvis C: *Physical examination and health assessment*, ed 2, Philadelphia, 1996, WB Saunders.

61. Johnson E: Shiatsu. In Tiran D, Mack S, editors: *Complementary therapies for pregnancy and childbirth*, ed 2, Edinburgh, 2000, Baillière Tindall.

62. Koehler N: *Artemis speaks: V.B.A.C. stories & natural childbirth information*, Occidental, Calif, 1985, Jerald R. Brown.

63. Kolasa KM, Weismiller DG: Nutrition during pregnancy, *Am Fam Physician* 56:205-212, 1995.

64. Kriebs JM, Burgin KB: Pharmacologic management of common musculoskeletal disorders in women, *J Nurse Midwifery* 42:207-227, 1997.

65. Kristiansson P, Svardsudd K, von Schoultz B: Back pain during pregnancy, *Spine* 21:702-709, 1996.

66. Lacroix R, Eason E, Melzack R: Nausea and vomiting during pregnancy: a prospective study of its frequency, intensity, and patterns of change, *Am J Obstet Gynecol* 182:931-937, 2000.

67. Lidstrom IM: Pregnant women in the workplace, *Semin Perinatol* 14:329-333, 1990.

68. Lockwood CJ: Applying new advances in OB ultrasound, *Contemp Ob Gyn* 46(6): 51-75, June 2001.

69. Mabey R et al, editors: *The new age herbalist*, New York, 1988, Collier Books.

70. MacPhail A et al: Maximal exercise testing in late gestation: fetal responses, *Obstet Gynecol* 96:565-570, 2000.

71. Malnory ME: Development of the pregnant couple, *J Obstet Gynecol Neonatal Nurs* 25:525-532, 1996.

72. Mayer IE, Hussain H: Pregnancy and gastrointestinal disorders, *Gastroenterol Clin* 27: 1-36, 1998.

73. McMurray RG et al: Recent advances in understanding maternal and fetal responses to exercise, *Med Sci Sports Exerc* 25:1305-1321, 1993.

74. Medina IM: *Issues in women's health care: nutrition and herbs from menarche to menopause 3/28-29/98*, Brooklyn, NY, 1998, State University of New York Health Science Center at Brooklyn College of Health Related Professions Midwifery Education Program (course syllabus).

74a. Meyer S et al: The effects of birth on urinary continence mechanisms and other pelvic-floor characteristics, *Obstet Gynecol* 92(4 part 1):613-618,1998.

75. Moerman ML: Growth of the birth canal in adolescent girls, *Am J Obstet Gynecol* 143:528-532, 1982.

76. Reference deleted in galleys.
77. Mozurkewich EL et al: Working conditions and adverse pregnancy outcome, *Obstet Gynecol* 95:623-635, 2000.
78. Murphy PA: Alternative therapies for nausea and vomiting of pregnancy, *Obstet Gynecol* 91:149-155, 1998.
79. Nelson WE, editor: *Nelson textbook of pediatrics*, ed 15, Philadelphia, 1996, WB Saunders.
80. Nissim R: *Natural healing in gynecology*, San Francisco, 1996, Pandora.
81. Ody P: *The complete medicinal herbal*, New York, 1993, Dorling Kindersley.
82. Orvos H et al: Is adolescent pregnancy associated with adverse perinatal outcome? *J Perinat Med* 27:199-203, 1999.
83. Page L: *Healthy healing*, ed 11, Carmel Valley, Calif, 2000, Healthy Healing.
84. Parvati J: *Hygieia: a woman's herbal*, Berkeley, Calif, 1985, Bookpeople.
85. *Physician's desk reference for herbal medicines*, Montvale, NJ, 1998, Medical Economics.
86. Perkins J, Hammer RL, Loubert PV: Identification and management of pregnancy-related low back pain, *J Nurse Midwifery* 43:331-340, 1998.
87. Perry LE: Preconception care: a health promotion opportunity, *Nurse Pract* 21:24-41, 1996.
88. Read J: Sexual problems associated with infertility, pregnancy, and ageing, *BMJ* 318:587-589, 1999.
89. RN: There's no reason to worry about caffeine addiction. In Acute care decisions: consult stat, *RN* 61:55-56, 1998.
90. Reifsnider E, Gill SL: Nutrition for the childbearing years, *J Obstet Gynecol Neonatal Nurs* 29:43-55, 2000.
91. Rose B, Scott-Moncrieff C: *Homeopathy for women*, London, 1998, Collins & Brown.
92. Sacher RA, McPherson RA: *Widmann's clinical interpretation of laboratory tests*, ed 10, Philadelphia, 1991, FA Davis Company.
93. Sahakian V et al: Vitamin B6 is an effective therapy for nausea and vomiting of pregnancy: a randomized double-blind placebo-controlled study, *Obstet Gynecol* 78:33-36, 1991.
94. Scholl TO et al: Weight gain during pregnancy in adolescence: predictive ability of early weight gain, *Obstet Gynecol* 75:948-953, 1990.
95. Singingtree DL: Herbal helps, *Midwifery Today* 26:16, Summer 1993.
96. Smith T: *Homeopathy for pregnancy and nursing mothers*, Worthing, England, 1993, Insight Editions.
97. Stapleton H, Tiran D: Herbal medicine. In Tiran D, Mack S, editors: *Complementary therapies for pregnancy and childbirth*, ed 2, Edinburgh, 2000, Baillière Tindall.
98. Stein J, editor: *Internal medicine*, ed 4, St Louis, 1994, Mosby.
99. Suitor CW: *Maternal weight gain: a report of an expert work group*, Arlington, Va, 1997, National Center for Education in Maternal and Child Health.
100. Summers L: Methods of cervical ripening and labor induction, *J Nurse Midwifery* 42:71-85, 1997.
101. Tarr K: *Herbs, helps, and pressure points for pregnancy and childbirth*, ed 3, Provo, Utah, 1984, Sunbeam.
102. Tellefson T: The chiropractic approach to health care during pregnancy. In Tiran D, Mack S, editors: *Complementary therapies for pregnancy and childbirth*, ed 2, Edinburgh, 2000, Baillière Tindall.
103. Tiran D: Massage and aromatherapy. In Tiran D, Mack S, editors: *Complementary therapies for pregnancy and childbirth*, ed 2, Edinburgh, 2000, Baillière Tindall.
104. Tiran D: Reflexology in midwifery practice. In Tiran D, Mack S, editors: *Complementary therapies for pregnancy and childbirth*, ed 2, Edinburgh, 2000, Baillière Tindall.
105. Ullman R, Reichenberg-Ullman J: *Homeopathic self-care*, Rocklin, Calif, 1997, Prima.
106. Varney H: *Varney's midwifery*, ed 3, Sudbury, Mass, 1997, Jones and Bartlett.
107. Vutyavanich T, Wongtra-ngan S, Ruangsri R: Pyridoxine for nausea and vomiting of pregnancy: a randomized, double-blind, placebo-controlled trial, *Am J Obstet Gynecol* 173:881-884, 1995.
108. Walker DS, McCully L, Vest V: Evidence-based prenatal care visits: when less is more, *J Midwifery Womens Health* 46:146-151, 2001.

109. Weed SS: *Wise woman herbal childbearing year*, Woodstock, NY, 1985, Ash Tree.
110. Williams RD: Healthy pregnancy, healthy baby, *FDA Consumer Magazine* [serial online] 33(2), 1999, accessed at *http://www.fda.gov/fdac/features/1999/299_ baby.html*.
111. Worthington-Roberts BS, Williams SR: *Nutrition and lactation*, ed 6, Madison, Wis, 1997, Brown & Benchmark.
112. Zhu BP et al: Effect of the interval between pregnancies on perinatal outcomes, *N Engl J Med* 340:589-594, 1999.

Chapter 2

Complications of Pregnancy and Their Management

Spontaneous Abortion

Spontaneous abortion (SAB) is the loss of a pregnancy at <20 weeks' gestation or weighing <500 g. An early abortion occurs before 12 weeks; a late abortion occurs between 12 and 20 weeks.[25]

Etiology: In 53% of first trimester SABs and in 36% of second trimester SABs, the fetus is abnormal. Most are chance mutations and not abnormalities that will repeat in future pregnancies.[25] SAB with normal chromosomes is seen more often with advanced maternal age.[95]

Incidence: The independent risk of SAB in any pregnancy is 14% to 19%.[95]

Risk Factors for SAB[95]:

Advanced maternal age
Anatomic abnormalities
Antiphospholipid antibodies
  (see p. 371)
Asherman's syndrome (see p. 462)
Autoimmune and alloimmune
  factors
Chronic medical problems
Cigarette smoking (risk doubled
  for ≥14 cigarettes/d)
Endocrine abnormalities

Environmental issues such as
  drugs, toxins, stress, and night
  shift employment
Infection
Luteal phase defect
Moderate or greater alcohol
  consumption
Polycystic ovarian syndrome
Poorly controlled diabetes
Systemic lupus erythematosus
  (see p. 370)

Complications[90]:

Anesthesia-related issues
Embolism

Hemorrhage
Infection

Prognosis for Pregnancy after SAB: Sixty percent to 75% of couples successfully achieve pregnancy after SAB without medical intervention.[95]

Differential Diagnosis: See p. 65 for vaginal bleeding. For abdominal pain, consider urinary tract infection (UTI), round ligament pain, placental abruption, preterm labor, and nonobstetric causes (see p. 328).

Types of Spontaneous Abortion

THREATENED ABORTION. Vaginal bleeding without passage of products of conception (POC). The presence of cramping is ominous. Bleeding usually begins 2 weeks after the pregnancy stopped developing.

INEVITABLE ABORTION. Vaginal bleeding (or loss of amniotic fluid) is present with cervical dilation, with or without abdominal pain.

INCOMPLETE ABORTION. Part but not all of the POC have been expelled from the uterus. Before 12 weeks, the abortion tends to be complete; after 12 weeks, POC tend to be retained.

COMPLETE ABORTION. All the POC have been passed.

MISSED ABORTION. Retention of the POC 4 to 8 weeks after fetal death. Uterine growth stops, then regresses. The fetal heart is not auscultated when expected by dates. No fetal movement is perceived, and breast changes regress. The mother may lose weight. Amenorrhea may continue, or spotting may be seen.

HABITUAL OR RECURRENT ABORTION. Three or more consecutive SABs. The likelihood of two recurrent SABs is 2.3%; the likelihood of three recurrent SABs is 0.34%. Etiology may be endocrine, genetic, immune, or medical factors; infection; uterine factors; an incompetent internal cervical os; or exposure to drugs, chemicals, radiation, or cigarettes.[32] No etiology is found in 50%.[95]

SEPTIC ABORTION. Any abortion occurring with a uterine infection.[32]

ⓜ Management of Spontaneous Abortion

1. **Determine whether the woman is hemodynamically stable.** Tachycardia, syncope, dizziness, or lightheadedness signal instability and the woman should receive urgent IV fluid replacement and evaluation for emergency intervention.[95]
2. Perform a gentle **pelvic examination,** noting blood in the vault, vaginal and cervical normalcy (ruling out causes of vaginal bleeding other than threatened abortion), whether the cervix is open, tenderness and size of the uterus, and/or masses in the adnexae.[53] Remove any **tissue in the os** and save for pathology. **Take cultures** if indicated.[95]
3. Assess the **viability** of the pregnancy. Box 2-1 lists the indicators of fetal viability. Krause and Graves[53] suggest the following regimen:
   <7 weeks: Serial human chorionic gonadotropin (hCG) or serum progesterone.

• *Box 2-1 /* Measures of Fetal Viability •

HCG

Positive 7-10 days after ovulation; levels double every 1.6 days during week 5, every 2 days during week 6, and every 2.5 days during week 7. Levels continue to rise more slowly, peaking at 10 weeks, plateauing at 24 weeks.[53]

ULTRASOUND FINDINGS[56]

- When the gestational sac is >10 mm, a yolk sac should always be visualized.
- A gestational sac of 18 mm (or 2.5 cm) should contain an embryo.
- An embryo >5 mm should have cardiac activity.
- A gestational sac should be visible by transvaginal ultrasound when the hCG is >2000 mIU/mL.
- A gestational sac should be visible by abdominal ultrasound when the hCG is >6500 mIU/mL.

ULTRASOUND CORRELATED WITH HCG AND DATING[32]

- At 34.8 (5 weeks) ± 2.2 days, the hCG is 914 mIU/mL ±106 and a fetal sac is identifiable.
- At 40.3 (5.8 weeks) ± 3.4 days, the hCG is 3783 mIU/mL ± 683 and a fetal pole is visible.
- At 46.9 days (6.7 weeks) ± 6 days, the hCG is 13,178 mIU/mL ± 2898 and fetal heart activity is seen.

SERUM PROGESTERONE

- ≥25 ng/mL: A viable pregnancy in >95% cases.[93]
- <10 ng/mL: An intrauterine pregnancy, if present, is nonviable.[32]

7 to 8 weeks: Serial hCG or serum progesterone; alternatively, transvaginal ultrasound followed by hCG measurement if no cardiac activity is present.

8 to 10 weeks: Transvaginal ultrasound followed by hCG or progesterone measurement if no cardiac activity is present.

≥10 weeks: Fetal heart tones (FHTs) by Doppler; if not heard, ultrasound.

4. Obtain **serial hCG measurements** every 2 to 3 days, transvaginal ultrasounds weekly, and weekly office visits until the prognosis of the pregnancy is certain. No medical therapy can prevent an SAB—even progesterone administration to women with known luteal phase defects does not decrease the risk.[95]

5. Give **RhoGAM** to the Rh-negative mother when h

6. When an incomplete SAB is diagnosed, present **ment** approaches and their **risks and benefits** make the plan together. Diffuse intravascular c rare complication that may not be prevented b vention, and concern regarding this complic management decisions.[95]

   a. **Expectant management** may be plan cotic pain relief are prescribed for c

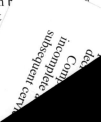

suggested. Medical or surgical treatment is generally conducted after 3 days without passage of the POC. Seventy-nine percent will pass the POC within 3 days.[53]

b. Medical and surgical interventions require **consultation** with a physician.

(1) **Medical management** may include administration of ergot alkaloids, ergots combined with misoprostol, or misoprostol alone or with methotrexate. The latter combination has a success rate of 45% to 95%. Side effects occur in 25% to 88% women and include nausea, vomiting, diarrhea, headache, dizziness, and hot flushes.[53]

(2) **Indications for a** dilation and curettage **(D&C)** include second trimester intrauterine death, septic abortion, failure of medication-induced abortion, failure of expectant management, or the client's choice.[53]

7. **Advise the woman** with an uncomplicated complete abortion to observe **pelvic rest** for 3 days. Prescribe **hormonal contraception** to be started after the SAB for the woman who desires it. Counsel the **woman who desires conception** to wait at least one cycle to allow for normalization of the endometrium, maximizing chances for success with the next pregnancy.[53]

8. **Follow-up with an office visit in 2 weeks** to examine the uterus; recheck urinary hCG levels in urine (85% will be negative; others should be checked again in 2 more weeks).[53]

9. **Address emotional concerns,** including concerns regarding the cause, whether to name the baby, whether to have a memorial service, and how to discuss the loss with other children. Grief counseling and religious counseling may be helpful for the couple who are having difficulty resolving their grief.[95]

10. The woman who experiences a **threatened abortion** but continues with a viable pregnancy is at increased risk for preterm labor, intrauterine growth retardation (IUGR), and oligohydramnios.[95]

Therapeutic Abortion

Surgical abortion techniques include menstrual extraction (aspiration of the endometrial cavity with a thin catheter and a syringe at 5 to 8 weeks), vacuum curettage (dilation of the cervix and suctioning of the uterus at <14 weeks), D&C (further dilation of the cervix and curettage with a metal curette at <14 weeks), or dilation and evacuation (D&E; wide dilation of the cervix followed by vacuum curettage after 16 weeks). Laminaria tents, Lamicel tents, and gemeprost pessaries are products that are inserted into the cervix to begin the dilation and [dec]rease the trauma to the cervix.[32]

[Comp]lications include bleeding, infection, uterine perforation, [ ]abortion, potentially fatal consumptive coagulopathies, and [cervi]cal incompetence or uterine synechiae.[32]

Medical induction of abortion is provided by a physician before 8 weeks' gestation. After 8 weeks' gestation, surgical abortion is preferred.[59] **Methotrexate** given in early pregnancy inhibits the action of folic acid, prevents synthesis of RNA and DNA, and leads to cell death, especially affecting rapidly proliferating tissues such as trophoblasts. HCG production stops, and the trophoblastic/decidual attachment is undermined within about 72 hours. **Misoprostol** (Cytotec) is a synthetic prostaglandin E1 analogue that increases amplitude of uterine contractions, assisting with the expelling of contents.[79] **Antiprogesterone RU 486 (mifepristone),** an oral antiprogesterone agent, may be given with misoprostol to terminate the pregnancy.[59] Medical induction of abortion after 8 weeks' gestation may include laminaria ripening, oxytocin induction, prostaglandins, and intra-amniotic hyperosmotic solutions.[32]

• ACUTE FATTY LIVER OF PREGNANCY

Fatty infiltration of the hepatocytes of unknown etiology, along with ammonia production by the hepatocytes, leads to hypoglycemia and coagulopathy from hepatic failure.[16,108] Usually occurring in the third trimester,[108] acute fatty liver of pregnancy (AFLP) is possibly a variant of severe preeclampsia.[40] The primigravida with preeclampsia is at increased risk.[65]

Hypertension, edema, and proteinuria are often present[108] as well as nausea or vomiting, abdominal pain (epigastric or RUQ), and anorexia.[65] Jaundice occurs as the disease advances.[16] DIC, hypoglycemia, and central nervous system (CNS) alterations are signs of worsening.[108] The maternal mortality rate is 10% to 18%[84]; the fetal mortality rate is 23%.[65]

Differential Diagnosis:

Preeclampsia	Hyperemesis gravidarum
HELLP* syndrome	Thrombotic thrombocytopenia
Acute viral hepatitis	Reye's syndrome
HSV hepatitis	Intrahepatic cholestasis or hemorrhage
Budd-Chiari syndrome	Hemolytic uremic syndrome
Systemic lupus erythematosus	Acetaminophen overdose

Diagnosis: Clinical and laboratory evidence of renal impairment, reduced hepatic metabolic activity, and coagulopathy diagnose AFLP. Liver biopsy is occasionally required to confirm the diagnosis, although viral serology is now available to distinguish AFLP from hepatitis.[26] Ultrasound, computed tomography (CT), and magnetic resonance imaging (MRI) may or may not show evidence of AFLP.[76]

Hypoglycemia is common in AFLP in contrast to other liver disorders. Many women with AFLP have preeclampsia, but women with preeclampsia who do not have AFLP are not usually jaundiced, nor do they develop hypoglycemia or reduced hepatic metabolic activity. DIC

---

*Hemolysis, elevated liver enzymes, low platelet.

is often seen with AFLP, but is only seen with preeclampsia when placental abruption is also present. The patient with acute hepatitis will have positive serology study findings and a higher serum transaminase level than the patient with AFLP.[108]

ⓜ Management

1. If a midwife suspects AFLP, immediate obstetric **consultation** is indicated. The goal is **early recognition and prompt delivery.**[26]
2. **Anticipatory guidance: Supportive intensive care** may involve gastroenterology, internal medicine, and nephrology experts.[26] If the patient is in labor and the fetal and maternal status is reassuring, **vaginal delivery** may be attempted. Otherwise, **correction of coagulopathy** should be followed by **cesarean section.**[16]

• ADVANCED MATERNAL AND PATERNAL AGE

As women age, their risk for congenital anomalies increases (see Table 2-1). Complications of pregnancy and delivery for the older gravida include hypertension, diabetes,[7] SAB, twinning, instrumental vaginal delivery, cesarean delivery, smaller birth weight, and lower gestational age.[41] The psychological tasks of pregnancy, however, may be accomplished more easily by older pregnant women. Problem-solving skills help them meet the challenges of pregnancy and birth. These woman are usually better educated, seek prenatal care earlier, and have higher incomes than younger women.[110]

Advanced paternal age increases the risk of new autosomal dominant mutations. The absolute risk of a new autosomal dominant defect in the infant of a 40-year-old father is at least 0.3%.[32]

Table 2-1 / Advanced Maternal Age and the Risk for Associated Anomalies

Maternal Age	Risk for Down's Syndrome	Total Risk for Chromosomal Abnormalities
20	1/1667	1/526
25	1/1250	1/476
30	1/952	1/384
35	1/378	1/192
40	1/106	1/66
45	1/30	1/21
49	1/11	1/8

Modified from Hook EB, Cross PK, Schreinemachers DM: Chromosomal abnormality rates at amniocentesis and in live-born infants, *JAMA* 249:2034-2038, 1983. 47,XXX was excluded from ages 20 to 32 (no data available).

> • *Box 2-2 /* **Differential Diagnoses for Antepartum**
> **Vaginal Bleeding** •
>
> - "Bloody show" at term
> - Cervical erosion, polyps (see p. 423), or cancer (see p. 418)
> - Cervicitis (see p. 423)
> - Circumvallate placenta (see p. 203)
> - Condylomata acuminata (see p. 439)
> - Ectopic pregnancy (see p. 71)
> - Hydatidiform mole (see p. 81)
> - Implantation bleeding (light, painless, 7 days after conception)
> - Incompetent cervix (see p. 69)
> - Placenta previa (see p. 102)
> - Placental abruption (see p. 102)
> - Preterm labor (see p. 150)
> - Hemorrhoids (see p. 36), rectal cancer, or polyps
> - Ruptured uterus (see p. 211)
> - Ruptured vaginal varicosities
> - Ruptured vasa previa (see p. 103)
> - Threatened SAB or SAB (see p. 59)
> - Urethritis or UTI (see p. 389)
> - Vaginal or cervical trauma
>
> From Scroggins KM, Smucker WD, Krishen AE: Spontaneous pregnancy loss, *Primary Care Clin Office Prac* 27:153-167, 2000.

• ANTEPARTUM VAGINAL BLEEDING

Incidence: Antepartum vaginal bleeding occurs in approximately 25% of all pregnancies during the first trimester.[25] Box 2-2 lists the differential diagnoses for bleeding during pregnancy.

Ⓜ Management

For **first trimester bleeding,** see management of SAB, p. 60. For **second and third trimesters,** see Figure 2-1 for midwifery diagnosis and management of antepartum bleeding.

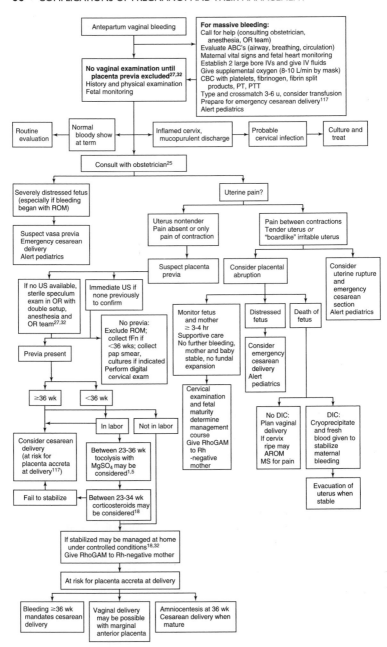

Figure 2-1 • Decision tree for midwifery management of antepartum bleeding. (Modified from Morrison EH: Common peripartum emergencies, *Am Fam Physician* Nov 1, 1998, published by The American Academy of Family Physicians at *http://www.aafp.org/afp/981101ap/morrison.html.*)

• BETA HEMOLYTIC STREPTOCOCCUS DISEASE

Infection of the fetus with the gram-positive diplococcus, beta hemolytic streptococcus (group B strep, or GBS), causes early- or late-onset neonatal disease, resulting in stillbirth, neonatal pneumonia, or sepsis and a neonatal mortality rate of 4%. The organism is present in 10% to 30% of all pregnant women, and colonization may be chronic, transient, or intermittent. Most often the woman is asymptomatic, although associated maternal morbidity may include urinary tract infection (UTI), chorioamnionitis, wound infection, or endometritis. Besides documented maternal GBS carriage, risk factors for early-onset neonatal GBS disease include gestational age <37 weeks, longer duration of membrane rupture before delivery, intraamniotic infection, young maternal age, black race, Hispanic ethnicity, and low maternal levels of anticapsular antibody. Transmission is perinatal, sexual, or by inoculation from rectal carriage.[91]

Intrapartum antibiotics are used to decrease the rate of early-onset neonatal disease. Before their use, 2 to 3 infants per 1000 live births contracted GBS early-onset disease. With the use of intrapartum prophylaxis, the rate fell to 0.5 infants per 1000 live births. Rates of maternal amnionitis and endometritis have also declined. Late-onset GBS neonatal disease is not, however, impacted by intrapartum antibiotics.[91] Until recently, intrapartum antibiotic prophylaxis was prescribed based on either a risk-based protocol or antepartum screening by GBS vaginal/rectal culture. A 2002 study found that the risk of early-onset disease was significantly lower for infants whose mothers had undergone screening and were treated accordingly (adjusted relative risk 0.46).[92] Eighteen percent of all deliveries are to women who are GBS positive but do not have obstetric risk factors.[91]

ⓜ *Management**

1. **Obtain vaginal rectal cultures for GBS from ALL women at 35 to 37 weeks' gestation.** The only **exceptions** are (1) the woman has had a **previous infant with invasive GBS disease and is not penicillin-allergic** and (2) the woman who has had documented **GBS bacteriuria in the current pregnancy and is not penicillin-allergic.** These women will receive intrapartum antibiotics regardless of current culture status. Penicillin-allergic women are tested for GBS resistance. The culture is taken from the vaginal introitus and through the anal sphincter, using one swab (culturing the vagina first) or two. Self-collected specimens after appropriate instruction yield similar results and are acceptable. If the woman is penicillin-allergic, the specimen should be labeled as such so that positive isolates can be tested for resistance to clindamycin and erythromycin.[91]

2. **Prescribe intrapartum antibiotics** (delineated later in this section) to the following women:
   a. Those with a positive antepartum GBS culture
   b. Those with GBS bacteriuria in any concentration (indicating heavy genital colonization) documented during the current pregnancy
   c. Those who have previously delivered a baby with invasive GBS disease
   d. Those whose culture results are not available at the time of delivery and who have an obstetric risk factor: delivery at <37 weeks' gestation; duration of ruptured membranes >18 hr, or temperature ≥100.4° F (≥38° C).[91]

3. The following women **do not** receive intrapartum antibiotics:
   a. Those with a negative antepartum screen within 5 weeks of delivery, even if they develop obstetric risk factors (delivery <37 weeks, prolonged rupture of membranes, or fever)
   b. Women who are GBS colonized undergoing planned cesarean section in the absence of labor or ruptured membranes
   c. Women known to have been GBS colonized in a previous pregnancy but who delivered an infant without GBS disease (unless GBS culture positive in the current pregnancy)
   NOTE: Women who are GBS colonized are not treated with antibiotics until the intrapartum period unless they have a GBS UTI.[91]

---

*As recommended by CDC (2002).

4. **Antibiotics recommended by CDC (2002):**
   a. Penicillin G, 5 million units IV initially, followed by 2.5 million units IV q4h until delivery
   b. Alternately, ampicillin, 2 g IV initially, followed by 1 g q4h until delivery
   c. Penicillin-allergic:
      (1) Women at low risk for anaphylaxis*: Cefazolin, 2 g IV initially, followed by 1 g q8h until delivery
      (2) Women at high risk for anaphylaxis*: Clindamycin, 200 mg IV q8h until delivery *OR* erythromycin, 500 mg IV q6h until delivery
      (3) GBS resistant to clindamycin or erythromycin or susceptibility unknown[†]: Vancomycin, 1g IV q12h until delivery

• CERVICAL INCOMPETENCE

Cervical incompetence is evidenced by painless, passive cervical dilation during the second or early third trimester followed by ballooning of the membranes into the vagina, rupture of membranes, and delivery of an immature fetus. The incompetent cervix is composed of more muscle fibers and less connective tissue than the normal cervix. Activity, multiple gestation, hormonal influences, and infection may play a part.[25] Cervical incompetence may account for as many as 20% of midtrimester abortions and preterm deliveries.[2] Women at risk for cervical incompetence include those with abnormal Müllerian duct formation or fusion, previous trauma to the cervix (conization, abortion, or obstetric laceration), Diethylstilbestrol (DES) prenatal exposure, or an unknown etiology.[25]

Diagnosis: Diagnosis is made by obstetric history or by observing cervical shortening and dilation during pregnancy. Serial ultrasonographic measurement of the cervix shows funneling, shortening, and a fully developed lower uterine segment. Funneling is normal after 30 to 32 weeks and may be normal as early as 24 weeks.[40]

Management

1. **Refer** the pregnant woman to an obstetrician.
2. **Anticipatory guidance:** Obstetric management may include surgical placement of a "purse-string" suture around the cervix (**McDonald cerclage,** or **Shirodkar procedure**). Bleeding, uterine contractions, or ruptured membranes are contraindications to the procedure. Emergency placement of a cerclage, especially when dilation has

---

*Women at high risk for anaphylaxis are those with a history of penicillin-related anaphylaxis and those with asthma or other conditions that would make treatment of anaphylaxis difficult.
[†]If possible, penicillin-allergic women at high risk for anaphylaxis should have clindamycin and erythromycin resistance testing of prenatal GBS isolate.[91]

already begun, is of little benefit. If it is too late to place the cerclage, the woman is managed as for preterm labor. Placement may be vaginal or abdominal. The procedure is delayed until after 14 weeks to allow for early pregnancy loss from other factors. At the beginning of the second trimester, the risk to the infant is 1% from this procedure. Later in the pregnancy, the risk is 2% to 5%.[40] The suture can be left in place until cesarean section, or it can be removed to allow vaginal delivery. Women usually go into labor normally after removal; however, cervical lacerations may occur at the site of scarring.

• CHORIOAMNIONITIS (AMNIONITIS, INTRA-AMNIOTIC INFECTION)

Chorioamnionitis usually results from ascending bacteria. Infection sometimes results from transplacental dissemination of microorganisms. Less commonly, the infection may be caused by obstetric procedures such as cervical cerclage, amniocentesis, intrauterine transfusion, or percutaneous umbilical blood sampling (PUBS).[31] Clinical findings include maternal fever, maternal and fetal tachycardia, and, in advanced cases, uterine tenderness, purulent amniotic fluid, and leukocytosis (although the latter may occur in normal labor as well).[40]

Risk Factors[40]:

Internal monitor use	Nulliparity
Lengthy labor	Pre-existing infection
Low socioeconomic status	Prolonged rupture of membranes
Meconium-stained amniotic fluid[1]	Young age
Multiple vaginal examinations	

Laboratory Findings: Elevated WBC count with shift to the left (see p. 591). In chorioamnionitis, amniocentesis will yield fluid that has a positive Gram stain or culture, WBCs $\geq 15,000$ cells mm^3, glucose ≤ 10 to 15 mg/dl, interleukin-6, ≥ 7.9 ng/mL, leukocyte esterase $\geq 1+$ reaction. Blood cultures are positive in 5% to 10% of patients.[40]

Incidence in Relation to Length of Ruptured Membranes: The infection rate for women who deliver within 24 hours of rupture of membranes at term is 1.6% to 29% depending on race, socioeconomic factors, receipt of prenatal care, and gestational age. In term pregnancies, the incidence of intrapartal fever rises with delivery later than 24 hours; if the latent period extends beyond 72 hours, the perinatal mortality rate is significantly increased.[117]

Three percent to 12% of infected women develop bacteremia. When cesarean section is performed, 8% develop wound infections and 1% develop a pelvic abscess. Maternal death is rare. Five percent to 10% of the fetuses develop pneumonia or bacteremia. Approximately 1% of term infants, and slightly more preterm infants, will develop meningitis. Mortality rates range from 1% to 4% in term infants to 15% in preterm infants.[41] The risk for cerebral palsy is increased for term and preterm infants.[96]

ⓜ *Management*

1. **Consult** the obstetrician.
2. Immediately initiate intrapartum **IV antibiotic treatment.** Ampicillin (2 g q6h) or penicillin (5 million U q6h) plus an IV aminoglycoside such as gentamycin (1.5 mg/kg q8h) are the most extensively tested combinations.[10] Antibiotics are continued until the patient has been afebrile and asymptomatic for 24 hours, when they can be discontinued and the patient can be discharged. An oral course follows only when the patient has had documented staphylococcus bacteremia.[40]
3. **Facilitate delivery.** Infection is not an indication for cesarean delivery.[23]
4. **Observe for dysfunctional labor,** which occurs more frequently with chorioamnionitis.[40]
5. **Closely observe the fetal heart rate (FHR).** Tachycardia and decreased variability occur in 75% of these infants.[40]
6. Notify the **pediatric** provider. **Prepare for a potentially ill infant.**

• ECTOPIC PREGNANCY

Ectopic pregnancy is the implantation of the fetus outside the uterus. Approximately 97% occur in the oviduct. Rupture of an ectopic pregnancy usually occurs within the first 8 to 12 weeks and may be fatal if the pregnancy is near uterine or ovarian arteries. Thirty-four women in the United States die each year from complications of ectopic pregnancy, accounting for 13% of all pregnancy-related maternal deaths.[113] Incidence is 1 in 100 to 200 pregnancies and 15% of all in vitro pregnancies. This rate is increasing because of sexually transmitted infections (STIs), intrauterine device (IUD) use, tubal surgery, and assisted reproduction.[25] Half of the women who have had an ectopic pregnancy eventually give birth to a liveborn baby. Of those who do become pregnant, 25% have a recurring ectopic pregnancy.[40]

Predisposing Conditions: Only 50% of women have any risk factors,[65] including history of pelvic inflammatory disease (PID), ectopic pregnancy, tubal surgery,[113] tubal pathology,[39] use of IUD, progesterone minipills, postcoital estrogens,[65] or assisted reproductive technology.[25]

Signs and Symptoms and Clinical Findings [25,40,63]:

Pain in the abdomen or inner thigh
Missed menses
Vaginal bleeding
Abdominal mass

Normal-sized uterus (66%)
Unilateral cervical motion
  tenderness (50%)

Once the ectopic pregnancy ruptures, the following signs of peritoneal irritation are present [25,65,69]:

Shoulder pain (referred
  phrenic nerve irritation)
Shock
Severe abdominal pain

Guarding
Rebound tenderness
Hypoactive bowel sounds
Fullness in the cul-de-sac

Diagnosis: See Figure 2-2 for the algorithm for diagnosis of ectopic pregnancy.

m *Management*

1. **Assess hemodynamic stability.** Immediately transport the woman who is hypotensive, tachycardic, short of breath, cyanotic, or disoriented to an emergency department.
2. If ectopic pregnancy is suspected, **refer** the woman to the obstetrician.[63]
3. **Anticipatory guidance:** If rupture of the ectopic pregnancy is suspected, immediate **surgical intervention** is required.[113] With an **unruptured ectopic pregnancy**, 47% to 100% spontaneously resolve and **management** may be **expectant.**[39] **Methotrexate** may be administered or **surgical intervention** (usually by laparoscopy) may be performed. **RhoGAM** is administered to the Rh-negative patient.[25]

• FETAL DEMISE

When fundal height plateaus and then regresses, breast changes regress, the woman loses or fails to gain weight, no FHTs are heard, and no fetal

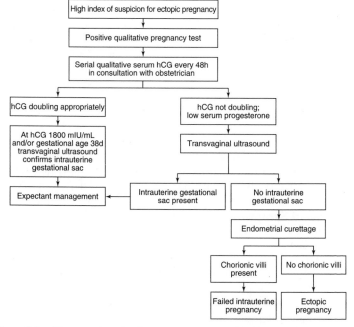

Figure 2-2 • Diagnosis algorithm for ectopic pregnancy. (Modified from Fylstra DL: Tubal pregnancy: a review of current diagnosis and treatment, *Obstet Gynecol Surv* 54:138-146, 1999.)

movement is felt, the midwife should suspect fetal demise. On vaginal examination, a collapsed skull may be palpated. Ultrasound shows Spalding's sign (overlapping of skull bones) and no cardiac or fetal movement. The spinal curve is exaggerated. Gas is seen in the circulatory system.[32]

m *Management*

1. **Consult** an obstetrician.
2. **Anticipatory guidance:** Two **treatment options are considered: induction** with pitocin, laminaria, or prostaglandin E_2,[40] or **expectant management.** Ninety percent of those managed expectantly deliver by 3 weeks. The woman is observed for ruptured membranes, fever (the patient checks her temperature twice a day), and uterine contractions. Coagulation studies are performed, including measurements of plasma thromboplastin (PT), partial thromboplastin time (PTT), fibrinogen, fibrin degradation products (FDP), and platelets. Abnormalities in these values indicate DIC and require immediate induction, although DIC rarely occurs sooner than 1 month after fetal death.[32]
3. **Facilitating the grieving process** is vital, including giving support through the birth, encouraging and preparing the woman and her support persons to view and hold the baby, assisting the family in making burial arrangements, and reviewing autopsy results. Varney[117] suggests pointing out even minor variations from normal in the baby, such as a nuchal cord, because the cause of death is often not determined and uncertainty is difficult to resolve. Primeau and Lamb[86] state that acknowledgement of the baby is the most helpful intervention. Acknowledgement includes being named, seen, touched, and held by the family; being recognized as a person who was born and who died; and being put to rest with dignity.
4. Resolution of grief is beneficial before **conceiving again** so that another baby will be appreciated for itself and not viewed as a replacement of the one who was lost. **Subsequent pregnancy** will, however, involve reliving the loss, working through fear of another loss, feeling guarded in attaching, letting go of grief for the lost child to embrace this one as an individual, and grieving the loss of oneself as parent to the first child. The woman grieves her body's inability to carry the first pregnancy. The couple may look for milestones of viability: completing the first trimester, hearing the FHTs, feeling fetal movement, and passing the gestational age of the previous loss. Anticipatory guidance regarding the normalcy of such fears and confusion facilitates the grieving and reattachment process. Providing clear information regarding the well-being of the pregnancy (whether positive or not) and possibly more frequent visits or other means of reassurance may decrease anxiety in future pregnancies.[29,116]

5. **Complementary measures:** Some experts suggest **homeopathic** remedies for grief after a birth.[47] **Acupuncture** may be used during expectant management after fetal demise.[22]

• INTRAUTERINE GROWTH RESTRICTION

Intrauterine growth restriction (IUGR, also known as fetal growth restriction and "small for gestational age") describes a fetus who has not reached its growth potential. The smallest tenth percentile for gestational age is used as a guideline to identify the growth-restricted fetus. However, up to 70% of these infants are simply constitutionally small because of maternal height, weight, and ethnicity.[56]

Fetal hypoxia occurs when there is a disturbance in the uteroplacental circulation. A long-standing interruption causes a low Po_2 level, reduced glucose availability, and reduced glycogen stores in the fetus. The fetus adapts by conserving energy by decreasing or stopping growth, decreasing activity, redistributing bloodflow to favor vital organs (heart, brain, and adrenals), increasing the number of RBCs (polycythemia: Hct >65%), and mobilizing stored fat and glycogen to increase hepatic gluconeogenesis and anaerobic metabolism of glucose, causing metabolic acidosis.[56]

The clinical pattern of IUGR depends on the causative factor and the timing and duration of the insult. In **symmetric IUGR** (20% to 30% of cases), the head and body are symmetrically decreased in size because fetal cellular hyperplasia was impaired in all organs. A mechanism causing IUGR before 30 weeks will probably result in a case of symmetric IUGR, the more severe restriction. In **asymmetric IUGR** (70% to 80% of cases), the abdomen is disproportionately small in relation to the head ("head-sparing") because of changes in fetal cellular growth and redistribution of cardiac output to favor the most vital organs.[56]

Maternal Risk Factors[32]:

Antiphospholipid antibodies
Environmental factors (high
altitude, stress)
Hypoxia from lung disease,
cardiac disease, or anemia
Infection
Multiple pregnancy

Poor nutritional status
Poor obstetric history
Renal conditions
Substance abuse
Vascular disease (hypertension,
preeclampsia, type I
diabetes mellitus)

Placental Risk Factors:

Inadequate penetration of the
spiral arterioles in the
placental attachment
Chronic abruption
Infarction of placenta

Infection of the placental villi
Small placenta
Tumor of placenta[81]
Umbilical abnormalities[56]

Fetal Risk Factors: Approximately 15% to 20% of IUGR pregnancies are caused by fetal factors, such as chromosomal abnormalities (7%).[56]

Prognosis: Infants with symmetric IUGR may have impaired visual-motor development, significantly lowered IQ,[112] and small but significant differences in academic achievement.[111] The adult is of smaller stature.[112] Later in life, the risk of cardiovascular disease is increased.[88]

🅜 *Management*

1. Carefully **establish dates** and observe fundal height growth.
2. Consider **ultrasound** at 16 to 20 weeks and again at 32 to 34 weeks to assess growth for the **woman at risk** for an IUGR infant. **Counsel the mother regarding lifestyle changes** that would benefit the baby's growth (such as ending substance abuse, changing diet, etc.).
3. **When the fundus is not growing**, **consult** the obstetrician. **Rule out descent** of the presenting part into the pelvis by Leopold's maneuvers and vaginal examination. Order **ultrasound evaluation** for lack of normal fundal growth, possibly by serial examinations, and to exclude oligohydramnios and congenital anomalies. Suggest **left lateral bed rest** to maximize placental perfusion (although there is no evidence that rest ameliorates IUGR). Conduct **antenatal surveillance.** When oligohydramnios develops and the fetus is greater than 34 weeks' gestation, **facilitate delivery.** At delivery, consider sending cord gases, placental cultures, and the placenta to pathology. Alert **pediatrics personnel,** who will observe and evaluate the infant for gestational age, anomalies, infection, hypothermia, hypoglycemia, polycythemia, and hyperviscosity.[32]

• FETAL SURVEILLANCE

The goal of antepartum testing is to prevent fetal death, although randomized, controlled trials have not provided evidence that it accomplishes this goal.[6]

The degree of hypoxemia and acidemia that will harm the fetus has not been determined. Fetuses with nonreactive NSTs have been shown to have an umbilical vein pH of 7.28 ± 0.11. Fetuses with abnormal movement counts have been shown to have an umbilical vein pH of 7.16 ± 0.08. A connection is implied between hypoxemia, FHR, and movement. Abnormal test results may occur in the presence of mild to severe acidosis as well as prematurity, fetal sleep cycle, medications, and fetal CNS abnormalities.[6] There is also a wide range of normal fetal behavior. Most clinicians use these tests to establish wellness rather than illness. Testing that is not reactive is called "nonreassuring."[73] A negative NST or biophysical profile (BPP) does not preclude an acute event such as placental abruption or a cord accident.[6] (See also FHR monitoring in the Intrapartum chapter, p.186.) Box 2-3 lists the signs of fetal compromise as they occur chronologically.

Initiation of Fetal Surveillance

Fetal surveillance begins for most indications at 32 to 34 weeks.[6] In multiple pregnancy or particularly worrisome high-risk conditions, the testing might begin earlier. Fetal testing begins after the fetus is viable

---

• *Box 2-3 / Chronologic Sequence of Fetal Deterioration* •

- Late decelerations appear on the CST
- Accelerations disappear on the NST
- Fetal breathing stops
- Fetal movement stops
- Fetal tone is absent
- Amniotic fluid decreases (hypoxia causes compensatory shifting of cardiac output from kidneys to brain and heart)

---

and when interventions could be made on the basis of findings—24 to 26 weeks at the earliest.[109]

Indications for Fetal Surveillance

Include Medical Conditions[6]:

Antiphospholipid syndrome
Cyanotic heart disease
Hemoglobinopathies
Hypertensive disorders

Hyperthyroidism
Systemic lupus erythematosus
Type I diabetes mellitus

Include Pregnancy-Related Conditions[6]:

Isoimmunization
IUGR
Multiple gestation
Oligohydramnios

Preeclampsia
Polyhydramnios
Postterm pregnancy
Previous fetal demise

Frequency of Testing: If the indication for a single test does not persist, no further testing is needed. If the condition persists, weekly testing is typically appropriate. In the presence of postterm pregnancy, type I diabetes, IUGR, or preeclampsia, some clinicians repeat testing twice a week. Any significant deterioration in the maternal condition requires reassessment of the fetus regardless of the interval since the last evaluation.[6]

Fetal Movement Counts (Fetal Kick Counts): At 20 to 30 weeks, movement becomes organized and rest/activity cycles are seen. Mothers perceive 80% of fetal movements.[32] Women are generally asked to rest on their left side 30 minutes after eating to count fetal movements. Three to five movements per hour is normal. Twelve hours without at least 10 movements requires investigation.[109] Maternal perception of decreased fetal movement is correlated with fetal death. Antepartum testing is suggested when fetal movement is absent to rule out fetal seizures and hypoxia when the fetus moves less than usual, more than usual, or when the quality of fetal movement has changed.[78]

m Management of Abnormal Findings

When abnormal findings are present, proceed to NST, contraction stress test (CST), modified BPP, or BPP.[6]

Nonstress Test

The NST tests the autonomic nervous system function—the sympathetic system that speeds the heart rate balanced with the parasympathetic system that slows the heart rate.[32] The normal fetus accelerates in response to movement. Hypoxia; neurologic depression (sleep, medications); maternal smoking; and fetal, cardiac, or CNS anomalies may cause a nonreactive NST.[78]

Fetal Age and Reactivity: From 24 to 28 weeks, up to 50% of fetuses are reactive; from 28 to 32 weeks, 85% are reactive.[6] Once the fetus has achieved reactivity, it should be reactive in future tests.[78]

Accuracy of Testing: The false-negative rate is 1.9 per 1000 (i.e., the number of stillbirths occurring within 1 week of a normal test result). The false-positive rate is up to 90% (nonreactive NST followed by a negative CST).[6]

Indication: Any fetus at risk for hypoxia.[78]

Technique: The woman is placed in a lateral tilt position and monitored externally. It may be necessary to continue for ≥40 minutes to take into account a fetal sleep cycle.[6]

Interpretation of Findings:

Reactive: ≥2 accelerations ≥15 BPM above the baseline at the nadir, of ≥15 seconds' duration from departure from the baseline to return to the baseline, whether or not associated with perceived fetal movement, within 20 minutes.

Nonreactive: 40 minutes of fetal monitoring failing to demonstrate the required accelerations.[6]

Variable Decelerations: Present in 50% of all NSTs, variable decelerations that last <30 seconds and are not repetitive do not represent fetal compromise that requires intervention. Three or more variable decelerations in 2 minutes, even if shallow, increase the risk for cesarean delivery.[6]

Eighty minutes of monitoring without demonstrating reactivity indicates an increased risk for oligohydramnios, IUGR, meconium-stained amniotic fluid, and/or placental infarction.[78] A pattern with waves of <5 BPM amplitude, no accelerations, and late decelerations with spontaneous uterine contractions is ominous.[32]

ⓜ Management of Abnormal Findings

Proceed to CST or full BPP.[6]

Contraction Stress Test

The CST assumes that fetal oxygenation is worsened by uterine contractions. The already compromised fetus will show late decelerations in the FHR when this stress is added to baseline compromise. Alternatively, umbilical cord compression, sometimes associated with oligohydramnios, may cause variable decelerations with contractions.[6]

Accuracy: The false-positive rate is 25% to 75% (i.e., a positive result occurring with a fetus who will tolerate labor). The false-negative rate is 0.3 per 1000 (stillbirth within 1 week of normal testing).[6]

Indications: A CST is indicated to further evaluate the fetus with a nonreactive NST; when a BPP is not available; to more fully evaluate the fetus in addition to the BPP; to evaluate a preterm fetus, an IUGR fetus, or the fetus of a diabetic woman for uteroplacental insufficiency; or when other tests are equivocal.[78]

Contraindications[6]:

Placenta previa	Previous classic cesarean section
PPROM	At risk for preterm labor

Techniques:

The CST can be performed in two ways:

1. **Nipple stimulation test:** The woman rests in the lateral recumbent position. She rubs one nipple through her clothing for 2 minutes or until a uterine contraction occurs. The nipple stimulation releases endogenous oxytocin, stimulating uterine contractions.[32] She then waits 5 minutes and resumes nipple stimulation unless the required three contractions, lasting at least 40 seconds each, have occurred within 10 minutes.[6] Alternative methods of nipple stimulation include using a breast pump, applying mineral oil and directly massaging the nipples, applying hot moist towels to the nipples, or rubbing a towel on the nipple. In all methods, stimulation is stopped when the contraction begins in order to avoid hyperstimulation.[78] Advantages include lower cost, noninvasiveness, and less time required in contrast to an oxytocin challenge test (OCT); contractions may begin 2 to 15 minutes after onset of stimulation.[32]

2. **Oxytocin Contraction Test (OCT):** IV oxytocin is initiated and titrated until three uterine contractions, lasting at least 40 seconds each, occur within 10 minutes.[32] ACOG[6] suggests beginning pitocin at 0.5 mU/min and doubling the rate every 20 minutes until an adequate contraction pattern occurs. Oxytocin is discontinued during the test if there is a tetanic contraction, a prolonged deceleration, two or more late decelerations in 10 minutes, or when three 40-second contractions have occurred within a 10-minute interval.[78]

Interpretation of Findings:

Negative CST: The absence of late or significant variable decelerations with three contractions of ≥40 seconds' duration each, occurring in 10 minutes.

Positive CST: Late decelerations following 50% or more contractions, whether or not the contraction pattern is adequate.

Equivocal suspicious CST: Intermittent late decelerations or significant variable decelerations occurring with contractions.

Equivocal hyperstimulatory CST: Decelerations occurring with uterine contractions that are closer than every 2 minutes or lasting >90 seconds.

Unsatisfactory CST result: A poor quality recording or the inability to establish an adequate contraction pattern.[6]

ⓜ *Management of Abnormal Findings*

Delivery is usually indicated for abnormal findings, taking into account fetal gestational age and the condition of the mother. Continually monitor the fetus during induction. Repetitive late decelerations should prompt cesarean delivery.[6]

Acoustic Stimulation Test (Vibroacoustic Stimulation)

The acoustic stimulation test involves applying a loud sound to the maternal abdomen to cause a fetal movement and acceleration. This measure may shorten overall testing time without compromising accuracy.[6] Acoustic stimulation may prevent a false nonreactive NST, but researchers recommend more study before routine implementation.[32] A fetus will occasionally respond to the sound with prolonged tachycardia or bradycardia, particularly if oligohydramnios is present.[109] The fetus is able to hear at 25 to 28 weeks' gestation, and acoustic stimulation may be used after this time.[78]

Technique: Apply a 1- to 2-second stimulation to the maternal abdomen in the vicinity of the fetal head. Results are best if the stimulus is applied when the FHR is at its baseline, and between contractions.[78] The stimulus may be repeated up to 3 times, increasing the duration of the stimulus to 3 seconds.[6]

Interpretation of Findings: Accelerations that occur as described in the reactive NST are reassuring.[6]

Variations: For decreased variability or in the absence of accelerations, Murray[76] suggests that scalp stimulation should be performed first, followed by acoustic stimulation if the cervix does not permit a finger to reach the scalp. The acoustic stimulus does not harm the fetus' hearing. The healthy fetus will respond to acoustic stimulus even if the mother has been given a narcotic. Once the membranes are ruptured and labor is underway, the response to acoustic stimulus lessens, possibly because of the loss of amniotic fluid decreasing the intensity of the sound or because hypoxia may cause a sensorineural hearing loss.[78]

ⓜ *Management of Abnormal Findings*

If abnormal findings are present, proceed with CST or BPP.[6]

Biophysical Profile

The BPP has been demonstrated to be a sensitive indicator of the immediate fetal condition, with considerable prognostic value and few false-positive (5% to 33%[78]) or false-negative results (0.8 in 1000).[23] The fetus scores 2 or 0 points for each of five variables. The perfect score of 10 indicates a well-oxygenated fetus. The five variables and requirements for a score of 2 include[6]:

1. **Amniotic fluid** (one pocket of >2 cm vertically)
2. **NST** (can be omitted without compromising the test if the other four variables are normal)

3. **Fetal tone** (one episode of extension and flexion of a fetal extremity or the opening or closing of a hand)
4. **Fetal movement** (at least three body or limb movements within 30 minutes)
5. **Fetal breathing movements** (sustained for at least 30 seconds within 30 minutes)

Amniotic Fluid Index

The amniotic fluid index (AFI) reflects long-term uteroplacental function.[6]

Technique: With the mother lying flat, mentally divide the uterus into four equal quadrants at the umbilicus and the linea nigra. The depth of the largest vertical pocket of fluid devoid of cord or fetal parts is measured in centimeters in each quadrant. The sum of the four measures is the AFI. Altitude and maternal hydration affect this measurement.[32]

Interpretation of Findings: An AFI of >24 cm (the 95th percentile) is considered polyhydramnios; <5 cm (the 5th percentile) is considered oligohydramnios. When determining the appropriate intervention for oligohydramnios, consider gestational age, maternal and fetal condition (as reflected in the other measures), and the AFI. Exclude ruptured membranes. Oligohydramnios occurs with increased frequency in postterm pregnancies and is an indication for delivery because of the association with meconium staining and cesarean section for nonreassuring FHR tracing.[6]

Fetal Breathing Movements

Two types of fetal breathing have been identified. Gasps or sighs may occur at a rate of 1 to 4 per minute. Irregular bursts may occur at rates up to 240 per minute. At approximately 33 to 36 weeks, when the lungs are beginning to mature, the fetus begins to slow its breathing rate and take in more volume. Variables that affect fetal breathing include labor, hypoglycemia, sound stimuli, cigarette smoking, amniocentesis, impending preterm labor, gestational age, time of day, and the FHR. Normal fetuses have been observed to go 122 minutes without a breathing movement.[32]

Interpretation and Management of Biophysical Profile Findings

A BPP of 8 is considered within normal limits unless the 2 points missed were for decreased amniotic fluid.[6] A BPP of 8 with oligohydramnios is considered high risk for perinatal asphyxia. Consider delivery for fetal indications. Conservative management includes maternal hydration and repeating the test in 24 hours. If the BPP is 6 of 10 with a normal AFI, the examination is considered equivocal. Consider delivery for fetal indications if the fetus is mature. If the fetus is immature, repeat the examination in 24 hours.[3]

A BPP of 6 in the mature infant is an indication for delivery if oligohydramnios is present. If the fetus is immature or if conditions for delivery are unfavorable, repeat the test in 24 hours. Consider corticosteroid administration for the fetus <34 weeks' gestation (see p. 156). If the second score is ≤6, initiate delivery regardless of maturity or favorability.[6]

Consult the obstetrician or refer the patient for medical management for a BPP of ≤6. For a BPP of 4, repeat the test the same day, and initiate delivery for a score of ≤6 on the second test. If the BPP is ≤2, initiate delivery.[3] Continuously monitor the fetus during induction. Repetitive late decelerations should prompt cesarean delivery.[6]

Modified Biophysical Profile

Researchers have found the NST and AFI in combination to be predictive. The false-negative rate of the modified BPP is lower than that of the NST and compares favorably with the CST and the complete BPP.[68] When measuring the AFI, minimum scanning criteria in limited third trimester ultrasound include placental location, AFI, identification of fetal number, fetal cardiac activity, fetal presentation, and indications of fetal well-being.[3]

Accuracy: The false-negative rate is 0.8 per 1000 and the false-positive rate is 60% (abnormal modified BPP followed by a normal full BPP).[6]

Percutaneous Umbilical Blood Sampling (Cordocentesis)

PUBS involves introducing a needle through the maternal abdomen to withdraw blood from either the vein or an artery of the umbilical cord of a fetus. Arterial sampling carries the risk of bleeding or fetal bradycardia. Indications for PUBS include prenatal diagnosis of blood dyscrasias, isoimmunization, metabolic disorders, fetal infection, fetal karyotyping, evaluation of fetal hypoxia, or the need to treat the fetus by monitoring drug levels or transfusing blood.[23] The fetal loss rate is approximately 1%.[32]

Umbilical Artery Doppler Velocimetry

The umbilical artery Doppler velocimetry measures the end-diastolic umbilical artery velocity, which is associated with increased vascular resistance in the fetoplacental circulation.[32] Normally growing fetuses show high velocity umbilical artery diastolic flow. IUGR fetuses show decreased, absent, or reversed umbilical artery diastolic flow, reflecting placental spiral artery obliteration, fetal hypoxia and acidosis, and the risk for fetal morbidity and death. In one study, the false-negative rate was zero.[6]

• HYDATIDIFORM MOLE (MOLAR PREGNANCY)

A molar pregnancy is one with abnormal chorionic villi and various degrees of trophoblastic proliferation, edema, and degeneration of the villous stroma. The chorionic villi form grape-like vesicles that hang in clusters from pedicles. With a fetus present, the mole is termed "incomplete"; with the fetus absent, the mole is termed "complete."[32] Symptoms of an incomplete mole (usually the result of a diploid sperm or two sperm fertilizing an ovum) are generally milder and slower to develop. A complete mole is made up of paternal genetic material only, with two sperm fertilizing an ovum that lacked genetic material from the mother. Complications include malignancy, pulmonary embolus, hyperthyroidism, and coagulopathy.[25] When the chorionic villi invade the local myometrium, the mole is termed "invasive." Such a mole rarely metastasizes, and the prognosis is good after chemotherapy. Choriocarcinoma may follow a molar pregnancy as well as a normal pregnancy or an SAB. Extremely malignant, this cancer has an affinity for arterial blood vessels, and the lung is the most common site of metastasis. Chemotherapy is required.

Older women are at increased risk for molar pregnancy.[32]

Signs and Symptoms: The uterus may be boggy, large for dates (50%), or small for dates (30%). Hyperemesis gravidarum may be present. Preeclampsia before 24 weeks is virtually diagnostic.[25] Ovarian theca-lutein cysts often coexist. Vaginal spotting or hemorrhage may occur. Bleeding may occur and be concealed in the uterus with maternal signs of hypovolemia. Grape-like vesicles may be expelled spontaneously between 16 and 28 weeks. In a complete molar pregnancy, no fetal parts are palpable and an FHR is not heard. The serum hCG is high for the number of weeks' gestation.[32]

Diagnosis: The serum hCG is elevated. Ultrasound is diagnostic.[32]

(m) Management

1. If a molar pregnancy is suspected, order an **ultrasound and a serum hCG** and **refer** the woman **to an obstetrician.**
2. **Anticipatory guidance:** The **physician evacuates the uterus** immediately by vacuum aspiration and gentle curettage, exploring the uterus, vagina, and vulva for malignancy. A **chest x-ray** is taken to identify lesions. **Pregnancy is prevented for 1 year. Serum hCG** levels are monitored. As long as the numbers regress, no further treatment is necessary. When testing has been normal for a year, follow-up is discontinued and pregnancy is allowed. If **serum hCG levels plateau or rise,** hysterectomy or chemotherapy is indicated.[32] In future pregnancies, the woman should have a **first trimester ultrasound** to rule out a recurrent mole.[40]

• HYDRAMNIOS (POLYHYDRAMNIOS)

Hydramnios is excessive amniotic fluid, diagnosed as mild when fluid pockets measure 8 to 11 cm in the vertical dimension on ultrasound, moderate when a pocket containing only small parts measures 12 to 15 cm, and severe when fluid pockets are >15 cm.[32] Alternatively, an AFI of >24 is considered hydramnios.[6] Two thirds of all cases are idiopathic. One third are associated with diabetes, erythroblastosis, or multiple pregnancy. The absence of fetal swallowing, excessive urination, transudation of fluid from exposed tissues, or impaired hormonal control associated with fetal abnormalities may cause excess fluid. Hydramnios seen with maternal diabetes may be osmotic diuresis of the hyperglycemic fetus. The clinical impression of hydramnios is confirmed by ultrasound.[32]

On examination, the uterus is large for dates or shows large interval growth, and there is difficulty palpating fetal parts or hearing FHTs. Maternal respiratory embarrassment, edema of the lower extremities and vulva, nausea and vomiting, and compression of the ureters causing oliguria all may occur with severe hydramnios. Fast accumulation of fluid (acute hydramnios) occurs earlier in pregnancy and is difficult for the pregnant woman to tolerate. Chronic hydramnios is a slow accumulation, usually occurring later in gestation and tolerated without difficulty. Preterm delivery, malpresentation, placental abruption as the uterus is emptied, uterine dysfunction, cord prolapse, increased risk for cesarean delivery, and postpartum hemorrhage (PPH) are potential complications.[32]

ⓜ Management

1. Order an **ultrasound** to assess fetal normalcy and the degree of hydramnios. **Screen for diabetes.**
2. **Consult** the obstetrician.
3. **Anticipatory guidance:** For severe hydramnios, **amniocentesis** may be performed for transient maternal relief. This intervention carries the risk that membranes will rupture or labor will begin. Some physicians prescribe **indomethacin** for hydramnios. Indomethacin apparently increases fetal lung absorption and/or decreases fetal lung fluid production, decreases fetal urine production, and increases the movement of fluid across the membranes. It may also may prevent closure of the fetal ductus arteriosus.[32]
4. During labor, slow removal of fluid during **amniotomy** is indicated to prevent cord prolapse.

• HYPEREMESIS GRAVIDARUM

Hyperemesis gravidarum is severe, intractable nausea and vomiting during pregnancy, usually peaking between 8 and 12 weeks and resolving by 16 weeks.[36] Hormonal changes and/or psychological and social stressors are probable causes of the condition.[32] Elevated T4 and decreased thyroid-stimulating hormone (TSH) levels are found in 50% of these women, and the thyroid is believed to be involved. These patients are not thyrotoxic, however, and should not be treated with antithyroid measures.[83] Occurring more frequently among younger women, the incidence is 0.5 to 10 per 1000 pregnancies.[36]

Signs and symptoms include weight loss, electrolyte imbalance (especially hypokalemia), ketonemia, and dehydration; possibly hepatic and renal damage, acidosis caused by starvation, and/or alkalosis due to the loss of hydrogen chloride.[128]

Diagnosis: Exclude pancreatitis, hepatitis, cholecystitis, pyelonephritis,[40] gastroenteritis, peptic ulcer, acute fatty liver of pregnancy,[32] appendicitis, diabetic ketoacidosis,[83] molar pregnancy, and pseudotumor cerebri.[40] Relevant laboratory studies include measurement of electrolytes, Hct, urine osmolality, liver function tests, urinalysis (UA), WBC (to rule out pyelonephritis), serum bicarbonate, urinary ketones, TSH (to exclude hyperthyroidism), and serum amylase/creatinine ratio (to exclude pancreatitis).[36]

🅜 *Management*

1. **Assess** the diet, the frequency of vomiting in relation to food retained, the nature of the vomitus, elimination, signs of infection, exposure to viral disease or contaminated foods, a history of eating disorders, abdominal pain, or a history of abdominal surgery. The physical includes weight, assessment of hydration, a thorough abdominal palpation, and noting whether there is a sweet odor to the breath (ketosis).
2. **Consult** the physician.
3. **Anticipatory guidance: Hospitalization** may be necessary for **IV fluid replacement**, caloric intake, and balancing of electrolytes. The patient should take nothing by mouth until vomiting has stopped for 48 hours.[40] Lactated Ringer's solution (possibly adding glucose), multivitamins, magnesium, pyridoxine, and/or thiamine are administered IV until the woman is able to tolerate fluids by mouth and the urine shows few or no ketones. **Parenteral nutrition** may be helpful[128] and **steroids** may be used for refractory hyperemesis. No **drugs** are FDA approved for the treatment of nausea and vomiting in pregnancy, and the risk of antiemetic antihistamines is weighed against the risk of prolonged starvation and dehydration.[36]
   - **Droperidol** (Inapsine), a pregnancy category C drug, may be used to reduce nausea, but it may cause extrapyramidal effects.[19]
   - Promethazine **(Phenergan)** (12.5 to 25 mg PO, PR, or IV q4h) is an antihistamine and an antiemetic with sedative properties. Contraindications include epilepsy, preeclampsia, seizure disorder, increased intracranial pressure, and hypotension. This drug potentiates other CNS depressants or anticonvulsants. Use with caution if the woman has glaucoma.[36] A low-dose continuous infusion of Phenergan may be helpful.[40]
   - **Doxylamine and pyridoxine** in combination (the components of Bendectin, provided by half of a 25-mg tablet of Unisom [a sleep

aid] and 25 mg vitamin B_6 qd or bid) may be recommended because it has been extensively studied and determined to be unrelated to birth defects and to be a safe combination during pregnancy. Doxylamine is an antihistamine and, like all antihistamines, is discontinued during preterm labor because of a risk of retrolental fibroplasia in premature babies who are delivered within 2 weeks of intrauterine exposure.

- Hydroxyzine **(Vistaril)** may be used in combination with metoclopramide, or may be used with pyridoxine instead of doxylamine.
- Oral dimenhydrinate **(Dramamine)** is used extensively in Canada but not in the United States. When given IV near term, it may have oxytocic effects.[19]
- Prochlorperazine **(Compazine)**—25 mg q12h PR or 5 to 10 mg IM, IV, or PO q6-8h prn—may be given for relief of nausea and vomiting. Contraindications include glaucoma, bone marrow suppression, and severe liver or cardiac disease. May be additive with other CNS depressants. Can cause dystonia, dyskinesia, pseudoparkinsonism, and neuroleptic malignant syndrome.[36]
- Selective serotonin receptor antagonists (dolasetron **[Anzemet]**, granisetron **[Kytril]**, and ondansetron **[Zofran]**) have not been extensively studied but do not appear to be teratogenic.[19]
- Prednisolone 10 mg tid PO, reduced gradually, may be prescribed for the woman who has lost weight.[71]

4. Addressing **social and psychological factors** may prevent relapse.[32]
5. **Complementary measures:**
   a. **Acupuncture** may improve the woman with hyperemesis.[22]
   b. **Reflexology:** Stimulation of the reflex zone for the endocrine system (pituitary, adrenals, thyroid, and ovaries zones) may relieve hyperemesis.[114] **See charts and information on reflexology, p. 567.**

• HYPERTENSIVE DISORDERS OF PREGNANCY

Pathophysiology of Preeclampsia

In preeclampsia, peripheral vascular resistance increases, elevating the blood pressure. Cardiac output is somewhat decreased from parasympathetic input.[23] Preeclampsia causes an **increased vascular reactivity to pressors**, including angiotensin II, and the vasospasm damages the blood vessels, causing local hypoxia and **subendothelial deposits of fibrinogen and platelets.** Hemorrhage, necrosis, and **end-organ damage** result. **Vasoconstriction, endothelial damage**, swelling, and fibrin deposits may reduce the glomerulofiltration rate by 25% and **increase permeability to protein.**[40] The **liver** may develop necrotic patches, increasing levels of aspartate aminotransferase (AST) and alanine aminotransferase (ALT).[32] **Acute fatty liver of pregnancy** may be a manifestation of preeclampsia (see p. 63). **Thrombocytopenia** exists with microangiopathic hemolytic anemia, and consumptive coagulation is present in fulminant preeclampsia. Cerebral hemorrhage, petechial as well as large hematomas, are seen, but cerebral edema is rare. The **CNS symptoms** of eclampsia are probably caused by the endothelial cell damage with platelet aggregation and fibrin deposits.[23]

Plasma volume is diminished by approximately 9% before hypertension is detected. The degree of volume reduction predicts the severity of IUGR and hypertension. Central venous pressure and pulmonary capillary wedge pressure remain normal or high, and volume replacement may lead to pulmonary edema.[23] Electrolytes do not vary appreciably from that of normal pregnancy.[32]

A variant of severe preeclampsia that occurs in 20% to 30% of women with preeclampsia or eclampsia, the **HELLP (h**emolysis, **e**levated **l**iver enzymes, **l**ow **p**latelet) **syndrome** is characterized by elevated liver enzymes and thrombocytopenia.[32] Hypertensive and renal indicators of preeclampsia may be absent in this variant. Table 2-2 describes hypertensive disorders and their management.

Theories regarding the etiology of preeclampsia include immunologic mechanisms, genetic predisposition, dietary deficiencies, the presence of vasoactive compounds, and endothelial dysfunction.[32] Some suggest that abnormal placentation plays a role. In normal pregnancy, the **spiral arteries of the placenta** extend through one third of the myometrial wall. In the preeclamptic pregnancy, the spiral arteries of the placenta inadequately invade the uterine wall. The number of well-developed arterioles in the placental vasculature is decreased, and umbilical artery resistance is increased. The myometrial segments of the spiral arterioles, left with their musculoelastic architecture, are responsive to hormonal influences and deliver reduced bloodflow.[56] **Hypoperfusion of the fetoplacental unit** results in the secretion of substances into the circulation that cause widespread changes in endothelial cell function. Endothelial injury occurs in the uteroplacental bed itself, and large placental infarcts, small placental size, and placental abruption are seen with increased frequency and are associated with fetal death.[32]

Experimental regimens have included **aspirin** and **calcium** administration, but neither has been found to prevent preeclampsia or related IUGR.[24,54] **Magnesium** supplementation has shown inconsistent results, and there are inadequate data regarding **zinc** supplementation.[40]

Maternal Complications: In severe preeclampsia, placental abruption, IUGR, thrombocytopenia, HELLP syndrome, and DIC may occur.[107] Hepatic and acute renal failure may also result.[80] Acute renal failure, pulmonary edema, ascites, pleural effusion, hepatic rupture, DIC, and placental abruption are seen in the HELLP syndrome.[40] In subsequent pregnancies, 19% of these women develop preeclampsia, 21% deliver prematurely, 12% develop IUGR, 2% experience placental abruption, and 4% of subsequent pregnancies result in perinatal death.[103] In addition, the

Text continued on p. 92

Table 2-2 / Hypertensive Disorders and Related Conditions: Description and Treatment

Hypertensive Disorder and Differential Diagnoses	Triad Symptoms: Proteinuria,* Edema, Blood Pressure	Additional Clinical Findings	Management
Chronic hypertension *Differential:* Essential hypertension (most common), aortic coarctation, collagen vascular disease, diabetes, hyperaldosteronism, hyperthyroidism, pheochromocytoma, renal vascular disease.[23]	**BP:** ≥140/90[115]; >170/110 termed "severe"[99]. 33% of women with chronic hypertension become normotensive in the second trimester.[117] **Proteinuria:** When present, baseline proteinuria increases risk of preterm delivery, IUGR, and NICU admissions.[102] **Edema:** Gestational edema may be present.	Known to predate pregnancy or identified before 20 weeks' gestation. Associated with vascular changes (e.g., retinal changes), cardiac enlargement, renal failure, or a history of gestational hypertension.[23] At increased risk for preeclampsia, placental abruption, IUGR, second trimester stillbirth.[23] 10% with mild hypertension develop superimposed preeclampsia; 32% of fetuses have IUGR. Otherwise perinatal outcome is like that of normal pregnancy.[98] 52% with severe hypertension develop superimposed preeclampsia with the risk greatest for those hypertensive more than 4 yr, with history of preeclampsia, or with a diastolic >100 in early pregnancy.[102]	1. **Co-manage** with or **refer** to physician. 2. **Diet and exercise** before pregnancy ideal; not advisable during pregnancy.[124] 3. Accurate **dating** essential. 4. **Baseline studies: Lab:** CBC with platelets, GTT, BUN, Creatinine, ANA, UA, urine C&S, 24-hr urine for protein and creatinine clearance; then follow serially. **Ultrasound:** Baseline study for dating; consider Doppler flow study, then follow serially. **ECG.**[45] **For severe hypertension or signs of cardiac disease:** Consider echocardiogram. **For wide BP fluctuation or elevated GTT:** Send 24-hr urine for vanilly mande-lic acid and metanephrines to rule out pheochromocytoma. **For severe hypertension or significant proteinuria:** Chest x-ray examination and serum complement.[40] 5. **Normal salt intake** unless salt sensitive or has renal disease.[124] 6. Counsel regarding **lifestyle:** negative impact of anxiety, nicotine, recreational drug use and caffeine. 7. Counsel regarding benefit of **rest** on BP, uteroplacental bloodflow, and perinatal outcome.[40] 8. **Antihypertensive therapy** decreases exacerbations, decreases proteinuria, and improves perinatal outcome.[23] 9. **Consult** with physician for hypertension and any two signs or symptoms of preeclampsia or one sign and hyperflexia.[117]

Table 2-2 / Hypertensive Disorders and Related Conditions: Description and Treatment—cont'd

Hypertensive Disorder and Differential Diagnoses	Triad Symptoms: Proteinuria,* Edema, Blood Pressure	Additional Clinical Findings	Management
Preeclampsia, mild	Diagnosis can be made with any one: **BP:** ≥140/90-160/110[23], alternately, a 30 mm Hg rise in the systolic BP or a 15 mm Hg rise in the diastolic BP. 14.5%-23% preeclamptic women **are not** hypertensive.[97,105] **Proteinuria:** 300-499 g protein/24 hr; or 1-2+ in 2 random specimens 6 hr apart.[117] 10%-19% preeclamptic women do **not** develop proteinuria.[97] **Edema:** >2 lb weight gain in 1 week with edema of hands and face.[117] 33% do **not** develop edema.[97]	**Risk factors:** Age extremes, primiparous (8 × risk)[32], family or personal history of preeclampsia[40], lower socioeconomic status (possibly due to nutritional factors or younger age at first pregnancy), diabetes (altered prostaglandin synthesis with preexisting vascular disease[32]); physically strenuous work,[75] fetal hydrops and multiple gestation (>2 × risk).[101] Usually present after 32 weeks' gestation; may occur until 7 days after delivery. May occur earlier with hydatidiform mole, renal disease or chronic hypertension.[23] Symptoms may include visual disturbances, anxiety[117] and IUGR.[32] **Lab:** Normal platelet count, renal studies, liver enzymes, and the absence of hemolysis.[23] Hemoconcentration may be present.[117]	1. **Accurately date** the pregnancy. 2. Educate woman regarding the nature of preeclampsia, importance of fetal movement counts, danger signs, bedrest slowing disease progression, and diet high in protein and calories with normal salt.[124] 3. Biweekly **fetal surveillance** for oligohydramnios; serial ultrasound for IUGR.[40] 4. **Exercise caution with parenteral fluid administration.** Constricted capillary bed may cause overload. 5. **Minimize bloodloss** because even a normal blood loss may be poorly tolerated due to diminished blood volume.[32] 6. **Consider in management:** severity of disease, maternal and fetal status, fetal gestational age, presence of labor, Bishop cervical score (≥6 desirable), and maternal wishes. 7. **Induce pregnancy** at term.[40] 8. **Observe for signs of worsening:** BP is an unreliable indicator[32], worsening proteinuria is not prognostic.[123] Upper abdominal pain and rising liver enzymes are usually indications for delivery as are a rising uric acid and thrombocytopenia (<100,000).[62]
Preeclampsia, severe	**BP:** ≥160/110 on 2 occasions ≥6 hr apart with woman at rest.[117] **Proteinuria:** ≥500 mg protein/24 hr[117] or persistently 3-4+.	**Symptoms:** Oliguria (<400 mL/24 hr),[32] hyperreflexia (especially clonus),[117] headache, visual changes, upper abdominal pain, IUGR, oligohydramnios,[45]	1. **Co-management with physician.** 2. **Administer MgSO₄** for anticonvulsant properties and to relieve cerebral vasospasm. Cunningham et al[32] protocol: MgSO₄ 20% 4 g IV no faster than 1 g/min.

Edema: May be present.[40]

development of HELLP syndrome or eclampsia.[117] pulmonary edema.[32]

Lab: Hemolysis (schizocytosis, spherocytosis, reticulocytosis, hemoglobinuria, hemoglobinemia). Elevated serum creatinine[32]: doubling indicates 50% reduction in GFR.

24-hr creatinine is decreased and is a more reliable indicator than a single serum creatinine. BUN is increased (doubling indicates 50% reduction in GFR).[117] Serum uric acid is inconsistent according to Gabbe.[40] Development of DIC: low fibrinogen, presence of fibrin split products, prolonged PT and PTT.[117]

Follow with 5 g 50% $MgSO_4$ deep IM into each buttock (with 1.0 mL 2% lidocaine for comfort).[32] Q4h thereafter give 5 g 50% $MgSO_4$ into one buttock, discontinue 24 hr after delivery. Gabbe et al[40] protocol: $MgSO_4$ 6 g over 15-20 min, followed by maintenance dose of 2 g/hr. $MgSO_4$ will prolong labor but not to a significant degree (16.5 vs. 17.8 hr in one study).[125] Serum Mg in 4 hr. See p. 93 regarding $MgSO_4$ administration.

3. **Antihypertensive therapy** to achieve the goal of a diastolic <110 mm Hg: hydralazine 5-10 mg IV in repeated doses as needed; **or** labetolol 20-40 mg IV (in 10-mg increments); **or** nifedipine 10 mg SL. Diuretics are indicated only for pulmonary edema.
4. **Delivery** for PPROM, severe IUGR (<5th percentile) or fetal or maternal distress, or anticipatory management.[40] Sibai et al[104] found perinatal outcomes to be equal, except those managed less aggressively were larger and more mature.[104]
5. **Continuous fetal monitoring**, serial fetal surveillance (BPP).
6. Continuous **monitoring of maternal condition:** vital signs, urine output, cerebral status, presence of danger signs, serial platelet counts, and liver enzyme measurements.[40]
7. **Mode of delivery** per routine obstetric criteria, but second stage may be facilitated.[123]

Eclampsia

Differential: For seizure not responsive to $MgSO_4$, rule out brain lesion, CVA, sickle cell crisis with hemolytic crisis, intracerebral bleed, epilepsy, metabolic causes (e.g., hypocalcemia,

BP: May be elevated.
Proteinuria: 4+ proteinuria may be present.
Edema: Generalized edema may be present.[40]

Generally, a grand mal tonic/clonic seizure lasts 60-90 seconds—despite interventions—due to cerebral edema, hemorrhage, or transient vasospasm. 3-4+ DTRs are present. 30% have IUGR, 65% have fetal distress during labor, 23% have placental abruption.

1. **Prevent injury** if possible (pad side rails), clear and protect airway as possible. Give oxygen. Do **not** force airway or tongue blade into mouth, which may cause injury or induce gagging and aspiration.[40]
2. Arrange immediate **physician management.**
3. **Treat for eclampsia** until another etiology is proven.[32]

Table 2-2 / Hypertensive Disorders and Related Conditions: Description and Treatment—cont'd

Hypertensive Disorder and Differential Diagnoses	Triad Symptoms: Proteinuria, * Edema, Blood Pressure	Additional Clinical Findings	Management
hypoglycemia, water intoxication, porphyria), infectious causes (meningitis, encephalitis), or hypertensive disease with encephalopathy.[125] If coma persists after seizure intracranial bleed.[40] (ominous sign) rule out Mg toxicity, cerebral edema, intracranial bleed.[40]		Hypertonicity of the uterus may follow the seizure for 2-14 min.[40] Fetal compromise is indicated by a brady-cardia >10 min, a sustained tachycardia >200 BPM, or by late decelerations and may indicate placental abruption.[32]	4. **Initiate MgSO$_4$** as described above for severe preeclampsia. In addition, Cunningham et al[32] protocol: For seizure persisting >15 min add MgSO$_4$ 2 g 20% IV—4 g for obese women—at rate no faster than 1 g/min. Using the protocol of Gabbe et al[40]: For seizure after loading dose, give additional MgSO$_4$ 2 g IV over 3-5 min. See p. 93 regarding MgSO$_4$ administration. 5. If MgSO$_4$ doesn't stop seizures, or if coma persists after seizure, **neuroimaging studies** are indicated.[125] 6. **Chest x-ray examination** after repeated seizures to rule out aspiration.[40] 7. Examine the woman for **injuries** and treat. 8. Draw blood gases; **correct acidemia.** 9. **Monitor electrolytes and serum Mg.**[40] See guidelines for therapeutic Mg levels, p. 93. 10. **Before 30 weeks,** give MgSO$_4$ and deliver by cesarean section. 11. After 30 weeks, **induce labor** after stabilization.[117]
Gestational or transient hypertension	**BP:** >140/90.[115] **Proteinuria:** None. **Edema:** None.	Begins late in gestation without accompanying signs of preeclampsia and without evidence of hypertensive vascular disease. Multiparous, obese	1. **Consult** with physician. 2. **See weekly.** 3. **Bedrest.** 4. **Antihypertensive medications** may be added.[23]

Gestational edema	**BP:** Normal. **Proteinuria:** None. **Edema:** Usually present in dependent extremities, but may also be present in hands and face.[32]	women with a family history of hypertension are at increased risk.[23] Thirst threshold rises, vasopressin secretion increases, plasma osmolality falls, and body fluids are increased by 6.5 L during normal pregnancy.[32]	**Left side lying** may improve dependent edema.
Gestational proteinuria	**BP:** Normal. **Proteinuria:** <500 g/24 hr.[32] **Edema:** None.	May occur because of normal renal changes of pregnancy.[32]	Rule out preeclampsia and renal disease.[32]
HELLP syndrome *Differential:* Acute fatty liver of pregnancy, hepatic encephalopathy, viral hepatitis, gastroenteritis, peptic ulcer, gallbladder disease, appendicitis, glomerulonephritis, hemolytic uremic syndrome, renal lithiasis, pyelonephritis, diabetes mellitus, hyperemesis gravidarum, idiopathic thrombocytopenia, SLE, thrombotic thrombocytopenia purpura.[40]	**BP:** Many are normotensive. **Proteinuria:** May be present. **Edema:** Generalized edema may be present.[40]	A variant of severe preeclampsia, HELLP syndrome is experienced by 20%–30% of women with severe preeclampsia or eclampsia.[32] Occurs, like preeclampsia, prenatally (often remote from term) or up to 7 days after birth.[40] **Symptoms:** Upper abdominal pain in 65%. Nausea and vomiting in 50%. Nonspecific viral-like symptoms such as malaise in 90%.[40] **Lab:** Elevated liver enzymes (LDH, AST, and ALT). Thrombocytopenia (<100,000). Bilirubin ≥1.2 m/dL. NOTE: The rate of change may be more indicative of severity than the absolute value.[40]	1. **Co-manage** with physician. 2. **Stabilize maternal condition,** especially correcting coagulation abnormalities by giving fresh frozen plasma. 3. **Evaluate fetal well-being.** 4. **Delivery is indicated regardless** of BP. If there is no evidence of DIC, and if the lungs are immature, may delay delivery for **corticosteroid administration.** 5. **Delivery mode** is determined according to routine obstetric indications. 6. **Postpartum monitoring** includes observation for bilirubin, creatinine, and LDH to normalize, hemolysis to be absent, platelet count to rise, as well as any sign of organ dysfunction. 7. **After 72 hr without resolution,** fresh frozen plasma is administered.[40]

*Excretion of protein varies over a 24-hr period[32] and is affected by contamination, exercise, pH, and specific gravity.[40] Urine dipsticks are unreliable and should not be used to make management decisions.[67,123] Investigate a ≥2+ dipstick with a 24-hr urine collection.[117]

woman who develops eclampsia may develop pulmonary edema from aspiration; congestive heart failure from severe hypertension and fluid overload; sudden death from cerebral hemorrhage; cerebral edema with or without uncal herniation, causing death; blindness from retinal detachment; occipital lobe ischemia or infarction (usually resolves spontaneously); or psychosis (also usually resolves). Electroencephalographic changes and neurologic sequelae are not permanent.[100,106] Women who experience hypertensive complications of pregnancy are at increased risk for chronic hypertension. Those who develop preeclampsia early in the pregnancy or who have underlying chronic hypertension are at greater risk for complications in subsequent pregnancies.[99a,100,103]

Mortality Rates: Normotensive women with preeclampsia have an overall perinatal mortality rate of 7.7%; hypertensive women with superimposed preeclampsia have a perinatal mortality rate of 13.5%.[107] In HELLP syndrome, perinatal mortality rate is 7.7% to 60%; maternal mortality rate is as high as 24%.[40] Maternal mortality rate in eclampsia ranges from <1% to 20%.[32]

Ⓜ Management

See Table 2-2 for management of preeclampsia. Box 2-4 outlines the procedure for $MgSO_4$ administration.

• INCARCERATION OF THE PREGNANT RETROVERTED UTERUS

When the pregnant retroverted uterus enlarges to approximately 12 weeks' size, it can become entrapped in the hollow of the sacrum, wedged under the sacral promontory. The lower segment of the uterus dilates to accommodate the growing fetus. Symptoms are abdominal pain, inability to void, or paradoxic incontinence (small amounts of urine passed involuntarily, with the bladder never completely emptying).[32] This condition is rare.

Ⓜ Management

1. **Evaluate** the woman with a retroverted uterus **early in the second trimester** for incarceration. If the uterus cannot be readily identified abdominally, confirm the incarceration by vaginal examination.[32]
2. **Consult** with the physician when an incarcerated uterus is identified.
3. **Anticipatory guidance:** The **bladder is emptied with a urinary catheter,** leaving it in place until bladder tone returns. With the woman **in knee-chest position, the physician places two fingers into the vagina and pushes the uterus forward into the abdomen.** Spinal or general **anesthesia** is occasionally required. A soft **pessary** may be used after the procedure to prevent reincarceration.[32]

• Box 2-4 / Magnesium Sulfate (MgSO₄) Administration* •

DOSAGE
Loading dose is 4-6 g IV over 20 min followed by a **maintenance dose** of 1-2 g/h.[40]

THERAPEUTIC MG LEVEL
4-6 mEq/L or 4.8-9.6 mg/dL.

SIGNS OF MgSO₄ TOXICITY IN ORDER OF INCREASING SEVERITY
- Loss of deep tendon reflexes
- Feeling of warmth and flushing
- Somnolence
- Slurred speech
- Muscular paralysis
- Respiratory difficulty
- Cardiac arrest[40]

ASSESSMENT FOR SAFE MgSO₄ ADMINISTRATION
- **Reflexes** present (reflexes are absent at Mg level of ≥8-10 mEq/L).
- **Respirations** are adequate (depression occurs at Mg level of ≥15 mEq/L).
- **Normal level of consciousness** (with normal **speech**).
- **Urine output** >100 mL/4 hr by indwelling urinary catheter.[32] MgSO₄ is excreted by the kidneys, so decreased urinary output prompts a reduced dose; a high output may mandate an increased dose.[40]

IF TOXICITY IS SUSPECTED
- Stop the MgSO₄ infusion.
- If respiratory depression is noted, give calcium gluconate 1 g IV over 3 min and administer oxygen. Endotracheal intubation and ventilation are performed when necessary.[32]

---

*The **ANTIDOTE** to MgSO₄ is calcium gluconate 1 g IV over 3 min. It is kept at the bedside at all times during MgSO₄ administration.[32]

• INTRAHEPATIC CHOLESTASIS OF PREGNANCY

Intrahepatic cholestasis of pregnancy (ICP) is a condition in which bile flow is suppressed or blocked resulting in destruction of the liver cell membrane by bile acids, releasing bile acids into the blood. Occurring in the third trimester (rarely before 25 weeks), ICP spontaneously resolves after delivery and biochemical evidence disappears within a month.[20] Etiology is unknown; the occurrence may be familial. Associated skin pruritus **(pruritus gravidarum)** without lesions begins on the soles of the feet and palms, spreading to the trunk and extremities. Approximately 20% of women with ICP have mild jaundice, dark urine, hyperbilirubinemia, anorexia, nausea, and vomiting. The liver is normal in size and nontender. Twenty percent of women with ICP experience PPH (due to altered coagulation),[33] and the incidence of UTI is increased.[20] The perinatal mortality rate is 35 in 1000 live births because of poor maternal weight gain and poor placental clearance of fetal bile acids. Complications include meconium passage (thick in 27% to 58%), preterm delivery (in 36% to 44%), and intrauterine fetal distress (in 36% to 44%). The fetal death rate is not related to severity of maternal disease.[33]

Laboratory Findings: Serum bile acid level is consistently 10 to 100 times normal. In 20% to 60%, **serum aminotransferase** (ALT) levels are 2 to 109 times normal, **alkaline phosphatase** levels rise variably, and **total and direct serum bilirubin** levels are slightly to moderately elevated.[20]

Differential Diagnosis: Gallbladder disease, hepatitis, acute fatty liver of pregnancy or preeclampsia, primary biliary cirrhosis.[33] Renal failure, anemia, and hyperthyroidism or hypothyroidism will also cause pruritus.[37]

ⓜ Management

1. **Consult** with an obstetrician.
2. **Anticipatory guidance:** Some women will experience relief from the pruritus with **rest and a low-fat diet.** Antihistamines, benzodiazepines, minor tranquilizers, phenobarbital, dexamethasone, cholestyramine, epomeidol, S-adenyl-methionine, or ursodeoxycholic acid may be used for pruritus. **Fetal surveillance** begins at 34 weeks. **Labor is induced at 38 weeks** with documented lung maturity unless the mother is jaundiced and the indices indicate maturity, in which case induction is conducted at 36 weeks.[33]

• ISOIMMUNIZATION

Isoimmunization is sensitization of the mother to a paternal antigen that she does not carry, causing fetal hemolytic anemia and hydrops to varying degrees.[32] Box 2-5 lists red cell antigens and their propensity to cause hemolytic anemia in the fetus. ABO incompatibility usually occurs in a mother with blood type O with anti-A or anti-B antibodies and a type A or B baby. This accounts for 60% of all hemolytic disease of the newborn. Most antibodies formed are immunoglobulin M (IgM), which does not cross the placenta, and the resulting hemolytic disease is mild. Fewer than 1% require exchange transfusion, and the hemolysis does not affect obstetric management.[40]

If untreated, approximately 16% of Rh-negative women will become isoimmunized by their first pregnancy with an Rh-positive fetus. Antepartum sensitization rarely occurs, however, before 28 weeks.[40] Isoimmunization causes CHF and anemia in the fetus. (See erythroblastosis fetalis, p. 289.) The incidence of isoimmunization is as high as 1 in 1000.[28]

Laboratory Studies: The pregnant woman with a positive antibody screen has an **antibody** identification and **titer.** If the antibody is one that causes hemolysis, if the titer is $\geq 1:8$, and depending on the homozygosity or heterozygosity of the father, amniocentesis is indicated and **serial amniocentesis** dictates the management only if the fetus is positive for the antibody.[28] The **Delta OD 450** value of amniotic fluid (spectrophotometric determination of the amniotic fluid bilirubin that is a byproduct of hemolysis) is an indirect measurement of fetal anemia.[40] Amniotic fluid samples are used to measure bilirubin concentration spectrophotometrically, the result being plotted on a graph divided into zones I, II, and III. Results indicate the degree of hemolysis occurring in the fetus.[87]

The **indirect Coombs'** test screens for abnormal antibodies in maternal serum. Once the "critical titer" is reached, indicating that an amniocentesis is required (the value varying between 1:8 and 1:32 in various laboratories), this value may plateau. This test is then no longer used to manage the sensitized woman.[40] The **direct Coombs'** test detects maternal antibodies in neonatal blood and is positive in the infant with hydrops.[32]

The pregnant woman is tested with an **antibody level** at 12 to 16 weeks, 28 to 32 weeks, and 36 weeks.[81] If the patient receives RhoGAM at 28 weeks, her antibody titer at 38 to 40 weeks should be <8 from the RhoGAM itself. A value >8 suggests active immunization. The acid-elution test identifies the percentage of fetal cells in maternal blood. The

---

- *Box 2-5 /* **Red Cell Antigens and Their Propensity to Cause Hemolytic Disease in the Fetus Whose Mother is Isoimmunized** •

- **Antigens not proven to cause hemolytic disease:** I, the Duffy family Fy^b, and Lewis antigens
- **Antigens that cause mild hemolytic disease:** N (of MNSs system); Lutheran family (Lu); Xg family; public antigens Yt^b, Lan, Ge, and Jr^a; private antigens Co^a and Co^b; Batty, Becker, Berrens, Evans, Gonzales, Hunt, Jobbins, Rm, Ven, and Wright^b
- **Antigens that cause moderate hemolytic disease:** Public antigens En^a, private antigens Biles, Heibel, Rain, Zd
- **Antigens that cause mild to moderate hemolytic disease:** C and e of the CDE family
- **Antigens that cause moderate to severe hemolytic disease:** Public antigen Yt^a
- **Antigens that cause mild to severe hemolytic disease:** c and E of the CDE (Rh) group, k of the Kell group, Jk^a and Jk^b of the Kidd group, M, S, s, and U of the MNSs group, the Diego family (Di^a and Di^b), and PP of the P group
- **Antigens that cause mild to severe hemolytic disease with hydrops fetalis:** D of the CDE (Rh) group, K of the Kell group, Fy^a of the Duffy group
- **Antigens that cause severe hemolytic disease:** Co^a and private antigens Good and Wright^a

Data from American College of Obstetricians and Gynecologists, *Management of isoimmmunization in pregnancy,* Technical Bulletin No. 90, Washington, DC, 1986, ACOG.

volume is then estimated and divided by 15 mL (the number neutralized by 300 μg RhoGAM). Enough RhoGAM is injected to detect free antibody in the maternal serum.[32]

ⓜ Management of the Rh-Negative Woman

1. **Test all women for their blood type and for the presence of antibodies** at registration and at 28 weeks. The **Rh-negative woman** receives an indirect Coombs' test; if the result is positive, she then receives antibody titers. If the indirect Coombs' test result is negative, it is repeated at 28 weeks. The putative paternal D-antigen status is helpful information (depending on whether he is the father) because if the father is negative, the fetus cannot be affected.[32]

2. **Carefully establish dates,** obtain a **careful obstetric history,** and obtain the history of any **blood transfusion.**[32]

3. If the patient's **antibody screens are negative:**

   a. At **28 weeks** and for any of the following events, offer the Rh-negative woman **RhoGAM.** RhoGAM is composed of IgG-passive antibodies that prevent the body from having an immune response. The amount that crosses the placenta to the baby during pregnancy is physiologically negligible. The standard RhoGAM dose, 300 μg, covers a 30-mL transfusion of fetal blood.[32] RhoGAM is given IM within 72 hours of possible or actual fetomaternal hemorrhage. **Events necessitating RhoGAM administration and the appropriate dosage are:**
      - SAB or therapeutic abortion before 12 weeks: 50 μg
      - First trimester chorionic villus sampling (CVS): 50 μg
      - Ectopic pregnancy before 12 weeks: 50 μg
      - Ectopic pregnancy after 12 weeks: 300 μg
      - Second or third trimester procedures: 300 μg
      - Second trimester amniocentesis: 300 μg
      - Second trimester CVS: 50 μg
      - Fetomaternal hemorrhage (e.g., second trimester bleeding, second or third trimester fetal demise, or trauma): 10 μg per estimated mL of fetal blood

      If delivery follows amniocentesis within 72 hours, RhoGAM is withheld until the fetal blood type is identified at delivery; and RhoGAM is given within 72 hours of the amniocentesis to cover both events. If delivery is delayed beyond the 72 hours, however, the RhoGAM is administered.[40]

   b. At delivery, **laboratory evaluation of the newborn** includes type and Rh and direct Coombs' test if the fetus is a different type than the mother. **If the infant is Rh positive,** the Rh-negative mother receives 300 μg **RhoGAM** within 72 hours of delivery. Offer the mother RhoGAM even if a tubal ligation is planned because of the high rate of tubal reanastamoses.

   c. Studies have shown that 1% of mothers receive more than 30 mL fetal blood at term delivery, in which case the standard 300 μg

RhoGAM dose is insufficient for the Rh-negative mother. Because there is not an identifiable risk factor for this larger fetomaternal hemorrhage, it is recommended that all Rh-negative mothers be tested at delivery with the **erythrocyte rosette test** or a similar test to identify which women need a greater dose of RhoGAM.[32]

   d. Test the **Rh-negative woman who has received repeated doses of RhoGAM** during the pregnancy, such as for repeated uterine bleeding in the second trimester, with an indirect Coombs' test to determine whether she requires more RhoGAM after delivery.[32]

4. **If the antibody screen is positive,** the patient is isoimmunized. **Refer** her to an obstetrician for prenatal care. **Anticipatory guidance:** Fetal Rh status can be identified by amniocentesis (without cordocentesis) or CVS. Management of isoimmunization is similar regardless of the antigen, except for the Kell antigen, which is discussed below. If the indirect Coombs' test is 1:16 or higher (varying by laboratory), further evaluation is required. Cordocentesis or a Delta OD 450 reading of amniotic fluid is required to further evaluate the fetus' condition. Lower zone II fetuses generally have a hemoglobin level of 11 to 13.9 g/dL; upper zone II fetuses generally have a hemoglobin level of 8.0 to 10.9 g/dL. Zone III fetuses are severely affected, and death is predicted within 7 to 10 days. Transfusion or delivery is indicated.[32] Ultrasound can also be used to monitor the fetus for signs of hydrops, although it cannot exclude the condition.[40] Transfusions may be given to the fetus by PUBS.[23] PPROM (0.4%), amnionitis (0.5%), fetal bradycardia (7%), hyperkalemia, porencephalic cyst formation, depressed neonatal erythropoiesis, and fetal death have occurred with this procedure. Intraperitoneal transfusion may also be performed during pregnancy, although increased mortality, lower Apgar scores, and an increased incidence of cesarean section are seen with this approach.[32]

The Delta OD 450 reading and the indirect Coombs' test do not appear to reflect the fetal condition in **Kell sensitivity,**[40] in which marrow suppression rather than hemolysis is the primary problem. In this case a normal OD 450 reading may be present with a severely anemic fetus, and means of directly detecting fetal anemia are more appropriate.[57] Eighty percent of Kell-positive fetuses have mild to moderate disease.[40]

• LARGE FOR DATES: DIFFERENTIAL

Differential Diagnoses[32]:

Closely attached adnexal mass
Fetal anomalies
Hydatidiform mole
Hydramnios
Inaccurate dating

Macrosomia
Multiple pregnancy
Placenta previa
Uterine fibroid

• MACROSOMIA (LARGE FOR GESTATIONAL AGE INFANT)

Definition: Macrosomia refers to an infant weighing ≥4500 g.[5]

Risk Factors: Risk factors include maternal diabetes or a positive 50 g glucose screen with a negative 3-hour glucose tolerance test, constitutionally large parents, maternal obesity, large pregnancy weight gain, multiparity, male fetus, history of macrosomia, ethnicity, postdatism, and maternal age <17 years. Sixty percent of women who deliver macrosomic infants have no risk factors.[5,32]

Diagnosis: The macrosomic growth of the diabetic woman's fetus can be identified ultrasonographically after 30 weeks' gestation by extra fat deposited in the abdominal and interscapular areas. Prediction of macrosomia by ultrasound is inaccurate, whether additional parameters are added to the equation or whether a series of ultrasounds is performed to extrapolate a rate of growth.[70] Clinician estimates and maternal guesses are equal to ultrasound in accuracy.[32]

Neonatal Complications: Shoulder dystocia, increased birth injuries (see p. 279), greater incidence of congenital anomalies,[81] higher rate of depressed 5-minute Apgar scores and admission to neonatal intensive care, and increased risk of being overweight in later life.[5]

Maternal Complications: Increased risk for dysfunctional labor, operative delivery, lacerations of the birth canal, PPH, and postpartum endometritis.[43]

ⓜ Management

1. Delivery of macrosomic infants is appropriately **managed by midwives with appropriate consultation** with a physician.[82]
2. **Route of delivery:** ACOG[5] concluded that labor and vaginal delivery are not contraindicated for infants of nondiabetic mothers whose estimated fetal weight (EFW) is ≤5000 g. Prophylactic cesarean delivery may be considered for infants of nondiabetic women with EFW >5000 g and for infants of diabetic mothers with EFW >4500 g.
3. **Induction** of labor **is not effective** in preventing poor maternal and infant outcomes with the suspected macrosomic infant and increases the risk of cesarean delivery.[5]
4. Suspected macrosomia is **not a contraindication** for attempting vaginal birth after cesarean section (VBAC).[5]
5. **Observe labor progress** because of the increased risk of cephalopelvic disproportion.
6. Practice **shoulder precautions** (see p. 184).
7. Women who have a prolonged second stage and then undergo midpelvic instrumental delivery have an increased risk of shoulder dystocia (0.16% to 4.57%).[40] The choice of **instrumental versus cesarean delivery** is made with great caution.

• MULTIPLE GESTATION

The number of multiple pregnancies is rising because of assisted conception and because childbearing is more often being delayed, and the likelihood of experiencing a multiple pregnancy increases after age 40 years.[61] Twins account for <1% of all deliveries yet account for 10% of perinatal deaths.[42] Screen women by ultrasound for one or more of the following factors for early identification of multiple pregnancy: large for dates uterus, rapid interval growth, history of fertility treatments, family history of fraternal twins, abdominal palpitation of three or more large parts and/or multiple small parts, and auscultation of more than one fetal heart different in rate from another fetal heart (and the maternal heart rate) by at least 10 BPM.[117] Although not diagnostic, hCG is elevated, as is the maternal serum alpha fetoprotein (MSAFP) level.[32]

Prenatal Testing: Monozygotic twins need only be tapped once. CVS can be done at 10 to 12.9 weeks by an experienced operator, although a specimen may be inadequate (1%) or contaminated with cells from the sibling (4% to 6%).[12] Amniocentesis can usually be done on twins by marking the first with indigo carmine dye.

Complications of Multiple Pregnancy: Higher rates of SAB (risk of congenital anomalies is twice that for singletons),[32] polyhydramnios, PPROM, intrauterine fetal demise, placental abruption, preeclampsia,[78] hyperemesis, pyelonephritis, PPH,[42] and prematurity occur with increased frequency. The infant mortality rate is increased.[61] Approximately 75% of all twins show evidence of growth problems.[42] IUGR is diagnosed when one twin falls below the tenth percentile or when there is a discordancy of 20% between the infants.[12] Intrauterine growth appears to stop at 39 weeks, and postdates characteristics have been seen in twins born at 40 weeks. Most clinicians therefore consider the 40-week twin gestation postdates. Monoamniotic twins have a 50% risk of dying from a cord accident. Vascular communication in twin placentas may result in underperfusion of one twin or neurologic damage.[32] Monozygotic twins more often have structural anomalies, such as conjoining and acardia.[12]

Prenatal Surveillance of Twins: Ascertain that both infants are actually being monitored. With the first NST, identify each fetus as twin A or twin B, identifying the baseline heart rate for each. Twin NSTs may be synchronous (accelerations occur within 15 seconds of each other) or nonsynchronous. Fetal movement counts are conducted bid and the woman should call if there are <10 movements/h. Approximately 25% of fetal movements are simultaneous in twins.[78]

Nutrition: During pregnancy, the woman carrying twins is counseled to eat about 300 extra calories per day and to gain an average 10 lb more than the mother of a singleton fetus.[12] Iron (60 to 100 mg/d) and folate (1 mg/d) are supplemented.[32] Reifsnider and Gill[86] suggest that the optimal weight gain for a twin gestation is 24 lb by 24 weeks then 1.25 lb weekly until delivery. For higher multiples, a weight gain of 36 lb by the twenty-fourth week followed by 1.25 lb until delivery is suggested.

Ⓜ Management

1. The midwife **may co-manage** the woman's care with a physician.
2. **Counsel regarding nutrition.**
3. **Prevention and management of complications:** Closely monitor the pregnancy for preterm labor. If preterm labor occurs, mothers of multiples have a greater risk for CHF with tocolytic agents (caused by anemia, greater volume, and decreased osmotic colloid pressure). Corticosteroid therapy does not differ from singleton pregnancies.[12] Closely observe the pregnant woman for preeclampsia. Hypertension tends to occur earlier and to be more severe.[32]
4. Patient **education and support** encompasses concerns and monitoring of the multiple pregnancy, physical discomforts, preparation for infant care, stresses related to body image, and financial burdens.
5. Conduct **fetal surveillance** as described above.
6. The position of twin A generally determines **mode of delivery,** although some physicians will deliver twins weighing <1700 g by cesarean section. In most cases, when twin A is vertex, vaginal delivery is attempted. If twin B is breech, the usual risks for breech delivery are present as well as the additional risk of locked twins (chins interlocking when twin B is vertex) and cord prolapse. Cesarean section is recommended for monozygotic twins because of the risk of cord entanglement. VBAC of twins does not carry increased risk for uterine rupture or maternal or perinatal morbidity and mortality.[97]
7. **Delivery** should occur by 40 weeks according to ACOG.[12]
8. **Conduct of delivery:**
   a. An obstetrician is present for the delivery.[117]
   b. Cunningham et al[32] suggest continuously monitoring each twin, establishing an IV with 5% dextrose in lactated Ringer's solution running, if needed, at 60 to 120 mL/h. Blood is typed and crossed.
   c. Anesthesia must be immediately available. Epidural anesthesia may be helpful in the delivery of twin B if there is a malpresentation (5% to 15%).[27] Many clinicians place an epidural catheter prophylactically.
   d. A pediatric team is ready for each twin.[97]
   e. Once delivery of the first twin is accomplished, there is no time limit for the delivery of the second twin.[12,97]
   f. Have an ultrasound machine available to image the second fetus after the first delivery.
   g. If twin B's vertex is in the birth canal or can be guided to it, rupture the membranes and conduct delivery. If the vertex is not engaged, use an oxytocin drip to start contractions and descent.

For fetal distress, cord prolapse, or placental abruption, prompt delivery of twin B is carried out by cesarean section or internal podalic version and extraction.[27]

• OBESITY RISKS DURING PREGNANCY

Obesity is defined as a 20% increase in body weight or a body mass index greater than the 85th percentile.[32] See p. 574 regarding calculation of body mass index. The obese pregnant woman is at increased risk for the following: hypertension, gestational diabetes, postterm pregnancy, multiple pregnancy, macrosomia, preeclampsia, and increased need for induction, oxytocin augmentation, and cesarean section. Extremely obese women have twice the risk for neural tube defects, cardiac defects, and other anomalies. They have more postpartum infections than other women.[72]

• OLIGOHYDRAMNIOS

Definition: An AFI of <5 or the absence of any vertical pocket >1 cm is considered oligohydramnios.[32] An AFI of 5 to 8 is considered borderline.

Signs and Symptoms: Decreased fluid may be palpated around the fetus on abdominal examination. Variable decelerations may be noted in the FHR.

Etiology: Placental insufficiency with IUGR, fetal renal obstruction or agenesis, chronic leakage of amniotic fluid, or an unknown etiology causes oligohydramnios.[51]

Predisposing Factors[32]:

Antihypertensive medications	Placental abruption
Congenital anomalies	Postmature syndrome
Diabetes	PPROM
Fetal demise	Preeclampsia
Hypertension	Twin-twin transfusion
IUGR	Uteroplacental insufficiency

Complications: Early in pregnancy (greatest risk for infant), deformities from compression or adhesions between the amnion and fetal parts and pulmonary hypoplasia may occur secondary to the oligohydramnios. During labor, the risk is increased for variable decelerations, meconium-stained fluid, and operative delivery.[32]

Ⓜ Management

1. In early gestation, **refer** the patient to the obstetrician.
2. **Anticipatory guidance:** Conservative management includes **bedrest,** good **nutrition,** and **fetal surveillance. Amnioinfusion** for the **second trimester** fetus with oligohydramnios (to prevent pulmonary hypoplasia) carries the risks of PPROM (1%), amnionitis (4%), and failed amnioinfusion (4%). Whether repeated

amnioinfusions during midtrimester for oligohydramnios improve the fetal outcome is unclear.[50] **Induction** and delivery are carried out when indicated.

3. In late gestation, **consult** with the physician.
4. **Maternal hydration** may improve AFI.[50]
5. **Induce** and deliver when indicated. **Intrapartum amnioinfusion** may relieve variables.[51]

• PLACENTAL ABRUPTION

Placental abruption is the premature separation of the normally implanted placenta. The abruption may be total, partial, or concealed (blood is trapped behind the placenta, membranes, or fetal head and no bleeding is visible externally). Signs and symptoms include vaginal bleeding (the amount does not necessarily reflect severity), fetal distress, back pain, uterine tenderness and rigidity, persistent uterine hypertonus, signs of hypovolemic shock, and a platelet count of $<60,000/mm^3$.[127] Often a diagnosis of exclusion, abruption is identified by ultrasound in only 50% of cases.[18] Postpartum hemorrhage, Couvelaire uterus (extravasation of blood into the uterine muscle), Sheehan's syndrome (see p. 485), and DIC (see p. 361) may complicate delivery. The incidence is 1 in 150[32]; the risk of recurrence is tenfold.[25] The perinatal mortality rate is 25% to 30%, increasing with the severity of the abruption.[18] An acute abruption of approximately 50% usually results in fetal death, but chronic abruption allows adaptation and is better tolerated.[17]

Risk Factors [32,117]:

African-American race
Cigarette smoking
Cocaine abuse
Delivery of placenta of twin
  B after twin A delivery
External version
Folic acid deficiency
History of abruption

Increasing parity
Preeclampsia
Chronic hypertension
PPROM
Short umbilical cord
Sudden uterine decompression
Trauma
Uterine leiomyoma located under
  placenta

ⓜ Diagnosis and Management

See Figure 2-1, decision tree for midwifery diagnosis and management of antepartum vaginal bleeding (p. 66).

• PLACENTA PREVIA

In placenta previa, the placenta is located over or adjacent to the internal cervical os. Variations include total placenta previa, partial placenta previa, marginal placenta previa (placental edge at the edge of the internal cervical os), and low-lying placenta (placental edge implanted in the lower uterine segment near the edge of the internal cervical os). Signs of total and partial placenta previa are usually absent until painless vaginal bleeding occurs as a result of placental separation as the lower uterine segment is being formed and cervical dilation begins (possibly with uterine contractions) at the end of the second or third trimesters.[18,32] Transabdominal ultrasound diagnosis is accurate in 93% of cases. If the condition is diagnosed before 20 weeks, 90% resolve by term. A total previa diagnosed during the second trimester will remain so in 26% of women. Partial and marginal previas will remain so in 2.5%[18] for an overall incidence of 0.3% to 0.7%. Fetal effects of hemorrhage include respiratory distress syndrome and anemia.[30] Maternal complications include hemorrhage and an increased risk for placenta accreta.

Vasa previa occurs with velamentous insertion of the umbilical cord into the placenta when the fetal blood vessels course through the membranes above the cervical os. Vasa previa is rare but is associated with often fatal fetal hemorrhage.[32]

Risk Factors:
Cigarette smoking (which doubles risk)[18]
Cocaine use (possibly from compensatory placental hypertrophy)[32]
Erythroblastosis[32]
History of cesarean section (after one, 1% to 4% risk; after ≥4, 10% risk)[18]
History of therapeutic abortion[32]
Increasing parity[32]
Maternal age >35 years[32]
Multiple pregnancy[32]

m Diagnosis and Management

See Figure 2-1, decision tree for midwifery diagnosis and management of antepartum bleeding, p. 66.

• POSTTERM PREGNANCY

Definition: Pregnancy exceeding 42 weeks' gestation—accounting for 10% of all gestations.[13] Seventy percent of "postdates" pregnancies are actually misdiagnoses due to delayed ovulation. Rarely, anencephaly and adrenal hypoplasia cause pregnancy to be prolonged.[32]

Maternal Complications[40]:
Hemorrhage due to uterine atony
Higher cesarean section rate
Increased frequency of induction of labor
Postpartum endometritis
Prolonged hospitalization
Wound complications

Neonatal Complications:
Increased perinatal mortality rate   Neonatal seizures

Oligohydramnios

Macrosomia

Meconium aspiration syndrome

Postmature syndrome

Shoulder dystocia

Postmature Syndrome: Occurring in 25% of postdates pregnancies due to diminished placental function, the postmature infant—who appears wrinkled, with peeling skin, no vernix or lanugo, alert facies, creases over the entire sole of the foot, long nails, and a thin, wasted-appearing body—is at risk for respiratory distress syndrome, hypoglycemia, polycythemia, and temperature instability.[32]

ⓜ Antepartum Management

1. Accurately **assess dates** at the first prenatal visit.
2. Teach the woman to do **fetal movement counts** in the third trimester.
3. Discuss risks and benefits of the postdates delivery, options for management, and make the **delivery plan** with the mother.
4. Some clinicians propose the **stripping of membranes** at prenatal visits every 3 days after 39 weeks decreases the number of women who exceed 42 weeks' gestation.[58] However, stripping of the membranes carries the risks of introducing infection, causing bleeding from an unsuspected low-lying placenta, and unintentionally rupturing the membranes. Gabbe et al[40] state that the method has unproven efficacy, and should not be used as a routine practice.
5. Other clinicians administer prostaglandin ε_2 gel on an outpatient basis.[35]
6. Some clinicians begin **antenatal testing** at 41 weeks, including biweekly AFI. Some prefer induction and perform antenatal testing only if the cervix is unfavorable. Antenatal testing has not improved outcomes in clinical trials, and ACOG[13] does not offer recommendations on timing, frequency, or which tests to conduct.
7. **Consultation** with the physician is required when **delivery is indicated** for any medical condition, such as diabetes or hypertension, that precludes conservative management, or for nonreassuring fetal testing.
8. ACOG[13] states that there is not enough information to determine whether the woman with a postdates pregnancy will have a better outcome with **expectant management** or with **induction at 42 weeks** (whether or not the cervix is favorable).
9. Some clinicians will **consider cesarean section** when the cervix is unripe and the baby is estimated to weigh ≥**4500 g** at 42 weeks.[32]

• PRETERM PREMATURE RUPTURE OF MEMBRANES

Rupture of membranes is considered preterm before 37 weeks' gestation. An infection and inflammatory process begins in the space between the amnion and the chorion. PPROM and preterm labor are caused by the enzymes and cytokines released. Infection may have preceded pregnancy, ascended through the cervix, or spread hematogenously. Organisms implicated include anaerobes, bacterial vaginosis, gonorrhea, chlamydia, trichomonas, and group B strep. The younger the gestational age, the more days precede delivery. When PPROM occurs before 26 weeks, 30% to 40% will gain a week before delivery; 20% will gain more than 4 weeks. Of patients with PPROM between 28 and 36 weeks' gestation, 70% to 80% will deliver within the first week. At term, 80% go into labor within the first 24 hours. Digital examination hastens delivery significantly compared with sterile speculum examination.[40]

Clinical chorioamnionitis occurs in 13% to 60%; the younger the fetus, the greater the risk. The incidence of fetal malposition is increased.[11] Abruptio placenta occurs in 4% to 12%. The greatest danger to these infants are the complications of prematurity—specifically respiratory distress syndrome. The belief that PPROM facilitates fetal lung maturity is controversial.[66] These infants are at higher risk for perinatal death (1% to 2% risk of stillbirth), intraventricular hemorrhage, and neonatal sepsis.[11] Other risks include cord prolapse, cord compression causing fetal heart variables and resulting in operative delivery, or cesarean delivery due to failure of induction.[40] Complications of midtrimester PPROM include fetal complications associated with midtrimester oligohydramnios (see p. 101): stillbirth (3.8% to 21.7%[11]), chorioamnionitis (39%), endometritis (14%), abruptio placenta (3%), retained placenta, PPH requiring D&C (12%), and maternal sepsis.[66] About half the survivors of midtrimester PPROM have normal development[38]; the other survivors show developmental delays and less commonly cerebral palsy, chronic lung disease, blindness, hydrocephalus, and mental retardation.[11]

Risk Factors[40]:

Bleeding in pregnancy   Low socioeconomic status
Coitus   Poor nutrition
Genital tract infection or colonization   Smoking

ⓜ Management

1. Perform a **sterile speculum examination (SSE)** to confirm rupture of membranes, and take a **culture for GBS.** (See p. 578 regarding SSE.) Observe for cervicitis, a prolapsed umbilical cord or fetal part, cervical dilation, and effacement. After 32 to 34 weeks, collect vaginal pool fluid, if possible, for fetal maturity testing.[66]
2. **Defer digital examination** because it increases the risk of neonatal infection and neonatal death and increases the likelihood of labor occurring sooner.[66]
3. **Refer** the woman for physician management.
4. **Anticipatory guidance:** If the diagnosis remains in question, indigo carmine may be introduced by amniocentesis and a perineal pad is observed or repeat SSE is performed to observe for dye passage within 30 minutes. **Ultrasound** is done to measure the AFI, to

determine fetal presentation, fetal size, gestational age, and fetal abnormality.[66] **Fetal well-being** is assessed. Determine the need for **GBS prophylaxis** (see p. 67).[11] Management is planned considering the gestational age and the risk for infection. The risk of neonatal prematurity tends to outweigh any other risks before 30 to 32 weeks' gestation, and conservative management is appropriate for these women. After 34 to 35 weeks, the risk of neonatal infection or neonatal compromise from oligohydramnios is the most threatening possibility.[40] The risks of cesarean delivery and neonatal infection are the same with induction or expectant management. Management decisions are made in concert with the mother with these risks kept in mind.[11] Options include **immediate delivery** of all infants beyond a certain gestation or a certain estimated weight (usually 1500 to 1800 g), resulting in more cesarean sections for failed induction; **conservative or expectant management;** or **delay of delivery long enough to administer steroids and antibiotics,** using tocolytics if necessary.[40]

a. **Antenatal corticosteroid therapy** administration is controversial in this setting because some suggest that PPROM itself facilitates lung maturity; because corticosteroids may increase the risks of infection; and because many PPROM pregnancies will deliver before receiving the benefit of corticosteroids. Corticosteroid therapy increases the risk of maternal and fetal infection only slightly (9.1% vs. 7.2%).[121] It reduces the risk of infant death by 30%, respiratory distress syndrome by 50%, and intracranial hemorrhage and periventricular leukomalacia by 70% (the latter two being predictors of long-term neurologic damage, including cerebral palsy).[55] The National Institutes of Health consensus panel and ACOG[9] recommend corticosteroids for PPROM before 30 to 32 weeks. The appropriate dose is betamethasone 12 mg q24h for 2 doses or dexamethasone 6 mg q12h for 4 doses.[121] See a further discussion on the risks and benefits of corticosteroid administration and repeated courses, p. 156.

b. In pregnancies before 35 weeks, **antibiotics** prolong pregnancy and reduce the incidence of chorioamnionitis, postpartum endometritis, neonatal sepsis, respiratory distress syndrome, pneumonia, necrotizing enterocolitis, and intraventricular hemorrhage, thereby reducing the perinatal mortality rate. Ampicillin and erythromycin IV for 48 hours followed by oral administration for 5 days has been used, as has IV ampicillin followed by oral amoxicillin or IV ampicillin/sulbactam followed by oral amoxicillin/clavulanate. Any of these dosages would treat GBS. Once labor begins, GBS prophylaxis is administered as recommended (see p. 67).[10]

c. **Conservative or expectant management** entails hospitalization and observation for fetal well-being and signs of infection. This approach results in fewer cesarean sections, but fetal surveillance must be performed daily. Signs of infection are sometimes missed.

NST alone does not predict subsequent amnionitis. A BPP of ≤6, however, is predictive. Once pulmonary maturity has been documented, expectant management may offer only brief prolongation of pregnancy at the risk of chorioamnionitis, cord compression, and neonatal sepsis workup.[66] Although some studies document similar outcomes for women with PPROM who are managed at home, ACOG[11] suggests further study, citing a less certain neonatal outcome. Delivery is facilitated if the mother develops clinical chorioamnionitis, placental abruption, or signs of fetal compromise. Signs of chorioamnionitis include a temperature of ≥101° F, uterine tenderness, or WBC count of ≥20,000 mm³. Amniocentesis may be performed to study the amniotic fluid for gram stain, amniotic fluid glucose levels (a low value of 16 to 20 mg/dL correlates with infection), and culture (only 1% to 15% of women with clinically evident chorioamnionitis have positive cultures). The presence of leukocytes in the amniotic fluid alone is not confirmation of chorioamnionitis.[66]

   d. Women with a history of **herpes simplex virus with PPROM** have a theoretical 19% risk of neonatal herpes simplex virus. Acyclovir may be administered prophylactically to these women.[40]

• PRURITIC URTICARIAL PAPULES AND PLAQUES OF PREGNANCY

Pruritic urticarial papules and plaques of pregnancy (PUPPP) (also called late prurigo of pregnancy and polymorphic eruptions of pregnancy) is a rash, usually occurring in the third trimester, of erythematous papules that coalesce into plaques. Small vesicles may develop on the plaques. The rash is intensely pruritic and usually begins in the abdominal striae. It may spread to the arms, legs, or buttocks within 2 to 3 days. The face and periumbilical area are not affected. PUPPP is not associated with systemic symptoms. It resolves spontaneously 10 to 14 days after delivery and usually does not recur in future pregnancies. PUPPP is not associated with increased fetal morbidity and mortality rates. It occurs in 1 in 200 to 240 pregnancies and is common in primigravid women with prominent abdominal striae, twins, or polyhydramnios. The cause is unknown. Diagnosis is made by identification of a papular eruption with laboratory exclusion of cholestasis.[40]

ⓜ Management

1. **Consult** the physician.
2. Topical or systemic **steroid** therapy may be prescribed,[118] and **antipruritic drugs** such as hydroxyzine and diphenhydramine may be helpful.[40]
3. Some researchers have suggested **increased antenatal testing,** but adverse outcomes have not been documented.[40]

4. In some women the discomfort of the pruritus may be sufficient to **induce labor** after fetal maturity is assured.[40]

• SUBSTANCE ABUSE DURING PREGNANCY

Experts have estimated that 15% to 21% of pregnant women use illicit drugs.[52] Most of these individuals are abusing more than one substance, which may act synergistically to increase risk to the fetus. Some drugs contain impurities that have adverse effects on the mother and/or the fetus. Often the woman who uses drugs is already at risk due to poor maternal health and nutrition and the presence of infectious diseases. The risks for a particular drug are therefore not calculable.[32]

Variables that determine how a fetus will be affected by a substance include the timing of the exposure, dosage, chronicity, and interactions of polydrug use. The lipid solubility, molecular size, protein binding capacity, degree of ionization, method of transport across the placenta, the placental structure and bloodflow, and the maternal/fetal pH gradient all affect how much of the drug the fetus receives. The fetal capacity to metabolize and excrete drugs is less than the mother's; thus, the dose is greater proportionately and lasts longer for the fetus than for the mother.[119] Box 2-6 lists those drugs that may result in addiction of the fetus.

• Box 2-6 / Drugs Associated With Neonatal Abstinence Syndrome •

- Alcohol (including nonprescription cough meds)
- Barbiturates
- Benadryl
- Caffeine
- Cocaine
- Codeine
- Darvon
- Diazepam
- Heroin
- Methadone
- Librium
- Lorazepam
- Marijuana
- Nicotine
- Other narcotics
- Phencyclidine
- Talwin

Data from Wagner CL et al: The impact of drug exposure on the neonate, *Obstet Gynecol Clin North Am* 25:169-194, 1998.

Recognizing Stages of Readiness for Change

Addicted individuals follow a process when changing their behavior. Health care providers need to assess the readiness of each client, avoiding alienating one who is not ready to change by using confrontational techniques, and encouraging one who has relapsed that she can be successful in the future. Stages to recognize include:

1. **Precontemplation:** Lack of interest in changing the behavior
2. **Contemplation:** A growing awareness of the negative aspects of the behavior and increased interest in changing
3. **Action:** Taking actual steps to change the behavior, often with backsliding and renewed efforts
4. **Maintenance:** Cessation of behavior with little temptation to return.[49]

Signs and Symptoms of Drug Abuse

Behavioral Indicators:

Emergency room visits
Failure to seek prenatal care
History of drug use, STIs, or
  prostitution
Insomnia
Marital and custodial issues
Missed appointments

Noncompliance
Persistent tobacco use
Problems with law enforcement
Requests for analgesics, tranquilizers, sedatives, or stimulants
Suicide attempts
Unexplained poor prenatal nutrition

Maternal Physical Indicators:

Needle tracks or tattoos to cover tracks
Unusual infections in unusual places
Withdrawal symptoms

Social Indicators:

Domestic violence
Family history of substance abuse
History of multiple injuries

Obstetric History:

Inadequate prenatal care
IUGR
Multiple pregnancy loss
Placental abruption
Neonatal withdrawal

Preterm labor
Unexplained neonatal neurologic complications such as intracranial hemorrhage, cerebral infarction, or seizures

Complications of Pregnancy[119]:

IUGR
Labile maternal BP
Unexplained fetal tachycardia

Unexplained placental abruption
Unexplained preterm labor

Laboratory Studies: Hepatitis B and C studies, VDRL, STS, HIV, 6C, and CT cultures, Pap smear, AST, ALT, UA, and toxicology studies will reveal evidence of substance use. Urine toxicology screening results may be false-positive if anesthetic lubricant was used to catheterize a patient or if a UTI is present.[23] See Table 2-3 for the timing of laboratory detection of various drugs.

ⓜ Management for All Substance-Abusing Pregnant Women

1. Because significant damage may be done to the infant before the woman knows that she is pregnant, **education and support before conception** are ideal.[89]

2. **Identify** the woman who is abusing substances by using history and physical clues as well as laboratory studies. Elicit a **drug history,** including drugs used, dose, route, when used, frequency, duration, where obtained, withdrawal symptoms, use of needles and whether they are sterile.

3. **Refer to special prenatal programs** tailored to the needs of the addicted woman, if one is available, including substance abuse programs, legal and social services. Refer to **self-help groups** such as Alcoholics Anonymous.

4. Establish a **trusting relationship** to ensure that the woman will continue to receive prenatal care even if she continues to use drugs.

5. **Counsel the woman regarding the risks to herself and to her fetus** from the substance abuse. Reinforce this concern at every prenatal visit. Counsel regarding the **benefits of reducing drug use during pregnancy:** IUGR may be improved, and the effect of drugs on brain development will be minimized throughout pregnancy.[89] **Encourage abstinence**, or even small reductions.[52]

6. **Withdrawal** from a narcotic during pregnancy may cause preterm labor. Uncontrolled barbiturate withdrawal may be fatal for mother and fetus. **Detoxification** is best carried out in a drug program during the second trimester when the risks of withdrawal-induced preterm labor are lowest. Cocaine, alcohol, amphetamine, and bar-

---

Table 2-3 / Timing of Detection of Drugs of Abuse by Urine Toxicology Testing

Drug	Window of Detection
Amphetamine	2-3 days
Methamphetamine	2-3 days
Cocaine as benzoylecgonine	2-3 days
Marijuana metabolites	2 days-3 weeks
Opiate metabolites	2-3 days
Phencyclidine	8 days-3 weeks
Benzodiazepines	≥3 days
Methadone	3 days
Methaqualone	2 weeks

Data from Dasgupta A: Urinary adulterants and drugs-of-abuse testing, *MLO Med Lab Obs*; 35(2):26-28, 30-31.

biturate addictions are managed by inpatient, controlled with-drawal; minor tranquilizer, marijuana, and tobacco addictions are managed by outpatient withdrawal; and narcotic dependence is managed by methadone maintenance.[23]

7. Provide **nutritional counseling** to prevent ketosis and provide calo-ries, vitamins, and protein.

8. **Ongoing prenatal care: Screen for STIs**, hepatitis, and HIV. **Screen periodically** for polydrug abuse. Monitor for complications: **IUGR** (baseline and periodic ultrasound), **preterm labor,** and **preeclampsia. Use alternatives** to support the woman's efforts: antidepressants for depression; acupuncture, biofeedback, and coun-seling to address the issues of substance-abusing women; and refer for social services, child care, and vocational and legal assistance. **Observe for depression or suicidal ideation** as well as signs of **physical abuse.** Be aware of resources available for these women.

9. If the woman is using a drug that may cause neonatal withdrawal, or if polydrug use is suspected, **deliver in a hospital with staff experienced** in recognizing and treating withdrawal symptoms.

10. Provide **appropriate pain management** during labor with anal-gesics and anesthesia while carefully noting maternal response to enable comfort without overmedicating.

11. Assist the mother in making the decision **whether to breastfeed**, considering the risks and benefits. Breastfeeding is contraindicated when the mother is abusing drugs. Other risk behaviors may expose the infant to HIV or hepatitis through the breastmilk.

12. **Long-term intervention** for this woman and her child is required to support her changed lifestyle.

Alcohol

History: A brief questionnaire can be used to indirectly assess alco-hol intake by asking about the woman's tolerance to alcohol.[89] To iden-tify women at risk, the interviewer may want to ask about alcohol intake before pregnancy to avoid any stigma regarding drinking during the pregnancy. The TWEAK test includes the following items[89]:

Tolerance: How many drinks can you hold? (The woman who answers more than 1 to 2 drinks is revealing a tolerance and excessive intake.)

Worry: Does your spouse (or parents) ever worry or complain about your drinking?

Eye-opener: Have you ever had a drink first thing in the morning to steady your nerves or get rid of a hangover?

Amnesia: Have you ever awakened the morning after drinking the night before and found that you cannot remember part of the evening?

Kut/cut down: Have you ever felt that you ought to cut down on your drinking?

Maternal Complications: Fertility is diminished with increasing alcohol intake.[48] Thiamine and other vitamin deficiencies occur in alcohol abuse. **Signs of alcohol withdrawal** involve tremulousness, irritability, and delirium tremens—a life-threatening condition manifested by sympathetic overactivity, fever, encephalopathy, visual hallucinations, seizures, and preterm labor in the pregnant woman.[23]

Complications of Pregnancy: First and second trimester bleeding occurs 3 times as often; infection and placental abruption occur with increased frequency. The risk of first and second trimester SABs is increased, and habitual abortion occurs twice as often.[23]

Fetal/Neonatal Complications: The most common cause of mental retardation in the neonate, **fetal alcohol syndrome** (FAS), is significantly related to alcohol intake in the first 2 months of pregnancy.[52] Women who drink more than 2 oz of 100-proof alcohol a day during the first trimester have a 30% to 40% risk of having a child with full-blown FAS[23]; women who drink 3 oz or more of 100-proof alcohol daily have a 71% risk. Binge drinking also causes FAS.[32] One in 300 to 2000 liveborn infants in the United States has FAS, with the frequency depending on the community. FAS is diagnosed when the fetus manifests one sign in each of three categories: IUGR, CNS involvement, and facial dysmorphology (microcephaly, micro-ophthalmia, short palpebral fissures, flat nasal bridge, small chin, epicanthic folds, poorly developed philtrum, thin upper lip, or flat maxillary area). Approximately 30% to 40% also have cardiac defects, minor defects of the hands and feet, neural tube defects, and other congenital anomalies.[119]

Lesser amounts of alcohol (1 to 4 drinks/d) are associated with **fetal alcohol effect,** which may affect 3 times as many children as FAS. Effects may include minor anomalies, moderate growth deficiency,[52] hyperactivity, sleep disturbances,[23] significantly lower IQ scores,[64] learning disabilities, memory problems, failure to thrive, recurrent otitis media, hearing and visual problems, and neurodevelopmental delays.[119]

Acute alcohol withdrawal may occur in the neonate, and there is an increased risk of alcoholism in the offspring.[23]

ⓜ Special Management for the Woman Who Has Used or Is Using Alcohol

Screen for alcohol-related hepatitis, pancreatitis, and neuropathy. Supplement with thiamine and other vitamins liberally. Women with pancreatitis, diabetes, and liver disease should be completely abstinent from alcohol because of special risks for their fetus.[23]

Amphetamines

Amphetamines are known by a wide variety of names, including "meth," "speed," "ice," "crystal," "tweak," "go," "chalk," and the so-called designer drugs: mescaline, TMA, STP (serenity, tranquility, and peace—the most potent), DOM, DOB, MDA, MDMA (methylene-dioxymethamphetamine, known as "ecstasy" or "Adam"), MDEA ("Eve"), and methcathinone.[85]

CNS stimulants that are taken IV or PO cause vasospasm of the uteroplacental vessels, dropping the fetal Pao_2, possibly causing preterm labor, placental abruption, and IUGR.[52] The anorexic effect of the drugs may contribute to malnourishment.[85] The woman who uses these drugs regularly develops a tolerance to them, is hyperactive, and is often paranoid with hallucinations.[23] Women addicted to amphetamines during pregnancy may develop hypertension, tachycardia, proteinuria, preterm labor, and placental abruption.[85] IV use is associated with maternal cardiac arrhythmias during obstetric anesthesia. Maternal withdrawal is manifested by lethargy and profound depression.[23]

Fetal/Neonatal Complications

The risk for symmetrical IUGR is increased with methamphetamines. Crystal methamphetamine, known as "ice" or "blue ice," is associated with reduced head circumference and stillbirth.[52] Fetal effects associated with amphetamines include cleft lip, cardiac defects, reduced head circumference, biliary atresia, prematurity, hyperbilirubinemia requiring exchange transfusion, cerebral hemorrhage, mongolian spots, systolic murmur, undescended testes, visual cognitive problems (processing what is seen), learning difficulties, and behavior changes. Growth may be accelerated in boys and delayed in girls; puberty may be accelerated in boys and delayed in girls.[85] Neonatal withdrawal is similar to that from cocaine.[23]

ⓜ *Special Management for the Woman Who Has Used or Is Using Amphetamines*

Detoxification is indicated. Advise anesthesia personnel if amphetamines have been used so that they will observe for cardiac arrhythmias if obstetric anesthesia is administered.[23]

Cigarettes

Pathophysiology: Cigarettes contain more than 2500 identified chemicals, including carbon monoxide, ammonia, acetone, formaldehyde, hydrogen cyanide, pyrene, and vinyl chloride.[120] In the body, nicotine releases acetylcholine, epinephrine, norepinephrine, and antidiuretic hormone, causing tachycardia, increased cardiac output, peripheral vasoconstriction, increased BP, and changes in fat and carbohydrate metabolism.[44] Vasoconstriction decreases uteroplacental bloodflow during pregnancy. Carbon monoxide crosses the placental barrier and binds with hemoglobin, reducing oxygenation of fetal blood.[120]

Maternal Complications: Smoking increases the risk of chronic obstructive pulmonary disease, cervical cancer, infertility, earlier onset of menopause, and ectopic pregnancy.[44] It is implicated in 29% of all cancers and is responsible for 55% of the cardiovascular deaths in women younger than 65 years.[120] **Withdrawal symptoms** include craving cigarettes, restlessness, anxiety, anger, difficulty concentrating, insomnia, depression, increased appetite or weight gain,[44] headaches, constipation, flatulence, mouth sores, thirst, coughing and hoarseness, sinus congestion, leg cramps,[50] and a decreased heart rate. Symptoms begin within a few hours and may last days to months.[120]

Complications during Pregnancy: Of the 23.5% of women in the United States who describe themselves as smokers, 24% to 40% quit smoking when they find out they are pregnant. Twenty percent to 50% smoke throughout pregnancy. Seventy percent of women who quit during pregnancy relapse within a year.[91] **SAB** and **placental complications** increase with smoking during pregnancy because of accelerated degeneration of placenta and membranes (abruption, previa, premature rupture of membranes, and prolonged ruptured membranes).[120] Smoking also carries a higher risk of stillbirth. **The perinatal death rate** is increased by 27%; if the woman smokes more than one pack/d, the rate is increased by 35%.[119]

Cigarette smoking decreases birth weight by an average of 200 g.[119] The risk for LBW is greater with increasing age; smoking after the age of 35 years increases the risk of IUGR fivefold.[120] Older women who smoke have more premature births than younger women who smoke.[122] The effects on the fetus of most of the 2500 identified chemicals in cigarette smoke are unknown.[50]

Risks of Maternal Exposure to Secondhand Smoke: Secondhand smoke is associated with a twofold risk of delivering a LBW baby in one study[34] and with a 192-g deficit in the birth weight in another study.[88]

Positive Effects of Quitting Smoking: Within 12 hours of quitting smoking, the levels of carbon monoxide and nicotine rapidly decrease, and the heart and lungs begin to repair damage caused by the smoke. Within a few days, taste and smell improve, and long term, the risk of life-threatening cancers and heart disease decreases.[8] Infants whose mothers quit smoking during pregnancy were 241 g heavier than those whose mothers continued to smoke in one study. Those whose mothers reduced their smoking during pregnancy were 92 g heavier than their counterparts. Pregnancy lasted 1 week longer for the mothers who quit. Although quitting by 16 weeks prevents many adverse affects, even quitting in the third trimester, when much fetal growth occurs, is beneficial.[52]

Risks of Smoking during Lactation: See p. 314.

Childhood Illness and Disease after Nicotine Exposure in Utero: The incidence of **childhood cancers** is doubled when the mother smokes during pregnancy; there is also an increased risk of childhood **asthma** and more episodes of **pneumonia and bronchitis** in the first year. **Strabismus, attention deficit-hyperactivity disorder, IQ scores** 10 points lower, and 1200 to 2200 cases of **sudden infant death syndrome** (SIDS) annually are related to cigarette smoking.[50,52]

ⓜ Special Management for the Woman Who Smokes Cigarettes

The CDC recommends that **hemoglobin and hematocrit** cutoffs for anemia be raised for smokers[52] (see p. 588). Determine whether the nutrients depleted by smoking—zinc, carotene, cholesterol, vitamin B_{12}, iron, amino acids, vitamin C, and folate—are sufficiently supplemented in the **prescribed prenatal vitamins.**

Smoking Cessation Treatments

Offer smoking cessation treatments. Offer nicotine replacement if the mother smokes more than 15 cigarettes a day and has previously experienced withdrawal symptoms that prevented her from quitting. The likelihood of smoking cessation must outweigh the risk of nicotine replacement and concomitant smoking. The serum nicotine level is less with nicotine replacement than with smoking.[120] Although some experts advise against nicotine replacement during pregnancy,[15] ACOG[14] recommends nicotine replacement for heavy smokers who have failed nonpharmacologic attempts to stop smoking and for whom the likelihood of cessation success outweighs the risks of the nicotine. The mother is instructed that nicotine replacement in pregnancy may jeopardize the fetus.[120] Abstinence rates, however, are 2 to 3 times greater with nicotine replacement.[14] Replacements include:

1. **Nicotine gum:** Available without a prescription in 2- and 4-mg doses. Two milligrams is used to replace two cigarettes. The gum is chewed a few seconds until it feels peppery, "parked" in the cheek until the sensation is gone, then repeat. The gum lasts about 30 minutes. After 1 to 2 months, the woman weans by decreasing 1 unit dose/wk.[120] Mouth irritation may occur.
2. **Nicotine patches** provide more constant levels of nicotine. They are available without a prescription in strengths that vary from 5 to 22 mg, are applied each morning, and are worn 16 to 24 hr/d.[15] Lighter smokers can use the 16-hour patch; heavier smokers can use the 24-hour patch, weaning to successively lower doses beginning in 2 to 4 weeks. Side effects include skin irritation and sleep disturbance.[120]
3. **Nicotine nasal spray** provides the most rapid rise in nicotine (10 minutes) but causes more dependency and has more adverse effects (nasal and throat irritation). One spray is taken per nostril 1 to 2 times/hr, with no more than 32 doses in 24 hours. Weaning is recommended during the third month of use. Contraindicated in women with asthma or chronic nasal, sinus, and bronchial disorders.[120]

Cocaine

Cocaine is taken orally, IV, or SQ and sniffed or smoked (known as "freebasing," which is particularly powerful). "Crack" is a pure form of the drug that is smoked, resulting in rapid blood levels and addicting euphoria. In some inner-city hospitals, it is estimated that 15% of the women deliver while on cocaine.[52] This sympathomimetic drug stimulates the peripheral sympathetic system and the CNS and is a vasoconstrictor.[23] It increases epinephrine and norepinephrine, causing tachycardia, BP elevation, vasoconstriction, a decreased need for sleep, and decreased uteroplacental bloodflow.[119]

Maternal complications of cocaine use may include cardiac and pulmonary disorders, chronic rhinitis, perforated nasal septum, seizures, renal insufficiency, stroke, bowel ischemia, hyperthermia, and sudden death.[32] Pregnancy complications include impaired fetal oxygenation; fetal hypertension; more frequent SABs; premature rupture of membranes in 20%; premature delivery in 25%; IUGR in 25% to 30%; meconium-stained amniotic fluid in 29%; stillbirth and placental infarction, insufficiency, or abruption (increased fourfold)[40]; congenital anomalies (affecting heart, brain, and other systems), and fetal CNS manifestations (seizures, abnormal electroencephalogram, neurobehavioral problems, and stroke).[23,52] Infants who are exposed to narcotics are at increased risk for SIDS.[119]

Neonatal withdrawal occurs in the infant of the cocaine addict.[23] Symptoms include irritability, tremulousness, gastrointestinal (GI) problems, inability to suck, and respiratory problems.[52] The intensity and length of withdrawal is generally less than that for other narcotics.[119]

Ⓜ Special Management for the Woman Who Has Used Cocaine

Detoxification is indicated.[23]

Heroin

Heroin is an injectable narcotic associated with maternal complications related to injection: cellulitis, abscess formation, endocarditis, hepatitis, and HIV infection.[52] Social complications related to illegal drug use include criminal behavior, overdose, and complications related to uncontrolled drug use. Chronic lung changes sometimes follow repeated insults by IV particulate matter[23] and contamination by filler substances or funguses, bacteria, or viruses (including HIV) in the drug.[23] Early **signs and symptoms of heroin withdrawal in the woman include** restlessness, rhinorrhea, piloerection, yawning, irritability, lacrimation, mydriasis, perspiration, vomiting, and diarrhea. Later signs are abdominal and uterine cramps, bone and muscle aches, and muscular irritability.[23]

During pregnancy, heroin use is associated with preterm labor, chorioamnionitis, an increased incidence of preeclampsia, and hemorrhage. Stillbirth, prematurity, and neonatal death are increased 3 to 7 times.[52] Although heroin does not increase the risk of congenital anomalies, IUGR, decreased head circumference, mild developmental delays, and behavioral disturbances are increased. It is unclear whether these complications are caused by the heroin itself or by the poor general health of the woman who abuses heroin.[32] Infants who are exposed to narcotics are at increased risk for SIDS.[119]

Neonatal withdrawal symptoms are seen in 50% to 80% of neonates born to addicted mothers, starting from 48 hours to 6 days.[119] Symptoms include a high-pitched cry, poor feeding, hypertonicity, irritability, sneezing, sweating, vomiting, diarrhea, tremors, and occasionally seizures.[52]

ⓜ Special Management for the Woman Who Has Used Heroin

Detoxification should take place after the pregnancy. Refer the pregnant woman for methadone maintenance to remove the patient from the high-risk lifestyle, to avoid overdose and contaminant exposure, and to prevent withdrawal. Use narcotic antagonists, such as Narcan, Talwin, Stadol, and Nubain, with caution to avoid putting the fetus into withdrawal, which may cause SAB or stillbirth.[23] NOTE: Heroin will cause a false-positive pregnancy test result.

Marijuana

One in three women uses marijuana (THC, *Cannabis sativa*) in their childbearing years.[119] Habitual smoking of marijuana affects the lungs similarly or more severely than cigarettes, causing bronchitis and elevated carboxyhemoglobin levels.[23] In pregnancy, precipitant labor, meconium staining, a reduction of birth weight, and shorter gestations have been associated with marijuana use in various studies.[98] No evidence exists to associate teratogenic effects and IUGR with marijuana use.[32] However, IUGR, lethargy, hypotonia, blunted response to stimuli, a lower neonatal light reflex, an increased Moro's reflex, tremor, dysmaturity of the visual pathways, and neurodevelopmental delays have been reported among infants of heavier users.[119]

Methadone

Methadone is a synthetic opiate narcotic with a half-life that is longer than heroin.[32] It has been used since the late 1960s to manage the opiate-addicted pregnant woman with the goal of preventing or reducing withdrawal symptoms and drug craving, to prevent relapse to the use of other addictive drugs, and to normalize any physiologic function disrupted by the drug abuse. The effectiveness of this management strategy is challenged because many women taking methadone are using multiple other substances.[21] Preterm birth, rapid labor, placental abruption, and meconium staining rates are significantly higher among mothers using methadone than among those using heroin.[32] Congenital anomalies are not increased. Reports vary regarding whether birth weight is decreased by methadone.[21] Methadone is metabolized more quickly than heroin during pregnancy, and some women may experience withdrawal symptoms by 24 hours. Withdrawal symptoms may include fetal hyperactivity, preterm labor, or fetal death. Heroin may be used to ameliorate these symptoms. Experienced clinics provide increased dosages split into morning and evening doses.[49]

The neonate is at risk for thrombocytosis within the first 4 months of life. As for all narcotic-exposed children, this child is at greater risk for SIDS.[119] The **neonatal withdrawal syndrome** occurs in 30% to 90% of infants whose mothers use opiates. Symptoms are the same as those for heroin. Methadone withdrawal may appear at 24 hours to 10 days after birth.[52] Withdrawal is prolonged (up to 3 weeks) because of methadone's longer half-life.[32] For this reason, some women avoid methadone.[49]

ⓜ Special Management for the Woman Taking Methadone

Gabbe et al[40] states the goal of management is to get the patient to a level of approximately 20 to 40 mg/d. Avoid manipulation of the dose in the third trimester because of the risk of fetal withdrawal in utero. Screen for other drugs periodically. Because withdrawal may occur after discharge from the hospital, inform the mother or caretaker of signs and symptoms.[52] NOTE: Methadone will cause a false-positive pregnancy test.

"Sniffing" ("Huffing")

Sniffing of organic solvents such as spray paint, glue, gasoline, thinners, or toluene causes maternal complications including renal tubular acidosis, pulmonary injury, and cardiac arrhythmias. During pregnancy, preterm birth, IUGR, and fetal death may occur. Developmental delays, and facial dysmorphism, much like the fetal effects of FAS, are identified among these infants.[40]

ⓜ Specific Management for the Woman Who Is Sniffing Solvents and Other Substances

Beta-mimetic tocolysis is contraindicated in these patients because these drugs potentiate the effects of the inhaled drugs.[23]

Tranquilizers and Sedatives ("Downers")

Benzodiazepines, barbiturates, glutethimide, and ethchlorvynol are often used in conjunction with other drugs (cocaine, amphetamines, and alcohol) to treat withdrawal symptoms. They produce tolerance and withdrawal symptoms themselves in the mother and fetus. Women who are abusing these drugs are often malnourished, avoid prenatal care, and are prone to traumatic injuries. Overdose may occur with resultant coma, hypoxia, and sometimes death. Withdrawal will manifest in the mother as restlessness, irritability, insomnia, and automatic stimulation to delirium, psychosis, and seizures and may be fatal if not treated.

There are no proven teratogenic effects, and barbiturates prescribed in controlled circumstances for the control of seizures do not result in IUGR. The fetal withdrawal syndrome is similar to that seen in cocaine-exposed infants. Infants of women taking phenobarbital for seizures also undergo withdrawal. Withdrawal from benzodiazepines is less severe; however, benzodiazepines do readily cross the placenta and withdrawal is better well before delivery to avoid a depressed baby at birth who must undergo neonatal withdrawal.[23]

• REFERENCES

1. Adair CD et al: Meconium-stained amniotic fluid-associated infectious mortality: a randomized, double-blind trial of ampicillin-sulbactam prophylaxis, *Obstet Gynecol* 88: 216-220, 1996.
2. Alexander GR et al: Preterm birth prevention: an evaluation of programs in the United States, *Birth* 18:160-169, 1991.
3. American College of Nurse-Midwives (ACNM): Limited obstetrical ultrasound in the third trimester, Clinical Bulletin No. 1, *J Nurse Midwifery* 42:344-348, 1997.
4. Reference deleted in galleys.
5. American College of Obstetricians and Gynecologists (ACOG): *Fetal macrosomia,* Practice Bulletin No. 22, Washington, DC, 2000, ACOG.
6. ACOG: *Antepartum fetal surveillance,* Practice Bulletin No. 9, Washington, DC, 1999, ACOG.
7. ACOG: Pregnancy later in life, *ACOG Woman's Health* 1999, accessed at *http://www.acog.com/from_home/publications/womans_health/wh6-2-7.htm.*
8. ACOG: When quitting spells success, *ACOG Woman's Health* 1999, accessed at *http://www.acog.com/from_home/publications/womans_health/wh11-10-7.htm.*
9. ACOG: *Antenatal corticosteroid therapy for fetal maturation,* Committee Opinion No. 210, Washington, DC, 1998, ACOG.
10. ACOG: *Antimicrobial therapy for obstetric patients,* Educational Bulletin No. 245, Washington, DC, 1998, ACOG.
11. ACOG: Premature rupture of membranes, Practice Bulletin No. 1, *Int J Gynecol Obstet* 63:75-84, 1998.
12. ACOG: *Special problems of multiple gestation,* Educational Bulletin No. 253, Washington, DC, 1998, ACOG.
13. ACOG: *Management of postterm pregnancy,* Practice Pattern No. 6, Washington, DC, 1997, ACOG.
14. ACOG: *Smoking and women's health,* Educational Bulletin No. 240, Washington, DC, 1997, ACOG.
15. Andrews J: Optimizing smoking cessation strategies, *Nurse Practitioner* 23:47-67, 1998.
16. Bacq Y: Acute fatty liver of pregnancy, *Semin Perinatol* 22:134-140, 1998.
17. Baergen RN: Macroscopic examination of the placenta immediately following birth, *J Nurse-Midwifery* 42:393-402, 1997.
18. Baron F, Hill WC: Placenta previa, placenta abruptio, *Clin Obstet Gynecol* 41:527-532, 1998.
19. Briggs GG: Nausea and vomiting of pregnancy. In Drugs, pregnancy, and lactation, *ObGyn NEWS* Aug 1, 2001.
20. Brites D et al: Correction of maternal serum bile acid profile during ursodeoxycholic acid therapy in cholestasis of pregnancy, *J Hepatol* 28:91-98, 1998.
21. Brown HL et al: Methadone maintenance in pregnancy: a reappraisal, *Am J Obstet Gynecol* 179:459-463, 1998.
22. Budd S: Acupuncture. In Tiran D, Mack S, editors: *Complementary therapies for pregnancy and childbirth,* ed 2, Edinburgh, 2000, Baillière Tindall.
23. Burrow GN, Ferris TF: *Medical complications during pregnancy,* Philadelphia, 1995, WB Saunders.
24. Caritis S et al: Low-dose aspirin to prevent preeclampsia in women at high risk: National Institute of Child Health and Human Development Network of Maternal-fetal Medicine Units, *N Engl J Med* 338:701-705, 1998.
25. Carter S: Overview of common obstetric bleeding disorders, *Nurse Pract* 24:50-73, 1999.

26. Castro MA et al: Reversible peripartum liver failure: a new perspective on the diagnosis, treatment, and cause of acute fatty liver of pregnancy, based on 28 consecutive cases, *Am J Obstet Gynecol* 181:389-395, 1999.
27. Chamberlain G, Steer P: ABC of labour care: unusual presentations and positions and multiple pregnancy, *BMJ* 318:1192-1194, 1999.
28. Chescheir NC, Hansen WF: New in perinatology, *Pediatr Rev* 20:57-63, 1999.
29. Côté-Arsenault D, Mahlangu N: Impact of perinatal loss on the subsequent pregnancy and self: women's experiences, *J Obstet Gynecol Neonatal Nurs* 28:274-282, 1999.
30. Crane JMG et al: Neonatal outcomes with placenta previa, *Obstet Gynecol* 93:541-544, 1999.
31. Creasy RK, Resnick R: *Maternal-fetal medicine principles and practice,* Philadelphia, 1994, WB Saunders.
32. Cunningham FG et al: *Williams obstetrics,* ed 20, Stamford, Conn, 1997, Appleton and Lange.
33. Davidson KM: Intrahepatic cholestasis of pregnancy, *Semin Perinatol* 22:104-111, 1998.
34. Dejin-Karlsson E et al: Does passive smoking in early pregnancy increase the risk of small-for-gestational-age infants? *Am J Public Health* 88:1523-1527, 1998.
35. Doany W: Outpatient management of postdate pregnancy with intravaginal prostaglandin E2 and membrane stripping, *Am J Obstet Gynecol* 174:351, 1996.
36. Edelman A, Logan JR: Pregnancy, hyperemesis gravidarum, *Emedicine* Dec 1999, accessed at *http://www.emedicine.com/emerg/topic479.htm.*
37. Errickson CV, Matus NR: Skin disorders of pregnancy, *Am Fam Physician* 49:605-610, 1994.
38. Farooqi A et al: Survival and 2-year outcome with expectant management of second-trimester rupture of membranes, *Obstet Gynecol* 92:895-901, 1998.
39. Fylstra DL: Tubal pregnancy: a review of current diagnosis and treatment, *Obstet Gynecol Surv* 54:138-146, 1999.
40. Gabbe SG, Niebyl JR, Simpson JL: *Obstetrics: normal and problem pregnancies,* San Francisco, 1996, Churchill Livingstone.
41. Gilbert WM, Nesbitt TS, Danielson B. Childbearing beyond age 40: pregnancy outcome in 24,032 cases, *Obstet Gynecol* 93:9-14, 1999.
42. Gordon JD et al: *Obstetrics gynecology & infertility,* Glen Cove, NY, 1998, Scrub Hill Press.
43. Gregory KD et al: Maternal and infant complications in high and normal weight infants by method of delivery, *Obstet Gynecol* 92:507-513, 1998.
44. Grimes DA, editor: Helping patients stop smoking: a new treatment option, *The Contraception Report* 9:12-14, 1998.
45. Hacker NF, Moore JG: *Essentials of obstetrics and gynecology,* ed 3, Philadelphia, 1998, WB Saunders.
46. Hewell SW, Hammer RH: Antiphospholipid antibodies: a threat throughout pregnancy, *J Obstet Gynecol Neonatal Nurse* 26:162-168, 1997.
47. Idarius B: *The homeopathic childbirth manual,* Talmage, Calif, 1999, Idarius Press.
48. Jensen TK et al: Does moderate alcohol consumption affect fertility? followup study among couples planning first pregnancy, *BMJ* 317:505-510, 1998.
49. Kearney MH: Drug treatment for women: traditional models and new directions, *J Obstet Gynecol Neonatal Nurse* 26:459-468, 1997.
50. Kilby JW: A smoking cessation plan for pregnant women, *J Obstet Gynecol Neonatal Nurse* 26:397-402, 1997.
51. Kilpatrick SJ: Therapeutic interventions for oligohydramnios: amnioinfusion and maternal hydration, *Clin Obstet Gynecol* 40:328-336, 1997.
52. King JC: Substance abuse in pregnancy, *Postgrad Med* 102:135-150, 1997.
53. Krause SA, Graves BW: Midwifery triage of first trimester bleeding, *J Nurse-Midwifery* 44:536-548, 1999.
54. Levine RJ et al: Trial of calcium to prevent preeclampsia, *N Engl J Med* 337:69-76, 1997.

55. Leviton LC et al: Methods to encourage the use of antenatal corticosteroid therapy for fetal maturation: a randomized controlled trial, *JAMA* 281:46-52, 1999.

56. Lin C, Santolaya-Forgas J: Current concepts of fetal growth restriction. Part 1. Causes, classification, and pathophysiology, *Obstet Gynecol* 92:1044-1055, 1998.

57. Lockwood CJ: Applying new advances on OB ultrasound, *Contemp OB/GYN* June: 51-75, 2001.

58. Magann EF et al: Can we decrease postdatism in women with an unfavorable cervix and a negative fetal fibronectin test result at term by serial membrane sweeping? *Am J Obstet Gynecol* 179:890-894, 1998.

59. Mackenzie SJ, Yeo S: Pregnancy interruption using mifepristone. *J Nurse-Midwifery* 42:86-90, 1997.

60. Magid MS et al: Placental pathology in systemic lupus erythematosus: a prospective study, *Am J Obstet Gynecol* 179:226-234, 1998.

61. Martin JA, Parks MM: Trends in twin and triplet births: 1980-97, *National Vital Statistics Reports* 47:99-120, 1997.

62. Martin JN et al: The spectrum of severe preeclampsia: comparative analysis by HELLP (hemolysis, elevated liver enzymes, and low platelet count) syndrome classification, *Am J Obstet Gynecol* 180:1373-1384, 1999.

63. Mashburn J: Ectopic pregnancy: triage do's and don'ts, *J Nurse-Midwifery* 44:549-557, 1999.

64. Mattson SN et al: Heavy prenatal alcohol exposure with or without physical features of fetal alcohol syndrome leads to IQ deficits, *J Pediatr* 13:718-721, 1997.

65. Mayer IE, Hussain H: Pregnancy and gastrointestinal disorders, *Gastroenterol Clin* 27: 1-36, 1998.

66. Mercer BM: Management of preterm premature rupture of membranes, *Clin Obstet Gynecol* 41:870-882, 1998.

67. Meyer NL et al: Urinary dipstick protein: a poor predictor of absent or severe proteinuria, *Am J Obstet Gynecol* 170:137-141, 1994.

68. Miller DA, Rabello YA, Paul RH: The modified biophysical profile: antepartum testing in the 1990s, *Am J Obstet Gynecol* 174:812-817, 1996.

69. Minnick-Smith K, Cook F: Current treatment options for ectopic pregnancy, *MCN* 22:21-25, 1997.

70. Moore TR: Fetal growth in diabetic pregnancy, *Clin Obstet Gynecol* 40:771-786, 1997.

71. Moran P, Taylor R: Management of hyperemesis gravidarum: the importance of weight loss as a criterion for steroid therapy, *Qual J Med* 95:153-158, 2002.

72. Morin KH: Perinatal outcome of obese women: a review of the literature, *J Obstet Gynecol Neonatal Nurs* 27:431-440, 1998.

73. Morrison EH: Common peripartum emergencies, *Am Fam Physician* 1998, available at: *http://www.aafp.org/afp/981101ap/morrison.html.*

74. Reference deleted in galleys.

75. Mozurkewich EL et al: Working conditions and adverse pregnancy outcome, *Obstet Gynecol* 95:623-635, 2000.

76. Murray M: *Antepartal and intrapartal fetal monitoring,* ed 2, Albuquerque, 1998, Learning Resources International.

77. Reference deleted in galleys.

78. National High Blood Pressure Education Program (NHBPEP): Report of the National High Blood Pressure Education Program Working Group on High Blood Pressure in Pregnancy, *Am J Obstet Gynecol* 183:S1-S22, 2000.

79. Nelson WE, editor: *Nelson textbook of pediatrics,* ed 15, Philadelphia, 1996, WB Saunders.

80. Nixon SA, Avery MD, Savik K: Outcomes of macrosomic infants in a nurse-midwifery services, *J Nurse-Midwifery* 43:280-286, 1998.

81. Payton RG, Gardner R, Reynolds D: Pharmacologic considerations and management of common endocrine disorders in women, *J Nurse-Midwifery* 42:186-206, 1997.

82. Pereira SP et al: Maternal and perinatal outcome in severe pregnancy-related liver disease, *Hepatology* 26:1258-1262, 1997.

83. Plessinger MA: Prenatal exposure to amphetamines, *Obstet Gynecol Clin North Am* 25:119-138, 1998.

84. Primeau MR, Lamb JM: When a baby dies: rights of the baby and parents, *J Obstet Gynecol Neonatal Nurs* 24:206-208, 1995.

85. Ramsay MM et al: *Normal values in pregnancy,* Philadelphia, 1996, WB Saunders.

86. Reifsnider E, Gill SL: Nutrition for the childbearing year, *J Obstet Gynecol Neonatal Nurs* 29:43-55, 2000.

87. Russell M et al: Detecting risk drinking during pregnancy: a comparison of four screening questionnaires, *Am J Public Health* 86:1435-1439, 1996.

88. Saraiya M et al: Spontaneous abortion-related deaths among women in the United States, 1981-1991, *Obstet Gynecol* 94:172-176, 1999.

89. Scheibmeir M, O'Connell KA: In harm's way: childbearing women and nicotine, *J Obstet Gynecol Neonatal Nurs* 26:477-484, 1997.

90. Reference deleted.

91. Schrag S et al: Prevention of perinatal group B streptococcal disease, revised guidelines from CDC, *MMWR Recomm Rep* 51(RR-11):1-22, 2002.

92. Schrag SJ et al: A population-based comparison of strategies to prevent early-onset group B streptococcal disease in neonates, *N Engl J Med* 347(4):233-238, 2002.

93. Scroggins KM, Smucker WD, Krishen AE: Spontaneous pregnancy loss, *Primary Care Clin Office Prac* 27:153-167, 2000.

94. Reference deleted in galleys.

95. Shachar IB, Weinstein D: High risk pregnancy outcome by route of delivery, *Curr Opin Obstet Gynecol* 10:447-452, 1998.

96. Sherwood RA et al: Substance misuse in early pregnancy and relationship to fetal outcome, *Eur J Pediatr* 158:488-492, 1999.

97. Sibai BM: Eclampsia: VI—maternal-perinatal outcome in 254 consecutive cases, *Am J Obstet Gynecol* 163:501-509, 1990.

98. Sibai BM, Abdella TN, Anderson GD: Pregnancy outcome in 211 patients with mild chronic hypertension, *Obstet Gynecol* 61:571-576, 1983.

99. Sibai BM, Anderson GD: Pregnancy outcome of intensive therapy in severe hypertension in first trimester, *Obstet Gynecol* 67:517-522, 1986.

99a. Sibai BM, Mercer B, Sarinoglu C: Severe preeclampsia in the second trimester: recurrence risk and long-term prognosis, *Am J Obstet Gynecol* 165(5 Pt 1): 1408-1412, 1991.

100. Sibai BM, Sarinoglu C, Mercer BM: Eclampsia. VII. Pregnancy outcome after eclampsia and long-term prognosis, *Am J Obstet Gynecol* 166:1757-1765, 1992.

101. Sibai BM et al: Hypertensive disorders in twin versus singleton gestations, *Am J Obstet Gynecol* 182:938-942, 2000.

102. Sibai BM et al: Risk factors for preeclampsia, abruptio placentae, and adverse neonatal outcomes among women with chronic hypertension, *N Engl J Med* 339:667-671, 1998.

103. Sibai BM et al: Pregnancies complicated by HELLP syndrome (hemolysis, elevated liver enzymes, and low platelets): subsequent pregnancy outcome and longterm prognosis, *Am J Obstet Gynecol* 172:125-129, 1995.

104. Sibai BM et al: Aggressive versus expectant management of severe preeclampsia at 28 to 32 weeks' gestation: a randomized controlled trial, *Am J Obstet Gynecol* 171:818-822, 1994.

105. Sibai BM et al: Maternal-perinatal outcome associated with the syndrome of hemolysis, elevated liver enzymes, and low platelets in severe preeclampsia-eclampsia, *Am J Obstet Gynecol* 155:501-509, 1986.

106. Sibai BM et al: Neurological findings and future outcome, *Am J Obstet Gynecol* 152: 184-192, 1985.

107. Sibai BM et al: Pregnancy outcome in 303 cases with severe preeclampsia, *Obstet Gynecol* 64:319-325, 1984.

108. Simpson KR, Luppi CJ, O'Brien-Abel N: Acute fatty liver of pregnancy, *J Perinat Neonat Nurs* 11:35-44, 1998.

109. Smith-Levitin M, Petrikovsky B, Schneider EP: Practical guidelines for antepartum fetal surveillance, *Am Fam Physician* 56:1981-1988, 1997.
110. Stark MA: Psychosocial adjustment during pregnancy: the experience of mature gravidas, *J Obstet Gynecol Neonatal Nurs* 26:206-211, 1997.
111. Strauss RS: Adult functional outcome of those born small for gestational age: twenty-six year follow-up of the 1970 British Birth Cohort, *JAMA* 283:625-632, 2000.
112. Strauss RS, Dietz WH: Growth and development of term children born with low birthweight: effects of genetic and environmental factors, *J Pediatr* 133:67-72, 1998.
113. Terraza HM, Moore RD: Gynecologic causes of the acute abdomen and the acute abdomen in pregnancy, *Surg Clin North Am* 77:1371-1394, 1997.
114. Tiran D: Reflexology in midwifery practice. In Tiran D, Mack S, editors: *Complementary therapies for pregnancy and childbirth,* ed 2, Edinburgh, 2000, Baillèrie Tindall.
115. Tobin LJ: Evaluating mild to moderate hypertension. *Nurse Practitioner* 24:22-43, 1999.
116. Todd L: After loss: journey of the next pregnancy, *Birth* 23:54-55, 1996.
117. Varney H: *Varney's midwifery,* ed 3, Sudbury, Mass, 1997, Jones and Bartlett.
118. Vaughn Jones SA, Dunnill MG, Black MM: Pruritic urticarial papules and plaques of pregnancy (polymorphic eruption of pregnancy): two unusual cases, *Br J Dermatol* 137:161, 1997.
119. Wagner CL et al: The impact of drug exposure on the neonate, *Obstet Gynecol Clin North Am* 25:169-194, 1998.
120. Ward S: Addressing nicotine addiction in women, *J Nurse-Midwifery* 44:3-18, 1999.
121. Weismiller DG: Preterm labor, *Am Fam Physician* 59:593-602, 1999.
122. Wen SW et al: Smoking, maternal age, fetal growth, and gestational age at delivery, *Am J Obstet Gynecol* 162:53-58, 1990.
123. Witlin AG: 7 myths about managing preeclampsia, *OBG Manage* 12:44-53, 2000.
124. Witlin AG: Counseling for women with preeclampsia or eclampsia, *Semin Perinatol* 23:91-98, 1999.
125. Witlin AG, Friedman SA, Sibai BM: The effect of magnesium sulfate therapy labor on the duration of labor in women with mild preeclampsia at term: a randomized, double-blind, placebo-controlled trial, *Am J Obstet Gynecol* 176:623-627, 1997.
126. Reference deleted in galleys.
127. Witlin AG et al: Risk factors for abruptio placentae and eclampsia: analysis of 445 consecutively managed women with severe preeclampsia and eclampsia, *Am J Obstet Gynecol* 180:1322-1329, 1999.
128. Worthington-Roberts BS, Williams SR: *Nutrition and lactation,* ed 6, Madison, Wis, 1997, Brown & Benchmark.

Chapter 3

The Intrapartum Period and Its Management

Ambulation and Position Changes During Labor

Allowing the woman in labor to ambulate and change position as desired provides distraction, muscular relaxation, and a sense of personal control and dignity, and it may promote the baby's progress down the birth canal. Two randomized clinical trials allowing such movement demonstrated greater uterine contractility, shorter labors, less need for oxytocin augmentation, less need for analgesia, fewer operative deliveries, and fewer indicators of fetal distress.[73,169] Another larger randomized clinical trial, however, found neither a benefit nor a disadvantage for the progress of labor when allowing the woman to ambulate and move as desired. This trial had methodologic problems—the walking group usually walking only briefly in early labor. The women did express satisfaction with being able to ambulate.[38] If studies lack clear outcomes, maternal comfort and preference remain the reason to reserve this freedom.

Intrapartum Nutrition

Common sense says that the woman in labor would require food and water to sustain efficient function. Prohibition of food or drink during labor began during the 1940s and 1950s when general anesthesia was frequently used during the second stage of labor. In 1949, a study by Mendelson detailed maternal morbidity and mortality from aspiration of gastric contents, termed Mendelson's syndrome. Decreased esophageal sphincter pressure and tone, decreased motility of the entire gastrointestinal (GI) tract, increased gastrin levels in the third trimester, and the mechanical effect of the enlarged uterus increasing intragastric pressure increase the risk for aspiration in the pregnant woman.[4] The use of narcotics further increases the woman's risk.[55] In Mendelson's time, however, the rate of this complication was 0.15%. The practice has continued in response to cesarean rate, which exceeds 20%, even though improvements in anesthesia techniques have dramatically reduced this risk.[4] The 1989 birth center study[174] showed 11,814 women who ate and drank during labor, with no incidence of gastric aspiration even though emergency cesarean sections were sometimes required. O'Reilly et al[154] studied 106 women who ate and drank during labor without morbidity or mortality. Aspiration occurs rarely, and even in those cases most have only mild symptoms. Serious aspiration usually occurs due to a lack of skill on the part of the anesthesiologist, not because of the laboring woman's intake. Moreover, fasting during labor does not guarantee an empty stomach—in fact, stomach contents become increasingly acidic and more caustic, increasing the danger when aspiration does occur.[4]

Indications cited for the use of IV hydration include prolonged or abnormal labor, epidural anesthesia, dehydration from vomiting, lack of oral intake, fever, and IV access for drug administration in anticipation of emergency medications.[199] The laboring woman requires approximately 50 to 100 kcals of energy each hour,[4] and when not fed, they undergo muscular exertion and enforced starvation. When glucose is not available, fat stores are used, resulting in ketosis and eventually ketonuria. Uterine activity may be diminished by the accumulation of ketone bodies.[65] Other effects of mild ketosis during labor are unknown. IV fluids are not an adequate substitute for oral intake (they are often inadequate in kcals; a liter of 5% dextrose in water [D5W] or normal saline [NS] provides only 225 kcals). Maternal fluid overload, hyponatremia, decreased motility, hemodilution, and lactic acidosis, as well as neonatal hyperglycemia, hyperinsulinemia with subsequent hypoglycemia, hyponatremia, acidosis, jaundice, and/or transient tachypnea, may result.[4] Ten percent glucose should be avoided.[65]

Many healthy women, when given the freedom to do so, will choose to eat and drink while in labor.[55] Many experience stress when they are denied food and drink. Stress causes catecholamine release, unfavorably affecting uterine contractions and uteroplacental circulation, lengthening labor, and contributing to fetal distress.[4] For some mothers, an IV confers an "illness" status to labor, resulting in a perceived loss of power. A more acceptable alternative to IV solutions as prophylaxis for emergencies may be the use of a heparin lock[199] or the treatment of nausea with remedies such as ginger tea or miso soup.[156]

The ACNM[4] encourages informed consent of the mother before labor. Factors that increase the risk of aspiration include poor physical status, obesity, emergency procedures, hypertension, embolism, and hemorrhage. Risk identification and selective management—such as limiting solid food or oral fluids for the selected at-risk client—are indicated. Share information regarding a woman's high-risk status with anesthesia personnel.

The Doula

A doula is an experienced laywoman who provides continuous emotional support to the laboring woman, including praise, reassurance, measures to improve physical comfort, physical contact, explanations of events in labor, guidance and emotional support of the partner, information (nonmedical advice, explanations of procedures, anticipatory guidance), facilitation of communication between the woman and staff, and companionship.[86,186,195]

Effect on Labor Outcomes: Gordon et al[86] reported that in the presence of doulas, women used epidural anesthesia significantly less often, were more likely to characterize the labor experience as positive, had a sense of having coped well with labor, felt that it reflected positively on their womanhood, and had a positive perception of their body's strength and performance. In three other meta-analyses, women reported that labor was shortened, less difficult and painful, and that the need for cesarean delivery, operative vaginal delivery, and oxytocin augmentation and analgesia were reduced. The presence of the father did not produce the same obstetric effect as a doula.[186]

Postpartum Effects: Reduced anxiety, positive feelings about the birth, and increased rates of breastfeeding initiation have been measured postpartum when a doula was present at birth. Three meta-analyses studying the doula's effect demonstrated less postpartum depression, improved self-esteem, exclusive breastfeeding, and increased sensitivity of the mother to her baby.[186]

Length of Labor

The curve of mean values shown in Table 3-1 are those of Friedman, who studied the labors of American, African, Asian, and European women and established parameters by calculating the ninety-fifth percentile of the data collected.

The use of rigid parameters for expected cervical dilation and/or fetal descent results in the overdiagnosis of dystocia.[173] The normal labor curve by definition smooths out the data, blurring the fact that individual labors progress with variation. Williams Obstetrics cites a study conducted by Sokol et al[198] in 1977 in which 25% of nulliparous labors and 15% of parous labors were "complicated by active phase abnormalities" while later admitting that dystocia is overdiagnosed.[60] Albers et al[26] measured the lengths of labor for 1473 low-risk women at term. As defined by the Friedman criteria, 20% had "prolonged" first stages and 4% had "prolonged" second stages. None suffered increased maternal or fetal morbidity. The authors concluded that expectations for the length of active labor should be lengthened. Diegmann et al[63] found the mean lengths of second stage among an African American group and a Puerto Rican group to be significantly shorter than the Friedman curve, suggesting that the curve may not apply equally to all ethnic groups.

Other researchers monitored 501 spontaneously laboring women who required pitocin augmentation for failure to progress. Two hundred Montevideo units of uterine activity were maintained for 4 hours

Table 3-1 / Length of Labor as Identified by Friedman

Time in Labor or Rate of Change	Mean	Limit
Primigravida		
Latent phase	6.4 h	20.1 h
Active phase	4.6 h	11.7 h
Deceleration	0.84 h	2.7 h
Maximum slope	3.0 cm/h	1.2 cm/h
Second stage	1.1 h	2.9 h
Multigravida		
Latent phase	4.8 h	13.6 h
Active phase	2.4 h	5.2 h
Deceleration	0.36 h	0.86 h
Maximum slope	5.7 cm/h	1.5 cm/h
Second stage	0.39 h	1.1 h

Used with permission from Friedman EA: *Labor: clinical evaluation and management,* ed 2, New York, 1978, Appleton-Century-Crofts.

without progress (rather than the usual 2 hours) before a cesarean section was performed. Sixty-one percent of the women who remained arrested for more than 2 hours delivered vaginally. Among these women, no infants sustained a serious complication, but the rates of chorioamnionitis and endometritis were both increased by 26%. These authors suggest that the Friedman curve may not be valid for oxytocin-augmented labor or for women who have received epidural anesthesia.[180]

• PAIN RELIEF IN LABOR

Natural Techniques

The following measures offer pain relief and comfort to women in labor. Offer suggestions, inviting the woman to alter the technique or to reject it if it does not help. A technique that does not work at one point may offer relief at another point.

- Offer **emotional comfort** in labor. Stress and fear release catecholamines, which shunt blood away from the uterus to the heart, brain, and skeletal muscles and reduce uterine contractions.[170,194] Studies have found that satisfaction with delivery is more affected by emotional care received during labor than by the physical process.[192]
  Prenatal Suggestions:
- Prepare to make the birthing place comforting to all the senses using music, scents, favorite clothing or pictures.
- Write a birth plan to communicate wishes.

- Invite only those individuals whose presence would be comforting. Educate the woman regarding the role of doulas.
  During Labor:
- **If not in the home, orient** the mother to the birthing area. **Discuss the birth plan** or parental wishes.
- Reassure with words and, as appropriate, with touch.[194] The **presence** of the midwife helps reduce anxiety. The quality of the woman's relationships and the support she perceives during labor are consistent predictors of childbirth satisfaction.[96]
- Offer **anticipatory guidance** regarding all procedures, tests, and findings.
- **Support coaches** with comfort suggestions: verbalizing contraction length, observing for relaxation of the body, supporting breathing techniques, massaging, wiping the face with a cloth, offering fluids, offering verbal encouragement and praise, assisting with hourly emptying of bladder. Model tolerance of the laboring woman's needs and verbalizations. Many comfort measures are most appreciated as suggestions for the support person to carry out.
- If not at home, offer the **amenities of the facility** that may help: shower, whirlpool bath, birth ball, hot or cold packs, mirror, rocking chair, fresh linens, positioning of a birthing bed.[194]
- Suggest **imagery** and **visualizations,** which may help some women.
- **Suggest music** (dancing), which may help some women.
- **Validate** the difficulty of labor. This may normalize the experience for the woman as well as relieve her of the need to communicate the intensity of her discomfort.
- Offer **hygiene measures** for comfort: assist with perineal care, freshen linens, brush and arrange hair, and assist with oral care.
- Encourage **mobility and frequent position changes** to facilitate the fetus' descent. Upright positions maintain good uteroplacental bloodflow and take advantage of gravity. Rhythmic movement such as rocking, dancing, and swaying may facilitate progress. Avoid restriction of maternal activity for fetal monitoring whenever possible.[194]
- Provide **heat.** Localized hot packs or compresses (including for the perineum during second stage), immersion in warm water, or application of a warm blanket may all provide comfort. Heat increases circulation, causes relaxation, and is calming.
- Provide **cold.** Localized cold packs, cool cloth to forehead, icepack for hemorrhoids during second stage and to the perineum after delivery may all provide comfort. Cold reduces swelling, muscle spasm, and slows transmission of pain.
- Provide **water.** Immersion in water provides buoyancy that relieves weight-related discomfort. Water delivered by shower or bath provides warmth, muscle relaxation, skin stimulation that reduces pain (according to the gate control theory of pain), and the decrease of anxiety, possibly decreasing catecholamine levels. Warm water may

slow contractions in preterm labor, with Braxton Hicks contractions, or in early labor. Warm water therefore is suggested after 5-cm dilation when labor is desired. The suggested temperature is body temperature or lower. Bathing during labor is not associated with an increased infection rate.[195]

- Offer **massage** for emotional and physical comfort. Massage includes **effleurage,** or light stroking, of the abdomen (reduces pain according to the gate control theory).
- Suggest **breathing and relaxation techniques,** which may be calming, may release tension, and offer a structured means of control.[194]
  For techniques specifically for **back labor,** see p. 142.

Complementary Measures for Pain Relief in Labor

1. Midwives skilled in **hypnosis** may offer it for pain relief during labor.
2. **Chinese medicine:** A number of acupoints are recommended for pain relief during labor.
   a. **For pain relief,** go from Spleen 6 to Bladder 60 to Large Intestine 4 and then to Gallbladder 21 until the woman feels that the pain has been reduced.[56]
   b. Large Intestine 4 and Spleen 6 are particularly useful when contractions are **excessively painful** and are not causing cervical dilation.[56]
   c. **To help pain during a prolonged labor,** apply firm pressure between contractions on Stomach 3; during contractions, apply firm pressure to Bladder 60.[108]
   d. **Back pain** may be reduced by applying firm pressure to Bladder 31 and 32. The woman can indicate the intensity of the pressure.[56,116,205]
   e. **During second stage,** support the mother's head by applying pressure with the hand around the occipital ridge (Bladder 10) while someone else applies pressure to Bladder 67, either squeezing between the thumb and index finger or using the fingernail to press into the point. This pressure blocks sensation during **sacral and pelvic pain.**[108]
   f. **For exhaustion,** the Stomach and Bladder meridians may be worked for some relief.[108]
   For charts and information on Chinese medicine see p. 559.
3. **Reflexology:** The uterus point, found on the heel, is less effective than other points but may be worked deeply (rubbed between the midwife's two palms) to **increase comfort during labor.**[116,205,210] Gentle stimulation of the entire sole of the foot, attending especially to zones for the uterus, pituitary gland, lymphatic system, and pelvic organs, will **ease labor pain.**[210] After episiotomy in a previous delivery, however, the nerve connections between the foot and the reproductive organs have been severed, and foot massage is not effective

in diminishing pain.[116,205] Stimulation of the fallopian tube and the reproductive lymphatic areas **relieves pelvic congestion and may ease and facilitate labor.**[210] **See charts and information on reflexology, p. 567.**

Systemic Analgesia

Systemic analgesia is generally given at the request of the mother for pain relief after the prodromal phase of labor—when analgesia can slow the contraction pattern—and before second stage, when the analgesia may depress the baby at birth. The fetus is the most depressed shortly after the analgesic effect peaks for the mother. Administration is thus preceded by a vaginal examination to assess the status of the labor. Analgesia given during the active phase of labor may actually increase uterine activity, probably by diminishing catecholamine levels. The fetal heart rate (FHR) is evaluated to avoid giving narcotics to a fetus depressed by physiologic events. The woman is less mobile after receipt of a narcotic, and FHR may show diminished beat-to-beat variability.

Examples of analgesics used during labor include meperidine (Demerol) 50 to 100 mg IM q3-4h (or maximum 50 mg IV), butorphanol (Stadol) 1 to 2 mg/h (antagonizes the action of other narcotics; may cause sinusoidal FHR pattern), fentanyl 50 to 100 μg/h, and nalbuphine (Nubain) 15 to 20 mg IV, which does not cause neonatal depression.[60] Sedatives and tranquilizers may be given with narcotics to potentiate the pain relief, prevent nausea, and relieve anxiety. Promethazine (Phenergan), 25 mg IM or 12.5 mg IV, and hydroxyzine (Vistaril) 50 mg IM are used in this capacity.[90]

Naloxone (Narcan) is a narcotic antagonist that may be administered to the neonate who is depressed because of a recent maternal dose of narcotic. The dose for a neonate is 0.1 mg/kg body weight. The medication, when administered into the umbilical vein, generally acts within 2 minutes. No response in 3 to 5 minutes is an indication for a second dose. The action of naloxone may expire before the action of the narcotic, and the infant must be observed for approximately 4 hours. The infant of an addicted mother may experience withdrawal symptoms after receiving naloxone.[60]

Meperidine has been shown to alter newborn suckling and hand movements at the breast.[168]

Inhalation Labor Analgesia: Nitrous Oxide

Inhalation analgesia is used by women in many countries around the world, including 50% to 75% of laboring women in the United Kingdom, but by virtually none in the United States. An anesthetic, usually nitrous oxide (NO_2), is administered with oxygen. By using less than anesthetic levels, laryngeal reflexes are preserved. NO_2 does not alter uterine contractions, minimally depresses the cardiovascular system, and is minimally toxic. NO_2 acts on the brain to provide analgesia that 90% of women describe as "partial pain relief" and may be used in conjunction with other analgesia. The gas is self-administered intermittently using a mouthpiece. Pain relief begins 50 seconds after inhalation, but continuous administration is sedating. Slow, deep breathing and beginning administration before the contraction starts may make the gas more effective. It may be used in both the first and second stages. Dreams, drowsiness, and hazy memory are occasionally reported. Perinatal mortality rate, Apgar scores, and fetal neurobehavioral outcome are not affected by the use of NO_2.[176]

Anesthesia

The types of anesthesia used during labor and delivery in the United States include epidural anesthesia, intrathecal anesthesia, general anesthesia, spinal anesthesia, paracervical block, pudendal block, and local anesthesia. Evolving techniques being used in some centers include patient-controlled epidural anesthesia and the combination of intrathecal and epidural anesthesia. Decisions about anesthesia use should include consideration of the following factors: the woman's preferences, maternal physical characteristics (such as thrombocytopenia, which excludes epidural anesthesia), maternal allergies, parity and history of previous labors, history of previous anesthesia, estimated fetal weight (EFW), progress in labor, cervical dilation, station of the presenting part, FHR pattern, time elapsed since the most recent food intake, maternal vital signs, the speed with which the anesthesia is needed, available clinicians, whether an episiotomy is planned, maternal exhaustion, the estimated length of labor remaining, and the expected length of the second stage.

Local Anesthesia

Local anesthesia may be used for episiotomy and repair of episiotomy and lacerations.[60]

Provider: Local anesthesia may be administered by the midwife.[214]

Procedure: When used shortly before delivery, 10 mL of 1% lidocaine (or another local anesthetic) is injected into the perineum with a 22-gauge 1½-cm needle attached to a 10-mL syringe. The needle is inserted from the fourchette down toward the rectum, aspirated to ensure the location is not intravascular, and a maximum of 10 mL injected as the needle is slowly withdrawn. The needle may also be inserted at the fourchette and infiltration performed in a fan-like fashion, injecting laterally and posteriorly as well as anteriorly. A visible and palpable wheal is created. If the episiotomy is intended to be mediolateral, the injection should be in that direction.

When given after delivery for the repair, the amount of anesthetic and needle size are chosen for the laceration site and size. The injection is made from one end of the laceration under the edge of the laceration, aspirating, and then injecting during withdrawal.

Pudendal Block

A pudendal block provides regional anesthesia of the pudendal nerve. Effective for spontaneous vaginal delivery, low forceps or vacuum delivery, or repair of episiotomy.[60]

Provider: A pudendal block may be administered by the midwife.[214]

Procedure: Administered shortly before delivery or after for repair, 10 mL of 1% lidocaine or 2% chloroprocaine is used with a 20- to 22-gauge needle through a tubular director (usually an Iowa trumpet)[60] (see Figure 3-1). *Before each injection, the needle is aspirated to be certain that the medication is not being given IV.*[60] Varney[214] suggests aspirating, rotating the needle 180 degrees, and aspirating again.

Cunningham et al[60] state that 1 mL is administered in a wheal just below the ischial spine; the needle is advanced until it touches the sacrospinous ligament, where 3 mL are injected; the needle is then advanced past the ligament into the loose areolar tissue behind, and 3 mL are injected at this point. The needle is removed from this area and moved to just above the ischial spine, where the remaining 3 mL is injected. The procedure is repeated on the other side. Varney[214] describes the procedure as palpation of the spine, placement of the needle guide medial to and just beneath the spine, insertion of the needle through the ligament into the space behind (feeling a slight give), aspiration, and injection of 10 mL of the local anesthetic. Repeat on the opposite side.

Anesthesia occurs within 3 to 4 minutes.[60] The level of anesthesia can be tested by scratching a sharp instrument along each side of the perineum and noting the lack of anal sphincter contraction. The anesthesia lasts for 1 to 2 hours. The pudendal's 20-mL dose provides 200 mg lidocaine.

Complications: If the anesthesia is ineffective, a local anesthetic may be administered to augment the pain relief to a maximum dose of

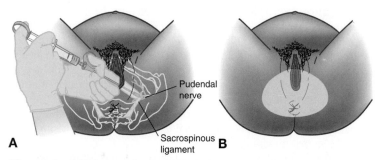

Figure 3-1 • **A,** Technique of pudendal block, showing the needle extending beyond the needle guard to inject into the pudendal nerve. **B,** The area anesthetized by a pudendal block. (From Matteson PS: *Women's health during the childbearing years; a community-based approach,* St Louis, 2001, Mosby.)

500 mg lidocaine. Inadvertent IV injection causes toxicity symptoms. A hematoma may occur, usually in women with a defective clotting mechanism. Rarely, infection may occur at the injection site, causing an abscess.[60] If the needle is injected too deeply, a sciatic nerve block may occur.[90] Pudendal block with mepivacaine has been associated with decreased infant suckling/hand massage movements at the breast immediately after birth.[168]

Epidural Anesthesia

Epidural anesthesia is local anesthetic administered by bolus and then continuously injected into the epidural space of the spine with an indwelling catheter. An epidural may be used for abdominal and vaginal analgesia or for complete anesthesia. Opiates may be added to the local anesthetic, reducing the amount of anesthetic required and maintaining motor function. The medication may be injected in boluses periodically (approximately every 2 hours) or given continuously by pump, or the woman may control the epidural dosage.[31] The epidural has been combined with an intrathecal block in some centers. The block may be administered through the lumbar vertebrae or caudally. The spread of the action of the anesthesia depends on the location of the catheter tip, the medication used, its potency and the dose given, and the maternal position.

Provider: An epidural is administered by an anesthesiologist.

Contraindications: Patient refusal, maternal septicemia or untreated febrile illness, coagulopathy, actual or anticipated serious maternal hemorrhage, infection near the site of potential injection, or evidence of neurologic disease.[215]

Benefits: With an epidural, the mother enjoys total or nearly complete pain relief without a change in mental status and without neonatal depression. If cesarean section is required, the anesthesia dose is easily given and general anesthesia may be avoided.[50] Fetal depression from parenteral narcotics is avoided.[91]

Women who may particularly benefit from this anesthesia include teens without prenatal preparation and poor coping skills and women with developmental disabilities who are unable to understand or cope with labor. Women at risk for emergent cesarean, such as with twins or breech presentation, may avoid general anesthesia with an epidural. The woman with preeclampsia may benefit from the peripheral vasodilation that occurs with regional blocks. The woman who is anxious and/or exhausted may also benefit, although whether labor progress is improved by epidural anesthesia and the reduction of maternal stress has not been proven.[113]

Complications: Bias is inherent in studies regarding the complications of epidural anesthesia because of the possibility that the woman who is experiencing a dysfunctional labor is more likely to request epidural anesthesia. Asking women to accept pain relief in labor according to randomization results in a high number of noncompliant patients, which confuses the statistical analysis. Variations in timing, placement, and choice of medications during the epidural procedure also confuse the picture.

1. The most common side effect is the increased risk of a **hypotensive episode** during labor.[91,189,215] Sympathetic blockade with resultant vasodilation of the lower peripheral vasculature decreases blood return to the heart. Hypotension results in 1.4% to 10% cases according to Gabbe et al[79] or in as many as 32% according to Cunningham et al.[60] Administration of 500 to 1000 mL isotonic crystalloid solution (without glucose) before the procedure and positioning with left uterine displacement prevent many cases of hypotension. If the hypotension occurs, Ephedrine, a vasoconstrictor unlikely to cause uterine vessel constriction, is given in 5- to 10-mg doses.[79] Check the blood pressure (BP) every 2 minutes for 20 minutes after injection of anesthesia into the epidural catheter.[60]

2. Transient bradycardia is seen in 14% to 74% of fetal heart tracings after an injection of local anesthetic.[113] Creasy and Resnick[58] state that **fetal distress** may be seen in as many as 20% of cases. Possible mechanisms include a small amount of the anesthetic crossing the placenta and affecting the fetal heart or, more likely, reduced uteroplacental flow due to hypotension. Placental vessels are not capable of constricting or relaxing in response to volume changes, and hypotension sufficient to affect the fetus may not be reflected in BP measured in the brachial artery.[215]

3. Significantly increases the risk of **malpresentation.** The resistance of the pelvic floor generally rotates the vertex into a favorable position. Anesthesia of sacral nerves 2, 3, and 4 relax the pelvic floor. Persistent occiput transverse or occiput posterior positions may thus result.[79,99,100,208] Epidural placement after engagement of the fetal head may prevent these malpresentations.[171]

4. Significantly **prolongs the first stage** of labor according to the majority of researchers.* However, Bofill et al[39] did not find this stage to be prolonged.

5. Significantly **increases** the need for **oxytocin** augmentation.[91,166,208,228]

6. Significantly **prolongs the second stage** of labor.[52,91,208] The woman's sensation of pressure on the pelvic floor provides stimulus for pushing in the second stage, and anesthesia of the sacral nerves prolongs this stage.[79] Bofill et al[39] did not find this stage to be prolonged. Delayed pushing and a lengthened second stage is not associated with FHR abnormalities, low Apgar scores, or poor cord gas levels.[129] However, it may increase the risk of anal sphincter injury.[78]

---

*References 52, 91, 166, 189, 207, 208.

7. Increases the need for **forceps or vacuum delivery** if the block is continued during the second stage.[39,91,121,189]

8. Whether the risk of **cesarean section** is increased remains controversial, and findings have been contradictory.* Mechanisms that could cause an increased risk of cesarean section include decreased uterine activity, relaxation of the pelvic floor, and decreased maternal urge and ability to push.[99] ACOG[5] and the American Society of Anesthesiologists find the present evidence to be inconclusive and state that in the absence of a medical contraindication, maternal request is sufficient indication for an epidural during labor.

9. Increases the incidence of **intrapartum fever,**[69,91,121,166,188] resulting in neonatal fever workup, antibiotic therapy, and prolonged hospitalization.[121] Halpern et al[91] state that the fever typically begins 2 to 5 hours after the epidural, resolves by about 6 hours after delivery, and rarely exceeds 38.5° C. Dashe et al[62] found fever to be present only when placental inflammation—and thus infection—was present, concluding that the fever was not caused by the anesthetic.

10. **Pruritis.**[79]

11. **Urinary retention** is treated by catheterization or by the placement of an indwelling urinary catheter if necessary.[215]

12. **Ineffective anesthesia** sometimes occurs. Perineal anesthesia may be inadequate at delivery.[60]

13. Inadvertent **complete spinal block** may occur. A high spinal block may cause hypotension and apnea, progressing to cardiac arrest. Treatment includes airway establishment and respiratory support, left lateral displacement, hydration, and the administration of ephedrine for BP maintenance.[60]

14. **Spinal headache** occurs in 1% to 3% of women after epidural anesthesia, occurring when cerebral spinal fluid drips out during the tap (a "wet tap"). A prone position is usually more comfortable for these women. Administration of epidural normal saline may diminish the headache. Oral analgesics, hydration, and caffeine may also be given, followed by an epidural blood patch if the headache persists. Fifteen milliliters of the patient's own blood is placed into the epidural space, coagulating over the hole in the dura to prevent further leaking.[79]

15. In 0.5% of epidural cases, the patient experiences **toxicity** of a systemically administered local anesthetic[215] usually caused by injection of the drug into a blood vessel instead of the epidural space or an overdose of the medication. Central nervous system (CNS) symptoms may occur and at higher doses and cardiovascular effects may also be seen. Eighty-three percent result in neurologic damage or death to the mother, neonate, or both. Bupivacaine 0.75% is particularly cardiotoxic and should be given with caution.[79]

---

*References 39, 52, 99, 121, 144, 166, 208.

16. **Epidural abscess or meningitis** is **extremely rare.**[215]
17. **Paralysis and nerve injury** such as foot-drop are **extremely rare** after epidural anesthesia, occurring in less than 1 in 10,000 cases.[79]

Neonatal Complications: Clinicians have reported that newborns whose mothers received epidural anesthesia have more **breastfeeding difficulties**, but studies are difficult because of the many confounding factors: oxytocin, instrumental delivery, maternal fever and neonatal workup, and the difficulty of randomization.[197] The drugs that are given by this route do pass into the placenta and are absorbed by the fetus. Fentanyl has been associated with depressed neonatal neurobehavior and delayed breastfeeding.[124]

m *Midwifery Management*

1. Women should be educated about the risks and benefits of epidural anesthesia well before labor to allow them to make an **informed choice.**[120]
2. Epidural anesthesia should be **administered when the patient is contracting regularly and the cervix is dilating.**[79]
3. A brief period of decreased uterine activity, possibly related to hydration, may follow initiation of epidural anesthesia. Longer periods of depressed uterine activity require **oxytocin** administration.[79]
4. Continued administration of epidural anesthetic during **second stage** is determined on a case-by-case basis.[79] See p. 172 regarding management of second stage with epidural anesthesia.

Intrathecal Anesthesia

Intrathecal anesthesia is also called labor intrathecal analgesia (LIA), or the "walking epidural." Fentanyl or morphine is placed into the spinal canal, directly affecting the opioid receptors on the spinal cord causing analgesia without interrupting motor function.[113] Intrathecal opioids inhibit the conduction of visceral pain, which is transmitted by slowly conducting nerve fibers. Pain of the first stage is the visceral type—dull and aching as the cervix thins and dilates. LIA is preferably administered at the onset of active labor (3 to 5 cm).[226] Although LIA is not as effective as an epidural during active labor, it provides significant pain relief that surpasses IV narcotic.[113] Second stage pain is sharp, somatic pain conducted by rapidly transmitting nerve fibers and is less effectively relieved by intrathecal anesthesia.[118] Local anesthesia is required for episiotomies.[226]

Provider: LIA is administered by anesthesiologists, credentialed family practice physicians, or obstetricians, who are not required to attend continuously after giving the anesthetic, thereby decreasing its cost.[118,226]

Procedure: After the mother's consent is obtained, the fetal heart monitor is placed and IV access is established before the spinal injection. If less than 4 hours of labor remain, Fentanyl is used. If more than

4 hours remain, fentanyl can be used with morphine. Other authors report using bupivacaine and sufentanil. Onset is within 5 minutes, peaking at 20 minutes. Duration of anesthesia is approximately 3 to 5 hours. Some authors note that a second intrathecal dosage might be used for a long labor.[226] Others limit administration to a one-time dose because of the risk of spinal headache.[113]

Side Effects and Treatment: No blood vessels are within the spinal column, and **no narcotic** reaches the maternal or placental circulation.[113] Fetal heart tracings show fewer accelerations after administration of LIA, similar to the effect of IV narcotic. Uterine hypertonus has been noted.[66]

For **inadequate relief,** one study noted giving half the usual dose of Stadol or Nubain with pulse oximetry monitoring for 1 hour.[226] **Pruritis** occurs in a dose-response relationship, as does the analgesic effect, when intrathecal fentanyl is given.[95] Vincent and Chestnut[215] report pruritus in one half; one third of these was sufficiently bothersome to be treated with 25 to 50 mg IV Benadryl. Kurokawa and Zilkoski[118] report early and late **maternal respiratory depression** with LIA. Twenty-five percent experience **nausea** and may need an antiemetic. Four percent will have **urinary retention,** and may be treated with in-and-out catheterization.[113] Postdural **headaches** (6%) are reported and require anesthesia consultation. All other side effects resolve spontaneously by 24 hours.[226]

Contraindications: Systemic infection, allergy to narcotics, and thrombocytopenia or coagulopathy.[226]

General Anesthesia

General anesthesia is rarely used for vaginal delivery in the United States because of fetal depression, the risk of aspiration of stomach contents, and pulmonary complications. General anesthesia may be used in emergencies such as shoulder dystocia, undiagnosed twins, or breech presentation.[90]

Paracervical Block

Local anesthesia of the paracervical nerves blocks the pain of the first stage of labor but not the perineal pain of delivery.[60] Its duration of action is brief.[177] The method has largely fallen out of use because of serious complications, but it is still used in some centers that do not have epidural anesthesia available.[58]

Procedure: Five to 10 mL lidocaine 1% or chloroprocaine 1% are injected just lateral to the cervix. Administration may have to be repeated because the anesthetics are short-acting.[60]

Provider: Paracervical blocks are administered by a physician.

Complications: Fetal bradycardia occurs in 0% to 40%, and fetal death occasionally occurs. In addition, peripheral vascular collapse, sacral neuritis, and hematoma may occur.[177]

Contraindication: Any situation in which potential fetal compromise exists or if delivery is imminent.[177]

Spinal Anesthesia

This anesthetic, also known as a "saddle block," administered into the subarachnoid space at the L4-L5 interspace, confers anesthesia extending down from the tenth thoracic dermatome (the level of the umbilicus)—appreciably more of the body than comes into contact with a saddle. Nearly all local anesthetics are used. A higher spinal block, extending up to the eighth thoracic dermatome (the level of the xiphoid) is necessary for a cesarean section.[60]

Complications:

1. **Hypotension** caused by vasodilation of peripheral vasculature (with secondary decreased uteroplacental blood flow) is counteracted with IV fluid administration.[90]
2. **Spinal headache** is seen more often when used in the pregnant patient than in the nonpregnant patient.[90]
3. **Pushing efforts may be diminished** with this anesthetic for vaginal delivery, frequently necessitating instrumental delivery.[58]

• MANAGEMENT OF THE FIRST STAGE OF LABOR

Documentation of Admission to Labor and Delivery

When the mother presents for delivery, collect and document the following information:

1. Age, race (if pertinent), gravidity, parity, weeks of gestation, and presenting concern.
2. Significant **family, medical, surgical, menstrual, gynecologic, and social histories.**
3. **Obstetric history,** including pregnancies in chronologic order, weeks of gestational age at delivery, method of birth, weight, current health, complications of pregnancy, deliveries, and postpartum or neonatal periods including the presence of urinary incontinence (reported as 21%) and fecal incontinence (reported as 5.5% to 22%).[78,139] For any cesarean deliveries, note also the type of incision, indication, when the surgery occurred during labor, anesthesia, and complications. For any abortions, note the gestational age, whether spontaneous or therapeutic, and complications.
4. **Present pregnancy:** Onset of prenatal care and number of visits, dating (ultrasounds, size/date correlations), BP baseline and range, weight baseline, total weight gained, 28-week testing results, tests of fetal well-being, complications and their management, lab results, exposures to teratogens and substances, and significant social factors.
5. **Labor history:** If and when membranes have ruptured, color and quantity of fluid, sterile speculum examination results if done; fetal movement; vaginal bleeding; contraction onset, current frequency, and strength; vaginal examination if done; patient's toleration of labor; nutrition; hydration; rest; support; and plan for pain management.

6. **Fetal evaluation:** FHR, movement, position, amniotic fluid index, EFW.
7. **Impression:** Gravidity, gestation, stage of labor, infant status, any problems.
8. **Management** plan: disposition, treatments, follow-up.

Labor Management Plan for the First Stage of Labor

Assess the following variables:
- The woman's emotional status and her self-assessment regarding comfort and physical and emotional stamina, support, and other factors
- Maternal birth plan or preferences
- Knowledge deficits
- Involvement of significant others
- Maternal vital signs
- FHR
- Hydration and nutrition
- Maternal energy
- Bladder and bowel status
- Uterine contraction pattern
- Labor progress, including position and station of vertex, cervical location, consistency, effacement, and dilation
- Status of membranes, color of fluid
- Complications

🅜 *Management Plan to Include:*

- Interventions to treat fetus for signs of fetal compromise
- Interventions to treat maternal exhaustion
- Interventions to treat lack of labor progress
- Comfort measures
- Position and ambulation
- Hydration and nutrition
- Interventions for bowel or bladder
- Plan of next assessment of progress: next vaginal exam
- Ongoing screening or interventions for complications and/or need for consultation
- Preparation for delivery: parental wishes, visualization of fluid before delivery, expected timing, expected precautions and procedures, pediatric attendance

Intrapartum Progress Note

Subjective: The woman's assessment of discomfort, coping, support, hydration, nutrition, and position.

Objective: Contraction pattern (rate and quality), FHR interpretation, vital signs, intake and output, nutrition, and position. Midwife's assessment of the woman's discomfort, coping, and support.

Assessment:

Gravidity and weeks of gestation

Phase of labor

Whether progressing

Fetal condition

Plan:

Expectant management

New or continued management

When the next formal assessment (possibly vaginal examination) is planned

Note consultation with physician and physician's concurrence with the plan if appropriate.

• VARIATIONS ON THE NORMAL FIRST STAGE OF LABOR

Posterior Presentation (Occiput Posterior)

The posterior presentation is a vertex presentation with the fetus' occiput facing the maternal spine. It is associated with back labor because of pressure of the occiput on the sacrum. This condition persists in 6% to 10% of labors, most often in women with an anthropoid or android pelvis.[214] Reasons include a poorly flexed head, flat sacrum, ineffective uterine contractions failing to facilitate descent and rotation, or epidural anesthesia causing diminished pelvic floor tone. Delivery from the posterior position is possible with adequate pelvic diameters, but labor is usually prolonged.[47]

Diagnosis: Posterior presentation is diagnosed by fetal skull landmarks on vaginal examination (see p. 581) and Leopold's maneuvers. On abdominal examination, a depression may be noted at the maternal umbilical area that looks like, and must be differentiated from, a full bladder.

ⓜ Management

1. The woman may feel the **premature urge to bear down** because of the pressure of the occiput against the rectum. She must be assisted not to push to avoid a protracted pushing period, exhaustion, edema, and laceration of the cervix.[170] Maternal positions that shift the occiput away from the sacrum may be helpful: knee-chest, hands and knees, or a semi-prone Sims' position supported by pillows. Encourage breathing techniques (blowing) through contractions. Analgesia or an epidural may be necessary to help the woman resist the urge to bear down.[194]

2. **When considering amniotomy,** be aware that preservation of the forewaters may increase the likelihood of rotation of the vertex to the occiput anterior position. Studies have not been conducted to

determine whether either rotation or progress in labor is enhanced with amniotomy under these circumstances.[194]

3. **Methods of facilitating rotation** to the occiput anterior position include:

   a. Vary maternal **position** to try to free the baby from the pelvis or use the fetus' own weight to facilitate rotation:

      (1) Position the mother with **back up, stomach hanging down** (widely open knee-chest position, on hands and knees). She can lean forward onto a birthing ball, lean on the elevated head of the bed, stand on the floor leaning forward with her arms folded on a raised bed, or stand leaning onto a partner.

      (2) The woman may **lie on her side with the baby's back down** to enlist gravity in rotating it around the back to the anterior position.[194] In addition, the Trendelenburg position (of 45 degrees or less) may encourage rotation.[211]

      (3) The woman may lie in **Sim's position**, moving forward until **semi-prone**, supported by pillows. She lies **with the fetal back up** to encourage the fetal weight to rotate the vertex around the front to the occiput anterior position.[69]

      (4) Duck walking, lunging, stair climbing with one leg abducted, and hula-style belly dancing have all been described as useful.[67]

      (5) Simkin and Ancheta[194] suggest that the **woman with a pendulous abdomen** may have better success in a semi-sitting position in which the baby relaxes back out of the pelvis and can rotate. Alternately, standing with hips in a pelvic tilt, holding the lower abdomen on either side below the umbilicus, and lifting it with contractions applies the baby's weight more effectively to the cervix.

   b. **Pelvic rocking** in these positions may encourage movement of the fetus.

   c. **Massaging** the **abdomen** in the direction you want the baby to turn may facilitate rotation.[103,170,194] Massage applied to the **sacrum** during and between contractions may facilitate rotation of the baby's head. Use firm circular motions with the heel of the hand or smaller circular motion with the thumbs, pointing up on either side of the spine.[209]

   d. **Intrathecal anesthesia** for the woman with persistent occiput posterior presentation allows the woman to relax and may allow rotation. Three to 4 hours may be required after administration of anesthesia for the fetus to rotate. The woman rests on her side, empties her bladder frequently, and maintains hydration. Oxytocin augmentation is required if contractions are inadequate to rotate the head. Await a strong urge to push before expulsive efforts are begun.[118]

   e. If membranes are intact when rotation occurs, rupture of the membranes may settle the vertex into the pelvis, stabilizing the anterior presentation.
4. **Comfort measures specific for back labor:** see general pain relief measures, p. 127.
   a. The **positions** described earlier provide comfort in addition to their therapeutic value. Movement and frequent position change will bring comfort to the woman with back labor.
   b. **Counterpressure** to the back is comforting in the location of the fetal occiput, as indicated by the woman. Lean into the hands using the weight of the body. Tennis balls, a rolling pin, or warm or cold objects placed under the recumbent woman's back are alternatives.
   c. **"Double hip squeeze":** The partner, with elbows out, stands behind the woman who is on hands and knees. The partner places his or her hands over the meatiest portion of the woman's gluteal muscles, fingers pointing at those of the opposite hand, and squeezes the hands and gluteal muscles together—pressing with the entire palm—during contractions. Excessive force is not useful.[194]
   d. **The "knee press":** The woman sits well back in a straight-backed chair with feet on the floor a few inches apart. Her partner kneels in front of her and places one hand on each knee. As the contraction begins, the partner, using his or her body weight, presses the knees toward the chair. This maneuver alters the pelvis, releasing the sacroiliac joints, and relieves low back pain.[194]
   e. A shower or whirlpool bath, with **water** directed at the back, may be comforting.
   f. **Transcutaneous electrical nerve stimulation (TENS) units** may be applied to the sacral area.[194]
   g. Use of a **birthing ball,** which assists the woman in assuming many positions, makes swaying and rocking effortless. The woman may lean against the ball when standing (ball on a bed) or kneeling, or she may sit on the ball. She should hold on with her hands for safety when sitting down.[194]
   h. **Sterile water papules** may be effective because hyperstimulation of the skin decreases perception of visceral pain as suggested by the gate control pain theory, because of an endogenous endorphin release, or because an acupuncture-type reaction may occur. Four intradermal injections of 0.1 mL sterile water (NOT saline) are administered. The first two sites are located over the posterior iliac spines (where the dimples are located). The other two sites are located 2 to 3 cm below, 1 to 2 cm medial to the first two sites (see Figure 3-2). Some women find the procedure easier when injections are given simultaneously by two nurses during a contraction. A sharp local pain is experienced for approximately 20 to 60 seconds,

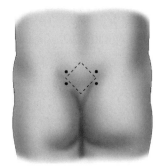

Figure 3-2 • Placement of sterile water papules. (From Walsh LV: *Midwifery: community-based care during the childbearing year,* Philadelphia, 2001, WB Saunders.)

and then back pain improves (after an average of 2 minutes, range 1 to 30 minutes, and lasting 1 to 3 hours). Researchers have not found the course of labor to be affected. The procedure may be repeated.[1,109,195]

5. **Complementary measures for posterior presentation** include:
   a. Some experts suggest **homeopathic** remedies for posterior presentations.[92,103] An **ice pack on the mother's lower back** may encourage the baby to turn.[164]
   b. **Chinese medicine: Acupressure** or **shiatsu** of sacral points is suggested for back pain. Sacral points **Bladder 31 and 32** are suggested. Work on the sacral foramen during contractions with the thumbs or palms. Place one thumb on each side of the spine in the lumbar area and apply pressure while applying pressure with the fingers on the iliac spine.[108,205,209] **See charts and information on Chinese medicine, p. 559.**

Premature Rupture of Membranes

Premature rupture of membranes (PROM) is rupture beginning 1 hour before the onset of labor at any gestational age.[79] Approximately 8% of all term pregnancies are complicated by PROM. Ninety-five percent of these women deliver within 28 hours.[17] The onset of labor depends on the gestational age. At term, 75% will go into labor spontaneously by 24 hours.[60] Regardless of gestational age, birth is likely to occur within 1 week.[17]

Complications: The most significant maternal risk is chorioamnionitis. Risks for the baby include cord compression and ascending infection.[17] The incidence of neonatal infection after 24 hours of ruptured membranes is approximately 1% (a 10-fold elevation). When clinical chorioamnionitis is present, the risk increases to 3% to 5%.[187]

Predictors of Neonatal Infection:

1. Clinical chorioamnionitis (the strongest predictor with 16% infants infected)

2. Group B streptococcus (GBS) colonization (neonatal infection occurs in 4% to 11%)
3. ≥7 or 8 digital vaginal examinations
4. Time from rupture of membranes to active labor >24 hours[187]

m *Management of the Woman at Term With PROM*

1. Confirm diagnosis by **sterile speculum examination (SSE)** and **take cultures.**[17] Leopold's maneuvers and ultrasonographic confirmation are used to determine that the fetal **position** is vertex.
2. **Induce** the mother who is beta strep positive or whose fetal testing is not reassuring. **Induction may be offered** with informed consent on confirmation of ruptured membranes. Alternately, **anticipatory management** for 24 to 72 hours awaiting spontaneous labor may be offered. **Anticipatory management** includes maintaining pelvic rest, checking the temperature every 4 hours,[17] doing kick counts, and being followed with nonstress tests (NSTs) and WBCs.
3. **Withhold digital vaginal examinations** for the woman who is not in active labor and for whom immediate induction is not planned.[17] See chorioamnionitis, p. 70.

Induction of Labor

Induction of labor is initiation of labor by artificial means.[90] Before term, induction is indicated only for the patient whose own health or fetal health is at risk if the pregnancy continues.

Possible Indication for Induction at Term[90]:

Abnormal fetal testing	Chorioamnionitis
Diabetes	Fetal abnormality
Intrauterine grown retardation (IUGR)	Maternal heart disease
Postdates pregnancy	Preeclampsia
PROM	Rh incompatibility

Contraindications to Induction[90]:

Active herpes lesion	History of classical cesarean section
Invasive cervical carcinoma	Placenta previa
Transverse fetal lie	Vasa previa

Relative Contraindications to Induction[90]:

Abnormal fetal position

History of uterine surgery, especially that involving complete transection of the uterus (myomectomy or reconstruction)

Overdistended uterus

Proceed With Induction With Caution[203]:

Maternal cardiac disease

Multiple gestation

Nonreassuring FHR tracing not presently requiring emergency delivery

Polyhydramnios

Presenting part is above the pelvic inlet

Complications: Elective induction doubles the risk of cesarean section, particularly for nulliparous and older women.[130]

Procedure:

1. Give the mother **informed consent.**
2. Review accuracy of **dates.**
3. Assess **fetal lung maturity** by amniocentesis if indicated and if delivery can wait until results are obtained.[90] See Box 3-1 for interpretation of tests of fetal maturity.
4. Evaluate the cervical **Bishop score** (see Table 3-2).[90] Bishop[35] suggested induction with a Bishop score of 9 or more. Gordon et al[85] state that successful induction occurs in 50% to 55% of those with scores 0 to 4, in 90% of those with scores 5 to 9, and in 100% of those with scores of 10 to 13.
5. Consider whether **cervical ripening** is indicated. Pharmacologic hormonal methods are available. Continuous electronic fetal monitoring (EFM) should accompany these interventions. GI side effects are minimal. Caution is recommended in using these products in women with asthma, glaucoma, or pulmonary, hepatic, or renal impairment.[203]

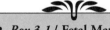

• *Box 3-1 / Fetal Maturity* •

Lecithin/sphingomyelin (L/S) ratio. Before 34 weeks, lecithin (phosphatidylcholine) and sphingomyelin are present in the amniotic fluid in similar concentrations. At approximately 34 weeks, lecithin begins to exceed sphingomyelin. By 35 weeks, the L/S ratio is approximately 2.0.[79]

L/S Ratio	Risk for RDS
≥2	Risk for RDS is low
1.5-1.9	50% of infants will develop RDS
<1.5	73% of infants will develop RDS[79]

NOTES: Meconium and blood invalidate the test.[79] When gestational diabetes is present, respiratory distress may occur despite an adequate L/S ratio, possibly because of sepsis or birth asphyxia. Values may differ among ethnic groups.[60]

Phosphatidylglycerol (PG). PG enhances the surface-active properties of surfactant, providing additional, though not absolute, reassurance of respiratory maturity. Appears at 35 weeks' gestation and then rises rapidly between 37-40 weeks. Blood, meconium, and vaginal secretions do not invalidate, but gardnerella, listeria, and *Escherichia coli* cause a false-positive result when the specimen is collected vaginally. Absence of PG does not preclude lung maturity, particularly in the presence of a mature L/S ratio.[60,79]

Lamellar body count of >30,000/mL reliably predicts fetal lung maturity; <10,000/mL is associated with significant RDS risk. Lamellar bodies are the storage bodies for surfactant. The test requires <1 mL amniotic fluid, is not altered by blood or amniotic fluid, and takes 15 minutes to perform.[79]

Table 3-2 / The Bishop Score: Evaluating Cervical Readiness

	Score*			
Factor	**0**	**1**	**2**	**3**
Dilatation (cm)	0	1-2	3-4	5-6
Effacement (%)	0%-30%	40%-50%	60%-70%	80%
Station	−3	−2	−1/0	+1/+2
Consistency	Firm	Medium	Soft	
Position	Posterior	Mid	Anterior	

From Bishop EH: Pelvic scoring for elective induction, *Obstet Gynecol* 24:267, 1964. Reprinted with permission from the American College of Obstetricians and Gynecologists.
*The score is the total of the scores for each factor. A maximum of 13 is possible.

- a. Pharmacologic hormonal methods for cervical ripening:
  - (1) **Prostaglandin E2 (PGE$_2$; dinoprostone, Prepidil, Cervidil)** applied locally causes dissolution of cervical collagen and an increase in water content of cervical tissues. Generally used for cervical ripening in the woman with a Bishop score of ≤4, PGE$_2$ may induce labor for those women with a Bishop score between 5 and 7.[60]
    - (a) **Prepidil,** a gel, causes little uterine activity and effectively ripens the unripe cervix when placed in the cervical canal just below the internal os. The woman should remain supine for 30 minutes. The dose is 0.5 mg q6h to a maximum 1.5 mg per 24-hour period. Once the cervix is ripened, oxytocin may be begun 6 to 12 hours later. Side effects include GI symptoms, back pain, vaginal warmth, and fever.[203]
    - (b) **Cervidil,** a vaginal insert, is placed in the posterior fornix of the vagina and releases 10 mg dinoprostone at a slower rate. It can be removed if hyperstimulation occurs.[203] Hyperstimulation has occurred from 1.5 to 9.5 hours after placement and resolves within several minutes of removal. ACOG[15] has recommended that EFM be used for as long as the dinoprostone is in place and for at least 15 minutes after removal. The medication is removed after 12 hours or when active labor begins.[203]
  - (2) **Prostaglandin E1 gel (PGE$_1$; misoprostol or Cytotec)** is less expensive than PGE$_2$ and is stable at room temperature. The 25- to 50-μg dose is placed into the posterior vaginal fornix.[203] However, misoprostol has been implicated in uterine rupture in women with a history of a cesarean[36,162] and is associated with fetal compromise.[117] The Food and Drug Administration (FDA)[74] has stated that Cytotec may be used in pregnancy but that it is associated with uterine rupture in

the following situations: later trimester pregnancies, higher doses of the drug (noting 100-µg tablets), prior cesarean delivery or major uterine surgery, or in the woman who has had 5 or more previous pregnancies. ACOG[10] states that misoprostol is safe and effective for cervical ripening and labor induction when used appropriately. They suggest an initial dose of 25 µg, a frequency no greater than q3h, initiation of oxytocin ≥4 hours after misoprostol administration, and reserving the drug for women with no history of cesarean or major uterine surgery.

6. Induction methods:

a. **Stripping of the membranes** releases prostaglandins in proportion to the area of membranes loosened, increasing the likelihood of labor beginning.[75] It is routinely implemented by some clinicians to decrease the number of postdates gestations.[128,203] Stripping of the membranes, however, entails the risks of introducing infection, bleeding from an unsuspected low-lying placenta, and unintentional rupture of the membranes. Gabbe[79] suggests that the method is unpredictable and its efficacy is unproven and that it should not be used as a routine practice.

b. Two ounces of **castor oil** in root beer or orange juice may be taken, ideally early in the morning after a good night's rest.[103,203] Onset of action is 2 to 6 hours. This technique is often used after PROM. Dosages used by surveyed nurse-midwives ranged from 5 to 120 mL.[133]

c. **Enemas** were previously routine but are now generally only used for the patient who feels constipated or to stimulate labor.

d. **Amniotomy,** or artificial rupture of the membranes (AROM), releases prostaglandin. Uterine activity results within 2 to 4 hours.[79] For induction, amniotomy may be performed initially, with or without oxytocin. It commits the woman to delivery; therefore, some practitioners use amniotomy after cervical dilation is underway. Other indications include need for the fetal scalp electrode (FSE), intrauterine pressure catheter (IUPC) placement or amnioinfusion, for visualization of amniotic fluid to facilitate preparation for delivery if meconium is present, to facilitate descent or to stimulate labor. **Conditions necessary for AROM by midwife** according to Varney[214] include active labor at term, 4 to 5 cm dilation, with the vertex at zero station. Many midwives will rupture the membranes when the head fills the pelvis and is well applied to the cervix. **Potential complications** include rupture of aberrant blood vessels, prolapse of cord or fetal extremity, compression of the umbilical cord, rapid descent with resultant fetal bradycardia, prolonged labor with resultant fetal and maternal infection.

Effect on labor and fetal outcomes: Three large studies were published in 1993 and 1994 regarding the effect of amniotomy.

The first studied 925 randomly assigned nulliparous women in labor who underwent amniotomy at ≥3 cm dilation. The amniotomy group had less dystocia (34% vs. 45%), a shorter labor by 136 minutes, and reduced need for oxytocin.[76] The second study randomly assigned 459 pregnancies and performed amniotomy at the mean of 5.5 cm cervical dilation. Among the women who underwent amniotomy, labor was shortened by 81 minutes, oxytocin was used less often, and although the occurrence of mild and moderate cord compression fetal heart patterns increased, the rate of cesarean section was not increased and neonatal outcomes were equivalent.[82] The third study was conducted with 1463 randomly assigned laboring women, with amniotomy performed at an average 5.1 cm cervical dilation. Labor was shortened a mean of 60 minutes, with no increase in oxytocin use, cesarean delivery, or change in neonatal outcomes.[212]

- e. **Mechanical dilators** such as balloon catheters, laminaria, and synthetic osmotic dilators have been used. Laminaria is a type of processed seaweed that is placed into the cervical os; as it expands, the Bishop score is increased.
- f. **Pharmacologic hormonal method: Oxytocin** is administered by either low-dose (1 to 4 mU/min) or high-dose (6 to 40 mU/min) protocols, but no regimen has been proven superior to others in shortening the length of labor.[203] Response depends on parity, cervical readiness, and gestation (development of uterine oxytocin receptors). Continuous EFM is indicated.[90] When an oxytocin infusion rate is initiated, 30 to 40 minutes are required to see the resultant uterine contraction pattern. Exogenous oxytocin causes contractions that rise in intrauterine pressure at a greater rate than do naturally occurring contractions.[79] Oxytocin is discontinued for more than 5 contractions in 10 minutes, contractions longer than 1 minute, or for FHR decelerations. The half-life of oxytocin is 5 minutes, and its effect is quickly cleared.[60] Side-effects are primarily dose related and include uterine hyperstimulation, uterine rupture, fetal distress, or water intoxication. The latter occurs from the antidiuretic effect of oxytocin when electrolyte-free fluids are being administered in large amounts.[203]

7. **Serial induction** Induction may be done "serially" when membranes are intact and fetal and maternal conditions can wait. Induction is typically continued approximately 10 hours or until dinnertime, when—if the cervix has not changed—oxytocin is discontinued, the patient eats and rests, and oxytocin administration is begun again in the morning. Prostaglandin preparations or low-dose oxytocin may be used during the night. Three days of induction is generally regarded as the maximum. Membranes may be ruptured the third day if the clinician is ready to commit the patient to delivery. If the induction is unsuccessful, a

cesarean may be performed. Alternately, induction may be repeated after an interval of a few days if membranes are intact.[90]

Determining the Adequacy of Labor

The adequacy of labor is measured in terms of Montevideo units, measured with the IUPC. It is calculated by multiplying the intensity of the contractions (millimeters of mercury above the baseline) by the number of contractions in a 10-minute period. Labor has been described as beginning when the Montevideo units total 80 to 120, increasing to three to five 50–mm Hg contractions every 10 minutes at the end of the first stage of labor.[60] ACOG[24] suggests that a woman have ≥200 Montevideo units in 10 minutes for a 2-hour period in active phase without cervical change before proceeding to cesarean delivery for an arrest disorder. See p. 126 regarding this controversy.

Complementary Measures for the Induction of Labor

1. **Chinese medicine: Acupuncture, acupressure, and shiatsu massage** have been used with success to stimulate labor. Labor induction may take several hours or a series of acupressure sessions. Stimulation is applied to **Spleen 6,**[103,108,203,225] **Liver 3** and **Liver 4,**[108,203] **Gallbladder 21,**[108] **Bladder 67,**[108] and **Large Intestine 4.**[108,225] **See charts and information on Chinese medicine, p. 559.**

2. **Reflexology:** Stimulation of the uterus and the pituitary zones may induce labor.[210] **See charts and information on reflexology, p. 567.**

3. **Homeopathy:** The homeopathic remedy most commonly used is **caulophyllum** (blue cohash),[59,103,203] 200x q30min for 2 hours to initiate labor.[219] **Cimicifuga** (black cohash) 30c or 200c q2h for 6 total doses can also be used. Skip a day, repeating the next day if needed. Cimicifuga may be alternated with caulophyllum. Even if labor does not begin, the remedy is beneficial for uterine tone.[59,103]

4. **Herbs:** For cervical ripening, 3 capsules of **evening primrose oil** can be taken daily for up to 1 week.[203] Idarius[103] gives the dose as 3 to 6 capsules per day, including during early labor. Sixty percent of nurse-midwives replying to a 1999 survey prescribe evening primrose oil, suggesting doses at term from 1 capsule PO qd to 6 capsules PO q4-6h for 3 days. Some pair it with calcium tablets. Some suggest vaginal administration by placing the oil of 1 capsule in a diaphragm, by placing 6 to 8 capsules in the posterior fornix, or by using the oil as lubricant during intercourse. Give with caution to women with epilepsy or those taking antidepressants, phenothiazines, or epileptogenic drugs.[133] **Black cohash** tincture 10 drops SL q1h affects the cervix in 3 to 4 hours and is continued until the cervix is fully soft and ripe.[29,133,203] **Blue cohash** tincture 3 to 8 drops in warm water or tea q30min for 4 hours can also be taken. If labor does not begin, administer 1 dropperful SL q1h for 4 more hours as needed,[219] or

5 drops tincture q4h, or 10 drops q2h in hot water.[88,133,203] **See information on herbs, p. 563.**

• INTRAPARTUM COMPLICATION: PRETERM LABOR

Definition: Labor between 20 and 37 weeks' gestation is considered preterm labor and includes approximately 10% of all deliveries in the United States. Despite preterm prevention programs, pharmacologic treatment for preterm labor, and recognition of risk factors for preterm labor, the rate has not changed over the last 40 years.[220]

Risk Factors: More than half of the pregnant women who deliver prematurely have none of the known risk factors for preterm birth[136]:

1. **Demographics:** black maternal race, low socioeconomic status, age <18 or >40 years.[79]
2. **General health:** high personal stress; poor nutrition; low prepregnancy weight; anemia; bacteriuria; medical conditions such as diabetes, asthma, and pyelonephritis[79]; maternal heart disease[202]; cigarette smoking (doubles risk); substance abuse (triples risk).[94]
3. **Employment:** physically demanding work, prolonged standing, shift and night work.[146]
4. **Uterine conditions:** anomalies, cervical injury or abnormality (including in utero diethylstilbestrol [DES] exposure, cervical conization, or a history of second trimester induced abortion), fibroids, excessive uterine contractility, infection.[79]
5. **Obstetric factors:** previous preterm delivery between 16 and 36 weeks (2 to 3 times the risk: the more preterm births, the earlier the gestational age, the greater the risk—the outcome of the most recent delivery being the most predictive), PPROM, placenta previa, incompetent cervix, abruptio placenta, preeclampsia, intrauterine growth retardation (IUGR), oligohydramnios, amnionitis, fetal anomalies, vaginal bleeding after the first trimester, little or no prenatal care.[79]

Identification of the Woman at Risk For Preterm Delivery: Many researchers have attempted to create risk-scoring systems to identify the woman at risk for preterm delivery. These scores have found variable success and are least predictive among inner-city populations.[220] The most valuable predictors are the presence of fetal fibronectin (fFN), a short cervix by ultrasound, a history of preterm birth, the presence of bacterial vaginosis (especially for black women), and BMI <19.8 (especially for non-black women).[181]

Etiology of Preterm Labor: The cause of preterm labor is unknown and appears to be multifactorial. Some cases may be unpreventable and related to IUGR.[158]

Clinical Findings: Findings may include menstrual-like cramps; dull, low backache; suprapubic pain or pressure; pelvic pressure or heaviness; change in character or quantity of vaginal discharge; diarrhea; uterine contractions every 10 minutes for an hour or more not relieved by rest; and/or PPROM.[214]

Diagnosis of Preterm Labor:

1. **Increase in uterine activity:** Maternal activity, time of day, and gestational age affect the number of contractions experienced during normal pregnancy. Recumbency reduces contractions, whereas coitus and exercise increase them. Emotional status has no effect. Women who deliver at term tend not to have more than four contractions an hour, and they have more contractions in the afternoon and evening. A change in this diurnal pattern may be as significant as the number of contractions an hour.[79] Home uterine monitoring of uterine activity for women at high risk does not, however, reduce preterm delivery rates.[220]

2. **Change in the effacement and/or dilation of the cervix:** Studies have shown that the woman who presents with her cervix 3 cm dilated is more likely to fail tocolysis and deliver within 24 to 48 hours. It is suggested that the patient with persistent contractions and a cervix 80% effaced and 2 cm dilated should receive tocolysis. Lesser degrees of cervical change represent a diagnostic difficulty. Softening of the lower segment and effacement are more predictive of preterm labor than the other signs. Serial digital cervical examinations are inconsistent in diagnosing preterm labor.[79]

3. **Transvaginal ultrasound measurement of the cervix** is more predictive and probably safer than digital examination.[181] A cervical length of ≥30 mm is reassuring that effacement has not begun (30 mm is the 25th percentile for cervical length).[79] Cervical length of <20 mm is predictive of preterm delivery in high risk or symptomatic patients, although less accurate in twin gestations. Cervical dilation (>1.5 cm) is useful only in evaluating multiparous women or when observed during tocolysis. Progressive funneling is an accurate predictive sign.[181]

4. **Fetal fibronectin** is an extracellular protein found in fetal membranes, decidua, and amniotic fluid that serves as an adhesive between the membranes and the decidua. Appearing in cervicovaginal fluid at implantation, infrequently after 20 weeks, and rarely after 24 weeks, it is not normally present at 24 to 37 weeks.[123] The presence of fFN ≥50 ng/mL in cervicovaginal secretions increases the risk that a woman with preterm contractions will deliver prematurely within 2 weeks. The negative predictive value of fFN (when fFN is absent) is 95% accurate, but the positive predictive value is only 15% to 46% accurate (when fFN is present).[8] fFN is present up to 96 hours after sexual intercourse, and a coital history is necessary to prevent false-positive readings.[190] Blood invalidates the findings.[79] fFN collection must precede digital vaginal examinations or follow them by 24 hours.

5. Identification of **causative factors** such as infection: Adjunctive treatment may be required, such as antibiotics in the presence of amnionitis,

Table 3-3 / Survival of Infants Born Prematurely

Reporting Authors	22 wk	23 wk	24 wk	25 wk	27 wk	28 wk	29 wk	34-37 wk
			No. Weeks' Gestation					
Gabbe et al[79]	–	15%	56%	80%	–	–	–	–
ACOG[22]	Rare	0%-8%	15%-20%	50%-60%	–	85%	90%	Within 1% term
Draper et al[64]	–	–	9%-21%*	–	55%-80%*	–	–	–

*Depending on weight.

or a diagnosis such as placental abruption may indicate that delivery is the treatment of choice.[79]

Fetal Complications of Prematurity: Respiratory distress syndrome (RDS), intraventricular hemorrhage, bronchopulmonary dysplasia, patent ductus arteriosus, necrotizing enterocolitis, sepsis, apnea, hyperbilirubinemia, and retinopathy of prematurity are fetal complications of prematurity. **Long-term sequelae** include developmental delays, chronic lung disease, visual and hearing impairments, reduced head size and height, cerebral palsy, increased risk of sudden infant death syndrome (SIDS), and disruption of maternal-infant bonding.[79]

Since the development of artificial surfactant, neonatal survival has dramatically improved. Black race at weights <3000 g, and female gender favor survival.[79] Table 3-3 provides survival rates quoted by three sources.

Antenatal Surveillance of the Preterm Infant: If EFM is used between 33 and 37 weeks, 90.6% will have reactive NSTs. Because of their immature autonomic nervous system, decelerations in the preterm infant are a more ominous sign than in the term infant. The clinician must be prepared to act on information gained with fetal testing, so viability is considered when ordering antenatal testing.[147]

📖 Management of Preterm Labor

1. **Patient education:** Because 50% of the patients who will deliver prematurely do not have any risk factors, all patients should be taught the signs and symptoms of preterm labor.[79]
2. **Identify** the woman with **risk factors** for preterm labor.
3. **Preventive care for the woman at increased risk for preterm labor:**
   a. Screen for and treat **infections.** Test women with a history of preterm birth and those with infection episodes for normalcy of vaginal flora throughout the pregnancy, and give antimicrobial therapy at a lower intervention threshold. Bacterial vaginosis and trichomonas are associated with preterm delivery and low birth

weight, and antibiotic treatment reduces the incidence.[181] Moreover, chorioamnionitis is associated with cerebral palsy in preterm infants.[155]

b. Screen monthly for **asymptomatic bacteriuria.** GBS bacteriuria is associated with preterm birth, and antibiotic treatment decreases preterm delivery.[181]

c. Give **nutritional counseling.**

d. Discuss **stress reduction.**

e. **Comanage or refer** the woman at increased risk to the obstetrician. **Anticipatory guidance:** Treatment strategies include **prophylactic tocolytics** (i.e., before cervical change), **progesterone supplementation** to women with a history of preterm delivery, **reduced maternal activity,** and **cervical examinations** after 20 to 26 weeks (recommended despite failure to consistently predict).[79] As of this writing, a study was reported by Meis et al in which progesterone injections (17-alpha-hydroxy progesterone caproate, or 17P) weekly from 16 to 36 weeks to women at risk for preterm labor reduced preterm labor by 34%. Publication and duplication of this study may provide a significant preventive treatment for high-risk women.[87]

4. To rule out preterm labor in the woman with signs and symptoms, **collect the following data:**

a. **Determine fetal status:** gestational age, EFW, FHR, fetal position.

b. Perform a **speculum examination:** SSE for determination of membrane status (see p. 578); collection of fFN (taken from the external os and the posterior fornix, avoiding blood before or >24 hours after digital vaginal exam and ≥24 hours after last intercourse); wet mount and cultures for GBS, chlamydia, and gonorrhea as appropriate; and visualization of cervix.

c. **Evaluate the signs and symptoms of preterm labor:** assess back and suprapubic pain, evaluate uterine activity, assess abdominal tenderness, observe changes in vaginal discharge, including bleeding, and if membranes are not ruptured, perform a digital vaginal exam.

d. **Rule out placental abruption.** (Urine toxicology may be useful in assessing the risk.)

e. **Rule out infection,** such as urinary tract infection (UTI) (urinalysis [UA] and culture and sensitivity), costovertebral angle tenderness (CVAT), vaginitis, cervicitis, sexually transmitted infections (SSI; by SSE), systemic viral or bacterial infection.

f. Identify factors that are **contraindications** for tocolysis or a specific tocolytic agent.

5. **Follow-up after negative findings:** Discharge home with instructions to limit activity, maintain pelvic rest, and return in 1 week for

follow-up. Review signs and symptoms of labor and high-risk activities such as substance abuse.[214]

6. Make the **diagnosis** when the cervical dilation is ≥3 cm or when the cervical exam shows 2 to 3 cm dilation with a positive fFN, persistent contractions, and/or cervical change during observation.[79] **Consult** the obstetrician if you suspect preterm labor.[214]

7. IV **hydration** with 500 mL of hypotonic solution is useful if the woman is dehydrated. Administration should not delay initiation of tocolysis. Excessive hydration, particularly with hypertonic solutions, may cause pulmonary edema if tocolysis is begun.[22]

8. **Tocolytic drugs** do not decrease the number of preterm births, but they do provide a delay of up to 48 hours, allowing transport to a tertiary care center and administration of corticosteroids and antibiotics if necessary.[220] Assessment of gestational age and reviewing the dating accuracy, fetal lung maturity assessment, EFW, family history of RDS, maternal medical conditions, and the wishes of the mother and her family are weighed in deciding whether to administer tocolysis to fetuses 34 to 37 weeks, whose survival rates are within 1% of the term infant.[22]

Contraindications to tocolysis include severe maternal hypertension, significant bleeding, fetal demise or lethal anomaly, chorioamnionitis, fetal distress, severe preeclampsia or eclampsia, advanced dilation and effacement,[79] or maternal hemodynamic instability.[216] Tocolytic drugs include:

a. **Beta-mimetic tocolytics** (ritodrine, the only FDA-approved drug for tocolysis, and terbutaline, approved by the FDA for asthma but long used for tocolysis as well).

(1) **Contraindications** include poorly controlled maternal diabetes, hypertension, thyrotoxicosis, or cardiac disease.[22]

(2) The body becomes desensitized to beta mimetics after continuous administration, and **pulsatile administration** may be more effective. When given with dexamethasone treatment, the tocolytic effect is preserved.[79]

(3) **Side effects** include an increase in maternal heart rate and contractility, restlessness, bronchodilation, nausea, and vomiting. Fetal tachycardia may be seen.[79]

(4) **Complications** include hypotension, pulmonary edema, cardiac complications, hypokalemia, and/or hyperglycemia may be seen in the mother.[22] Hypoglycemia, hyperbilirubinemia, and respiratory depression may be seen in the neonate.[214]

(5) **Treatment plan:** Once oral administration is begun, it is usually continued through 35 to 37 weeks gestation. Dosage is adjusted according to uterine contractions and maternal side effects. Some titrate to achieve a maternal pulse of 90 to 105 BPM.[22]

(6) **Ritodrine** significantly reduces the number of deliveries that will occur within the first 48 hours without a demonstrated improvement in perinatal mortality rate, prolonging pregnancy, or birth weight.[22] If ritodrine use is anticipated, do not hydrate the patient in an attempt to stop the contractions because this will increase the likelihood of side effects.[79] I & O are monitored, fluids are restricted, vital signs are taken frequently, and the lungs are auscultated frequently for rales. Dosage is 0.05 to 0.35 mg/min.[220] The onset of action is 75% maximum within 20 minutes of the beginning of a continuous infusion.[79] The rate is decreased for a heart rate persistently >130 BPM, when an electrocardiogram (ECG) is performed to rule out ischemia. Twelve to 24 hours after the contractions have been controlled, she is weaned onto oral ritodrine 20 mg PO q2-4h. A pulse rate slightly above the normal resting rate correlates with control of contractions. The therapeutic drug level has not been established.

(7) **Terbutaline:** The IV dose for treatment of preterm labor is continuous infusion of 2.5 µg/min, increasing by 2.5 µg every 20 minutes as needed until the maximum dose, 17.5 to 20 µg/min, is reached. Onset of action is 1 to 2 minutes with IV boluses.[79] The SQ dose is 0.25 mg q3h. Onset of action is 3 to 5 minutes.[79] The PO dose is 2.5 to 5.0 mg q4-6h, titrated to the heart rate, and is begun 30 minutes before discontinuing the parenteral therapy.[90]

b. **Magnesium sulfate:**

(1) The mode of tocolytic action is uncertain, but replacement of calcium ions with magnesium ions may reduce contractility.

(2) Contraindications include renal failure, hypocalcemia, and myasthenia gravis.[22]

(3) Side effects for the mother include nausea, vomiting, visual changes, weakness, lethargy, urinary retention, and magnesium toxicity. The neonate may show drowsiness and hypotonia.[214]

(4) Complications include pulmonary edema. With toxic levels, respiratory depression, cardiac arrest, maternal tetany, profound muscular paralysis, and profound hypotension occur rarely.[22]

(5) Dose: 100 mL IV solution with 40 g magnesium sulfate, 4 to 6 g loading dose followed by 2 to 4 g hourly maintenance.[220] See p. 93 regarding administration of magnesium sulfate.[95]

c. **Indomethacin (Indocin):** Indomethacin may be used by some physicians before 32 weeks. It is useful with polyhydramnios because it restricts fetal urine output. After 32 weeks, its use may cause premature closure of the ductus arteriosus and pulmonary hypertension.[202]

    d. **Nifedipine (Procardia):** Nifedipine is a calcium channel blocker. Contraindications include maternal liver disease. Its efficacy as a tocolytic is superior to ritodrine with fewer side effects.[157] Complications include transient hypotension.[22] Dose is 5 to 10 mg SL every 15 to 20 minutes up to 4 times, then 10 to 20 mg PO q4-6h.[220]

9. Consider **antenatal corticosteroids.**

    a. **Benefits:** Infant mortality rate is reduced by 30%. Administration decreases RDS by 50%, decreases necrotizing enterocolitis, and decreases intracranial hemorrhage and periventricular leukomalacia by 70%—the latter two being predictors of long-term neurologic damage, including cerebral palsy. Nearly all women 24 to 34 weeks' gestation who are likely to deliver are candidates. Benefits begin 24 hours after administration and continue for 7 days. Because treatment for <24 hours is still associated with improved fetal outcomes, corticosteroid therapy is indicated unless delivery is imminent.[13]

    b. **Drugs and dosage:** Equally efficacious, betamethasone is generally preferred to dexamethasone because its 12-mg dose is administered at two 24-hour intervals, whereas the dexamethasone 6-mg dose is administered 4 times at 12-hour intervals.[79]

    c. **Side effects:** Maternal glucose intolerance is a common side effect of these drugs, especially when used in combination with beta-mimetic drugs. Significantly decreased FHR variability, decreased accelerations, and decreased fetal movement and fetal breathing all return to normal 96 hours after drug administration.[181] Research has not demonstrated an increased risk of infection for the neonate. The risk of maternal infection after corticosteroid administration is small, and benefits are considered to outweigh the risks.[13] No cognitive or neurologic effects have been demonstrated in children who were treated antenatally with one dose of corticosteroids when evaluated at 3, 6, and 12 years of age. **Repeated doses of steroids** after 7 days have not been shown to benefit the fetus but are associated with significant risks for the neonate.[101] Some clinicians believe that in PPROM the acceleration of pulmonary maturity that may occur is an adequate substitute for the corticosteroids, and that risks outweigh the benefits.[135]

10. **Antibiotics** may prolong pregnancy, but there is no improvement in neonatal morbidity or maternal outcome. The exception is GBS.[181] According to 2002 CDC guidelines, the woman whose GBS culture is positive is treated with antibiotics. The woman who has not been cultured needs a vaginal/rectal culture to be collected, and she is treated with antibiotics until the culture results are received (see p. 67).[183]

11. **Transfer** of the baby **in utero** to a high-risk perinatal center improves outcome in very low birth weight infants.

12. **Outpatient management after treatment for preterm labor:** Once labor has been arrested, the woman can go home to reduced activity, pelvic rest, stress reduction, and weekly vaginal examinations.[214]

m *Management of Premature Delivery*

1. Delivery of the preterm infant is managed by an **obstetrician** or by the midwife in collaboration with an obstetrician. The **pediatric** team is present at delivery.[202]
2. **Mode of delivery:** Spontaneous vaginal delivery is the preferred route. The baby in a nonvertex presentation is delivered by cesarean section.[79]
3. The **active phase** of labor in preterm births **may be rapid.** Maintain close observation to prevent precipitous delivery after a short second stage.[79]
4. **FHR interpretation** is the same as for term infants.[79]
5. **Pain relief:** Parenteral narcotics are undesirable because of the unpredictable rate of premature labor and the risk of respiratory depression. Avoiding asphyxia at birth results in a substantially higher survival rate in these infants. Epidural anesthesia reduces the tone of the perineal floor and may benefit the softer preterm infant's head.[79]
6. **Episiotomy** may be performed by some physicians in the case of a primigravida's resistant perineum. Take care to support a **gradual reduction of pressure on the fetal head.**[79]

• COMPLICATIONS OF THE FIRST STAGE OF LABOR

Cord Prolapse

Cord prolapse is frank or occult presentation of the umbilical cord in front of the presenting part (funic presentation) with subsequent cord compression. An unengaged presenting part or a presenting part that does not fill the pelvis predisposes the mother and fetus to this complication, which is diagnosed by repetitive FHR decelerations and/or palpation of a pulsatile cord during vaginal examination.[165]

m *Management*

1. If the funic presentation has been noted before rupture of the membranes, some physicians may assemble the surgical team and perform an **amniotomy in the operating room**, observing whether the cord slips to one side of the head. Cesarean delivery is conducted if the cord is occluded.[48] This practice may result in an emergency cesarean delivery and is **controversial.**
2. If the cord is palpated during vaginal exam, the examiner **lifts the presenting part up off the umbilical cord** vaginally, not removing the hand until the baby is delivered by cesarean section. This step may improve neonatal outcome even if delivery is delayed. **Distend the bladder** with 500 to 700 mL normal saline to decrease cord com-

pression. Administer a **tocolytic** to diminish uterine contractions while preparing for emergency cesarean section.[165] Wrap **warm saline compresses** around the cord if it protrudes beyond the introitus. **Minimize manipulations** to avoid causing spasm of the cord.[214] Place the woman in **knee-chest** or **Trendelenburg** position.[48]

3. **Alert staff, anesthesia personnel, and the consulting physician** regarding the need for an **emergency cesarean section. Summon a pediatric team** to be present at delivery and ready for resuscitation.

Dystocia of Labor in the First Stage

Dystocia is abnormal labor or difficult childbirth usually caused by malposition of the fetal head (asynclitism or extension), inadequate expulsive forces, fetal size or presentation, a contracted pelvis, or an abnormality of the birth canal.[60]

Predisposing Factors for Cesarean Section[34,93,179]:

Advanced gestational age
Arrest of dilation early in the
active phase
Current obstetric practices
Familial tendency
Greater maternal age
Greater prepregnancy body
mass index (BMI)

Insurance coverage
Large birth weight
Large pregnancy weight gain
Occiput posterior position
Short maternal stature
Use of oxytocin

Arrest of Labor Related to the Presenting Part

CEPHALOPELVIC DISPROPORTION. Factors associated with cephalopelvic disproportion (CPD) include macrosomia, shape and size of the maternal pelvis, inadequate uterine forces, a poorly flexed head, malpresentation, and arrest of internal rotation and descent. Increasing molding and caput without descent of the vertex may indicate CPD.

Evaluate and document the "three Ps": passageway, passenger, and power. Assess EFW, clinical pelvimetry, fetal position, FHR, and uterine contractions by palpation, external monitor, and IUPC. Assess maternal energy, hydration, and vital signs. Note status of membranes and consider rest and hydration.

m *Management Options*

1. Use **position** changes to take advantage of gravity in rotation and descent.
2. **Consider epidural** for rest.
3. Consider AROM and/or oxytocin to **augment labor.**
4. **Plan anticipatory management** with timely physician consultation for intervention, including cesarean section if necessary.

DEEP TRANSVERSE ARREST. Arrest of labor with the vertex in the right or left occiput transverse position is most often seen in platypelloid or android pelves caused by diminished anteroposterior diameter, prominent spines, and convergent sidewalls. Hypotonic uterine forces and regional anesthesia also predispose to this condition by altering the tone of the pelvic floor. Prolonged second stage, diminished strength of uterine contractions, and increased molding and caput may indicate deep transverse arrest.[60] Deep transverse arrest may be anticipated with clinical pelvimetry and confirmed by palpation of fetal position.

m *Management Options*

1. If it is desired, **administer epidural anesthesia after descent of the fetal head.**[79,99,100,208]
2. Ideally, begin the second stage with a **well-rested and hydrated** mother.
3. **Maximize effectiveness of pushing efforts** to minimize maternal exhaustion, such as pushing at the peak of uterine contractions. Use positions to facilitate descent.
4. The left lateral position **maximizes the uterine contraction pattern.** Oxytocin augmentation is used if indicated to maximize the uterine contraction pattern.
5. **Plan anticipatory management** with timely physician consultation for intervention, including instrumental delivery or cesarean section if necessary.[60]

PERSISTENT ASYNCLITISM. This condition is lateral flexion of the head whether the vertex is anterior or posterior. It tends to occur more often with epidural anesthesia.[218] May result in CPD in the infant (see Figure 3-3).

m *Management Options*

1. For asynclitic presentation, forward-leaning **positions** (see those suggested for posterior positions p. 141) and asymmetric positions may improve alignment of the vertex. Asymmetric positions enlarge the

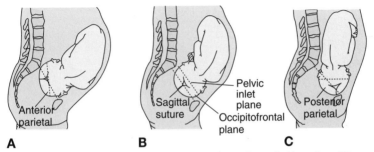

Figure 3-3 • Synclitism and asynclitism. **A,** Anterior synclitism. **B,** Normal synclitism. **C,** Posterior synclitism. (From Lowdermilk DL, et al: *Maternity and women's health care,* ed 7, St Louis, 2000, Mosby.)

pelvis on the side where the leg is raised, and the leg should be raised on the side of the occiput:
   a. Duck walking or stair climbing
   b. Sitting in a chair with one foot pulled up onto the chair
   c. Standing beside a bed with one foot up on the bed (at about knee height)
   d. Kneeling with one foot projected laterally resting the sole on the ground (leg alongside arm)
   e. Leaning forward onto partner, birthing ball, or head of bed with one leg drawn forward, resting the sole on floor or bed[69,194]

2. **Vaginal manual rotation** of the asynclitic vertex to a synclitic position may sometimes be accomplished, although it has not been tested for safety or effectiveness.[69,194]

3. When considering **amniotomy,** be aware that the asynclitic fetus may benefit from having intact forewaters in which to rotate. Studies have not been conducted to determine whether rotation or progress in labor is enhanced with amniotomy under these circumstances.[194]

4. **Plan anticipatory management** with timely physician consultation for cesarean section if indicated.

Arrest of Labor Related to Uterine Dysfunction

HYPOTONIA. Hypotonia is manifested by infrequent, mild contractions in the active phase or second stage of labor with failure to progress.

Assess the labor progress, frequency of contractions by external monitor, quality of contractions by palpation and possibly IUPC, maternal exhaustion, FHR, clinical pelvimetry, EFW, presentation and position, signs of chorioamnionitis, and status of membranes.

m *Management Options*

1. **Allow sedation or analgesia,** which may induce a hypotonic uterus, especially during early labor, **to subside.**
2. **Decrease stress** and fear.
3. Suggest **ambulation or nipple stimulation.**
4. Consider an **enema** to stimulate contractions.
5. Consider **AROM** to stimulate labor.
6. Consider **oxytocin** augmentation if progress is inadequate.
7. **Consult** the physician. Oxytocin stimulation may be indicated.

HYPERTONIA. Hypertonia is a disorganized uterine contraction pattern without progress in cervical dilation, effacement, or descent of the fetus. Maternal exhaustion and fetal intolerance of labor may occur. Contractions may be disproportionately painful.[214]

m *Management Options*

1. Provide **hydration.**
2. Stop labor by providing **therapeutic rest** (IM morphine).

3. **Plan anticipatory management.**
4. **Consult** the physician if labor continues and no progress is made.

Complementary Measures for Dystocia

1. **Homeopathy:** Many homeopathy experts recommend their remedies during labor.*
2. **Chinese medicine: Acupuncture** may be used to treat **dystocia.**[43] **Shiatsu** massage and **acupressure** may also be used.[108] For **dystocia,** apply acupressure to **Gallbladder 21, Spleen 6, Large Intestine 4,** and **Bladder 67.**[108] **If labor slows** during the first stage, apply strong thumb pressure to **Spleen 6, Large Intestine 4, Bladder 31, Liver 3,** and **Gallbladder 21,** as well as palm pressure on the sacral points **(Bladder 31 and 32).**[108] To **regulate labor (precipitous or no progress),** stimulate **Bladder 67, Spleen 6,** and **Bladder 60.**[56] **For exhaustion,** work the **Stomach and Bladder meridians** for some relief.[108] **See charts and information on Chinese medicine, p. 559.**
3. **Reflexology:** Massage the pituitary point to **coordinate uterine contractions that have been inadequate or excessive.**[116,205,210] Vigorous rubbing of the heel (the uterus point) between the midwife's two palms, and the mother or another briskly massaging the top of the ankles (the Fallopian tubes and the reproductive lymphatics) for 2 minutes every hour **relieves pelvic congestion, assists pain, and enhances uterine action.**[210] **See charts and information on reflexology, p. 567.**
4. **Herbs suggested for use during labor: Black cohash** aids uterine activity in labor, making contractions more productive and less painful.† One half to 1 tsp herb/1 cup water boiled for 15 minutes, or 2 to 4 mL tincture, tid is recommended.[98] **Blue cohash** in capsules, tincture (1 to 2 mL tincture), or as tea (1 tsp dry root/1 cup water simmered for 10 minutes) tid enhances the effectiveness of contractions. An antispasmodic, it may stop false labor.‡ **Raspberry leaf** tones uterine tissue and assists contractions. It may ease false labor and exhaustion in labor and prevent postpartum hemorrhage (administered as tea with a little honey).[97,153,156,160,201] **Squawvine** is a uterine toner that, taken as a tea, may help a prolonged first stage of labor.§ **See information on herbs, p. 563.**
5. **Miscellaneous:** Simkin and Ancheta[194] recommend **touching** the woman or suggesting that her support persons do so to increase endogenous oxytocin. They also suggest **warm compresses** to the fundus (augmented uterine contractions in one study).

---

*References 59, 92, 103, 163, 175, 196, 203.
†References 97, 127, 134, 156, 161, 163.
‡References 29, 88, 97, 116, 134, 152, 156, 161, 205.
§References 29, 88, 97, 98, 127, 153, 156, 205.

Arrest of Labor Related to a Contracted Pelvis

Contracted pelves are associated with 3 times the incidence of face and shoulder presentations, 4 to 6 times the occurrence of cord prolapse, and a higher incidence of prolonged labor, inefficient contractions, chorioamnionitis, and fetal distress.[60] Variations include:

1. **Contracted inlet:** Diagnosed by pelvimetry when the obstetric conjugate is <11.5 cm, a contracted inlet prevents the presenting part from descending into the pelvis before labor, if at all. Labor is prolonged, contractions are inefficient, chorioamnionitis may occur, and fetal distress may ensue. Molding and caput of the fetal vertex may occur and should not be confused with descent of the vertex. This variation is associated with umbilical cord prolapse.[60]

2. **Contracted midpelvis** may be detected during pelvimetry by noting prominent ischial spines, convergent sidewalls, and a narrow sacrosciatic notch. It is frequently a cause of deep transverse arrest.[60]

3. **Contracted outlet** is noted during pelvimetry by a biischial tuberous diameter of <8 cm. It usually occurs with a contracted midpelvis, but if the posterior portion of the outlet is large enough, delivery may occur. Perineal injury is increased with the contracted outlet because the vertex is forced downward.[60]

🅜 *Management Options*

1. **Assess pelvis** early in labor.
2. With all exams, assess **fetal position.** Monitor the **adequacy of labor.**
3. **Use measures to encourage rotation** to favorable positions if necessary. (See posterior presentation, p. 141, and persistent asynclitism, p. 159.)
4. Maintain adequate **rest and hydration** of the mother.
5. **Augment** with oxytocin if necessary.
6. **Consult** the physician regarding surgical intervention when the pelvis prevents descent.

Arrest of Labor Described by the Time in Labor Where Progress Is Impaired

PROLONGED LATENT PHASE OF LABOR. This phase begins when the woman perceives regular uterine contractions. The 95th percentiles for length of the latent phase are >14 hours in the multigravida and >20 hours in the primigravida according to Friedman.[77] An unripe cervix, excessive sedation, conduction analgesia, or Braxton Hicks contractions may prolong this phase.[60] Prolonged latent phase is associated with greater frequency of labor abnormalities, maternal fever, cesarean deliveries, neonatal resuscitation, thick meconium, neonatal intensive care unit admissions, lengthened hospital stays, and blood loss.[49]

Assess cervical change. Share all signs of progress such as station, cervical position, and consistency with the mother. Acknowledge her disappointment[194] and assess her discomfort and exhaustion level.

m *Management Options*

1. If the woman is anxious but rested, **do not admit** her to the birthing unit and encourage activities of distraction and mobility, continuous support, nutrition and hydration, and cessation of contraction timing until they are more intense. The bathtub may quiet contractions and provide rest at night.[194]
2. **Decrease stress** to diminish catecholamines that may delay progress.[194]
3. **Do not perform amniotomy** because 10% are actually in false labor.
4. Provide **therapeutic rest** with morphine IM. One of three outcomes occurs on awakening: no contractions (10%), contractions that cause cervical dilation (85%), or continued slow progress (5%).[218] Consider augmentation, in conjunction with the woman, if she awakens from therapeutic rest and continues slow progress.[77]
5. The woman who has had cervical procedures, such as loop electrosurgical excision, may be fully effaced without dilating due to **cervical scarring.** The cervix may feel like a buttonhole, with stenotic scarred edges felt on exam. Digitally loosening such scarring is not painful and may allow dilation.

PROTRACTED ACTIVE PHASE. Cervical dilation occurring <1.2 cm/h in primigravidas and <1.5 cm/h in multiparas during active phase is considered protracted. ACOG[24] suggests that the diagnosis of active phase arrest requires that the woman is in active phase (≥4 cm) and that uterine contractions have been sustained at ≥200 Montevideo units in 10 minutes for 2 hours without cervical change. Other researchers and clinicians resist rigid parameters in defining normalcy. See discussion, p. 126. Excessive sedation, conduction analgesia, and fetal malposition may contribute to a slow active phase.[60]

Evaluate and document the "three Ps": passageway, passenger, and power. Assessment includes maternal energy, hydration, vital signs, whether membranes are ruptured, clinical pelvimetry, EFW, fetal position, FHR, and uterine contractions.

m *Management Options*

1. In the case of the **occiput posterior** presentation, see p. 141 for measures to assist with rotation.
2. In the case of **asynclitic presentation,** see pp. 159 and 160 for measures to encourage rotation.
3. Allow **sedation** to subside.[218]
4. Consider **stress reduction** measures to decrease catecholamine levels and enhance contraction pattern, such as putting the woman into water and discussing privately with the woman whether she is comfortable with those who are present.[170] Simkin and Ancheta[194] describe **"emotional dystocia,"** evidenced by the woman who is anxious, fearful, who seems to have exaggerated responses to contractions or exams, is needy, extremely modest, angry, resentful, highly controlling or con-

trolled, or "out of control" during contractions (writhing, screaming, unreceptive to help). A fear of labor (possibly death), historic factors such as a previous difficult birth, a traumatic hospitalization, abuse in childhood, domestic abuse, substance abuse, dysfunctional family situations, or cultural factors may contribute to this woman's state.

a. Facilitate the woman's expression of her concerns (possibly fear of pain, disfigurement, loss of control and dignity; fear for her own or the baby's life; the presence of strangers; invasive procedures; fear of motherhood or abandonment).

b. Use reflective listening to be certain that you understand, and validate her fear.

c. When possible, problem solve to reduce anxiety. For example, provide privacy, discuss pain options, or suggest postpartum referrals. Provide information about labor and delivery. Correct any misunderstandings that are causing fear.

d. Offer massage, hydrotherapy, or another physical coping assistance.

e. Suggest visualizations to reduce fears.

f. Spend time with this woman to reduce her fearfulness.

5. Consider **nipple stimulation** to release endogenous oxytocin.

6. Consider **amniotomy** to augment labor. However, a fetus who is in an unfavorable position (occiput posterior or asynclitic) may benefit from having intact forewaters in which to rotate. Studies have not been conducted to determine whether rotation or progress in labor is enhanced with amniotomy under these circumstances.[194]

7. Augment labor by **oxytocin** administration when necessary to achieve an adequate labor pattern.[218]

8. The woman who is becoming exhausted should assume positions of comfort where she can **rest** between contractions.

9. **Plan anticipatory management** with timely physician consultation if no progress is made.

SECONDARY ARREST. Secondary arrest is defined as 2 hours without progress in dilation once cervical dilation has begun. This condition may be stressful for the fetus. Inadequate uterine contractions, excessive sedation, conduction analgesia, and fetal malposition may be causes.[60]

m Management Options

See measures for protracted active phase, p. 163.

PROLONGED DECELERATION PHASE. A prolonged deceleration phase is defined as dilation from 8 to 10 cm lasting >3 hours in the primigravida and >1 hour in the multiparous woman.[77]

m Management Options

1. See measures for protracted active phase, p. 163.
2. Measures for a **persistent cervical lip** include:

a. **Implement the position changes** suggested for occiput posterior or asynclitic presentations (see pp. 141 and 159).
b. The buoyancy of a deep **bath** may reduce weight on the cervix, allowing dilation.
c. **Crushed ice,** applied to the cervix in the finger of a sterile glove, may reduce swelling.[194]
d. Working with the mother to **manually reduce** the cervix during her bearing-down efforts may complete cervical dilation.

Malpresentations

The presentations illustrated in Figure 3-4 are considered malpresentations. Each presentation is identified by a certain point, called the *denominator.* The presentation and position are described by stating the location of the denominator in relation to the maternal pelvis. The denominator for the breech is the sacrum; for the brow, the frontum (forehead); for the face, the mentum (chin); and for the shoulder, the acromion.

Breech Presentation

The breech fetus is at increased risk for cord prolapse and head entrapment with vaginal delivery. Many clinicians will suggest the breech exercise and other techniques to encourage the fetus to turn. Should these fail, external cephalic version may be attempted. If this also fails, although maternal morbidity is greater with cesarean delivery, most breech babies are delivered by cesarean section in the United States.[27] Some authors have concluded that with prudent selection of appropriate cases, a significant number of patients can safely deliver breech infants vaginally.[47,61,107] ACOG[25] states that a woman can safely proceed with vaginal breech birth with a care provider experienced in vaginal breech deliveries, in a facility capable of emergency cesarean section, and with anesthesia present when the following conditions are present: the EFW is <4 kg, the fetus is in a frank breech position, the pelvis is adequate by pelvimetry, and labor progresses normally in effacement, dilation, and descent. The use of oxytocin is controversial.

Breech Exercise or "Tilt Position.": When the fetus is in the breech position at 33 to 34 weeks, the woman may be instructed to lie on the side opposite the fetal back, with her feet higher than her head, for 10 to 20 minutes 2 to 3 times per day when the fetus is active. (Lying on a collapsed ironing board with the narrow end securely propped against the seat of a sofa is one method. Another is to lie on the floor with knees flexed and pillows placed under the hips, but the woman cannot lie on her side with this method.) Concurrent relaxation exercises, deep breathing, and visualizations may be helpful. If she cannot tolerate the position, she should not do it. If she feels that the baby has turned, she should stop the exercise until seen by the clinician to check the position. If she is certain the baby has turned, a long walk may help the baby stabilize head down in the pelvis.[103,193]

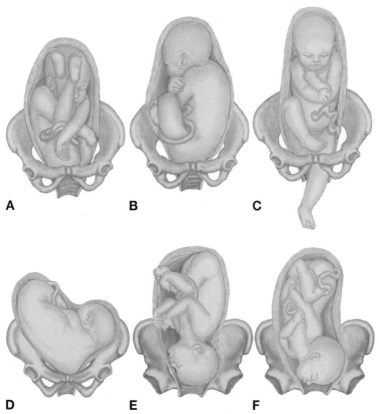

Figure 3-4 • Malpresentations. **A,** Frank breech; **B,** complete breech; **C,** incomplete breech (footling breech, one leg extending below buttocks); **D,** shoulder presentation (transverse lie); **E,** brow presentation; **F,** face presentation. (From Murray SS, McKinney ES, Gorrie TM: *Foundations of maternal-newborn nursing,* ed 3, Philadelphia, 2002, WB Saunders.)

Complementary Measures to Turn the Breech Fetus

1. **Homeopathy:** Some experts recommend **homeopathy** remedies for turning the breech baby.[59,103]
2. **Chinese medicine: Acupressure** may be used to stimulate **Bladder 67** with firm pressure for 10 to 15 minutes. **Moxabustion** or **acupuncture** is used for stronger stimulation of the point.[43,103] **See charts and information about Chinese Medicine on p. 559.**

External Cephalic Version: Current practice is to offer external cephalic version in the latter weeks of gestation, with tocolytics to relax the uterus in nulliparous women. At 38 weeks' gestation, external version is successful in 40% of nulliparous women and 60% of multiparous women.[47] RhoGAM is given prophylactically or when feto-maternal hemorrhage is suspected. Twenty-five percent of fetuses show transient

FHR changes such as bradycardia, decelerations, and reduced beat-to-beat variability. Emergency delivery is rare (one in 3151 cases in a literature review).[84]

Breech Extraction:

1. **Pediatrics and anesthesia** personnel should be present, and an **assistant** to the birth assistant is advisable.
2. The **bladder is emptied.**[47]
3. An **episiotomy** may be advisable.[25]
4. **Progress in labor, even if slow, should be left undisturbed** while the presenting part is well engaged, on the perineum, or protruding, as long as FHR is normal. Slow dilation assists the delivery of the aftercoming head. Rapid delivery may result in nuchal arms over an extended head.[25]
5. The **cervix must be fully dilated and the breech, legs, and abdomen should deliver spontaneously** (the legs are assisted by lateral pressure to flex away from the midline and deliver), at which time the umbilical cord is compressed.[60]
6. Hold the baby by the pelvis with a towel to avoid damage to soft parts, with hands around thighs and thumbs on buttocks; apply **gentle downward traction until the lower halves of the scapulae are delivered.**[60]
7. When one axilla is visible, encourage the **shoulders to deliver by rotating the trunk,** first bringing the bisacromial diameter of the baby into the anteroposterior diameter of the pelvis so that the anterior shoulder delivers out from under the pubis. Rotate the body in the reverse direction to deliver the posterior shoulder and arm. Alternately, deliver the posterior shoulder first by grasping the baby's ankles and drawing them up and over the maternal thigh of the mother until the posterior shoulder delivers; then apply posterior leverage with the baby's body to deliver the anterior arm.[47]
8. Delivery of the head is accomplished manually or with **Piper forceps.**[47] Piper forceps should always be on the table and an assistant prepared to help.[25] Manual delivery is conducted by the Mauriceau maneuver. The assistant applies **suprapubic pressure to maintain flexion of the baby's head;** the baby's body is placed over the left arm, the fingers of which are on the maxilla, maintaining flexion. Two fingers of the other hand are placed on the baby's shoulders on either side of the neck, and **downward traction is applied until the suboccipital region is seen** emerging under the symphysis pubis. **The body is then lifted toward the maternal abdomen** as the mouth, nose, brow, and finally occiput are delivered over the perineum.[60] To avoid injuring the fetal neck, the neck is not elevated above the horizontal plane, **avoiding hyperextension.**[25]

Brow Presentation

In a brow presentation, the vertex is partially extended. The denominator is the forehead, or frontum. Brow presentation may occur with CPD;

anomalies, tumors, or loops of cord preventing flexion of the head; or high parity.[60] The largest diameter of the head (mento-vertex, 13 cm) is presenting, and unless the head flexes, delivery can occur only if the fetus is very small or the pelvis large.[47] Most often, the brow presentation is unstable and the head converts to either occiput or face presentation and delivers. Incidence is <1%.[60]

Compound Presentation

Compound presentation is present when an extremity presents alongside the presenting vertex or breech. The denominator is stated according to the vertex or breech. The incidence is 1 in 700 deliveries. This condition occurs when the presenting part does not completely occlude the pelvic inlet, such as with a small infant. The risk of prolapsed cord is increased. The extremity may be left alone, or it may be pushed up into the uterus.[60]

Face Presentation

In the face presentation, the vertex is hyperextended, and the occiput is in contact with the back. The incidence is approximately 0.2%. Causes include anomalies, tumors, loops of cord preventing flexion of the head, CPD, anencephaly, or high parity. Vaginal delivery will follow if the head rotates to the mentoanterior position and the pelvis and contractions are adequate.[47]

Shoulder Presentation

The shoulder usually presents when the fetus is in a **transverse or oblique lie.** The position is expressed in terms of the maternal side toward which the shoulders are oriented, as well as dorsoanterior or dorsoposterior indicating the orientation of the fetal back. Unless the infant is very small in relation to the maternal pelvis, vaginal delivery does not occur from this position. External version may be successful before the onset of labor. Internal podalic rotation is rarely attempted, and cesarean delivery is the usual management.[47]

Meconium Staining of Amniotic Fluid

Meconium is fetal stool, rarely seen before 36 weeks. Meconium passage may stain the amniotic fluid (MSAF) after an episode of hypoxemia with resultant sphincter relaxation, or with acidemia caused by uteroplacental insufficiency. For most infants, however, meconium passage is maturational and not a sign of fetal distress. MSAF is present in 25% of pregnancies that deliver between 36 and 42 weeks,[80] 35% of postdates pregnancies,[200] and up to 50% of those after 42 weeks.[80]

Particulate meconium identified early in labor is associated with increased perinatal morbidity, low Apgar scores, meconium aspiration syndrome (MAS), and perinatal death.[147] MSAF may predispose the fetus to ischemic injury in utero by having a vasoconstrictive effect on the vasculature of the cord and placenta, or by diffusion of meconium components into fetal circulation where vasoconstriction then occurs in the brain, lungs, or other organs. Meconium increases the risk of chorioamnionitis because meconium inhibits neutrophil phagocytosis.[32] Preterm labor in the presence of MSAF is less likely to respond to tocolytics.[54]

Meconium Aspiration Syndrome: Neonatal aspiration of meconium may occur during fetal breathing, during vagal-mediated gasping related to fetal distress, or with first respirations at birth.[80] Asphyxial damage and in utero gasping—rather than the actual action of meconium on the lung parenchyma—is theorized to cause MAS.[110] Despite obstetric suctioning on the perineum and pediatric intubation immediately after birth, a 2% rate of meconium aspiration persists because of in utero aspiration. Only 5% to 10% of the infants with meconium below the cords develop MAS, for an incidence of 0.2%.[80] Of the infants who develop MAS, 7.3% to 35% are born through thin meconium and 4.9% to 37% die.[54]

The onset of signs and symptoms of MAS is immediate in severe cases but more typically occur within several hours of birth. Obstruction of the airways with atelectasis and pneumonitis may occur. Hypoxemia, acidosis, and hypercapnea may develop, sometimes causing pulmonary constriction, right-to-left shunting, and persistent pulmonary hypertension of the newborn.[200] These infants are at risk for adverse neurologic outcomes such as cerebral palsy, seizures, mental retardation, and neurodevelopmental delays.[223]

m *Management*

1. **Exclude breech** presentation as the origin of the meconium.
2. Note the **color and consistency** of the meconium.
3. **Maternal left side-lying, fluid resuscitation, and oxygen** administration optimize fetal oxygenation.
4. Take the **maternal temperature** every 2 hours because of the increased risk for chorioamnionitis.[147]
5. **Internal monitoring of the FHR** is preferable, and fetal assessment is factored into ongoing management decisions.
6. **Amnioinfusion** (instillation of sterile normal saline or Ringer's lactate through an IUPC into the uterus) is used to buffer the umbilical cord (reducing cord compression, variable decelerations, and the vagal stimulation that causes a fetus to gasp in utero) and to dilute the fluid to reduce the toxicity of aspiration should it occur. Studies have borne out that amnioinfusion reduces the number of MAS cases.[222] See p. 577 for the amnioinfusion procedure.
7. Suction the **oral pharynx and nares after delivery of the head and before delivery of the body.**[200]
8. **Pediatrics** personnel should be present at birth to receive the infant and continue resuscitation as needed. Intubation of all vs. selected infants is controversial because it may not improve the outcome for

affected infants to a greater degree than the risks inherent in the intubation process itself. Complications of intubation are transient and infrequent.[224] The following is a suggested **protocol for intubation of the infant** as described previously:

   a. Intubate once, taking no longer than 20 seconds. If unsuccessful, begin other resuscitation efforts and return to reintubate later. Meconium may be suctioned from the trachea for up to 1 hour after birth.

   b. Use 5 seconds of negative pressure without withdrawing the endotracheal (ET) tube.

   c. If meconium is still being withdrawn at the end of the 5-second interval, follow with another 5-second interval of suction.

   d. If meconium is still being withdrawn at the end of the additional 5-second interval, position the ET tube to be left in place for possible resuscitation while assessing further. The ET tube is used for positive pressure if necessary.[223]

   e. Irrigating the trachea with saline does not improve removal of meconium.[204]

9. When thick meconium is present, when the infant has shown FHR abnormalities, or when the infant is depressed at birth, **consider sending cord gases and the placenta to pathology** to determine in utero effects.[80]

• SECOND STAGE MANAGEMENT

The second stage of labor is defined as beginning with complete dilation and ending with delivery of the infant. Second stage may be divided into two parts: the period from complete dilation until the urge to bear down is felt and the stage of active pushing until delivery.[170,194]

A premature urge to push is felt by some women. Note the position of the presenting part. If the fetus is occiput posterior, see p. 140. If the vertex is at least +1, the position occiput transverse to occiput anterior, the cervix dilated 8 to 9 cm, the cervix soft and giving with contractions, the woman may be coached to push at the peak of the contractions—or only when and how her body directs her—and she will most often progress to full dilation.[170,194]

The Two Phases of the Second Stage of Labor

The first phase of second stage, the phase of passive fetal descent, may be characterized by a slowing of contractions and a lack of the urge to bear down. During this stage, the presenting part is rotating to the most favorable position and descending to the point in the pelvis where the stretching of the muscles and nerves results in Ferguson's reflex, which causes an increased release of oxytocin and an involuntary urge to push. The second phase—the active or expulsive phase—begins at this point, when conditions are optimal, allowing forceful bearing-down efforts to be effective and resulting in delivery of the fetal head.[170,194]

Pushing Techniques

Traditionally, when total dilation of the cervix is noted on vaginal examination, the woman is coached to begin pushing—whether or not she has the urge and regardless of fetal station or position. This may result in maternal fatigue, maternal dependence on the direction of others rather than following her own body messages, need for instrumental delivery, and increased perineal trauma—including neuromuscular injury predisposing to pelvic floor prolapse. The traditional coaching—taking a deep breath, closing the glottis, and counting down to 10 three times per contraction—is called Valsalva pushing. This technique decreases maternal venous return, cardiac output, arterial BP, and oxygenation of the mother and the placenta. Gasping for breath then causes a sudden increase in BP and results in petechial hemorrhages. Fetal hypoxia and acidosis may result.[170,172,194] Prolonged breath holding may also cause pelvic muscles to tighten, altering normal fetal descent.[172]

The coached pushing technique described above is very different than the natural pushing that occurs when most women follow their own body signals, in which pushing is accompanied by air release. As the first involuntary urges begin, the pushes are brief. The contraction must reach a certain intensity before the urge to push is felt and then the uncoached woman will push several times over the course of the contraction, for 5 to 7 seconds, usually taking several breaths between. While pushing she combines holding her breath and letting the air out; she may moan or make other sounds. As the baby descends the pushes become more forceful and more frequent. Women who push according to their body's signals have slightly longer second stages; however they may have fewer FHR decelerations, less fatigue, and equal Apgar scores as women who are pushing with the Valsalva technique.[170,194]

Maternal Position in the Second Stage

A Cochrane review of 18 trials regarding maternal position in the second stage of labor states that although the studies were variable in their methodologic quality and are to be interpreted with caution, the use of any upright or lateral position, compared with supine or lithotomy positions, was associated with shorter duration of second stage, a small reduction in assisted deliveries, a reduction in episiotomies, a smaller increase in second-degree lacerations, reduced reports of severe pain, fewer FHR abnormalities, but a greater incidence of estimated blood loss >500 mL.[89]

Mobility is another important aspect of second stage mangement. Studies have demonstrated the maternal preference to vary position and move about. Upright positions are often preferred by the mother and may maximize uterine perfusion, fetal alignment and descent, resulting in a shorter second stage, fewer episiotomies, fewer lacerations, fewer abnormal FHR patterns, and less severe pain. Squatting increases the capacity of the pelvis and avoids vena caval compression.[170,194] See p. 141 for positions that encourage rotation of the occiput posterior vertex and pp. 159 and 160 for positions that favor rotation of the asynclitic vertex.

At delivery, the lateral position is associated with fewer perineal lacerations, and side-lying results in good placental perfusion providing good fetal oxygenation. Birthing chairs, however, are associated with more edema, perineal lacerations, and greater blood loss.[170]

Optimal Management in the Second Stage

The stress of labor—pain, fear, and sustained muscular activity—results in catecholamine release, which decreases uterine contractility. Emotional support and addressing pain needs during the second stage is associated with decreased need for pain medication, a shorter labor, and less need for instrumental or cesarean delivery, and it supports the woman's biologic functions.[170]

Encourage the woman to delay pushing until conditions are optimal (vertex at +1 to +2 station in the anterior position). Only direct the woman's pushing efforts when necessary. Encourage the woman to follow her urge or coach her to let air out as she pushes. Assist her to the position of her choice, changing every 20 to 30 minutes. Emphasize simultaneous relaxation of the perineum. Reassure her of the normalcy of the intense perineal sensations she is experiencing.[194] Describe her progress (including rotation that may be not be obvious externally). Offer a mirror or suggest that she touch the baby's head to experience the progress. Pushing on the toilet has the advantage of being upright and may be a more natural and comfortable location for the woman.

The woman whose pushing is diffuse, undirected, and not resulting in progress should try another pushing position in which gravity assists in directing pressure toward the vagina. The increased pressure may help her push more effectively. If not, have the woman open her eyes and look toward her vagina. Called "self-directed pushing," this often focuses and improves the woman's pushing efforts.[194]

Epidural Anesthesia and the Conduct of the Second Stage

The woman with epidural anesthesia who does not have the urge to bear down may benefit from a delay in pushing of 1 to 2 hours (if mother and baby are tolerating it well) until the woman has an urge to push or until the vertex is visible at the perineum. The epidural may interfere with the perception of the need to bear down, and some providers may turn the epidural down or off. This practice must be done with informed consent. The return of pain may cause a surge of catecholamines that suppresses uterine activity, increasing the likelihood of instrumental delivery.[170,194] The lengthening of the second stage may be associated with increased risk of anal sphincter damage.[78]

Length of Second Stage

The ideal length of second stage has been arbitrarily set at 1 hour for the multigravida and 2 hours for the primigravida. It is unclear how long the woman should wait in the first phase for the urge to push. The phase of active pushing, rather than the entire length of the second stage, is related to maternal and infant outcomes. How long a woman can safely push in the active phase has also not been determined. One determinant is the FHR, which is observed for reactivity and variability, increasing fetal tachycardia, and the return to baseline of the decelerations that occur as expected with pushing. Consider intervention after 1 hour for multiparas and 2 hours for primiparas (adding an hour to each for regional anesthesia).[170]

Management Plan for the Second Stage of Labor

Assess second stage variables:
- The woman's preferences (position, location of delivery, disposition of baby, cutting of cord, collection of cord blood, placental delivery technique)
- Vital signs
- FHR and fetal tolerance of the second stage
- Whether fluid is meconium-stained
- Productivity of pushing (technique, energy, impact of anesthesia)
- Maternal emotional status
- EFW and comparison to previous vaginal deliveries
- Pelvimetry
- Maternal bladder status
- Anticipated length of second stage
- Involvement of significant others

Ⓜ Management Plan to Include:

1. Comfort measures: position; massage, counterpressure; complementary measures such as acupressure
2. Care of the perineum: compresses to perineum, perineal massage, and support (see p. 177).
3. Hydration
4. Preparation for delivery: timing, place, type, expected procedures, pediatric attendance
5. Need for episiotomy, consent, anesthesia
6. Ongoing screening for complications and/or need for consultation
7. Ongoing assessment of progress of rotation and/or descent of the vertex
8. Clamping and cutting of the cord

See third stage management, p. 197.

Complementary Measures for Second Stage Management

During the second stage, support the mother's head by applying pressure with the hand around the occipital ridge **(Bladder 10).** Someone else should apply pressure to **Bladder 67,** either squeezing between the thumb and index finger or using the nail and pressing into the point. This pressure blocks sensation of **sacral and pelvic pain.**[108]

Management of Normal Vaginal Delivery

See Figure 3-5 for illustrations of normal spontaneous vaginal delivery.

1. Before the delivery, **assemble necessary staff** (consider backup obstetrician, extra nurses if required, anesthesia and pediatrics personnel). Be certain that all **equipment and instruments** are assembled. If shoulder dystocia is anticipated, take **shoulder precautions:** be certain staff are alerted and are prepared for necessary maneuvers. Be aware of the woman's **bladder status** and consider emptying with a catheter.

2. Assist mother to the **position** of comfort, ensuring that the inferior vena cava is not compressed. Drape the mother if desired.

3. **Prepare the mother to work with you** at delivery to prevent perineal damage. When the head is crowning, coach the mother regarding when and how hard to push. Take into account the FHR, perineal resistance, previous scarring, the forcefulness of the uterine contractions, and the forcefulness of the voluntary muscle efforts. Respecting the rhythm that she has established in pushing will enhance her ability to work with you as well as her sense of success. Voicing awareness of the intense maternal sensations at this point may reassure the mother that the sensations are normal and that you are aware of her discomfort.

   The mother may need to be coached to bear down throughout, even between contractions if delivery is urgent. Alternately, ask the mother to blow through contractions or to bear down between contractions. This separates uterine and maternal voluntary efforts, thereby slowing delivery and possibly enhancing control. If delivery is proceeding rapidly, ask the mother to moan or make noises from her mouth as she pushes to slow her voluntary pushing efforts.

4. If an **episiotomy** is required (see p. 178), cut it when the vertex is expected to be born during that contraction. Local or pudendal anesthesia may be used (see pp. 131 and 132). Cut the episiotomy at the peak of the contraction, when the perineum is thinned and natural anesthesia prevents normal maternal sensation. Guard the apex of the episiotomy carefully by drawing the perineum together from either side to prevent damage to the rectal sphincter.

5. Measures to **protect the perineum** are discussed on p. 177. Provide warm compresses, perineal massage, or any other measures requested by the mother for her comfort.

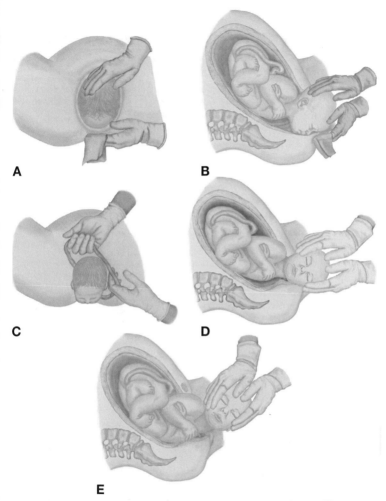

Figure 3-5 • Normal spontaneous vaginal delivery. **A,** Crowning of vertex. The vertex is prevented from emerging too quickly, and from rising to damage anterior structures. The perineum is supported during delivery. **B,** The head is born by extension. **C,** The assistant feels for the umbilical cord, reduces it if possible, clamping and cutting the cord too tight to reduce. **D,** The anterior shoulder is delivered. **E,** The posterior shoulder is delivered, and the baby is delivered into the maternal abdomen. (From Murray SS, McKinney ES, Gorrie TM: *Foundations of maternal-newborn nursing,* ed 3, Philadelphia, 2002, WB Saunders; McKinney ES et al: *Maternal-child nursing,* Philadelphia, 2000, WB Saunders.)

6. Accomplish three tasks simultaneously while managing the birth of the head:
   a. Flex the head to deliver with the **smallest presenting diameter.** In the occiput anterior position, for example, fingers on the lower

aspect of the emerging vertex push harder than those on the upper vertex.

b. Displace the vertex slightly **downward,** away from the delicate anterior perineal structures, which cannot stretch like the posterior tissues, and where injury is least desirable. Maintain this pressure until the head has passed through the introitus and can be extended without the occiput pressing back against the anterior structures.

c. Apply **counterpressure** to the emerging head as necessary to slow its movement and allow tissue stretching.

7. When immediate delivery is required for fetal safety, the **Ritgen maneuver** speeds delivery of the head. When the head is crowning about halfway, use one hand to manage the occiput, preventing it from rising into the anterior structures. Use the other hand to apply pressure forward and outward to underneath the baby's chin, pressing through the tissue just behind the maternal rectum, extending the baby's head for delivery. This maneuver is painful for the mother and predisposes to periurethral lacerations.

8. When the head is delivered, if meconium is present, use a DeLee to thoroughly **suction** the mouth and then the nares. If the fluid is clear, some midwives suction the mouth and then the nares with the bulb; others wipe the face with a towel or gauze to clear external debris and stimulate respirations less intrusively.

9. Feel around the baby's neck for the **umbilical cord.** If a loose loop is found, slip it over the head. If there is a tight loop, place two clamps side by side and cut the cord between the clamps, unwind the cord and complete the delivery. Alternately, the baby may be delivered through an intact loop by slipping the cord past the shoulders as they emerge, keeping the baby's body close to the mother's body to avoid traction on the cord.

10. Look for restitution of the fetal head on the shoulders that precedes delivery of the shoulders. While holding the baby's head between the hands, ask the mother to bear down. Pull downward to deliver the **anterior shoulder.** Delivery of the anterior shoulder is complete when the axillary crease is visualized. If this maneuver is unsuccessful, see management of shoulder dystocia, p. 184.

11. Still grasping the baby's head, pull the head upward to deliver the **posterior shoulder,** slipping your hand under the posterior shoulder to support the trunk as it comes and to keep the posterior hand from tearing the perineum by pressing it to the infant's trunk until fully delivered.

12. **Lift the baby's body** in the direction of the curve of Carus, the upward curve of the birth canal. The baby with meconium-stained amniotic fluid is kept unstimulated, the cord is cut and clamped immediately, and the baby is handed to pediatric staff for endotracheal suctioning before stimulation (see p. 162). Assess color, res-

pirations, tone, reflex, and heart rate. If the baby has poor color, respiratory effort, or tone, clamp and cut the baby's cord immediately and hand the baby to pediatric support staff for resuscitation. The vigorous baby with good tone and heart rate may be placed on the maternal abdomen if she desires. The baby is dried (stimulating respirations), suctioned if needed, and covered with a warm blanket.

13. Management of the third stage of labor is discussed on p. 197.
14. Examination and repair of episiotomy and lacerations is discussed on p. 178.

Care of the Perineum During the Second Stage

The muscles of the perineum are shown in Figure 3-6.

1. Daily **perineal massage** with an oil for 5 to 10 minutes from about 34 weeks by the nulliparous woman or her partner decreases the risk of perineal trauma.[68] This intervention was tested in a randomized, controlled study of 1034 women with no previous vaginal birth and 493 women with a history of a vaginal birth. The study group began massage at 34 to 35 weeks with sweet almond oil for 10 minutes daily. After doing perineal massage, 9.2% more nulliparous women delivered over an intact perineum. The more massage done, the better the result. The advantage was not significant for multiparous women.[119]

2. During the second stage, willingness of the birth assistant to **allow the mother to push as she desires,** avoiding the extended Valsalva pushing, maximizes the opportunity of the woman to deliver with minimal perineal injury.[68,170]

3. To achieve a controlled descent, use **positions that promote or delay progress**—gravity-neutral (side-lying, hands and knees) or gravity-enhancing (semi-sitting, squatting, standing), depending on

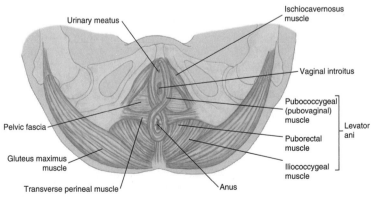

Figure 3-6 • Muscles of the perineum. (From Murray SS, McKinney ES, Gorrie TM: *Foundations of maternal-newborn nursing,* ed 3, Philadelphia, 2002, WB Saunders.)

the rate of the delivery. For delivery, the lateral position is associated with fewer episiotomies and lacerations.[170]

4. Enhance **relaxation of the perineum** by applying hot compresses.[68]
5. **"Iron out" the perineum** as the vertex descends, performing perineal massage with oil before delivery.[68]
6. Provide **perineal support** as the vertex emerges, bracing the perineum with the whole hand or drawing the perineum inward from the sides.[68,132,170]
7. Early in the second stage, remind the mother of the advantage of slow delivery. Prepare her to cooperate in slowing her pushing efforts when needed. Breathing techniques, a mirror, or placement of her hand on the baby's head may help.[116]
8. **Slow the delivery of the head** by applying a degree of counterpressure.[68]
9. **Flex the fetal head** as it emerges, minimizing the presenting diameter.[68]
10. **Avoid routine episiotomy.**[68]
11. **Avoid operative delivery** (forceps are worse than vacuum deliveries on perineal integrity).[68]
12. Use aseptic technique to cut an episiotomy if it is indicated. Repair the episiotomy and lacerations with aseptic, minimally traumatizing technique. Achieve hemostasis, close dead space, and approximate tissues with precision.

Episiotomy

Indications: Episiotomy is indicated when special maneuvers are anticipated for delivery (shoulder dystocia, breech delivery), for maternal exhaustion, maternal preference after informed consent, or nonreassuring fetal status.

Procedure: An incision is made into the perineum when delivery is anticipated during that contraction.

Principles of suturing:

1. Use strict aseptic technique. Clean away clots and debris before suturing.
2. Use appropriate-sized suture with atraumatic needles.
3. Minimize needle punctures and stitching.
4. Close dead space.
5. Approximate with care.
6. Do not pull suture too tight.
7. Handle tissue gently and minimally.[214]

Repair of the Midline Episiotomy: Repair of the midline episiotomy is conducted after the third stage, or during third stage with the clamped umbilical cord draped up out of the way, and a taped sponge in the vagina above the laceration. See Figure 3-7 for illustration of episiotomy repair.

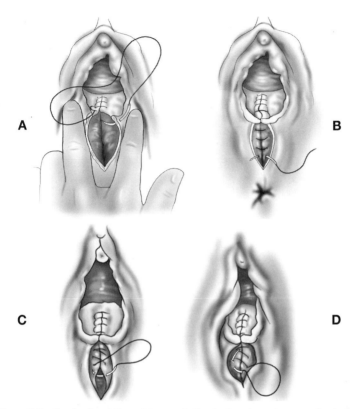

Figure 3-7 • Repair of a midline episiotomy. **A,** Starting just above the apex of vaginal laceration, using locked stitches, close the vaginal mucosal and submucosal layers, approximating the hymenal ring and stopping before it. **B,** If a tissue defect is present under the mucosal stitches, 3-4 uninterrupted stitches are placed to close the defect. **C,** The suture from the vaginal mucosa is placed behind the hymenal ring to emerge in the subcutaneous tissue of the perineum. Continuous stitches are used to close the subcutaneous tissue, ending at the posterior perineal apex. **D,** From the posterior apex, subcuticular stitches are used to approximate the perineal skin. A crown stitch may be placed at the juncture of skin and vaginal mucosa. The suture is placed through tissue under the hymenal ring where one more stitch is placed to enable tying off. (From Walsh LV: *Midwifery: community-based care during the childbearing year,* Philadelphia, 2001, WB Saunders.)

1. Differentiate the tissues, noting where each side should meet the other. Be certain that rectal structures are intact.
2. Provide adequate anesthesia. (See anesthesia, p. 131.)
3. With 3-0 absorbable suture, start just behind the vaginal apex of the laceration and place locked, continuous (blanket) stitches approximately every centimeter, moving toward the hymenal ring. Place the suture under the hymenal ring so that no suture lies across the hymenal ring.

4. Palpate the space underneath the laceration and if a small finger can be admitted, place approximately three deep sutures to close this space. Note that these sutures are placed in the horizontal plane. Some practitioners will use a separate suture for these stitches and place interrupted stitches.

5. Bring the suture into the subcuticular tissue below the skin anteriorly. Close the subcuticular tissue starting at the front top of the laceration and suturing with continuous stitches toward the anal apex.

6. Close the skin with subcuticular stitches.

7. Place the crown stitch at the entry to the vaginal introitus, biting into the bulbocavernosus muscle on the first side from above and coming out below in the incision and going across to the second side; go in below and come out above the muscle, still in the laceration.[214]

8. Suture to the vaginal tissue behind the hymenal ring and then take one final stitch to tie off the suture.[90]

9. Remove sponge if used.

10. Teach the woman about the nature of the injury and care of the laceration and comfort measures, including medications, that will be available for her.

Repair of the Third-Degree Laceration: A third-degree laceration is defined as a laceration of the anal sphincter not involving the anterior rectal wall.[90] See Figure 3-8 for an illustration of repair of the third-degree laceration.

ROLE OF THE MIDWIFE. To repair a third-degree laceration, the midwife is required to provide documentation of training, to give a demonstration of competency, and to be privileged for the procedure in the institution. Otherwise, repair of this laceration is conducted by the physician.

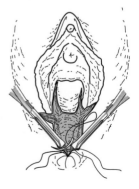

Figure 3-8 • Repair of third-degree laceration. Allis clamps grasp sphincter while interrupted or figure-of-eight sutures are placed. (Redrawn from Lowdermilk et al: *Maternity and women's health care,* ed 7, St Louis, 2000, Mosby.)

TECHNIQUE

1. Proper repair of the third-degree laceration begins with **differentiation of the tissues.** A depression on either side of the laceration indicates lacerated sphincter muscle fibers that have retracted. Palpate the rectum to identify the sphincter. The woman with a third-degree laceration cannot retract the sphincter.

2. Provide **anesthesia. Use Allis clamps to grasp the sphincter muscle** on each side.

3. **Carefully approximate** the **rectal sphincter.** Using 2-0 suture, execute repair with several figure-of-eight stitches or interrupted stitches—three along the posterior wall and three along the anterior portion of the muscle. Inclusion of the fascia will strengthen the repair. Rule out the presence of sutures in the rectum by rectal exam.[60] (Sutures found in the rectum must be removed to prevent fistula formation.)

4. Repair the second-degree laceration. Some midwives anchor a 3-0 suture in the inferior apex of the skin extension of the laceration and place a few subcuticular stitches at the lower apex of the laceration so that the now more anterior apex is easier to close when doing the final subcuticular layer of the repair.[214]

5. **Postpartum orders** may include a stool softener. Enemas are contraindicated. Iron supplementation may be deferred until laceration healing is well underway.

6. At the 6-week postpartum visit, inquire about the presence of fecal incontinence, present in 22% of women after their first delivery. Incontinence that persists after 6 months is an indication for referral to a gynecologist. Management is controversial, but some authors suggest anal sphincter repair and cesarean section for subsequent pregnancies.[78]

Disadvantages of Episiotomies:

- Increased incidence of third- and fourth-degree perineal lacerations.
- Increased pain immediately and 3 months postpartum compared with women who deliver intact or who sustain spontaneous perineal lacerations, preserving sexual function.
- Pelvic floor strength is strongest among women who deliver intact and weakest among women who deliver over episiotomies.[115]

Advantages of Episiotomies:

- Shortens second stage for the baby with fetal distress, or for the exhausted mother.
- Provides room for emergency maneuvers.
- Decreases the incidence of labial and urethral lacerations, according to Cunningham et al.[60]

Types of Episiotomy:

- **Median or midline episiotomy** cuts into the central tendinous point of the perineum, separating the two sides of the bulbocavernosus and superficial transverse perineal muscles and sometimes the deep transverse perineal muscle. Associated with less blood loss, the midline episiotomy heals well with a good anal outcome and causes decreased dyspareunia compared with other types of episiotomies.[60] The disadvantage is that extensions involve the rectal sphincter.[79]

• **Mediolateral episiotomy** cuts into the central tendinous point of the perineum in the direction of the ischial tuberosity, through the bulbocavernosus, superficial and deep transverse perineal muscles, and into the pubococcygeus muscle. The incision must begin centrally to avoid the Bartholin's glands and to leave at least 1 cm lateral to the rectal sphincter to allow for the repair.[214] The repair is more difficult, 10% heal with faulty anatomy, more have prolonged healing, and more have dyspareunia (location causes increased tension on the wound) and greater blood loss. Fewer rectal sphincter extensions result.[60]

Complementary Measures for Care of the Perineum During Second Stage

Herbs: Some herbalists suggest that various herbs—applied to the perineum during pregnancy by sitz bath, perineal massage, or compress—increase the flexibility of the tissue.[103,116,205] **See information on herbs, p. 563.**

Documentation of Vaginal Delivery

The following information may be included in a delivery note. Consistency with a computer-generated delivery note is important for medico-legal reasons:
• Age, gravidity, parity, weeks of gestation
• Length of stages of labor and period since rupture of membranes
• If bladder was emptied by catheter before delivery
• That delivery was spontaneous
• Fetal position, whether infant was viable, weight, sex, Apgar score, resuscitation, and response
• DeLee suctioning for meconium on the perineum, if done
• Nuchal or other cord, if present, and management
• Delivery of shoulders and any maneuvers required
• Anesthesia, if any
• Delivery of the placenta, whether spontaneous or assisted, Schultz or Duncan method
• Description of cord and placenta, including number of cord vessels and whether placenta was intact
• Fourth stage: status of the uterus, estimated blood loss, status of cervix, vagina, perineum, and rectum
• Repair of any incision or laceration and suture material used
• How tolerated by woman
• Bonding behaviors and breastfeeding observed
• Condition of mother and infant at the end of the delivery

• COMPLICATIONS OF THE SECOND STAGE OF LABOR

Dystocia of Second Stage

A rule of uncertain origin in American obstetrics has been that a second stage lasting longer than 2 hours is considered prolonged.[60] See p. 126 regarding the length of the second stage. Regional analgesia usually lengthens the second stage (see epidural anesthesia, p. 133).

Hypotonic Uterine Forces

A "lull" in contractions at the beginning of the second stage is normal. The fetus will rotate and descend, stimulating the mother's urge to push and stimulating endogenous oxytocin release in the expulsive phase of the second stage. Starting oxytocin and beginning pushing during the early part of the second stage is often unproductive, increases maternal exhaustion, decreases the woman's sense of working with her body, and may cause fetal hypoxia[170] (see p. 171). The appropriate length of the interval while waiting for contractions to resume has not been identified.

m *Management Options*

1. Simkin and Ancheta[194] suggest waiting 20 to 30 minutes, talking with the mother, then instituting measures to enhance descent and contractions: upright positions, trial expulsive efforts, and nipple stimulation.
2. For hypotonia that persists, see measures suggested for hypotonia during active phase, p. 160.
3. **Consider oxytocin** augmentation if necessary.

Arrest of Descent

Arrest of descent is defined as 1 hour without fetal descent.[77]

m *Management Options*

1. Use **pushing techniques** (non-Valsalva) that may be sustained with less maternal exhaustion and fetal distress, as described on p. 171.
2. Change pushing **positions** every 20 to 30 minutes. (See those suggested on p. 171.)
   a. **Squatting** widens the pelvic outlet and may allow descent.
   b. Pushing on the **toilet** has the advantage of being upright and may be a comfortable and familiar position for the mother.
   c. Simkin and Acheta[194] suggest **dangling** positions that use the woman's own weight to lengthen her spinal column and allow the fetus more vertical room for repositioning. The pelvis, free of external pressure, may change in shape.

(1) The woman may stand with her back to a partner's front. The partner stands with one foot forward and holds his or her hands under the woman's arms and above her breasts. She bends her arms and is supported under the arms, allowing her lower body to dangle.

(2) Alternately, an apparatus may be secured to the ceiling and attached to a sling into which the woman backs up, resting her shoulders into the sling, holding on with the hands. With contractions, she dangles the lower part of her body.

3. The **"pelvic press"** may help when malpositions and failure to rotate have delayed the second stage. With the woman in a squatting position, someone behind her places each hand on an iliac crest (fingers pointing toward umbilicus), and presses inward. In effect, inward tilting of the upper pelvis may cause outward tilting of the mid- and lower pelvis, allowing space for turning.[194]

4. See management of the second stage with **epidural** anesthesia, p. 172.

5. Although the ideal time to **intervene instrumentally or surgically** for delivery is unknown, the decision is at the discretion of the birth assistant in consultation with the mother, factoring in fetal condition. ACOG notes guidelines of 1 hour for multiparas and 2 hours for primiparas, adding an hour to either for regional anesthesia.

Shoulder Dystocia

Shoulder dystocia is diagnosed when maneuvers and extra time are required to achieve delivery of the shoulders.[19] The clinical picture is that of prolonged second stage and delivery of a head that restitutes without descent (the "turtle sign").[143]

Predisposing Factors: No risk factors are present in 50% of shoulder dystocia cases.[60,151,167]

Abnormal pelvic shape	Maternal obesity
EFW of 1 lb larger than previous babies	Postterm pregnancy
Excessive maternal weight gain	Prolonged first and second stages of labor
Gestational diabetes	Short maternal stature
Increasing parity	Vacuum- and forceps-assisted births (rate increased by 35% to 45%)[60]
Induction of labor	
Macrosomia (current, obstetric, or family history)	

Incidence: Reports vary from 0.15% to >4%.[167]

Maternal Complications:

Bladder injury[217]

Fourth-degree lacerations with subsequent wound dehiscence, infection, and fistula formation[217]

PPH from uterine atony and lacerations of the cervix and vagina[60]

Fetal Complications[217]:
Fractured humerus or clavicle
Brachial plexus injury
Asphyxia with neurologic sequelae
Death

🄜 *Management*

1. **Anticipation**
   a. ACOG[9] states that prophylactic cesarean delivery may be chosen as a delivery route for the diabetic woman whose infant's EFW is suspected to be >4500 g or for the nondiabetic woman's infant whose EFW is >5000 g.
   b. When risk factors are identified before vaginal delivery (only 50% of infants who experience shoulder dystocia are identifiable by risk factors), make and document preparations. The woman should participate in any decision-making before the delivery.[217] Appropriate **personnel** are alerted and are present for the delivery; the **bladder is emptied, anesthesia** is administered, and an **episiotomy** may be performed to allow maneuvers.
   c. When anticipating shoulder dystocia, some practitioners will take advantage of the momentum of the descent that occurs with the delivery of the head, immediately continuing with the delivery of the anterior shoulder, attempting to prevent restitution of the shoulders to the anteroposterior diameter (10.6 cm), and **deliver the shoulders through the oblique diameter** (12.75 cm).
2. **Attempt delivery** with maternal expulsive efforts.
3. For "snug shoulders," turning the woman into a **hands-knees position** facilitates delivery of the posterior (now uppermost) shoulder. This position may not be useful in true shoulder dystocia, however, and will prevent other measures from being used.[214]
4. **McRoberts'** position (pronounced flexion of legs onto maternal abdomen) is implemented.[217] This maneuver flattens the sacrum, rotates the symphysis pubis to a more favorable angle,[83] and lessens the traction necessary to deliver the infant.
5. **Suprapubic pressure** by an assistant may dislodge the shoulder from under the suprapubic bone.[217]
6. **Call for help:** Summon the obstetrician, extra nurses, anesthesia and pediatrics personnel.[60] Have attendants prepare for a PPH.
7. **Rubin's maneuvers:** Vaginally, push behind the anterior shoulder to **rotate the shoulders into an oblique pelvic diameter.** An assistant uses **oblique suprapubic pressure** (behind anterior shoulder) to decrease the bisacromial diameter of the shoulders.[167]
8. Reaching into the vagina, attempt to **exclude the following causes:** short umbilical cord, enlarged abdomen or thorax, locked or conjoined twins, and Bandl's retraction ring as the cause of dystocia (the

latter three possibilities suggesting neglect to make appropriate diagnoses earlier). If the cause is an enlarged thorax or abdomen, the Zavanelli maneuver is performed (see the list that follows) and the mother proceeds to cesarean birth.[214]

If the dystocia appears to be caused by the shoulders, perform the following maneuvers in any order:

1. **Woods screw maneuver:** Place the fingers of one hand on the posterior surface of the anterior shoulder; place the fingers of the other hand on the anterior surface of the posterior shoulder. Always keeping the spine anterior, rotate the shoulders 180 degrees by pushing them in a clockwise direction so that the baby faces the opposite direction. Attempt delivery. If unsuccessful, turn the shoulders back counterclockwise, 180 degrees, and again attempt delivery. Repeat 3 to 4 times if necessary, attempting delivery after each turn.[167]
2. Deliver the **posterior arm** by grasping the hand vaginally. If necessary, press into the antecubital space to move the hand into reach, grasp hand, and sweep arm across chest and above the head.[217]
3. **Rubin maneuver:** Suprapubically, **rock the impacted shoulder from side to side.**[217]
4. **Hibbard maneuver: Flex the fetal jaw or neck toward the mother's rectum** while an assistant applies fundal pressure.[60]
5. **Fracture the clavicle** by pressing it against the ramus of the pelvis. The risk is pneumothorax. This procedure may be technically difficult to accomplish.[217]
6. **Zavanelli maneuver:** Replace the fetal head by placing the head in occiput anterior or occiput posterior position, depressing the posterior vaginal wall and returning the head into the vagina. Cesarean delivery follows. Terbutaline or uterine-relaxing anesthesia will increase the likelihood of success.[182]
7. As for any difficult delivery, send **cord gases** to the laboratory and document each maneuver.[217]
8. Be prepared for PPH, for which this woman is at risk.

• MEASURES OF FETAL/INFANT WELL-BEING

Fetal Heart Rate Interpretation

In the United States, EFM is used in 75% of labors.[206] ACOG[21] recommends that in the woman with a high-risk pregnancy, FHR should be auscultated after a contraction every 15 minutes during the first stage of labor and every 5 minutes during the second stage. This protocol results in outcomes comparable to those pregnancies continuously electronically monitored. Studies have not demonstrated the necessary frequency of auscultation in a low-risk pregnancy to maintain safety. The greatest risk of continuous EFM, ACOG states, is the increased cesarean section rate that has been observed in both retrospective trials and in the majority of prospective, controlled studies.

In 1997, a National Institute of Child Health and Human Development (NICHHD) Research Planning Workshop determined a set of definitions in an attempt to standardize FHR pattern interpretation to facilitate evidence-based interpretation and treatment of intrapartum EFM and to enable better research.

Concepts From National Institute of Child Health and Human Development

All FHR patterns must be interpreted in light of the gestational age of the fetus, the maternal medical condition, medications, prior assessments of the fetus, and other relevant factors. A full description of any FHR pattern includes a description of the **baseline rate, the baseline variability, the presence of accelerations, periodic or episodic decelerations, and changes or trends in patterns over time.**[149]

UTERINE ACTIVITY. Note contraction frequency, duration, pattern (such as "doubling"), resting tone, and, if an IUPC is in place and internal monitoring is being done, the amplitude of contractions. Evaluate the FHR as the fetus responds to changes in the uterine environment. ACOG[24] defines an adequate active labor pattern as a uterine pattern of 200 Montevideo units or more in 10 minutes.

FETAL HEART RATE BASELINE. To determine the FHR baseline, the approximate mean FHR is rounded to the nearest 5 BPM during a 10-minute segment, excluding periodic and episodic changes, periods of marked variability, or segments of the baseline that vary by 25 BPM. At least 2 of the 10 minutes must be at the baseline rate or the baseline is defined as indeterminate.[149] Determined by the sympathetic and the parasympathetic nervous systems, the FHR baseline decreases with gestation as the nervous system matures and the parasympathetic system begins to dominate. At term and postterm, the normal baseline ranges from 100 to 160 BPM. The preterm fetus averages 120 to 160 BPM.[147]

Variability: Variability describes the fluctuations in the baseline FHR of ≥2 cycles/min. Irregular in amplitude and frequency, the fluctuations are visually judged in BPM from the peak to the trough: if there is no amplitude, variability is absent. If the amplitude ranges from undetectable to 5 BPM, there is minimal FHR variability. If the amplitude ranges from 6 to 25 BPM, there is moderate FHR variability. If the amplitude is >25 BPM, there is marked FHR variability. This description rules out the sinusoidal rhythm, which has a smooth, regular wave-like pattern of amplitude and frequency.[149]

NICHHD determined that "beat-to-beat variability" and "long-term variability" are determined visually as a unit based on the amplitude of the complexes, and thus determine only "variability."[149] Variability is a function of cerebral oxygenation and cardiac response and reflects the maturity and oxygenation of the autonomic system. Rapid changes are mediated by the vagus; slow changes are sympathetically influenced.[147] Variability increases with gestation. After 30 weeks, variability increases with activity and decreases with sleep. Drugs (analgesics, narcotics, barbiturates, phenothiazines, beta-adrenergic agents such as ritodrine or terbutaline, and anesthetics), hypoxia and acidosis, and anomalies may decrease the variability. Loss of variability is probably caused by the effect of metabolic acidemia on the fetal brain stem or on the fetal heart itself.[60] Variability will decrease after decelerations occur.[21]

Evaluation of decreased variability may include vibroacoustic stimulation or fetal scalp stimulation. Fetal acceleration in response indicates a fetus with a pH >7.25.[147] When decreased variability is accompanied by other signs of fetal distress, such as meconium, decelerations, or tachycardia, consider accelerated delivery.[90]

Tachycardia: Tachycardia is a FHR baseline >160 BPM,149 which indicates increased sympathetic tone or depressed parasympathetic tone and is therefore associated with decreased variability.[147] Identified as an isolated finding in the healthy term infant, tachycardia does not usually indicate a poor outcome.[125] In the preterm or postdates infant, closely observe tachycardia. When associated with meconium-stained amniotic fluid, late or prolonged variable decelerations, and decreased variability, tachycardia indicates fetal distress. A rate between 161 and 180 BPM is considered mild tachycardia. A rate >180 BPM is considered severe tachycardia.[60] Tachycardia may occur after decelerations when the fetus is hypoxic.[21]

The most common cause of fetal tachycardia is chorioamnionitis—when the tachycardia may precede maternal fever. The newborn may be septic, however, without tachycardia. Tachycardia may also occur from early hypoxia, systemic maternal fever, maternal dehydration with or without fever, thyrotoxicosis, drug effects, prematurity (<28 weeks' gestation as sympathetic tone develops before parasympathetic), congenital anomalies (particularly cardiac), or fetal anemia. The hypoxia and increased catecholamine levels associated with maternal cigarette smoking may cause tachycardia. Maternal anxiety, which also causes increased maternal catecholamine levels, may cause fetal tachycardia. Fetal tachyarrhythmias may also cause a tachycardia.[147]

Bradycardia: Bradycardia is a FHR baseline <110 BPM.[149] A rate of 100 to 119 BPM is normal in the term and postterm fetus but is considered bradycardia in the preterm fetus.[147]

A rate of 80 to 100 BPM is moderate bradycardia; <80 BPM for ≥3 minutes is severe bradycardia. Forty percent of infants with bradycardia of <90 BPM are acidotic. Observation for the presence or absence of variability and decelerations assists in evaluating whether the bradycardia indicates distress. Bradycardia may be seen with maternal use of drugs, fetal hypothyroidism, cardiac anomalies or heart block, or serious fetal compromise such as placental abruption, maternal hypotension, or maternal hypoglycemia. It may occur reflexively with stimulation of the vagal nerve and is sometimes caused by an occiput transverse or posterior presentation.[60]

Accelerations: An acceleration is a visually apparent abrupt increase in FHR above the baseline with the onset-to-peak lasting <30 seconds. The acme is ≥15 BPM above the baseline. The acceleration lasts ≥15 seconds but <2 minutes from the onset to return to the baseline. Before 32 weeks' gestation, an acceleration is defined as having an acme ≥10 BPM above the baseline lasting ≥15 seconds. A prolonged acceleration lasts between 2 and 10 minutes. An acceleration ≥10 minutes is a baseline change.[149] The presence of two or more accelerations during a 20-minute period, at least 15 BPM in amplitude and lasting for at least 15 seconds, is described as reactive and is reassuring.[60] Accelerations indicate a normal pH.[21]

Transient increases in the FHR occur either as a sympathetic impulse in response to fetal movement (called a spontaneous acceleration) or as a normal baroreceptor-stimulated response to hypotension and decreased cardiac output when a uterine contraction partially occludes the umbilical cord (called a uniform acceleration). The very premature or the IUGR fetus may not have accelerations. A beta-blocking drug, a CNS depressant drug, hypoxia, neurologic or cardiac anomaly, or brain death may cause the absence of accelerations.[147]

Decelerations: Decelerations are FHR changes associated with uterine contractions that are classified as early, late, or variable. Decelerations are described as either periodic (associated with uterine contractions) or episodic (unrelated to uterine contractions). A **prolonged deceleration** is a decrease in the baseline measured from the most recent baseline ≥15 BPM, lasting ≥2 minutes, but <10 minutes from onset to resolution. **Recurrent decelerations** are those occurring with ≥50% of uterine contractions in any 20-minute period.[149]

Early decelerations are a gradual decrease (from onset to nadir, ≥30 seconds) from and return to the baseline in the FHR associated with a uterine contraction in such a way that the nadir of the deceleration occurs at the same time as the peak of the contraction. The beginning and ending of the deceleration usually occur with the beginning and end of the contraction. The depth is calculated from the most recent baseline.[149] The rate does not usually drop below 100 BPM and does not require intervention. The early deceleration is believed to be a vagal reflex caused by head compression.[90] When the deceleration has an accompanying shoulder (see definition, p. 191), or is present with a vaginal exam that finds the presenting part high, without caput or molding, and a cervix ≤3 cm dilated, the deceleration is considered not early but rather a blunted variable deceleration. It may be part of a reassuring pattern when no other signs of hypoxia or asphyxia are present and may occur during a labor with CPD.[147] Umbilical cord compressions, which often coincide with uterine contractions, slow the heart with an abrupt onset and return, are of variable depth, length and shape, and are frequently preceded and followed by small accelerations.[21]

Late decelerations are a gradual decrease and return to baseline associated with a uterine contraction, with the onset of the deceleration to the nadir of ≥30 seconds. The nadir of the deceleration occurs after the peak of the contraction, and the onset, nadir, and recovery of the deceleration usually follow the beginning, peak, and end of the uterine contraction.[149] Late decelerations are the result of decreased oxygenation caused by uteroplacental insufficiency. They are usually shallow, 10 to 30 BPM, and in milder cases may be reflexive. In more severe cases, they may reflect myocardial depression. Occasional late decelerations are not uncommon during labor.[21]

Most important in the analysis of the rhythm with late decelerations is whether variability and accelerations are present. The absence of these indicates a more ominous prognosis.[147] Low et al[125] noted, however, that although accelerations were more frequent among infants who were not asphyxiated, they were sometimes noted among infants who were undergoing asphyxia. Persistent late decelerations are nonreassuring regardless of depth. Late decelerations that are reflexive generally become deeper the more severe the fetal distress.[21]

Late decelerations are believed to be caused by uteroplacental insufficiency, with a decreased oxygen supply stimulating an alpha adrenergic response in the fetus, causing fetal hypertension. A baroreceptor and parasympathetic response are stimulated in turn by the hypertension. As hypoxia worsens, however, and metabolic acidosis occurs, late decelerations occur with direct myocardial depression and, in this case, the depth will not reflect the severity of hypoxia. Maternal hypotension, uterine hyperactivity, or placental dysfunction can cause late decelerations.[60]

Variable decelerations are an abrupt (onset of deceleration to beginning of nadir of <30 seconds) decrease in FHR below the baseline. Depth is calculated from the most recent baseline. The decrease in the baseline must be ≥15 BPM, lasting ≥15 seconds, and <2 minutes from onset to return to baseline.[149] Variables have been identified in 40% of tracings by 5 cm dilation and in 83% of tracings by the end of the first stage of labor.[60]

Variable decelerations are believed to occur when the cord is compressed, causing umbilical artery occlusion, thereby causing hypertension and/or decreased oxygenation.[60] This stimulates the baroreceptors and causes fetal hypoxemia, which in turn stimulates fetal chemoreceptors that slow the FHR. Fetal head compression and fetal seizure may also cause variable decelerations.[147] Common during labor, variable decelerations indicate cord compression. They are of concern when they are persistent and progressively deeper (≤70 BPM) and last ≥60 seconds. When evaluating the seriousness of the variables, note the frequency, depth, rate of return to baseline (a slow return indicates myocardial depression), and the variability of the pattern. Consider the baseline rate and the presence of variability and accelerations when formulating a management plan in this situation,[21] which will include a vaginal exam to rule out cord prolapse.[143]

Shoulders represent an acceleratory phase of a deceleration pattern, not an acceleration. They occur before and/or after a variable deceleration in a well-oxygenated fetus.[147] These accelerations are baroreceptor-mediated changes in the heart rate to compensate for varying degrees of cord compression.[60]

Overshoot is the phase of a variable deceleration involving a rebound increase in the FHR that occurs after a variable deceleration with absent variability and a slow return to baseline. It is not an acceleration. The overshoot is a further sign of fetal decompensation.[147]

SINUSOIDAL PATTERN. The sinusoidal pattern is composed of undulating, repetitive, and uniform oscillations with a frequency of 3 to 5 cycles/min, an amplitude of 5 to 15 BPM above and below the baseline, with absent short-term variability. This pattern is associated with CNS abnormalities, gastroschisis, amnionitis, fetomaternal hemorrhage, severe chronic anemia, or severe hypoxia and acidosis. Medications (Demerol, Phenergan, and Nubain) may cause this pattern and do not indicate fetal compromise. Other benign causes of sinusoidal rhythm include rhythmic sucking and breathing clusters.[60]

Scalp stimulation or acoustic stimulation (see p. 79) may be performed to bring about an acceleration differentiating pseudosinusoidal from sinusoidal patterns. If oxygenation brings about fetal movement, the fetus is probably anemic and not asphyxiated. In the preterm fetus, seek and treat the cause of the sinusoidal rhythm. At term, immediate delivery with pediatric support is indicated to prevent fetal death.[147]

LAMBDA PATTERN. A lambda pattern is a benign pattern associated with both cord compression and fetal movement in which an acceleration is followed immediately by a deceleration, irrespective of the timing of the deceleration. This pattern is not associated with an adverse outcome but is believed to be a baroceptor/vagal response to a BP variation.[147]

WANDERING BASELINE. The wandering baseline is a pattern devoid of variability in which the baseline wanders between a rate of 120 and 160 BPM. A late sign of fetal distress, this pattern has been identified before fetal death and should prompt immediate cesarean delivery.[147]

SALTATORY BASELINE. A saltatory baseline describes rapidly recurring couplets of an acceleration and a deceleration associated with umbilical cord compression. Without other findings, it is not ominous.[60]

Fetal Arrhythmia

The differential of an irregular heartbeat includes premature atrial contractions, fetal tachycardia, and heart block. Definitive diagnosis is made by fetal echocardiogram.[57]

Ectopic systoles are as common in fetuses as they are in adults. In the absence of hydrops, fetal outcome is not improved by intervention and spontaneous delivery is usually well tolerated. Ventricular arrhythmias are uncommon in fetuses.[60] Atrial extrasystoles do not appear to be hemodynamically harmful. More aggressive management has been suggested for atrial extrasystoles, including the use of cardiac arrhythmia drugs, but the benefits have not been shown to outweigh the risks. A conservative reason to identify the fetus with complete heart block would be to ensure that it is delivered in a medical center with a pediatric cardiology department where a pacemaker could be placed. In utero corticosteroid administration has been proposed for the fetus with recent onset high-grade heart block to slow the progression from second-degree to complete heart block and to reduce the severity of fetal hydrops.[57]

Copel et al[57] identified 614 fetuses with an irregular heart rhythm from among 4838 fetuses. Normal rhythms were found in 55.4%; 42.9% had extrasystoles and 2.4% had hemodynamically significant rhythms. Structural heart anomalies occurred within this group with the same frequency as in the general population (0.3%). They concluded that atrial extrasystoles can precipitate runs of atrial tachycardia, which may result in fetal hydrops. Pharmacologic therapy may be indicated.

Fetal Scalp Stimulation

Fetal scalp stimulation is used to evaluate a fetus for metabolic acidosis and may prevent or precede fetal scalp blood sampling or operative delivery. Indications for scalp stimulation include diminished variability, the absence of accelerations, late decelerations, severe variable decelerations, tachycardia, decreased fetal movement, sinusoidal pattern, a new tachycardia or bradycardia of unknown significance, or any other fetal abnormality of uncertain significance. Perform the stimulation between contractions and decelerations when a baseline FHR has been determined. The goal of scalp stimulation is to elicit a sympathetic response in the form of an acceleration. An acceleration after scalp stimulation is associated with a scalp blood pH of greater than 7.19, indicating a nonacidotic fetus. The lack of an acceleration in response, however, is a poor predictor of fetal acidemia.[147]

Nonreassuring Fetal Status

In 1998, ACOG issued a Committee Opinion stating that the term "fetal distress" was imprecise and nonspecific—pointing out that the term has a low positive predictive value, even in a high-risk population, and that often the infant delivered expeditiously for "fetal distress" has good Apgars and/or good cord gases. The committee suggested that the term "nonreassuring fetal status" be used instead, followed by a specific description about the pattern of concern. Metabolic acidemia is the only term that ACOG[14] endorses as "fetal distress." The term "asphyxia" is used only for the infant who has acidemia, hypoxia, and metabolic acidosis. Figure 3-9 describes midwifery management of the woman with a nonreassuring FHR tracing.

Fetal Scalp Sampling

To evaluate fetal oxygenation, a cone is used to visualize the fetal scalp, and a physician punctures the scalp to collect a fetal scalp blood sample (FSS) in a heparinized capillary tube.[90] Interpretation and management of FSS values are delineated in Table 3-4. Fetal pH reflects maternal pH as well as fetal hypoxia. Contributing factors include respiratory rate, nutritional status, vomiting, dehydration, or ketoacidosis. To differentiate, maternal ABGs are drawn and sent simultaneously.[147]

Contraindications: Coagulopathy, intact membranes and rupture undesirable, vaginal bleeding (contamination of sample), and infection of the genital tract.[147] Cunningham et al[60] state that HIV transmission has not been increased by FSS. Anticipated vacuum delivery is a relative contraindication.[142]

Complications: Lancet breakage, bleeding from the scalp, infection, laceration of scalp, and perinatal transmission of a communicable disease.[147]

Cord Blood Gases

Collection of blood gases from a double-clamped length of umbilical cord reflects the oxygenation and acid-base balance of the newborn. Table 3-5 lists normal cord blood gas values.
Umbilical artery pH is classified by Murray[147] as the following:

7.10-7.20	Lower limit of normal
7.15	Moderate acidemia
7.10	Significant acidemia
7.05	Severe acidosis
<7.00	Severe acidosis, severe intrapartum asphyxia

Arterial Versus Venous Values

Umbilical arterial blood flows directly from the fetus and most accurately reflects the fetal status. Blood from the umbilical vein has just returned from the placenta and reflects the combination of maternal acid-base status, placental function, and fetal acid-base status.[184] Mixed values are not useful.[147]

Analysis of Findings

A cord blood pH <7.0, a base deficit ≤10 mEq/L, and a 5-minute Apgar ≤3 identifies the term or near-term infant at risk for multiorgan system

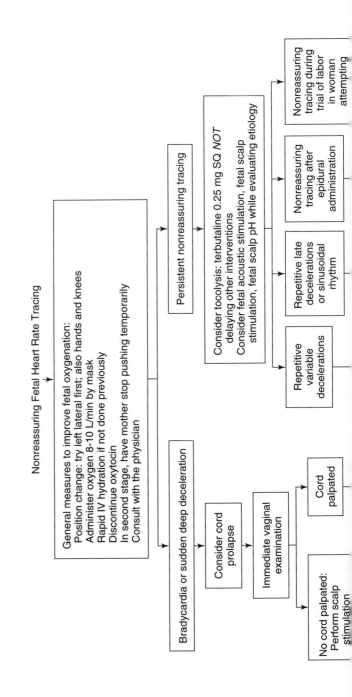

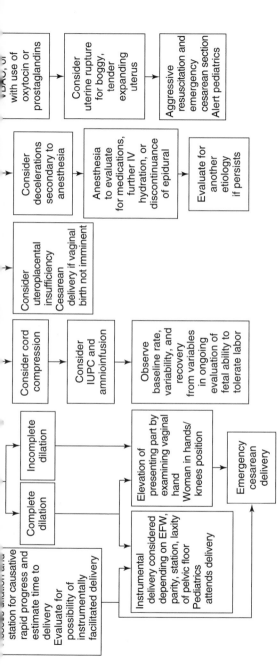

Figure 3-9 • Decision tree for midwifery management of nonreassuring fetal heart rate. (Adapted from Morrison EH: Common peripartum emergencies, *Am Fam Physician* Nov 1, 1998, published by the American Academy of Family Physicians at *http://www.aafp.org/afp/981101ap/morrison.html*.)

morbidity after acute perinatal asphyxia.[45] An umbilical artery base deficit of 12 mmol/L is the threshold of metabolic acidosis.[125]

Collection of Specimen

Clamp the umbilical cord before the infant's first breath, double-clamp and cut a length of cord, and draw the gases from the cord vessels within 60 minutes (within 30 minutes from placental vessels). With 1 to 3 mL heparinized (with 1000 U/mL heparin) syringes, enter the vessel tangentially and draw a sample. Venous blood is pinker than arterial blood. Draw and differentiate two samples and send the arterial sample to the lab for analysis (ice unnecessary). If the two samples appear similar, send both.[147]

Apgar Score

The Apgar score provides an objective way to evaluate the condition of the newborn. Five characteristics are rated at 1 and 5 minutes. In cases of resuscitation, clinicians may determine an Apgar at 3 minutes, as well as every 5 minutes for the duration of the resuscitation.[37,122] Table 3-6 describes the assignment of points to determine the Apgar score.

Factors that influence the Apgar score include infant maturity, neuromuscular or cerebral malformations, cardiorespiratory conditions, infection, maternal medications, and other conditions.[20]

Neither asphyxia nor hypoxia can be equated with a low Apgar score. Tone, reflex irritability, and color are in part a reflection of physiologic fetal maturity and do not reflect an anoxic event or cerebral depression.[20] Color is the least important of the signs, acrocyanosis (cyanosis of hands and feet) being normal for several hours. Pulse oximetry has been proposed as a better alternative.[122]

A 1992 ACOG Technical Bulletin stated that all the following criteria must be present to determine that a neurologic deficit was caused by perinatal asphyxia: umbilical metabolic or mixed acidemia (pH <7.0); Apgar score of 0 to 3 for >5 minutes; neonatal neurologic sequelae such as seizures, coma, or hypotonia; and multiorgan dysfunction (cardiovascular, renal, GI, pulmonary, and/or hematologic).[23] In 1996, ACOG issued another statement regarding the Apgar score. A low 1-minute Apgar score indicates a neonate who needs resuscitation, and it is not predictive of neonatal outcome. The 5-minute Apgar score is useful in evaluating the effectiveness of resuscitation efforts, but is still not predictive of future neurologic state. An Apgar score of 0 to 3 at 5 minutes is associated with an increased risk for cerebral palsy of 0.3% to 1.0%. The Apgar score does not clearly correlate with morbidity in low-birth-weight (LBW) infants and is not predictive, although it does reflect success of resuscitative measures and of the newborn's transition to extrauterine life.[122]

Table 3-4 / Normal Fetal Scalp Capillary Blood Gas Values

	Normal[79]	Respiratory Acidosis[79]	Metabolic Acidosis[79]
pH	7.25-7.40	Decreased	Decreased
Po_2	18-22	Usually stable	Decreased
Pco_2	40-50	Increased	Usually stable
Base deficit	0-11	Usually stable	Increased

Management[60]

pH >7.25	Observe closely; note CO_2 (metabolic acidosis is more dangerous than respiratory acidosis)
pH 7.20-7.25	Repeat FSS in 30 min, possibly after sending maternal ABGs and correcting acid/base balance
ph <7.20	Repeat immediately, preparing for immediate cesarean section if hypoxia confirmed

Apgar Scores and Fetal Scalp pH[147]

pH <7.2	Low Apgar scores
pH >7.25 in second stage	Apgar score of 8-10 at 2 min in 92%
pH 7.15-7.25	Not predictive of Apgar score
pH <7.15 in second stage	2-min Apgar of <6 in 80%

Table 3-5 / Normal Umbilical Cord Blood Gas Values

	Vein	Artery
pH	7.34±0.15	7.28±0.15
Po_2	30±15	15±10
Pco_2	35±8	45±15
Base deficit	5±4	7±4

Used with permission from Gabbe SG, Niebyl JR, Simpson JL: *Obstetrics: normal and problem pregnancies,* ed 3 New York, 1996, Churchill Livingstone.

• THIRD STAGE MANAGEMENT

The third stage of labor begins with delivery of the fetus and ends with the complete delivery of placenta, cord, and membranes. The length of third stage is <10 minutes in most births and <15 minutes in 95% of births.[79]

Cord clamping and infant placement vary among midwives. Placement of the newly delivered infant relative to the placenta, length

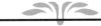

Table 3-6 / The Apgar Score

	Score		
Neonatal Characteristic	**0**	**1**	**2**
Color	Pale blue	Body pink, blue extremities	Completely pink
Respiratory effort	No respiratory effort	Slow, irregular	Good crying
Heart rate	Absent heart rate	<100 BPM	>100 BPM
Muscle tone	Flaccid	Some flexion of extremities	Active motion
Reflexes	Absent reflexes	Grimace	Vigorous cry[60]

of time before cord clamping, and oxytocics affecting placental attachment affect how much of the placental blood flows into the infant. Immediate cord clamping can reduce the red cell mass of the infant by 50% and has been demonstrated to increase neonatal anemia. Other theoretic concerns, such as underperfusion of organs during the transition to life, have not been shown in human beings. Delayed clamping has been theorized to cause polycythemia and increased viscosity, hyperbilirubinemia and transient tachypnea, but randomized controlled studies of significant numbers have not clearly demonstrated these associations.[137]

Expectant management is favored by many who consider natural physiology to be best and who are cautious with interventions. It includes delayed cord clamping and observation of maternal blood loss and maternal vital signs while watching for signs of placental separation. The placenta then drops into the upper vagina and is spontaneously expelled.[42]

Active management of the third stage is favored by other clinicians because it shortens the length of the third stage (by an average of 9.8 minutes), decreases blood loss (by an average of 79 mL), and decreases the incidence of PPH although increasing maternal discomfort. Active management involves **early cord clamping, cord traction,** and administration of **prophylactic oxytocics** before completion of the third stage (as early as at the delivery of the anterior shoulder).[42] The need for manual removal of the placenta does not differ significantly between expectant and active management techniques. Common principles are as follows:

1. Collect cord gases and cord blood.
2. **Draining the umbilical cord** theoretically decreases the volume of the placenta, encouraging separation, is innocuous, and has been shown to shorten the third stage and reduce blood loss.

3. **Prophylactic intraumbilical oxytocin** (10 to 20 IU oxytocin in 10 to 20 mL saline) has been shown to shorten the third stage and to decrease blood loss in some studies.[42]

4. **Suckling** and **nipple stimulation** immediately after birth have not been shown to significantly reduce blood loss or the frequency of PPH.[44,106]

5. During any maneuvers that put traction on the cord, one hand **guards the uterus,** preventing prolapse of the uterus into the vaginal vault with suprapubic pressure.

6. **Signs of placental separation:** A gush of **blood** comes from the vagina, the **cord lengthens,** the **uterine shape** (assessed without massage) changes from discoid to globular, and the **uterus rises** in the abdomen as it is freed from the weight of the placenta. The **modified Brandt-Andrews maneuver** entails holding the cord taut at the introitus with one hand, pressing fingers of the other hand into the lower abdomen straight downward just above the symphysis pubis. If the cord shortens, it is still attached. If the cord length remains the same, it is separated.[214] If the placenta can be **felt in the vagina,** it is separated. To determine whether the placenta is separated, use the right hand to pull on the clamped cord, place the left hand palm down against the uterus, and give **quick, short tugs** on the cord. A "stitch" can be felt in any area where the placenta remains attached.

7. **Excessive kneading** of the uterus impedes the physiologic mechanism of placental detachment, causing incomplete placental separation and increasing blood loss.[60]

8. An **upright maternal position** facilitates the delivery of the placenta by engaging the force of gravity.[214]

9. **Asking the mother to bear down** may aid delivery of the placenta by increasing intra-abdominal pressure.[60]

10. Maintain steady pressure on the cord until the placenta is visualized at the introitus. **Gently lift the placenta** out of the vagina, following the curve of Carus.[79] When the amniotic side of the placenta presents at the introitus, the placenta is described as a Schultz placenta ("shiny **Schultz**"). A retroplacental clot has formed, and the placenta extrudes with membranes encasing that clot. When the maternal side of the placenta presents at the introitus, the placenta is described as a Duncan placenta ("dirty **Duncan**"). Separation has begun at the edge of this placenta, and the placenta descends into the vagina sideways.

11. If **membranes trail** behind the placenta, the weight of the placenta itself will usually deliver the membranes. If not, apply a Kelly clamp and gently rock the clamped membranes up and down and from side to side. Alternately, twist the membranes around and around in the same direction, eventually peeling the membranes off

the uterine wall. Observe for a "giving" sensation when membranes deliver completely, versus a "tearing" sensation when a portion is left behind. When membranes tear, immediately attempt to clasp the tail of membranes receding up the vagina with a clamp. If membranes may still be present in the uterus, a course of Methergine (0.2 mg PO q4h for 24 hours) may be given to enhance uterine expulsion of the remaining fragments.

12. If the **placenta is retained, intraumbilical** administration of 10 to 20 IU **oxytocin** mixed in 10 to 20 mL saline is believed by many researchers to be useful.[42]

13. If there is no bleeding, the best time for manual removal has not been established. The need for manual removal of the placenta does not differ significantly between expectant and active management techniques. Manual removal that is not emergent is associated with maternal discomfort, infection, and trauma. When the uterus is bleeding, however, **manual removal** is necessary: with the abdominal hand, grasp the fundus. Pass the other hand through the vagina and cervix into the uterus. Locate the edge of the placenta and move the ulnar side of the hand—with the back of the hand toward the uterine wall—under the edge of the placenta, shearing it off the wall like separating the pages of a book. Grasp and slowly withdraw the now-separated placenta. Many clinicians will explore the uterus again with a sponge to be certain all remnants are removed.[60]

14. **Complementary measures for the third stage of labor:**
   a. **See PPH complementary measures if indicated.**
   b. Some experts suggest **homeopathic** remedies in the third stage of labor.[92,103]
   c. **Chinese medicine:** Johnson[108] suggests **shiatsu** stimulation of the following points to facilitate delivery of the placenta: **Gallbladder 21, Bladder 60, Large Intestine 4,** and **Spleen 6. See charts and information on Chinese medicine, p. 559.**
   d. **Reflexology:** Stimulation of the uterine and pituitary zones on the feet may facilitate delivery of the placenta.[210] **See charts and information on reflexology, p. 567.**

Placental Inspection and Variations

Inspect the placenta and membranes soon after delivery to assess whether any part is retained, allowing immediate uterine exploration (see Figure 3-10). The appearance of the placenta and cord changes as it dries. Submit the placenta to pathology for examination and documentation for the following indications:

Maternal Indications: Infection or maternal systemic disease.

Fetal Indications: Multiple gestation, IUGR, hydrops, oligohydramnios, and stillbirth.

Placental Indications: Abnormalities noted on the examination.[28]

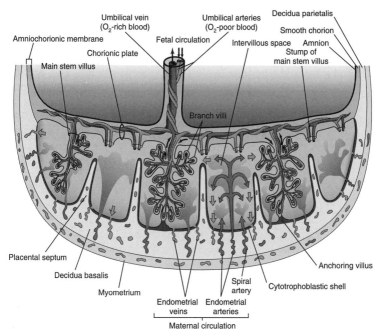

Figure 3-10 • A schematic drawing of a transverse section through a full-term placenta. The umbilical vein carries well-oxygenated blood to the fetus. The umbilical arteries carry poorly oxygenated fetal blood back to the placenta. Cotyledon consist of two or more main stem villi and their branches and are separated from each other by septa, which are projections of decidua basalis. (From Moore K, Persaud TVN: *Before we are born: essentials of embryology and birth defects,* ed 6, Philadelphia, 2003, Saunders.)

Description of the Normal Placenta

The placenta consists of 10 to 40 cotyledons, or lobes, divided by septa, or grooves, in a discoid shape, normally 1.5 to 3 cm thick. The average placental weight (without cord or membranes) is 480 ± 135 g (those delivered by cesarean section may weigh 100 mL more).[185] Fibrous, calcified areas where the spiral arteries have occluded because of age or impairment of placental circulation are normally present at term. Calcification, visualized by ultrasound, occurs in more than half of term placentas.[60] Beginning at the twenty-ninth week, these calcifications are not reliable indicators of placental maturity.[185] The marginal ring, at the edge of nearly every term placenta, is a dense, yellowish fibrous ring—an area of degeneration and necrosis.[60] Patches of white plaques 1 to 2 mm in size on the fetal side at the base of the cord are called squamous metaplasia (not a metaplastic process).[28] Present in 25% of placentas at term, these patches are thought to represent maturity. Subchorionic fibrin patches occur with maturity and are not clinically significant (2-mm spots or bosselations and plaques up to several centimeters in width) may be noted under the amnion on the fetal side of the placenta.[185]

Abnormal Variations on the Placenta

1. **Placental infarcts:** Initially dark red, then yellow, tan, and whitish in color. Infarctions in the placenta of a premature baby, on the maternal floor of the placenta (a recurring syndrome), or in the center of a placenta are abnormal.[28]

2. **Meconium staining, odor, paleness** (may accompany fetal anemia), or **dark redness** (may suggest polycythemia), **large sized placenta** (associated with diseases such as syphilis, diabetes, and erythroblastosis fetalis).[60,185]

3. **Succenturiate lobes:** May be indicated by torn blood vessels in the membranes. Part of the implantation site was less than optimal and atrophy occurred, isolating a lobe.[28]

4. **Edema, induration, or cysts:** Many lesions are palpable but not visible, so palpate the placenta for homogeneity.[185]

5. A **grossly disrupted placenta:** May suggest placenta accreta (see p. 204), which must be diagnosed from a uterine specimen after hysterectomy.[185]

6. Extensive **blood clots** (>200 cm^2) on the maternal surface: Stringy, gray, or gray-red-brown areas evolving to white and suggesting placental abruption, especially if they overlie an area of placental induration.[185]

7. **Misshapen placenta:** Occurs when implantation site is in the cornua or over a myoma or a uterine anomaly.[28]

8. **Thrombosis** of the fetal vessels: White streaks in the veins of the placenta. This is usually seen with a hypercoiled or an excessively lengthy cord.[28]

9. **Chorioangioma or hemangioma of the placenta:** A well-circumscribed hemorrhagic or fibrous mass bulging on the fetal side of the placenta. Small growths are generally asymptomatic; large growths are associated with hydramnios, antepartum hemorrhage, premature delivery, fetal to maternal hemorrhage, shunting in the fetal circulation (which can cause fetal heart failure), or consumptive coagulopathy and microangiopathic hemolytic anemia in the fetus.[28]

10. **Placenta bipartite or bilobed placenta:** Two placental masses exist for one fetus, with fetal blood vessels extending from one lobe to the other before uniting in the umbilical cord (or in the case of three masses, **tripartite or trilobed**). **Placenta duplex:** When the placenta has formed in two parts and the fetal vessels of each lobe remain distinct from the other lobes (or in the case of three parts, *triplex*).[90]

11. **Ring-shaped placenta:** A ring of placental tissue, sometimes horseshoe in shape, associated with antepartum and postpartum bleeding, as well as IUGR.[60]

12. **Membranaceous placenta or placenta diffusa:** Entire chorion is covered by a thin layer of chorionic villi. Often associated with antepartum hemorrhage. Separation may not occur, and hysterectomy may be necessary to stop hemorrhage.[90]

13. **Fenestrated placenta:** The central portion of a discoid placenta does not form, although the chorionic plate is usually intact.[60]

14. **Placenta extrachorialis:** Early in the pregnancy, when the chorionic villi regress from the whole chorionic plate, too much regression will cause compensatory proliferation of villi. These placentas are associated with a greater risk for early spontaneous abortion, antepartum hemorrhage, preterm delivery, perinatal death, and fetal malformations.[185]

   a. **Circumvallate placenta:** The chorionic plate (on the fetal side) is larger than the basal plate (on the maternal side). The center of the fetal side has a central depression surrounded by a raised, thick, grayish ring (a double fold of chorion and amnion with degenerated decidua and fibrin).[185]

   b. **Circummarginate placenta:** When the ring is flat, occurs at the edge of the placenta; it is also composed of degenerated decidua and fibrin.[185]

Description of the Normal Umbilical Cord

The normal cord is **inserted** centrally in the placenta. The average **cord length** is about 55 cm.[60] The **vessels** are normally two arteries and a vein. The vessels should be counted at least 3 cm away from the insertion into the placenta because 96% of cords have a fusion between the umbilical arteries near the placental insertion. **False knots** are a normal variation created by coiling. Average thickness is uniform and about 2 cm, reflecting the amount of water in the Wharton's jelly.[185] The mean **umbilical coiling** index is 0.21 ± 0.07 (standard deviation) per centimeter. Thirty percent of cords uncoiled early in gestation become coiled by delivery.[184]

Abnormal Variations on the Cord

1. **Length:** Long cords (>75 cm) carry a greater risk for true knots, thrombus formation, oligohydramnios, and cord compression. Short cords may be associated with abdominal wall defects and carry a greater risk for placental abruption and uterine inversion.[28]

2. **Vessel number:** Approximately 1% of infants are born with one artery and one vein. This is the most common congenital anomaly, and it does not have a genetic component. Other congenital anomalies will be present in 25% to 50% of these infants.[185] Four-vessel cords are of unknown significance.[60]

3. **Coiling:** Hypercoiled umbilical cords accompany more meconium staining, preterm birth, and operative delivery for fetal distress. Absence of coiling carries a greater risk for nuchal entanglement and suboptimal perinatal outcomes.[184]

4. True **knots, tumors, and calcifications: Constrictions** in the cord, usually located near the umbilicus, may be seen with intrauterine demise.[28] One- to 2-mm **yellow-green spots in the Wharton's jelly** may indicate candidiasis.[185] **Hematoma** is caused by the rupture of a dilated area of the vein or as a complication of cordocentesis. **"True" cysts** are small and form from remnants of tissue during the formation of the cord. **"False" cysts** are liquefactions of Wharton's jelly. **Edema** is present with an edematous fetus or a macerated stillborn fetus.[60] The cord is **thinner** in the presence of oligohydramnios, when the Wharton's jelly contains less water.[185]

5. **Cord insertion: Marginal insertion** of the cord or **battledore placenta** are insertions within 1.5 cm of the margin of the placenta.[185] **Velamentous insertion** of the cord is present when umbilical vessels travel through the membranes before uniting in the umbilical cord.[28] These vessels are vulnerable to pressure, tearing, or crossing in front of the presenting part (vasa previa), and there is an increased likelihood of the cord separating from the placenta during the third stage.[185] **Furcate insertion** occurs when the cord divides before insertion. **Interposition of the cord** exists when the cord runs between the amnion and chorion for a time before insertion.[28]

Description of Normal Membranes

The normal amnion and chorion are translucent, fused together, and appear to deliver completely.

Abnormal Variations on the Membranes

1. **Color variations: Opaqueness** may indicate chorioamnionitis. **Greenish staining** may indicate meconium staining, chorioamnionitis, or chronic hemorrhage. **Red-brown discoloration** may indicate an old abruption.[185] **Dusky-pink membranes** indicate hemolysis; may be seen after fetal demise.[28]

2. **Amnion nodosum:** One- to 5-mm fine, brownish yellow nodules on the membranes that can be rubbed off (occurs after prolonged oligohydramnios).[185]

3. **Absence of amnion:** When the amnion ruptures before fusing with the chorion, shrivels, and contracts as the fetus continues to grow inside the chorion. Remnants of amnion may become bands that can become tangled with the cord or fetus, causing anomalies called **amniotic band syndrome.**[185]

• COMPLICATIONS OF THE THIRD STAGE OF LABOR

Placenta Accreta

In placenta accreta, chorionic villi implant directly into the myometrium because of a deficiency of decidual tissue, causing abnormal adherence to the uterine wall.[28] When the chorionic villi actually invade the uterine wall, the condition is called *placenta increta.* When the villi go through the wall to the serosal layer, the condition is called *placenta percreta.* Placenta accreta is suspected at vaginal or cesarean delivery when the placenta cannot be manually removed. Heavy bleeding may occur after manual removal of fragments, and remaining fragments may be identified by ultrasound.[102]

Predisposing Factors: Unexplained elevated second-trimester MSAFP, advanced maternal age,[102] or two or more previous cesarean sections and an anterior or central placenta previa (40% risk).[7]

(m) *Management*

1. For a strong suspicion of placenta accreta (two or more previous cesarean sections and an anterior or central placenta previa), ACOG[7] suggests that the woman be informed of the risks of hysterectomy and blood transfusions and that preparations be made, including consideration of delivery location and timing; the ordering of blood products, clotting factors, and cell saver equipment; and obtaining a predelivery anesthesia consultation.
2. After a vaginal delivery when placenta accreta is suspected, immediately **consult** the physician and **prepare for hemorrhage and surgery.** Curettage or hysterectomy may be necessary.[102]
3. **Complementary measures for the retained placenta: see third stage measures listed previously.**
   a. Some experts recommend **homeopathic remedies** for the retained placenta.[59,103]
   b. **Acupuncture** may be used in the treatment of retained placenta.[43]

Postpartum Hemorrhage

A PPH is defined as a blood loss of 500 mL or more at delivery and within 24 hours. Bleeding may be caused by uterine atony (80%), episiotomy or lacerations of vagina and cervix, a ruptured or inverted uterus, retained products of conception, placenta accreta, and/or coagulation defects. PPH occurs in 4% of all deliveries.[90] Vaginal bleeding and a rising fundus are present. A contracted uterus and bright red vaginal bleeding indicate a genital tract laceration. The BP and pulse may not show alterations until a large amount of blood has been lost. Tachycardia and hypertension may develop in the normotensive woman as she compensates for lost volume. The hypertensive woman may appear normotensive while actually decompensating from blood loss.[60] Complications include maternal hypotensive shock and its attendant risks, the potential risks of blood transfusion, and Sheehan's syndrome (see p. 485). Worldwide, PPH is responsible for 30% of pregnancy-related deaths.[16]

Predisposing Factors[16,60]:

Amniotic fluid embolus	$MgSO_4$ administration
Coagulation disorders	Overdistended uterus

Conduction anesthesia

Episiotomy

High parity

Oxytocin use

History of PPH

Low implantation of the placenta
(decreased musculature in
lower uterine segment)[16]

Placental abruption

Precipitous labor

Prolonged labor

Prolonged or mismanaged third-
stage

Chorioamnionitis[60]

Uterine fibroids

Uterine rupture

Lab Findings: The average woman can lose 20% to 30% of her blood volume without a significant decrease in hct, whereas the woman with decreased volume, such as the woman with pregnancy-induced hypertension (PIH), may not tolerate a "normal" blood loss. The hb level decreases 1 to 1.5 g/dL and the hct 2% to 4% for every unit of blood lost. At 3 to 5 days, the plasma volume has begun to normalize. A hct reading on day 3 to 5 is suggested, with consultation for a value of ≤30 or symptoms (tachycardia, hypotension, pallor, and vertigo initially; fatigue, cool and clammy skin, impaired cognition, impaired lactation, and depression after 24 hours).[2]

ⓜ Management

See Figure 3-11, a decision tree for management of PPH.

Complementary Measures for Postpartum Hemorrhage

1. Experts recommend **homeopathy** remedies for PPH.[59,92,103,213]
2. **Chinese medicine:**
   a. **Acupuncture** may be used for hemorrhage.[43] Brucker[42] suggests **Spleen 1** to stop bleeding.
   b. **Acupressure** points to use for hemorrhage are on both sides of the lower ankle near the tendon **(Bladder 60** and **Spleen 6);** pinch firmly on both ankles.[205]
   See charts and information on Chinese medicine, p. 559.
3. **Herbs:** See p. 53 for herbs that are suggested prophylactically during the last months of gestation to tone the uterus and decrease the risk of PPH. The following herbs may be used singly or in combination at the time of bleeding: **bayberry (myrtle)**[42,156,160,205]: ½ tsp in tea[205] or 2 capsules[156]; **nettles**[42,156,160,201]: 1 to 4 mL tincture.[98] **Shepherd's purse** is known as a remedy for bleeding wounds*: ¼ cup steeped in 1 to 2 cups boiling water with honey, strain and give sips after placenta or at onset hemorrhage[205]; or 20 to 40 drops of the tincture of the fresh plant in flower to stop bleeding in 5 to 30 seconds by promoting contractions.[2] **See information on herbs, p. 563.**

---

*References 2, 42, 71, 81, 116, 127, 156, 160, 161, 205.

Uterine Inversion

Uterine inversion after delivery of the infant causes life-threatening hemorrhage without prompt treatment.[60] Infectious morbidity is common.[188]

Predisposing Factors[188]:

Fundal pressure	Short cord
Injudicious use of oxytocin	Strong traction on a cord attached
Macrosomia	to an unseparated placenta
$MgSO_4$ administration	implanted in the fundus
Placenta accreta	Uterine anomalies
Primiparity	Uterine atony

Uterine inversion may occur despite the absence of risk factors.[16]

ⓜ Management

1. Immediately **summon the obstetrician and anesthesia** personnel.
2. **DO NOT separate the placenta before replacement** (increases blood loss).[188]
3. To **attempt immediate replacement, push the fundus up** through the vagina and cervix using the palm and fingers; hold in place for several minutes.[143]
4. If the uterus was not successfully replaced in step 3, the **uterus with placenta attached is placed into the vagina.**[60]
5. Secure **two large-bore IV lines** and administer lactated Ringer's solution and whole blood.[143]
6. Administer **anesthesia. Tocolytics** may be used to relax the uterus so that it can be repositioned more easily. The **obstetrician** assumes management.[60]
7. **Oxytocin** is given after the uterus is replaced.[60]
8. Continue to **observe vaginally for recurrence** of the inversion.[60]
9. Consider **blood replacement** and **antibiotic** coverage.[188]
10. Inversion may recur with **subsequent deliveries,** and **caution** is advised in third stage management of those **labors.**[188]

• THE FOURTH STAGE OF LABOR

Newborn Behavior

When the unmedicated newborn is placed directly onto the mother's breast, it gives a birth cry that lasts from 30 seconds to 7 minutes, opens its eyes, and gradually (within the first hour) moves toward the mother's areola, massages the breast with his or her hands, finds the nipple and sucks. The hand massage, skin-to-skin contact and sucking releases oxytocin in the mother, which enhances attachment and milk production. At about 2 hours after birth, the infant falls asleep.[131,168] How the baby attaches to the areola this first time may predict the success of subsequent feedings and the duration of breastfeeding.[111] The less separation from the mother in the first 90 minutes of life, the less the infant cries.[51]

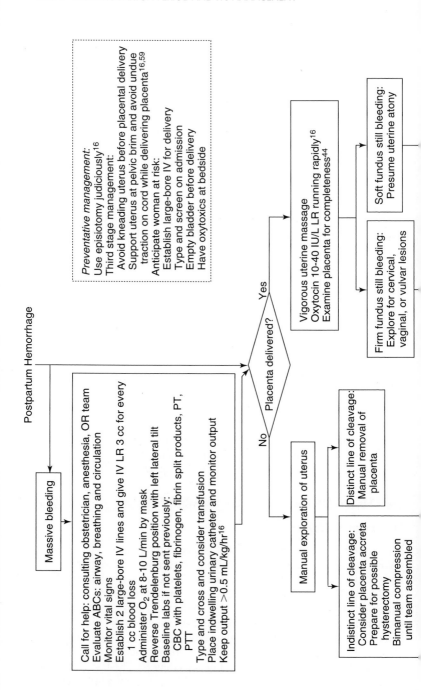

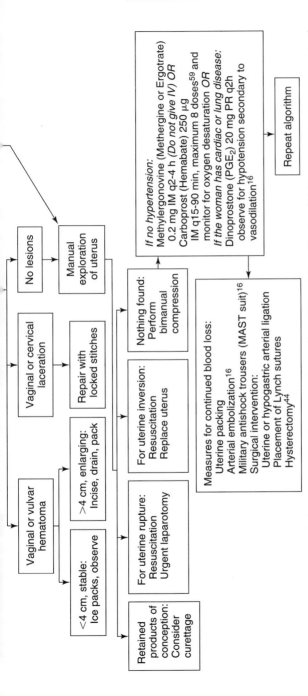

Figure 3-11 • Decision tree for midwifery management of postpartum hemorrhage. (Adapted from Morrison EH: Common peripartum emergencies, *Am Fam Physician* Nov 1, 1998, published by The American Academy of Family Physicians at *http://www.aafp.org/afp/981101ap/.morrison.html.*)

The first hours after birth are believed to be a sensitive period during which the mother and father may bond with the newborn. If immediate bonding is prevented, however, the human is felt to be highly adaptable, and bonding may occur in many other ways. Bonding is noted to occur in as many ways as there are mother-baby pairs.[114]

Maternal-Infant Attachment

Maternal-infant bonding or attachment determines the ability of the infant to form healthy attachments in the future. The consistency and emotional availability of the mother, her sensitivity to the infant and ability to offer appropriate stimulation influence the bonding process. Response from the newborn, such as movements and eye contact, also facilitate this attachment. Recent research has identified oxytocin as one of the hormones involved in attachment.[105] Skin-to-skin contact, infant hand massage of the breast, and suckling releases oxytocin and may enhance bonding.[131,168] The father's positive feeling about the infant positively affects maternal-infant attachment, as does parity, maternal confidence, and social support.[148]

Maternal behaviors shortly after delivery may predict the quality of the relationship a year later. Positive attachment behaviors include close contact with the baby, eye contact, holding the baby "en face," examining the baby, touching the child lovingly as an expression of caring and not just to examine, talking lovingly to the baby in tone and contact, and appearing happy much of the time.[41] Obstetric units must prioritize enhancement of maternal-infant attachment by encouraging skin-to-skin contact, breastfeeding as soon as possible after birth, encouraging rooming-in, and maintaining flexible visiting hours for the father. Parental bonding behavior is observed. When the attachment process appears to be at risk, notify pediatrics and arrange home visits.[138]

Neonatal behavioral states reflect the function of the autonomic and central nervous systems. Behavioral states of the normal newborn include deep sleep, REM sleep, drowsiness, alert with eyes open, focusing and following objects (about 10% of the first week of life[114]), active alert with eyes open and thrusting extremities, and crying. The Brazelton Neonatal Behavioral Assessment Scale may be performed at 2 weeks and reflects the ability of the infant to habituate, attend and respond to the environment, self-quiet, interact socially, and display various behavioral states and motor function maturity.

• COMPLICATIONS THAT MAY OCCUR THROUGHOUT THE INTRAPARTUM PERIOD

Amniotic Fluid Embolism

The most common cause of peripartum death, amniotic fluid embolism (AFE) may result when a breach occurs between the maternal and fetal circulations. Amniotic fluid and debris escape into the maternal circulation. This event, which is not uncommon, is usually innocuous. In some women, however, it causes an anaphylactic-like reaction rather than being an embolic-like event. Clinical and hemodynamic findings in AFE, anaphylactic shock, and septic shock suggest a similar physiologic mechanism.[53] The body releases catecholamines to maintain pressure and perfusion, and uterine hypertonus, previously considered the cause of the AFE, occurs.[60] Predisposing factors include an allergy history and male fetus. Neither prolonged labor nor oxytocin use increases the risk.[53]

AFE is heralded by the abrupt onset of hypotension, hypoxia, and consumptive coagulopathy, fetal distress, seizures, and/or uterine atony.[60,79] It may occur during labor, after vaginal delivery, or during cesarean section after delivery of the baby. Maternal mortality rate is 60%; 92% of the survivors are profoundly neurologically impaired. Neonatal survival is 70%, with almost 50% being neurologically impaired.[53]

Ⓜ Management

1. **Summon emergency help.** Immediately **consult and refer** to the physician.
2. Initiate **CPR.**[60]
3. The obstetrician and medical team provide **supportive treatment** and emergency **cesarean section** as soon as possible if the fetus is viable.[53]

Postdates Pregnancy Intrapartum Management

Pregnancy exceeding 42 weeks is considered postdates. About 10% of all pregnancies deliver after 42 weeks.[18] This situation may be recurrent. Complications include an increased perinatal mortality rate, oligohydramnios, cord compression, meconium-stained amniotic fluid,[60] and postmaturity syndrome in 25% (abnormal FHR tracings; IUGR due to placental insufficiency).[150]

Ⓜ Management

ANTEPARTUM MANAGEMENT. See p. 103.
INTRAPARTUM MANAGEMENT
1. **Admit early** in labor.[60]
2. **Monitor continuously.**[60]
3. **Visualize the fluid** (by AROM if necessary) well before delivery to allow controlled management of meconium-stained amniotic fluid, for which this mother is at risk.[60]
4. **Amnioinfusion** may ease some of the cord compression, reducing variables. It will also dilute meconium if present, decreasing meconium aspiration.[79] (See p. 577.)

Uterine Rupture

Uterine rupture, or separation of the uterine wall, represents the reopening and extension of an old uterine scar in 59%. The classical uterine scar that will rupture will do so before labor in 33%. Uterine incisions located in the noncontractile portion of the uterus rarely rupture before labor. Rupture of a classical incision is more likely to result in severe hemorrhage and perinatal morbidity and mortality than is rupture of a low transverse scar.[60] The bladder ruptures in 0.05% to 11.7%. Dehiscence may occur with prolapse of the umbilical cord through the ruptured uterine wall, and the fetus as well as the placenta may be extruded into the abdomen.[147] One in 8000 to 15,000 women have a spontaneous rupture of an unscarred uterus.[140] One in 200 women attempting vaginal birth after cesarean section (VBAC) will have a uterine rupture.[12] A fetal mortality rate of 50% to 75% is seen with rupture and expulsion from the uterus into the abdomen.[60]

Sudden, severe FHR decelerations are generally the most reliable sign of uterine rupture. The IUPC may lose pressure; contractions may stop, and sudden sharp abdominal and/or rectal pain may be felt by the mother. Abdominal or vaginal palpation of fetal parts, loss of fetal station, change in dilation, and vaginal bleeding are found on vaginal exam. Maternal anxiety, decreased level of consciousness, and circulatory collapse (hypotension and tachycardia) follow.[60]

Risk Factors[33,60]:

Breech version and extraction
Congenital anomaly of the uterus
High parity
History of invasive
 hydatidiform mole
Hypertonicity
Midforceps delivery
Midpregnancy termination
Midtrimester version
Oxytocin use
Placenta accreta

Previous cesarean section (classical
 cesarean scar increases risk
 by several times)
Prolonged labor
Prostaglandin gel use
Shoulder dystocia
Trauma to the uterus
Use of forceps
Uterine curettage
Uterine perforation during surgery

In many cases, women have no risk factors.[140]

m *Management*

1. When uterine rupture is suspected during labor, notify the **obstetrician and anesthesia and pediatrics staff** and prepare for **immediate cesarean delivery.**[143]
2. Give the mother **oxygen,** place her in the **left lateral tilt position,** elevate her legs, and start **two large-bore IV lines.**
3. **Type and crossmatch blood** or order O-negative blood from the blood bank.
4. **Prepare for maternal hypovolemic shock** and for possible **hysterectomy.**
5. **Antibiotic therapy** is administered after delivery.[60]
6. Uterine rupture found on intrauterine exploration to be the source of **bleeding after delivery** also requires **immediate surgical intervention.**[143]

Vaginal Birth After Cesarean Section

ACOG[11] recommends that the mode of delivery should be chosen based on the clinical circumstances and the patient's choice after appropriate counseling of potential risks. At this time, many VBAC consents warn that the fetus may suffer permanent injury or death. Delivery of the woman attempting VBAC should be confined to medical centers where emergencies can be quickly handled, weighing into the analysis the fact that some women may opt to deliver at home rather than travel far to deliver.[72] The ACNM[3] has issued a position statement strongly supporting the practice of VBAC for appropriately selected women and stating that midwives are qualified to care for these women. The midwife provides heightened surveillance of FHR patterns, medical consultation, emergency care, and informed consent.

Vaginal Birth After Cesarean Section Success Statistics:
- Sixty percent to 80% of women will have a successful VBAC.
- After a cesarean section for a nonrecurring indication (e.g., breech), women deliver vaginally at the same rate as if they had never had a cesarean.
- A history of vaginal birth before a cesarean birth increases the likelihood of vaginal delivery.[30]
- The woman delivered by cesarean at full dilation in the previous pregnancy has a 73% likelihood of vaginal delivery.[104]
- The woman whose first cesarean was for dystocia has a 50% to 70% probability of delivering vaginally.[191]
- The woman who has had a cesarean section followed by a successful VBAC has a shorter labor and a better chance of delivering vaginally with a third pregnancy than does the woman who has delivered vaginally first and then by cesarean.[46]
- Successful VBACs are experienced by 75% of women with more than one previous cesarean delivery.[178]
- Of 92 patients with twin pregnancies who had a history of cesarean section in one study, 70% delivered both twins vaginally, with no uterine ruptures and no increase in maternal or perinatal morbidity or mortality.[141]

Benefits of Vaginal Birth After Cesarean Section: The woman who delivers vaginally has less morbidity, fewer blood transfusions, fewer postpartum infections, shorter hospital stay, and no increase in perinatal morbidity,[11] and she may experience emotional satisfaction from achieving vaginal birth.

Maternal Complications: A meta-analysis of 15 studies and 47,682 women done in 2000 found that women undergoing a trial of labor (TOL) were more likely to have a uterine rupture than women undergoing an elective repeat cesarean section (odds ratio [OR] 2.10). Maternal mortality rate was the same in both groups. Fetal or neonatal death (OR 1.71) and 5-minute Apgar scores <7 (OR 2.24) occurred more often in the TOL group. Women who underwent elective cesarean were more likely to have fever (OR 0.70), require transfusion (OR 0.57), and undergo hysterectomy (OR 0.39).[145]

A retrospective study in 2001 found a uterine rupture rate of 1.6 per 1000 among women undergoing repeat cesarean section without labor. Among women attempting VBAC undergoing prostaglandin induction, 24.5 of 1000 had uterine rupture (relative risk, 15.6); among women attempting VBAC undergoing oxytocin induction, 7.7 of 1000 women had a ruptured uterus (relative risk, 4.9); among women attempting VBAC undergoing spontaneous labor, 5.2 of 1000 women had a ruptured uterus (relative risk, 3.3).[126] Uterine rupture occurs in 4% to 9% of women who have a classical uterine scar, in 4% to 9% of those with a T-shaped scar, and in 0.2% to 1.5% of those with a low transverse scar. Uterine rupture potentially results in death or hysterectomy for the mother.[227] The more time that has elapsed since the cesarean, the lower the chance of uterine rupture.[70] Hysterectomy and operative injury occur more often among those women who fail a TOL than among those who choose a repeat cesarean delivery.[11]

Neonatal Complications: Respiratory morbidity is significantly higher among infants born by elective repeat cesarean section, with 6% suffering from transient tachypnea—apparently because fetal maturity is not proven before the surgery is performed. Those born after a TOL have significantly more sepsis. Uterine rupture may result in death or neurologic damage for the fetus; however, the neonatal outcomes ultimately do not differ from those of infants born by repeat cesarean section without labor.[40]

Contraindications to Vaginal Birth After Cesarean Section: According to ACOG,[11] contraindications include prior classical or T-shaped incision or other transfundal uterine surgery, a contracted pelvis, inability to perform emergency cesarean birth facility, and other medical or obstetric contraindications for vaginal delivery.

Relative Contraindications to Vaginal Births After Cesarean Section: According to ACOG,[11] VBAC in the woman with multiple previous low transverse cesarean sections, an unknown uterine scar, breech presentation, twin gestation, postterm pregnancy, or suspected macrosomia is controversial.

Ⓜ Management

1. When possible, obtain **old records** and document that the uterine scar was in the lower uterine segment. **Discuss risks and benefits** with the woman, and she decides whether she will attempt a TOL. Obtain a signed **consent** and document the discussion. Inform the woman with an **unknown scar** of the risks and benefits of a TOL, and she and the backup physician or practice protocol will determine delivery route.[11] The physician is involved in this process according to practice protocol.

2. **External cephalic version** can be conducted successfully on the woman with a uterine scar whose fetus is breech.[11]
3. Delivery should occur in a **facility** where OR and anesthesia personnel are immediately available to provide emergency care.[11]
4. **Early admission** is required for spontaneous rupture of membranes or contractions.[11]
5. Consider **continuous EFM.**
6. Consider establishing a **heparin lock.**[11]
7. **Induction** is not contraindicated, although oxytocin has been associated with higher rates of uterine rupture. Induction with prostaglandins, however, is contraindicated in the woman with a history of cesarean section.[6]
8. **Epidural anesthesia** is not contraindicated.[11]
9. Closely observe **labor progress.**[11]
10. Observe for **signs and symptoms of uterine rupture** (fetal distress, abdominal pain, ascent of the fetus, vaginal bleeding).[11]
11. After delivery, **exploration of the uterus** for scar integrity is controversial. There is no evidence that a uterine dehiscence heals better if it is surgically repaired. If the woman is bleeding heavily after a delivery, both the old scar and the entire genital tract must be closely evaluated and repaired as appropriate.[11] When a **nonbleeding uterine dehiscence** is noted on intrauterine examination after VBAC, repair is not necessary but future deliveries should probably be by cesarean section.[60]

• REFERENCES

1. Ader L, Hansson B, Wallin G: Parturition pain treated by intracutaneous injections of sterile water, *Pain* 41:133-138, 1990.
2. Akins S: Postpartum hemorrhage: a 90s approach to an age-old problem, *J Nurse Midwifery* 39:123S-134S, 1994.
3. American College of Nurse-Midwives (ACNM): Position statement: Vaginal birth after cesarean delivery, *Quickening* 32:16, 2001.
4. ACNM: Intrapartum nutrition, *J Nurse Midwifery* 44:124-128, 1999.
5. American College of Obstetricians and Gynecologists (ACOG): *Analgesia and cesarean delivery rates,* Committee on Obstetric Practice, Committee Opinion No. 269, Washington, DC, 2002, ACOG.
6. ACOG: *Induction of labor for vaginal birth after cesarean delivery,* Washington, DC, Committee on Obstetric Practice, Committee Opinion No. 271, 2002, ACOG.
7. ACOG: *Placenta accreta,* Committee on Obstetric Practice, Committee Opinion No. 266, Washington, DC, 2002, ACOG.
8. ACOG: *Assessment of risk factors for preterm birth,* Washington, DC, Practice Bulletin No. 31, 2001, ACOG.
9. ACOG: *Fetal macrosomia,* Washington, DC, Practice Bulletin No. 22, 2000, ACOG.
10. ACOG: *Response to Searle's drug warning on misoprostol,* Washington, DC, Committee on Obstetric Practice, Committee Opinion No. 248, 2000, ACOG.
11. ACOG: *Vaginal birth after previous cesarean delivery,* Washington, DC, Practice Bulletin No. 5, 1999, ACOG.
12. ACOG: *ACOG strongly supports VBAC, but urges caution,* Washington, DC, 1998, ACOG (news release) *http://www.acog.com/from_home/publications/press_releases/998 vbac.htm.*

13. ACOG: *Antenatal corticosteroid therapy for fetal maturation,* Committee on Obstetric Practice, Committee Opinion No. 210, Washington, DC, 1998, ACOG.

14. ACOG: *Inappropriate use of the terms fetal distress and birth asphyxia,* Committee on Obstetric Practice, Committee Opinion No. 197, Washington, DC, 1998, ACOG.

15. ACOG: *Monitoring during induction of labor with dinoprostone,* Committee on Obstetric Practice, Committee Opinion No. 209, Washington, DC, 1998, ACOG.

16. ACOG: *Postpartum hemorrhage,* Educational Bulletin No. 243, Washington, DC, 1998, ACOG.

17. ACOG: Premature rupture of membranes, *Int J Obstet Gynecol* 63:75-84, 1998, ACOG.

18. ACOG: *Management of postterm pregnancy,* Practice Patterns No. 6, Washington, DC, 1997, ACOG.

19. ACOG: *Shoulder dystocia,* Practice Patterns No. 7, Washington, DC, 1997, ACOG.

20. ACOG: *Use and abuse of the Apgar score,* Committee on Obstetric Practice, Committee Opinion No. 174, Washington, DC, 1996, ACOG.

21. ACOG: *Fetal heart rate patterns: monitoring, interpretation, and management,* Technical Bulletin No. 207, Washington, DC, 1995, ACOG.

22. ACOG: *Preterm labor,* Technical Bulletin No. 206, Washington, DC, 1995, ACOG.

23. ACOG: *Fetal and neonatal neurologic injury,* Technical Bulletin No. 163, Washington, DC, 1992, ACOG.

24. ACOG: *Dystocia,* Technical Bulletin No. 217, Washington, DC, 1989, ACOG.

25. ACOG: *Management of the breech presentation,* Washington, DC, Technical Bulletin No. 95, Washington, DC, 1986, ACOG.

26. Albers LL, Schiff M, Gorwoda JG: The length of active labor in normal pregnancies, *Obstet Gynecol* 87:355-359, 1996.

27. Albrechtsen S et al: Perinatal mortality in breech presentation sibships, *Obstet Gynecol* 92:775-780, 1998.

28. Baergen RN: Macroscopic examination of the placenta immediately following birth, *J Nurse Midwifery* 42:393-402, 1997.

29. Balch JF, Balch PA: *Prescription for nutritional healing,* ed 2, Garden City Park, NY, 1997, Avery.

30. Ben Shachar I, Weinstein D: High risk pregnancy outcome by route of delivery, *Curr Opin Obstet Gynecol* 10:447-452, 1998.

31. Benhamou D: Epidural anesthesia during labor: continuous infusion or patient-controlled administration? *Eur J Obstet Gynecol Reprod Biol* 59:S55-S56, 1995.

32. Benirschke K: Fetal consequences of amniotic fluid meconium, *Contemporary OB/GYN* 46:76-83, 2001.

33. Benito CW et al: A case control study of uterine rupture during pregnancy, *Am J Obstet Gynecol* 174:485, 1996.

34. Berg-Lekas ML, Hogberg U, Winkvist A: Familial occurrence of dystocia, *Am J Obstet Gynecol* 179:117-121, 1998.

35. Bishop EH: Pelvic scoring for elective induction, *Obstet Gynecol* 24:267, 1964.

36. Blanchette HA, Nayak S, Erasmus S: Comparison of the safety and efficacy of intravaginal misoprostol (prostaglandin E1) with those of dinoprostone (prostaglandin E2) for cervical ripening and induction of labor in a community hospital, *Am J Obstet Gynecol* 180:1551-1559, 1999.

37. Bloom R, Cropley C: *Textbook of neonatal resuscitation,* Elk Grove Village, Ill, 1996, American Heart Association and American Academy of Pediatrics.

38. Bloom SL et al: Lack of effect of walking on labor and delivery *N Engl J Med* 339: 76-79, 1998.

39. Bofill JA et al: Nulliparous active labor, epidural anesthesia and cesarean delivery for dystocia, *Am J Obstet Gynecol* 177:1465-1470, 1997.

40. Boyers SP, Gilbert WM: Elective repeat caesarean section versus trial of labor: the neonatologist's view, *Lancet* 351:155, 1998.

41. Britton HL, Gronwaldt V, Britton JR: Maternal postpartum behaviors and mother-infant relationship during the first year of life, *J Pediatr* 138:905-909, 2001.

42. Brucker MC: Management of the third stage of labor: an evidence-based approach, *J Midwifery Womens Health* 46:381-392, 2001.

43. Budd S: Acupuncture. In Tiran D, Mack S, editors: *Complementary therapies for pregnancy and childbirth,* ed 2, Edinburgh, 2000, Baillière Tindall.

44. Bullough CH, Msuku RS, Karonde L: Early suckling and postpartum haemorrhage: controlled trial in deliveries by traditional birth attendants, *Lancet* 342:522-525, 1989.

45. Carter BS, McNabb F, Merenstein GB: Prospective validation of a scoring system for predicting neonatal morbidity after acute perinatal asphyxia, *J Pediatr* 132:619-623, 1998.

46. Caughey AB et al: Trial of labor after cesarean: the effect of previous vaginal delivery, *Am J Obstet Gynecol* 179:938-941, 1998.

47. Chamberlain G, Steer P: ABC of labour care: unusual presentations and positions and multiple pregnancy, *BMJ* 318:1192-1194, 1999.

48. Chamberlain G, Steer P: ABC of labour care: obstetric emergencies, *BM J* 318:1342-1345, 1999.

49. Chelmow D, Kilpatrick SJ, Laros RK: Maternal and neonatal outcomes after prolonged latent phase, *Obstet Gynecol* 81:486-491, 1993.

50. Chestnut DH: Epidural anesthesia and the incidence of cesarean section, *Anesthesiology* 87:172-175, 1997.

51. Christensson K et al: Separation distress call in the human neonate in the absence of maternal body contact, *Obstet Gynecol Survey* 51:86-87, 1996.

52. Clark A et al: The influence of epidural anesthesia on cesarean delivery rates: a randomized, prospective clinical trial, *Am J Obstet Gynecol* 179:1527-1533, 1998.

53. Clark SL et al: Amniotic fluid embolism: analysis of the National Registry, *Am J Obstet Gynecol* 172:1158-1169, 1995.

54. Cleary GM, Wiswell TE: Meconium-stained amniotic fluid and the meconium aspiration syndrome, *Pediatr Clin North Am* 45:511-527, 1998.

55. CNM Data Group: Oral intake in labor: trends in midwifery practice, *J Nurse Midwifery* 44:135-138, 1999.

56. Cook A, Wilcox G: Pressuring pain, *AWHONN Lifelines* 1:36-41, 1997.

57. Copel JA et al: The clinical significance of the irregular fetal heart rhythm, *Am J Obstet Gynecol* 182:813-819, 2000.

58. Creasy RK, Resnick R: *Maternal-fetal medicine principles and practice,* Philadelphia, 1994, WB Saunders.

59. Cummings B, Tiran D: Homeopathy for pregnancy and childbirth. In Tiran D, Mack S, editors: *Complementary therapies for pregnancy and childbirth,* ed 2, Edinburgh, 2000, Baillière Tindall.

60. Cunningham FG et al: *Williams obstetrics,* ed 20, Stamford, Conn, 1997, Appleton and Lange.

61. Daniel Y et al: Outcome of 494 singleton breech deliveries in a tertiary center, *Am J Obstet Gynecol* 174:485, 1996.

62. Dashe JS et al: Epidural analgesia and intrapartum fever: placental findings, *Obstet Gynecol* 93:341-344, 1999.

63. Diegmann EK, Andrews CM, Niemczura CA: The length of the second stage of labor in uncomplicated, nulliparous African American and Puerto Rican women, *J Midwifery Womens Health* 43:67-71, 2000.

64. Draper ES et al: Prediction of survival for preterm births by weight and gestational age, *BMJ* 319:1093-1097, 1999.

65. Dumoulin JG, Foulkes JEB: Ketonuria during labour, *Br J Obstet Gynaecol* 91:97-98, 1984.

66. Eberle RL et al: The effect of maternal position on fetal heart rate during epidural or intrathecal labor anesthesia, *Am J Obstet Gynecol* 179:150-155, 1998.

67. Edmunds J: Prolonged labor: past & present, *Midwifery Today* 31:13-14, 1998.

68. Edson E et al: Preventing perineal trauma during childbirth: a systematic review, *Obstet Gynecol* 95:464-471, 2000.

69. El Halta V: Preventing prolonged labor, *Midwifery Today* 31:22-27, 1998.

70. Esposito MA, Menihan CA, Malee MP: Association of interpregnancy interval with uterine scar failure in labor: a case-control study, *Am J Obstet Gynecol* 183:1180-1183, 2000.

71. Feral C: Natural remedies, *Midwifery Today* 26:35-38, 1993.
72. Flamm BL: Once a cesarean, always a controversy, *Obstet Gynecol* 90:312-315, 1997.
73. Flynn AM et al: Ambulation in labor, *BMJ* 2:591-593, 1978.
74. Food and Drug Administration (FDA): Major changes to Cytotec labeling, *http://www.fda.gov/medwatch/SAFETY/2002/cytotec_changes.PDF.*
75. Foong LC et al: Membrane sweeping in conjunction with labor induction, *Obstet Gynecol* 96:539-542, 2000.
76. Fraser WD et al and the Canadian early amniotomy study group: Effect of early amniotomy on the risk of dystocia in nulliparous women, *N Engl J Med* 328:1145-1149, 1993.
77. Friedman EA: *Labor: clinical evaluation and management,* ed 2, New York, 1978, Appleton-Century-Crofts.
78. Fynes M et al: Effect of second vaginal delivery on anorectal physiology and faecal continence: a prospective study, *Lancet* 354:983-986, 1999.
79. Gabbe SG, Niebl JR, Simpson JL, editors: *Obstetrics: normal & problem pregnancies,* ed 3, New York, 1996, Churchill Livingstone.
80. Galan H: Meconium-stained amniotic fluid: meaning and management, *OBG Manage* July 1999, *http://www.obgmanagement.com/799/cme799.html.*
81. Gardner J: *Healing yourself,* ed 7, Trumansburg, NY, 1982, Crossing Press.
82. Garite TJ et al: The influence of elective amniotomy on fetal heart rate patterns and the course of labor in term patients: a randomized study, *Am J Obstet Gynecol* 168: 1827-1832, 1993.
83. Gherman RB et al: Analysis of McRoberts' maneuver by x-ray pelvimetry, *Obstet Gynecol* 95:43-47, 2000.
84. Ghidini A, Korker V: Fetal complication after external cephalic version at term: case report and literature review, *J Mat-Fetal Med* 8:190-192, 1999.
85. Gordon JD et al: *Obstetrics gynecology & infertility,* Glen Cove, NY, 1998, Scrub Hill Press.
86. Gordon NP et al: Effects of providing hospital-based doulas in health maintenance organization hospitals, *Obstet Gynecol* 93:422-426, 1999.
87. Grady D: Premature birth treatment hailed, *The Press Democrat* (Santa Rosa, Calif) Feb 7, 2003.
88. Griffith HW: *Healing herbs: the essential guide,* Tucson, Ariz, 2000, Fisher Books.
89. Gupta JK, Nikodem VC: Women's position during second stage of labour, *Birth* 28:62, 2001.
90. Hacker NF, Moore JG: *Essentials of obstetrics and gynecology,* ed 3, Philadelphia, 1998, WB Saunders.
91. Halpern SH et al: Effect of epidural vs. parenteral opioid analgesia on the progress of labor: a meta-analysis, *JAMA* 280:2105-2110, 1998.
92. Hanafin MJ: *An introduction to homeopathy,* San Francisco, 1998, ACNM, lecture handout and notes.
93. Handa VL, Laros RK: Active-phase arrest in labor: predictors of cesarean section delivery in a nulliparous population, *Obstet Gynecol* 81:758-763, 1993.
94. Heffner LJ et al: Clinical and environmental predictors of preterm labor, *Obstet Gynecol* 81:750-757, 1993.
95. Herman NL et al: Analgesia, pruritis, and ventilation exhibit a dose-response relationship in parturients receiving intrathecal fentanyl during labor, *Anesth Analg* 89:378-383, 1999.
96. Hodnett ED: Pain and women's satisfaction with the experience of childbirth: a systematic review, *Am J Obstet Gynecol* 186:S160-S172, 2002.
97. Hoffmann D: *The complete illustrated holistic herbal,* Boston, 1996, Element Books.
98. Hoffmann D: *The holistic herbal,* Findhorn, Scotland, 1985, Findhorn Press.
99. Holt RO, Diehl SJ, Wright JW: Station and cervical dilation at epidural placement in predicting cesarean risk, *Obstet Gynecol* 93:281-284, 1999.
100. Hoult IJ, MacLennan AH, Carrie LES: Lumbar epidural analgesia in labor: relation to fetal malposition and instrumental delivery, *BMJ* 1:14-16, 1977.

101. Huang WL et al: Effect of corticosteroids on brain growth in fetal sheep, *Obstet Gynecol* 94:213-218, 1999.
102. Hung TH et al: Risk factors for placenta accreta, *Obstet Gynecol* 93:545-550, 1999.
103. Idarius B: *The homeopathic childbirth manual,* Talmage, Calif, 1999, Idarius Press.
104. Impey L, O'Herlihy C: First delivery after cesarean delivery for strictly defined cephalopelvic disproportion, *Obstet Gynecol* 92:799-803, 1998.
105. Insel TR: Toward a neurobiology of attachment, *Rev Gen Psychol* 4:176-185, 2000.
106. Irons DW, Sriskandabalan P, Bullough CH: A simple alternative to parenteral oxytocics for the third stage of labor, *Int Gynaecol Obstet* 46:15-18, 1994.
107. Ismail MA et al: Comparison of vaginal and cesarean section delivery for fetuses in breech presentation, *J Perinat Med* 27:339-351, 1999.
108. Johnson E: Shiatsu. In Tiran D, Mack S, editors: *Complementary therapies for pregnancy and childbirth,* Philadelphia, 2000, Harcourt.
109. Jonquil SG: Sterile water blocks for back pain in labor, *Midwifery Today* 30:18-19, 1997.
110. Katz VL, Bows WA: Meconium aspiration syndrome: reflection on a murky subject, *Am J Obstet Gynecol* 166:171-183, 1992.
111. Kennell J, McGrath S: What babies teach us: the essential link between baby's behavior and mother's biology, *Birth* 28:20-21, 2001.
112. Kilpatrick SJ: Therapeutic interventions for oligohydramnios: amnioinfusion and maternal hydration, *Clin Obstet Gynecol* 40:328-336, 1997.
113. King T: Epidural anesthesia in labor, *J Nurse Midwifery* 42:377-388, 1997.
114. Klaus M, Kennel J, Klaus PH: *Bonding: building the foundations of secure attachment and independence,* New York, 1995, Addison-Wesley Longman.
115. Klein MC et al: Relationship of episiotomy to perineal trauma and morbidity, sexual dysfunction, and pelvic floor relaxation, *Am J Obstet Gynecol* 171:591-598, 1994.
116. Koehler N: *Artemis speaks: V.B.A.C. stories & natural childbirth information,* Occidental, Calif, 1985, Jerald R. Brown.
117. Kolderup L et al: Misoprostol is more efficacious for labor induction than prostaglandin E2, but is it associated with more risk? *Am J Obstet Gynecol* 180:1543-1550, 1999.
118. Kurokawa JS, Zilkoski MW: Use of intrathecal analgesia in a rural hospital: case studies, *J Nurse Midwifery* 41:338-342, 1996.
119. Labrecque M et al: Randomized control of prevention of perineal trauma by perineal massage during pregnancy, *Am J Obstet Gynecol* 180:593-600, 1999.
120. Leiberman E: No free lunch on labor day, *J Nurse Midwifery* 44:394-398, 1999.
121. Leiberman E et al: Association of epidural anesthesia with cesarean section in nulliparas, *Obstet Gynecol* 88:993-1000, 1996.
122. Letko MD: Understanding the Apgar score, *J Obstet Gynecol Neonatal Nurs* 25:299-303, 1996.
123. Lockwood CJ, Kuczynski E: Markers of risk for preterm delivery, *J Perinat Med* 27: 5-20, 1999.
124. Loftus JR, Hill H, Cohen SE: Placental transfer and neonatal effects of epidural sufentanil and fentanyl administered with bupivacaine during labor, *Anesthesiology* 83:300-308, 1995.
125. Low JA, Victory R, Derrick EJ: Predictive value of electronic fetal monitoring for intrapartum fetal asphyxia with metabolic acidosis, *Obstet Gynecol* 92:285-291, 1999.
126. Lydon-Rochelle M et al: Risk of uterine rupture during labor among women with a prior cesarean delivery, *New Engl J Med* 345:3-8, 2001.
127. Mabey R et al, editors: *The new age herbalist,* New York, 1988, Collier Books.
128. Magann EF et al: Can we decrease postdatism in women with an unfavorable cervix and a negative fetal fibronectin test result at term by serial membrane sweeping? *Am J Obstet Gynecol* 179:890-894, 1998.
129. Maresh M, Choong KH, Beard RW: Delayed pushing with lumbar epidural anesthesia in labour, *Br J Obstet Gynaecol* 90:623, 1983.
130. Maslow AS, Sweeny AL: Elective induction of labor as a risk factor for cesarean delivery among low-risk women, *Obstet Gynecol* 95:917-922, 2000.

131. Matthiesen A et al: Postpartum maternal oxytocin release by newborns: effects of infant hand massage and sucking, *Birth* 28:13-19, 2001.

132. McCandlish R et al: A randomized controlled trial of care of the perineum during second stage of normal labor, *Br J Obstet Gynaecol* 105:1262-1272, 1998.

133. McFarlin BL et al: A national survey of herbal preparation use by nurse-midwives for labor stimulation, *J Nurse Midwifery* 44:205-216, 1999.

134. Medina IM: *Issues in women's health care: nutrition and herbs from menarche to menopause,* course syllabus 3/28-29/98, State University of New York Health Science Center at Brooklyn College of Health Related Professions Midwifery Education Program.

135. Mercer BM: Management of preterm premature rupture of the membranes, *Clin Obstet Gynecol* 41:870-882, 1998.

136. Mercer BM et al: The preterm prediction study: effect of gestational age and cause of preterm birth on subsequent obstetric outcome, *Am J Obstet Gynecol* 181:1216-1221, 1999.

137. Mercer JS: Current best evidence: a review of the literature on umbilical cord clamping, *J Midwifery Womens Health* 46:402-414, 2001.

138. Meyer K, Anderson GC: Using kangaroo care in a clinical setting with fullterm infants having breastfeeding difficulties, *MCN* 24:190-192, 1999.

139. Meyer S et al: The effects of birth on urinary continence mechanisms and other pelvic-floor characteristics, *Obstet Gynecol* 92(4, Part 1):613-621, 1998.

140. Miller DA, Paul RH: Rupture of the unscarred uterus, *Am J Obstet Gynecol* 174:345, 1996.

141. Miller DA et al: Vaginal birth after cesarean section in twin gestation, *Am J Obstet Gynecol* 175:194-198, 1996.

142. Mityvak product enclosure, San Antonio, Tex, 2002, Prism Healthcare.

143. Morrison EH: Common peripartum emergencies, *Am Fam Physician* 1998, The American Academy of Family Physicians, *http://www.aafp.org/afp/981101ap/morrison.html.*

144. Morton SC et al: Effect of epidural analgesia for labor on the cesarean delivery rate, *Obstet Gynecol* 83:1045-1052, 1994.

145. Mozurkewich EL, Hutton EK: Elective repeat cesarean delivery versus trial of labor: a meta-analysis of the literature from 1989 to 1999, *Am J Obstet Gynecol* 183:1187-1197, 2000.

146. Mozurkewich EL et al: Working conditions and adverse pregnancy outcome, *Obstet Gynecol* 95:623-635, 2000.

147. Murray M: *Antepartal and intrapartal fetal monitoring,* ed 2, Albuquerque, 1997, Learning Resources International.

148. Nagata M et al: Maternity blues and attachment to children in mothers of full-term normal infants, *Obstet Gynecol Survey* 55:545-546, 2000.

149. National Institute of Child Health and Human Development (NICHHD): Electronic fetal heart monitoring: research guidelines for interpretation, *Am J Obstet Gynecol* 177:1385-1390, 1997.

150. Nelson WE, editor: *Nelson textbook of pediatrics,* ed 15, Philadelphia, 1996, WB Saunders.

151. Nesbitt TS, Gilbert WM, Herrchen B: Shoulder dystocia and associated risk factors with macrosomic infants born in California, *Am J Obstet Gynecol* 179:476-480, 1998.

152. Nissim R: *Natural healing in gynecology,* San Francisco, 1996, Pandora.

153. Ody P: *The complete medicinal herbal,* New York, 1993, Dorling Kindersley.

154. O'Reilly SA, Hoyer PJP, Walsh E: Low risk mothers: oral intake and emesis in labor, *J Nurse Midwifery* 38:228-236, 1993.

155. O'Shea TM et al: Trends in mortality and cerebral palsy in a geographically based cohort of very low birth weight neonates between 1982 and 1994, *Pediatrics* 101:642-647, 1998.

156. Page L: *Healthy healing,* ed 11, Carmel Valley, Calif, 2000, Healthy Healing Publications.

157. Papatsonis DNM et al: Nifedipine and ritodrine in the management of preterm labor: a randomized multicenter trial, *Obstet Gynecol* 90:230-234, 1997.

158. Papiernik E, Grange G: Prenatal screening with evaluated high risk scores, *J Perinat Med* 27:21-25, 1999.

159. Parilla BV, McDermott TM: Prophylactic amnioinfusion in pregnancies complicated by chorioamnionitis: a prospective randomized trial, *Am J Perinat* 15:649-652, 1998.

160. Parvati J: *Hygieia: a woman's herbal,* Berkeley, Calif, 1985, Bookpeople.

161. *Physician's desk reference (PDR) for herbal medicines,* Montvale, NJ 1998, Thomson Medical Economics.

162. Plaut MM, Schwartz ML, Lubarssky SL: Uterine rupture associated with the use of misoprostol in the gravid patient with a previous cesarean section, *Am J Obstet Gynecol* 180:1535-1542, 1999.

163. Polone K: Nature in your birth bag, *Midwifery Today* 26:34, 1993.

164. Polone K: Pass the peas: tricks of the trade, *Midwifery Today* 26:10, 1993.

165. Prabulos AM, Philipson EH: Umbilical cord prolapse: is the time from diagnosis to delivery critical? *J Reprod Med* 43:129-132, 1998.

166. Ramin SM et al: Randomized trial of epidural versus intravenous analgesia during labor, *Obstet Gynecol* 86:783-789, 1995.

167. Ramsey PS et al: Shoulder dystocia: rotational maneuvers revisited, *J Reprod Med* 45: 85-88, 2000.

168. Ransjo-Arvidson A et al: Maternal analgesia during labor disturbs newborn behavior: effects on breastfeeding, temperature, and crying, *Birth* 28:5-12, 2001.

169. Read JA, Miller FC, Paul RH: Randomized trial of ambulation versus oxytocin for labor enhancement: a preliminary report, *Am J Obstet Gynecol* 139:669-672, 1981.

170. Roberts JE: The "push" for evidence: management of the second stage, *J Midwifery Womens Health* 47:2-15, 2002.

171. Robinson CA et al: Does station of the fetal head at epidural placement affect the position of the fetal vertex at delivery? *Am J Obstet Gynecol* 175:99-104, 1996.

172. Roodt A, Nikodem VC: Pushing/bearing down methods used during the second stage of labour, *The Cochrane Database of Systematic Reviews* Issue 3, 2002, last updated Oct 25, 2001.

173. Rooks J: Evidence-based practice and its application to childbirth care for low-risk women, *J Nurse Midwifery* 44:355-369, 1999.

174. Rooks JP et al: Outcomes of care at birth centers: the National Birth Center Study, *New Engl J Med* 321:1804-1811, 1989.

175. Rose B, Scott-Moncrieff C: *Homeopathy for women,* London, 1998, Collins & Brown.

176. Rosen MA: Nitrous oxide for relief of labor pain: a systematic review, *Am J Obstet Gynecol* 186:S110-S126, 2002.

177. Rosen MA: Paracervical block for labor analgesia: a brief historical review, *Am J Obstet Gynecol* 186:S127-S130, 2002.

178. Rosen MG, Dickinson JC: Vaginal birth after cesarean: a meta-analysis of indicator for success, *Obstet Gynecol* 76:865-869, 1990.

179. Roshanfekr D et al: Station at onset of active labor in nulliparous patients and risk of cesarean section, *Obstet Gynecol* 93:329-331, 1999.

180. Rouse DJ et al: Active phase labor arrest: revisiting the 2-hour minimum, *Obstet Gynecol* 98:550-554, 2001.

181. Sawdy RJ, Bennett PR: Recent advances in the therapeutic management of preterm labour, *Curr Opin Obstet Gynecol* 11:131-139, 1999.

182. Sandberg EC: The Zavanelli maneuver: 12 years of recorded experience, *Obstet Gynecol* 93:312-317, 1999.

183. Schrag S et al: Prevention of perinatal group B streptococcal disease, *MMWR* 51(RR11):1-22, 2002, *http://www.cdc.gov/mmwr/preview/mmwrhtml/rr5111al.htm.*

184. Schuler-Maloney D: Letter to the editor, *J Midwifery Womens Health* 45:437-438, 2000.

185. Schuler-Maloney D: Placental triage of the singleton placenta, *J Midwifery Womens Health* 45:104-113, 2000.

186. Scott KD, Klaus PH, Klaus MH: The obstetrical and postpartum benefits of continuous support during childbirth, *J Womens Health Gender-Based Med* 8:1257-1264, 1999.

187. Seaward PGR et al: International Multicenter Term PROM Study: evaluation of predictors of neonatal infection in infants born to patients with premature rupture of membranes at term, *Am J Obstet Gynecol* 179:635-639, 1998.

188. Shah-Hosseini R, Evrard JR: Puerperal uterine inversion, *Obstet Gynecol* 73:567-570, 1989.

189. Sharma SK et al: A randomized trial of epidural versus patient-controlled meperidine analgesia during labor, *Anesthesiology* 87:487-494, 1997.

190. Shimoya K et al: Effect of sexual intercourse on fetal fibronectin concentration in cervicovaginal secretions, *Am J Obstet Gynecol* 179:255-256, 1998.

191. Shipp TD et al: Labor after previous cesarean: influence of prior indication and parity, *Obstet Gynecol* 95:913-916, 2000.

192. Simkin P: The experience of maternity in a woman's life, *J Obstet Gynecol Neonatal* 25:247-252, 1996.

193. Simkin P: *Turning a breech baby to vertex,* 1987. Handout available from Pennypress, Inc., Seattle, Wash.

194. Simkin P, Ancheta R: *The labor progress handbook,* Boston, 2000, Blackwell Science.

195. Simkin P, O'Hara M: Nonpharmacologic relief of pain during labor: systematic reviews of five methods, *Am J Obstet Gynecol* 186:S131-S159, 2002.

196. Smith T: *Homeopathy for pregnancy and nursing mothers,* Worthing, England, 1993, Insight Editions.

197. Smith JW, Tully MR: Midwifery management of breastfeeding: using the evidence, *J Midwifery Womens Health* 46:423-438, 2001.

198. Sokol RJ et al: Normal and abnormal labor progress, I. A quantitative assessment and survey of the literature, *J Reprod Med* 18:47-53, 1977.

199. Sommer PA, Norr K, Roberts J: Clinical decision-making regarding intravenous hydration in normal labor in a birth center setting, *J Midwifery Womens Health* 45:114-121, 2000.

200. Srinivasan HB, Vidyasagar D: Meconium aspiration syndrome: current concepts and management, *Comp Ther* 5:82-89, 1999.

201. Stapleton H, Tiran D: Herbal medicine. In Tiran D, Mack S, editors: *Complementary therapies for pregnancy and childbirth,* ed 2, Edinburgh, 2000, Baillière Tindall.

202. Steer P, Flint C: Preterm labour and premature rupture of the membranes, *BMJ* 318:1059-1062, 1999.

203. Summers L: Methods of cervical ripening and labor induction, *J Nurse Midwifery* 42:71-85, 1997.

204. Taeusch HW, Sniderman S: Neonatal resuscitation. In Taeusch HW, Christiansen RO, Buescher ES: *Pediatric and neonatal tests and procedures,* Philadelphia, 1996, WB Saunders.

205. Tarr K: *Herbs, helps, and pressure points for pregnancy and childbirth,* ed 3, Provo, Utah, 1984, Sunbeam.

206. Thacker SB, Stroup DF, Peterson HB: Efficacy and safety of intrapartum electronic fetal monitoring: an update, *Obstet Gynecol* 86:613-620, 1995.

207. Thorp JA, Breedlove G: Epidural analgesia in labor: an evaluation of risks and benefits, *Birth* 23:63-83, 1996.

208. Thorp JA et al: The effect of intrapartum epidural analgesia on nulliparous labor: a randomised controlled prospective trial, *Am J Obstet Gynecol* 169:851-858, 1993.

209. Tiran D: Massage and aromatherapy. In Tiran D, Mack S, editors: *Complementary therapies for pregnancy and childbirth,* ed 2, Edinburgh, 2000, Baillière Tindall.

210. Tiran D: Reflexology in midwifery practice. In Tiran D, Mack S, editors: *Complementary therapies for pregnancy and childbirth,* ed 2, Edinburgh, 2000, Baillière Tindall.

211. Tritten J: Tricks of the trade, *Midwifery Today* 31:7, 1998.

212. UK Amniotomy Group: A multicentre randomised trial of amniotomy in spontaneous first labor at term, *Br J Obstet Gynaecol* 101:307, 1994.

213. Ullman R, Reichenberg-Ullman J: *Homeopathic self-care,* Rocklin, Calif, 1997, Prima.

214. Varney H: *Varney's midwifery,* ed 3, Sudbury, Mass, 1997, Jones and Bartlett.

215. Vincent RD, Chestnut DH: Epidural analgesia during labor, *Am Fam Physician* 58:1785-1792, 1998.
216. Von Der Pool BA: Preterm labor: diagnosis and treatment, *Am Fam Physician* 57: 2457-2464, 1998.
217. Wagner RK, Nielsen PE, Gonik B: Shoulder dystocia, *Obstet Gynecol Clin North Am* 26:371-383, 1999.
218. Warenski JC: Managing difficult labor: avoiding common pitfalls, *Clin Obstet Gynecol* 40:525-532, 1997.
219. Weed SS: *Wise woman herbal childbearing year*, Woodstock, NY, 1985, Ash Tree.
220. Weismiller DG: Preterm labor, *Am Fam Physician* 59:593-602, 1999.
221. Weismiller DG: Transcervical amnioinfusion, *Am Fam Physician* 57:504-510, 1998.
222. Wenstrom K, Andrews WW, Maher JE: Amnioinfusion survey: prevalence, protocols, and complications, *Obstetrics Gynecol* 86:572-576, 1995.
223. Wiswell TE, Fuloria M: Management of meconium-stained amniotic fluid, *Clin Perinatol* 26:659-668, 1999.
224. Wiswell TE et al: Delivery room management of the apparently-vigorous meconium-stained neonate: results of the multicenter, international collaborative trial, *Pediatrics* 105:1-7, 2000.
225. Yelland S: *Acupuncture in midwifery*, Cheshire, England, 1996, Books for Midwives Press.
226. Zapp J, Thorne T: Comfortable labor with intrathecal narcotics, *Military Med* 160: 217-219, 1995.
227. Zelop CM et al: Effect of previous vaginal delivery on the risk of uterine rupture during a subsequent trial of labor, *Am J Obstet Gynecol* 183:1184-1186, 2000.
228. Zhang J, Klebanoff MA, DerSimonian R: Epidural anesthesia in association with duration of labor and mode of delivery: a quantitative review, *Am J Obstet Gynecol* 180: 970-977, 1999.

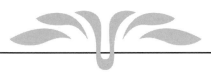

Chapter 4

The Puerperium

• POSTPARTUM ROUNDS AFTER VAGINAL DELIVERY

Components of hospital postpartum rounds include the following:

1. Review the chart (antepartum, intrapartum, postpartum notes) noting the following: vital signs, elimination, activity, mother-infant interaction, and care of baby.
2. Greet the woman and review birth experience.
3. Ask the woman for her assessment of her comfort level, emotional state, infant condition and care, and breastfeeding.
4. Perform a physical examination, including the following:
   a. **Breasts:** Firmness (filling), support, nipple condition
   b. **Uterine fundus:** Height (after voiding) and location, as well as firmness, tenderness, and presence of cramping
   c. **Lochia:** Color, odor, amount, whether expressed with fundal massage
   d. **Perineum:** Lacerations approximated and wound edges clean; edema, ecchymosis, hematoma, bleeding, varicosities, hemorrhoids
   e. **Extremities:** Edema, redness, Homans' sign, tenderness, clonus
5. Check postpartum CBC if drawn and results of other laboratory tests ordered.
6. Assess maternal psychological state and mother-infant interaction.
7. Assess breastfeeding.
8. Confirm RhoGAM status of the Rh-negative mother and determine whether the rubella immunization has been offered to the nonimmune mother.
9. Create a discharge plan with the woman.
10. Teaching includes the following topics:
    a. Comfort suggestions: Medications, ice packs then sitz baths
    b. Normal course of recovery: Healing of perineum, resumption of bowel movements, resolution of hemorrhoids, expected course of vaginal bleeding, normalcy of postpartum blues and s/s of postpartum depression, resolution of edema of extremities

   c. Self-care measures: Fluid intake and nutrition, continuation of vitamins and other supplements, breast care for the breastfeeding mother and lactation suppression for the bottlefeeding mother, Kegel exercise, decreased activity, and help at home

   d. Breastfeeding: Frequency, length of time at each breast, normal number of wet diapers, rotation of breasts, positioning, nipple care and measures for relief of soreness, growth spurts, breast lumps

   e. Infant care: Cord care, circumcision care, feeding, jaundice, nighttime regimen

   f. Pelvic rest and resumption of sexual intercourse: Need for use of lubricants while breastfeeding, contraception planning

   g. Danger s/s and when to call the health care provider: Fever, malaise, s/s mastitis, endometritis, postpartum hemorrhage (PPH), postpartum depression

11. Plan postpartum visit and baby's pediatric appointment.

12. Document findings and plan.

• POSTPARTUM ROUNDS DOCUMENTATION

Use the SOAP (**S**ubjective, **O**bjective, **A**ssessment, and **P**lan) method to document postpartum rounds.

Postpartum Day #_____

S: Subjective: Description of general emotional state, her assessment of physical discomforts, infant feeding and care, and concerns.

O: Objective: Vital signs, laboratory test results, whether voiding or has had bowel movement, urinary or fecal incontinence, RhoGAM or rubella status. Physical examination: breasts, fundus, diastasis recti, perineum (bruising, edema, approximation and healing of episiotomy or lacerations), lochia (color, quantity, and odor), hemorrhoids, costovertebral angle tenderness (CVAT), extremities (edema, tenderness, redness, warmth, Homans' sign, deep tendon reflexes [DTRs] if indicated).

A: Assessment: Primipara or multipara, number of days after delivery, whether stable, status of infant feeding. Problem diagnoses if any.

P: Plan for discharge and follow-up postpartum and pediatric appointments.
  • Comfort or other measures instituted.
  • Teaching done.

• POSTPARTUM HOME VISIT FORMAT

During the postpartum home visit, which takes place during the first week after delivery, assess the following:

Baby

1. Sleep: Where? time intervals? position?
2. Nutrition: When? any problems with burping or spitting up? perceived infant satisfaction?

3. Breast: How often and for how long on each? use of supplements? appropriate nipple care? maternal satisfaction?
4. Bottle: Formula type, style, preparation method, bottle care?
5. Behavior: Observe mother's interpretation of and response to crying and the baby's response to the mother.
6. Clothing: Appropriate? method of laundering? diaper type?
7. Bath: Where given, soap used, care of umbilicus, whether oil or powder is used.
8. Elimination: Stool (color, consistency, frequency, problems, how infant is washed after stool) and urine (color, frequency, amount; any problems? skin condition?).
9. Physical examination: Have mother undress baby; weigh and examine baby (see p. 249).
10. Follow-up: Pediatric appointment.

Mother

1. Discuss birth experience.
2. Perform physical examination, noting vital signs, breast condition, fundus, episiotomy, lochia, and edema.
3. Ask about appetite, rest, and exercise.
4. Ask about urinary and fecal incontinence. Discuss frequency of occurrence and Kegel exercise. Persistent incontinence should be discussed at the 6-week visit.
5. Observe for signs of fatigue, nervousness, depression, or anxiety.
6. Evaluate parenting: Response to new responsibilities, knowledge needed, relationship between parents, relationship between father and baby, response of siblings to baby, and presence of any additional significant other who assumes any care of baby.
7. Note any social problems and determine need for referral (e.g., need for more food, fuel, rental assistance, better home, or counseling regarding family relationships or other problems).
8. Make appointment for postpartum follow-up visit.

• POSTPARTUM OFFICE VISIT FORMAT AT 6 TO 8 WEEKS

1. Chart review: Social, family, medical/surgical, obstetric, and gynecologic histories; antepartum, intrapartum, and postpartum records; results of laboratory tests; and any subsequent problems.
2. Take postpartum history:
   a. Social: Support and assistance
   b. Emotional: Depression?
   c. Menstrual: Since delivery, including lochia
   d. Postpartum: Birth review, problems, treatments, data to evaluate success of treatment, urinary incontinence, fecal incontinence, urinary tract infection (UTI) symptoms, fever, chills, flu symptoms

e. Sexual: Since delivery; dyspareunia? satisfaction?

f. Contraception: Method used since delivery, method desired; contraindications?

g. Subjective appraisal: State of health, sleeping, eating and fluid intake, infant feeding, voiding and bowel movements, mothering, other family relationships

h. Pediatric care established?

i. Postpartum exercise, including Kegel exercises

j. Questions

k. If significant other has accompanied mother to visit, his or her perceptions and concerns

3. Perform a complete physical examination, including the following items relevant to the postpartum period:

a. Thyroid (see p. 345)

b. Breasts, nipples, support, review of breast self-examination

c. Abdomen: Diastasis recti and inguinal lymph nodes

d. Extremities: Edema, varicosities, Homans' sign, DTRs

e. Pelvic:

(1) External: Bartholin's, urethral, and Skene's glands; episiotomy or laceration healing; hemorrhoids

(2) Speculum: Cervical healing, secretions, inflammation, vaginal secretions and inflammation, Pap, GC and CT cultures

(3) Bimanual: Tenderness of perineum, cervix, and uterus; size, shape, and position of cervix and uterus; adnexa; pelvic and perineal support (Kegel exercises)

(4) Anus: Hemorrhoids, assessment of sphincter

(5) Rectovaginal: Integrity of the rectovaginal septum, mass, or strictures

f. Rule out contraindications to use of desired contraceptive

g. Perform physical examination of infant per practice protocol

4. Laboratory tests: Urinalysis (UA), Hct and Hb, thyroid function tests if appropriate (see p. 346). Diabetic screening for women who had gestational diabetes mellitus (GDM) (see p. 343).

5. Initiate contraception (see p. 495).

6. Make next appointment.

7. Referrals may include a breastfeeding support group, parenting group, counseling, medical treatment for medical complications, or a smoking cessation program. Women who are experiencing urinary or fecal incontinence should be seen at 6 months and referred to a gynecologist if the condition has persisted.

• NORMAL POSTPARTUM INVOLUTION

Breast Changes

See p. 229 regarding nonlactating breasts and care and p. 303 regarding lactating breast changes and care.

Uterine and Perineal Changes

The uterus descends into the pelvis by 2 weeks and returns to normal size by about 4 weeks after delivery. For a few days after delivery, the cervix will admit two fingers. It contracts slowly and retains a wider size with depressions where lacerations occurred during delivery. Vaginal rugae reappear by the third week, and the vagina shrinks but rarely returns to its pregravid dimensions.[15] Urinary incontinence and fecal incontinence may persist after the puerperal period.[43] (See pp. 470 and 471.)

Endometrial Changes

The endometrium is restored by 16 days after delivery in all areas except the placental site, which continues to show signs of healing at the cellular level for as long as several months. Lochia persists for 3 to 8 weeks: it begins as a heavy flow of bright red blood *(lochia rubra)*, slows to dark red by days 3 to 4, and changes to paler, pink *(lochia serosa)* for an average of 3 weeks. Fifteen percent of women still have lochia serosa at the 6-week visit. *Lochia alba*, a yellowish white discharge, follows.

There may be a brief (lasting <2 hours) self-limiting episode of heavier vaginal bleeding during the second week, when the placental eschar sloughs. Neither the use of oral contraceptives nor breastfeeding alters the length of lochial flow.[22]

Abdominal Wall

A two-fingerbreadth (FB) diastasis recti may be resolved by the 6-week postpartum visit. A wider one will take longer. Resolution is facilitated by abdominal exercise. Failure to correct this musculature separation contributes to back problems later.

Weight Loss

An average of 12 lb is lost at delivery. Further weight loss is seen in the first 6 weeks after delivery, although 6 months is usually required for those women who do return to their prepregnancy weight.[69] See p. 241 for further discussion regarding weight loss.

Hemodynamics

The woman who delivers vaginally loses an average of 5 Hct points; the woman who is delivered by cesarean section loses an average of 6 points.[22] Approximately 200 to 500 mL of blood is lost during a normal delivery; and the total lochial loss is approximately 240 to 270 mL. The leukocytosis seen when labor begins may remain for about 2 days after delivery and may be elevated to 25,000 to 30,000 cells/μL if the woman had a prolonged labor.[69]

• VARIATIONS IN BREAST INVOLUTION

Lactation Suppression

Engorgement and breast pain begin on postpartum days 1 to 4 and may continue beyond day 4 in women who are not breastfeeding.[61] Since 1988, the Food and Drug Administration has recommended that no pharmacologic agents be used to suppress lactation. Suggestions for lactation suppression have been poorly researched. Among women who receive these instructions, moderate engorgement occurs in 21% to 52%, and severe engorgement, in 1% to 44%. Moderate pain is reported by 29% to 68% of women, and severe pain by 10% to 33% of women.[61]

ⓜ Management of the Nonlacting Woman

Instructions for the nonlactating mother, though not supported by research, include:

1. Wear a **tight-fitting bra,** an ace wrap, or a towel tightly safety-pinned down the front. Elevate pendulous breasts as you wrap them.
2. **Apply ice** and avoid heat application to breasts.
3. **Avoid all stimulation to nipples,** including keeping the back to the shower.
4. **Do not express milk** to relieve pressure; this will only increase milk production.
5. **Restrict fluid intake.**
6. Be aware that the **most uncomfortable period** reaches its peak and lasts for approximately **24 to 48 hours** after delivery.
7. Take a **mild analgesic** for the discomfort.
8. **Complementary measures:**
   a. **Miscellaneous:** Wear **cool cabbage leaves** in the bra to reduce engorgement.[55,59]
   b. **Herbs: Sage** decreases the milk supply* and is a uterine stimulant.[28] Sage is suggested in the following forms: 1 to 2 tsp of dried leaf tea, 1 to 8 times/d; 5 to 40 drops of fresh leaf tincture, 1 to 3 times/wk[70]; or tea made with 2 Tblsp leaves and flowers/L water, 3 cups/d. Alternately, 30 to 40 drops of tincture bid.[46] **Parsley** is suggested. It is a diuretic and also a uterine stimulant.† Boil 1 tsp of the plant in 1 cup of liquid for 10 minutes: 1 cup tid.[46] **See information on herbs, p. 563.**

Mastitis

Mastitis is cellulitis of the interlobular connective tissue in the breast, ranging from local inflammation to abscess to septicemia.[45a] Mastitis is most often caused by *Staphylococcus aureus* but may also be caused

---

*References 23, 24, 27, 34, 38, 46-49, 55.
†References 24, 28, 34, 38, 46, 48.

by other bacteria originating from the infant's nose and throat, from the mother's or other caregivers' hands, or from the environment. Bacteria may enter through a fissure, small laceration, or possibly the lactiferous ducts.[15] Initially, the woman may be afebrile and feel well but notes a firm, warm, painful, red, swollen area if the duct is close to the skin—or if it is deeper—a palpable lump with defined margins, caused by milk stasis from a plugged duct as a result of incomplete emptying. Noninfectious inflammation may occur. After symptoms have persisted for 48 hours, they are unlikely to abate without medication. Mastitis presents as the rapid onset of severe pain in a localized area of the breast. The area, possibly wedge-shaped, is tender, swollen, and hard and may be red. Chills, malaise, fatigue, headache, tachycardia, and a fever of 100.4° to 104° F accompany the local symptoms.[5]

An abscess may form if treatment is delayed or inadequate (incidence 10%). An abscess should be suspected if high fevers last >48 hours, chills continue, suppuration or a hard fluctuant mass is observed, or mastitis does not resolve within a few days of initiation of antibiotic therapy. Ultrasound examination may confirm the diagnosis.[5]

Predisposing Factors

1. **Poor general health:** Stress, fatigue, poor nutrition, anemia.
2. **Demographics:** Age 30 to 34 years, employment outside the home.
3. **Physical factors:** Fissured nipples, constriction by a tight bra, engorgement, milk stasis during sleep, abrupt change in frequency of feedings, plugged ducts, infant latching difficulties.[59]
4. **Strenuous exercise:** Interstitial leakage of milk may occur during an exercise that is strenuous for the upper body. During lactation, such exercise should only be undertaken after the breasts have been emptied.[45a]

🅜 Management

1. Teach **prevention** of mastitis by means of meticulous handwashing; early, frequent feedings; good positioning of infant at breast; gentle handling of breasts; use of a supportive, nonconstricting bra; cleansing nipples with water rather than drying agents; avoidance of individuals with staphylococcal infections; observation of the baby for skin or cord infections; and examination of the breasts for lumps.[5]
2. **Once a lump is detected,** teach the mother: **Empty the breasts frequently** by feeding the baby or, if the breast is too tender, by using a pump. Apply moist **heat and massage** the breast before and during feedings.[55] **Begin feeding on the affected side.**[37] Use **different positions** than usual. Point the baby's nose toward the affected area for best drainage of that area.[5] **If the infant refuses the affected breast,** it is probably because of the engorgement rather than a change in the taste of the milk, and pumping a small amount will

relieve the problem.[15] These measures and **increased rest** will often relieve a blocked duct within 48 hours.[5]

3. Should the lump worsen or fail to resolve in 48 hours, or should constitutional symptoms begin, prescribe **antibiotics.** The standard antibiotic is a penicillinase-resistant penicillin or cephalosporin that covers *S. aureus* for 6 to 10 days (cloxacillin, 250 to 500 mg PO q6h; dicloxacillin, 125 to 250 mg PO or IM q6h; oxacillin, 500 mg to 1 g PO or IM q4-6h; cephalexin, 250 to 500 mg PO q6h; cephradine, 250 to 500 mg PO q6h; or cefaclor, 250 to 500 mg PO q8h).[55] Courses of 10 to 14 days are suggested by some authors to reduce the risk of abscess and recurrence.[45a]

4. Instruct the mother: Increase **fluid intake. Bed rest.** Take **analgesics** for comfort. Apply **cold or warm packs** for pain relief.

5. **Improvement should be seen in 48 hours.** If it is not, or if a palpable mass or fluctuation develops, **consult** a physician, who will rule out an abscess. **If an abscess is suspected, refer** to a surgeon for drainage (by needle or left open to heal by second intention).[55] The infant can continue to be fed on the affected side. If the wound is too close to the nipple and the mother cannot tolerate breastfeeding on that side, unilateral weaning is an option.[5]

6. If the mastitis occurs while a woman is **pumping** her **milk for a hospitalized baby,** the milk should be discarded until clinical symptoms are resolved.[45a]

7. **Chronic cases** are sometimes treated with erythromycin, 250 to 500 mg q6h, or trimethoprim-sulfamethoxazole (Bactrim, Septra) for an extended period.[55]

8. **Complementary measures:**
   a. **Miscellaneous: Cabbage leaves** are anti-inflammatory, and a slightly softened fresh leaf tucked into the bra may be used to treat mastitis and may prevent recurrences.[47,65] A **grated potato and/or onion** poultice will draw out an obstruction (wrap the onion in a porous cloth to protect the skin).[50]
   b. **Homeopathy** experts recommend remedies for mastitis.[13,56,60,68]
   c. **Acupuncture** may be used in the treatment of mastitis.[7]
   d. **Nutritional suggestions:** The woman with repeated infections may want to try **eliminating cow's milk** from her diet for a few weeks to see whether the infections decrease.[65] Maternal intake of **garlic** is known to increase the amount of milk a baby will consume, and garlic is antibacterial.[3] Four or more **garlic** capsules (or fresh garlic) may be taken daily.[65]

      Vitamin C is suggested in large doses as soon as breast soreness is noted.[48,65,68] To acidify the body, making it less hospitable to bacteria, the woman may take 1 Tblsp of apple cider **vinegar** in one glass of water every hour until symptoms resolve.[65]
   e. **Herbs: Comfrey leaf** may be used externally as a poultice.[34,50,65] Comfrey should be washed off the nipple before the baby is

breastfed. **Echinacea** stimulates the immune system, is a natural antitoxin for internal and external infections, and may help heal wounds.[24,50] Two dropperfuls of tincture in water tid or six capsules daily are suggested.[68] Tincture of **goldenseal** may also be used: two dropperfuls in water tid or six capsules daily are suggested.[50,65,68] **See information on herbs, p. 563.**

• VARIATIONS IN INVOLUTION OF THE UTERUS

Subinvolution

Usually diagnosed at the 4- to 6-week postpartum examination, prolonged involution or failure of involution may be caused by fibroids, retained products of conception, infection, or abnormal placental implantation. Symptoms include prolonged lochia; leukorrhea; irregular, heavy bleeding; and an enlarged, boggy uterus, which may be tender. Adnexa may be tender.[15]

Management

1. Obtain a lochia sample for **culture.**
2. **Ultrasound** examination may be done to identify retained fragments.[22]
3. **Methergine** (methylergonovine) or Ergotrate (ergonovine maleate), 0.2 mg every 3 to 4 hours for 3 days, may be prescribed. Broad-spectrum antibiotics may be added if the uterus is tender after 2 weeks.[69]
4. Some practitioners recommend initial treatment with **antibiotics**, finding infection to be a common factor in delayed involution.[15]
5. **Complementary measures:**
   a. **Acupuncture** is used in the treatment of excessive lochia.[7]
   b. **Reflexology:** Treatment of the pituitary and uterine zones of the feet may relieve subinvolution, preventing the need for medical intervention.[66] **See charts and information on reflexology, p. 567.**

Endometritis

Infection of the endometrium caused by bacteria ascended from the birth canal is the most common cause of puerperal fever. Endometritis is also called *endomyometritis*, *endoparametritis*, and *metritis*. Clinical findings include jagged temperature elevation between 101° and 104° F (38.3° and 40° C), chills, anorexia, malaise, tender uterus, uterine cramping, subinvolution, slight abdominal distention, leukocytosis ranging from 15,000 to 30,000 cells/μL, tachycardia, and a moderate amount of foul lochia or a scant, odorless lochia (the latter seen with β-hemolytic *Streptococcus* infection).[15]

Predisposing Factors

Obstetric: Severe pregnancy-induced hypertension (PIH), premature rupture of membranes (PROM), preterm premature rupture of membranes (PPROM), chorioamnionitis, colonization of the genital tract with pathogenic bacteria, preterm delivery, fetal distress, cesarean delivery, cervical or vaginal lacerations, retained products of conception, low Apgar scores, neonatal mortality.

Iatrogenic: Multiple cervical examinations, internal fetal monitoring, instrumental delivery, manual removal of the placenta.

General Health: Anemia, poor nutrition and hygiene, GDM.

Demographic: Young age, low socioeconomic status.[10]

Differential Diagnoses: See puerperal fever, p. 244.

Complications: Salpingitis and oophoritis rarely occur 9 to 15 days postpartum as a flare-up of a preexisting colonization. (See pelvic inflammatory disease [PID], p. 425.) **Pelvic cellulitis** is infection of the broad ligament when bacteria have spread through the lymphatic system (see p. 237). A **pelvic abscess** rarely forms when metritis results in a parametrial pus-forming inflammation, which forms a mass in the broad ligament (see p. 237). **Septic pelvic thrombophlebitis** occurs when the veins in an infected placental site become thrombosed and bacterial growth extends to these thromboses (see p. 244).

Ⓜ Management

1. Hacker and Moore[25] state that the woman who has puerperal fever and cessation of lochial flow should undergo a **pelvic examination,** and any pelvic remnants or clots from the lower uterine segment should be removed.

2. **Consult** with the physician and prescribe **antibiotics:** After a vaginal delivery, a penicillin in combination with an aminoglycoside; after cesarean delivery, gentamycin, 1.5 mg/kg q8h, mixed with clindamycin, 900 mg q8h. Ampicillin may be added in some circumstances.[2] An oral agent may be used in mild cases. IV antibiotics are given for moderate to severe cases.[15] Should an infection develop after a prophylactic antibiotic has been given, change antibiotics.[2]

3. Advise the patient to **rest**, drink lots of **fluids,** maintain good **nutrition**, perform good **perineal care**, and take **analgesics.**

4. The infection **should respond within 48 to 72 hours.** If it does not, **consult** with the physician again. Cellulitis, abscess, hematoma, septic pelvic thrombophlebitis, or resistant bacteria should be ruled out. If fever persists, ultrasound, computed tomography (CT), or magnetic resonance imaging (MRI) may be used to detect retained placental tissue, a pelvic abscess, or ovarian vein thrombosis.[22]

5. The woman may be **discharged** when she has been afebrile for 24 to 48 hours. Extended antibiotic therapy is indicated for staphylococcal infection.[22]

6. **Complementary measures:**
   a. Some experts recommend **homeopathic** treatment for endometritis.[29]
   b. **Acupuncture** is used in the treatment of puerperal fever.[7]

Delayed Postpartum Hemorrhage

Hemorrhage that occurs 1 to 30 days after delivery is called *delayed postpartum hemorrhage*. When the PPH is of short duration and is self-limiting in nature, it probably represents the shedding of the placental eschar. PPH is associated with retained products of conception in 40% of cases.[22] Other possible causes include placental site endometritis and thrombosis with delayed involution, hematoma, or a previously undiscovered laceration of the birth canal.

ⓜ Management

1. **Consult** with the physician regarding curettage or other treatment.
2. **Antibiotics** reduce the risk of developing uterine adhesions.[22] IV antibiotics are needed if the woman has sepsis.[11]

• PERINEAL CARE AND VARIATIONS IN NORMAL INVOLUTION AND HEALING

Care of the Perineum

After vaginal delivery:

1. **Examine** the woman who is experiencing severe perineal pain for hematoma or infection.[22] (See p. 236 regarding hematoma and p. 235 regarding infection.) Assess the episiotomy wound as it heals for redness, approximation, ecchymosis, discharge, and edema.[69] Suture material will dissolve in 2 weeks, and the woman can expect the episiotomy to be healed in 3 to 4 weeks.
2. **Teach** the woman who has delivered vaginally to care for her perineum by:
   a. Washing her hands before and after perineal care.
   b. Using a squirt bottle filled with warm water to spray away lochia and stool from the perineum after using the toilet. Pat the area dry, moving from front to back, using a fresh tissue for each wipe.
   c. Applying a new perineal pad that has not been handled on the wound surface.
   d. Refraining from sexual intercourse or the use of tampons or other devices in the vagina until the perineum is comfortable.[22]
   e. Soaking in a bathtub, which is safe after a vaginal delivery.[15]
3. Teach the following **comfort measures:**
   a. Ice packs for 24 to 48 hours.
   b. Topical anesthetics such as Dermaplast (benzocaine) or Nupercaine (dibucaine).[15]
   c. Sitz bath bid to tid. Early baths may be cold; warm baths may be taken after 24 to 48 hours. Cold sitz baths are conducted by having the woman sit in a bath at room temperature and adding ice cubes to gradually cool the water.[22]
   d. **Use of witch hazel** compresses or Tucks.

e. **Analgesia:** Ibuprofen, acetaminophen, Vicodin (hydrocodone and acetaminophen), or codeine.

f. Kegel exercises.

g. For hemorrhoids, see p. 36.

4. **Complementary measures to enhance healing of the perineum:**

a. **Homeopathy** experts recommend their remedies for healing of the perineum.*

b. **Acupuncture** may be useful in the treatment of perineal discomfort after delivery.[7,72]

c. **Herbs: Chamomile** is an antibacterial, antifungal, and anti-inflammatory agent and may help heal wounds.[28,33a,38,52]

The remaining herbs suggested for healing of perineal wounds are contraindicated during pregnancy. They should be used with caution by the lactating mother. Comfrey has a constituent named *allantoin* that encourages cell proliferation. Allantoin is easily absorbed through the skin and is recommended for healing wounds†; however, it is not recommended for the treatment of deep wounds because it may heal superficial layers prematurely, causing abscesses.[28] **External use during lactation is acceptable only in small doses of limited duration because of its hepatotoxicity.**[52] It may be added as tea to a sitz bath; used in a perineal spray bottle; or used externally as a poultice, lotion, or infused oil.[47,50] **Calendula,** a major remedy for facilitating healing of perineal wounds, has antifungal, antiseptic, and anti-inflammatory properties and moisturizes skin.‡ Calendula may be taken orally as tea (1 tsp/cup tea) or 60 to 120 drops of tincture per day,[46] or it may be applied locally as a lotion, in a compress or poultice (made with diluted tincture), or in an infused oil added to a sitz bath.[47] **St. John's wort** has anti-inflammatory, healing, astringent, and antibacterial properties and is also useful when applied externally to healing wounds.[24,38,47,52] Infused oil of St. John's wort may be added to a sitz bath.[47] **Slippery elm** is soothing when applied externally to healing wounds.[24,28,38,62] **Yarrow** is an anti-inflammatory agent and is used fresh in a poultice or in an ointment to heal wounds.[24,28,33a,38,52] **Goldenseal** is an antiseptic useful in facilitating wound healing.[28,33a,38,52,62] **See information on herbs, p. 563.**

Episiotomy and Genital Laceration Breakdown and Infection

Genital wound breakdown may involve dehiscence with parametrial extension and lymphangitis. Infection of cervical lacerations may extend into the broad ligament, causing parametritis and peritonitis. Such infec-

---

*References 13, 14, 29, 48, 56, 60.
†References 3, 24, 28, 38, 46, 48, 62, 69.
‡References 3, 14, 28, 38, 41, 46, 47, 52, 60, 62.

tions follow episiotomy in 0.05% to 0.5% of cases; fourth-degree lacerations are observed in 5.4% of cases. Wound breakdown and infection usually manifest 4 to 5 days after delivery with local pain, edema, dehiscence, redness, inflammation, purulent discharge, dysuria, and a low-grade fever or a spiking fever with chills.[15]

Predisposing Factors: Poor hygiene and nutrition, cigarette smoking, fourth-degree laceration, coagulation disorders, human papilloma virus.[15]

ⓜ Management

1. **Consult** with the physician.
2. **Anticipatory guidance:** Physician management includes **debridement** of the wound, **daily cleansing** with Betadine (povidone-iodine) and **sitz baths**, IV broad-spectrum **antibiotics**, ensuring proper nutrition and rest, analgesia, treatment of anemia, and the use of peri-lamps. When a negative culture has been obtained, the wound is reapproximated with the use of regional anesthesia and is followed by sitz baths, use of stool softeners, and pelvic rest.[15]
3. **Complementary measures:**
   a. Some experts recommend **homeopathic** remedies for wound infection.[13,29]
   b. **Nutritional suggestions:** Make sure that the mother has enough **zinc** in her diet, or suggest a supplement to support healing of the perineum.[62]
   c. **Herbs:** See complementary measures for perineal care, noting that several are mentioned for infection. **Thyme,** applied externally in a poultice or lotion, is an antiseptic that is valuable for the treatment of infected wounds.[24,28,38] **This herb is not recommended for use during pregnancy and should be used with caution by the breastfeeding mother. See information on herbs, p. 563.**

Pelvic Hematoma

Hematomas may develop in the vulva or vulvovaginal or retroperitoneal areas immediately after delivery or over the course of 1 to 2 days, usually after a difficult vaginal delivery.[30] They present with seemingly disproportionate pain, or pressure in the bladder, rectum, urethra, vagina, or perineum, and they may cause urinary retention. A discolored, tense, fluctuant swelling may project into the vagina. The tissue overlying the hematoma may give way, causing hemorrhage, and hemorrhage into the peritoneum may be massive and fatal. Retroperitoneal dissection may result in a mass reaching as far as beneath the diaphragm, which may be palpable in the abdomen or may become evident as the woman becomes anemic or an infection develops.[15] Alternately, the woman may present with hemodynamic instability and abdominal pain after delivery.[44]

Predisposing Factors: Episiotomy, forceps delivery, pudendal block, incomplete hemostasis with repair, rough handling of the tissues during repair.

Diagnosis: By clinical examination or MRI.[30]

m *Management*

1. A hematoma ≤4 cm in size and not enlarging is **managed expectantly.** Apply **ice** for 24 hours, then apply heat. Order broad-spectrum **antibiotics**. Prescribe good **perineal care**, iron supplementation to **correct anemia, good nutrition and fluid intake, analgesia, and rest.**[44]
2. The hematoma >4 cm, or one that continues to enlarge, requires **consultation** with the physician. **Anticipatory guidance: Incision and drainage** is performed with ligation of bleeding vessels and closure and packing of the wound. **Antibiotics** may be given.[44] Blood loss is usually greater than suspected. Hypovolemia and anemia must be assessed and corrected.[15]

Pelvic Cellulitis

Bacteria from an infected uterus or cervix invade connective tissue extending through the broad ligament. Endometritis and subinvolution are present. The degree of fever generally reflects the degree of infection, and high fever suggests cellulitis. Chills suggest bacteremia.[15]

m *Management*

1. **Consult** with the obstetrician.
2. **Anticipatory guidance: Antibiotics** are prescribed. Surgical incision and drainage may be required if an abscess has formed.[15]

Pelvic Abscess

A pelvic abscess forms when endometritis results in a parametrial pus-forming inflammation, forming a mass in the broad ligament. Rupture can cause life-threatening peritonitis.[15] The woman's fever persists after antibiotics are given. Malaise and tachycardia are present. The woman has lower abdominal pain and tenderness; and a pelvic mass is palpable anterior, posterior, or lateral to the uterus. The WBC count is elevated with a shift to the left.[22]

Diagnosis: Ultrasound examination, MRI, and CT may be used to confirm the diagnosis.[22]

m *Management*

1. **Refer** the woman to an obstetrician when the fever and other symptoms of endometritis do not subside after 48 hours of antibiotic prophylaxis.
2. **Anticipatory guidance:** Physician management includes **surgical drainage** (by colpotomy, needle aspiration, or open laparotomy) and administration of **antibiotics** until the woman has been afebrile and asymptomatic for 24 to 48 hours.[22]

• PSYCHOLOGICAL CHANGES OF THE PUERPERIUM

Postpartum Blues ("Maternity Blues" or "Baby Blues")

This normal, mild, self-limiting depression usually peaks between days 3 and 5, typically resolving within 24 to 72 hours or by day 10, although it may recur over the next several weeks.[32] Occurring in up to 70% women after delivery, the depression may be related to lowered tryptophan levels and will resolve spontaneously.[15] Recent research has shown that the maternal hypothalamic-pituitary-adrenal (HPA) axis is suppressed during the third trimester as a result of the placental output of corticotropin-releasing hormone. Delivery of the placenta with abrupt discontinuance of the placental hormones may affect mood until the maternal HPA axis resumes full function in days to weeks.[19,39] Weeping, depression, anxiety, restlessness, headache, elation, mood lability, forgetfulness, irritability, depersonalization, insomnia, appetite disturbances, and negative feelings toward the infant may be observed.[32]

m *Management*

1. **Offer support**[22] and reassure the woman about the normalcy and the transient nature of the depression. Encourage verbalization of what may seem like socially unacceptable feelings.
2. Encourage **skin-to-skin mother-infant contact** that stimulates hormonal secretion and may stimulate earlier resumption of HPA axis function, preventing depression.[19]
3. Evaluate the woman's fatigue and assist her in problem-solving if she is **sleep-deprived.**[22]
4. Observe for **resolution vs. development of neurosis or psychosis.** See postpartum neurosis, below, and postpartum psychosis, p. 240.
5. **Complementary measures:**
   a. **Homeopathy** experts recommend remedies for postpartum depression.[29,48,56]
   b. **Acupuncture** and **shiatsu** may be used in the treatment of postpartum depression to bolster a mother's energy and spirits.[31,72]
   c. **Nutritional measures:** Suggest **vitamin B** supplementation[48] if intake appears to be inadequate.
   d. **Reflexology:** A general treatment, with special attention given to any areas of discomfort, may lift the spirits.[66] **See information on reflexology, p. 567.**
   e. **Herbs: St. Johns's wort** is known to be useful in the treatment of mild to moderate but not severe depression.[24,28,38,48,52] **See information on herbs, p. 563.**

Postpartum Depression (or Neurosis)

Major postpartum depression begins about 10 days to 30 weeks after delivery, lasts as long as 1 year, and is different from the baby blues described previously.[4] Postpartum depression occurs in 8% to 15% of new mothers[54] and may recur.[22] In addition to signs of depression, the new mother may feel that "no one understands," she may think obsessively about being a "bad mother," and she may have thoughts of harming the infant associated with guilt and fear.[4] Most new mothers do not seek help for depression, and only about 25% of cases are recognized.[6] The role of hormones is unclear, but they are probably influential.[26] The relationship with the infant may be impaired, and long-term effects on child development and behavior may be seen.[58] Depressed mothers talk less to their infants, display less affection, and are less responsive to infant cues than nondepressed mothers. Infants of depressed mothers show more negative facial expressions and fewer positive facial expressions at the age of 3 months, have more eating and sleeping difficulties, and are more withdrawn than infants of nondepressed mothers.[35]

Predisposing Factors:
- **Psychiatric factors:** A negative birth experience; history of psychiatric illness; low self-esteem[54]; stressful life events[51]; a history of prenatal depression, postpartum "blues," or prenatal anxiety[4]
- **Demographic factors:** Teenaged unmarried, medically indigent, family of origin of ≥ 6 children, economic difficulties, dissatisfied with education
- **Relationship factors:** Separation from one or both parents in childhood; poor parental support and attention in childhood; poor family support during pregnancy[45]; sexual, emotional, and/or physical abuse in childhood[8,9]; poor relationship with partner
- **Cultural factors:** The degree of religiosity, role definition, and community support and rituals are associated with decreased depression (explaining the varying incidence among populations)[16]

Differential Diagnoses:
- Sleep deprivation[35]
- Puerperal hypothyroidism[22]
- Other underlying medical illnesses[71]
- Psychosis (see p. 240)[243]

Pharmacologic Treatment for the Lactating Mother

During lactation, lithium crosses into breastmilk. Some infants experience lithium toxic effects. Valproate also crosses into the breastmilk. Thrombocytopenia and anemia were reported in one infant. Carbamazepine also crosses into breastmilk in amounts that have been reported to be sufficient to result in hepatic dysfunction. Historically, valproate and carbamazepine—but not lithium—have been considered safe for use during breastfeeding. Authors suggest that the research is inadequate, and these recommendations are based on insufficient evidence.[12] Paroxetine, fluoxetine, and sertraline have been shown to be safe for use by the lactating mother.[35]

m *Management*

1. Include questions for **identification of risk factors** for postpartum depression in the initial prenatal history.[22]
2. **Conduct postpartum "debriefing"** (counseling, support, and understanding regarding the birth experience), which may reduce postpartum depression.[36]
3. Identify the problem early by maintaining a high index of suspicion. Schedule a postpartum visit before the standard 6 weeks for a patient at risk. **Carefully explore any sign** of depression, because the mother may be embarrassed to seek help, feeling that she is failing in her new role.[22]
4. **Consult or refer** the woman for psychologic and pharmacologic treatment.
5. **Pharmacologic intervention:** Tricyclic antidepressants or selective serotonin reuptake inhibitors (SSRIs) are prescribed.[20] According to Epperson,[20] plasma concentrations of the medications are usually low in the serum of breastfed babies and most drugs can be used without adverse affects on the infant. Suri et al[64] suggest that the infant's serum levels be closely monitored. They add that the drugs that have been studied in a limited way include tricyclic antidepressants, SSRIs, benzodiazepines, lithium, carbamazepine, and divalproex. Schou[57] suggests that the tricyclic antidepressants, lithium, or the SSRIs may be used after delivery if required.
6. **Education and support of the woman's family** is essential.
7. **Identify suicidal risk.** The woman at risk may require hospitalization.[71]
8. See **complementary measures** noted under Postpartum Blues and Psychosis, on pp. 238 and 241.

Puerperal Psychosis

The diagnosis of puerperal psychosis is made when the depressed woman expresses suicidal ideation or becomes delusional.[22] Previously diagnosed mental illness may recur. In most of these women, puerperal psychosis manifests as manic or depressive episodes with confusion and disorientation. Threats of violence toward herself or the children are dangerous signs to be taken seriously.[15] The incidence of psychosis is 1 to 2 per 1000; and it recurs in 50% to 75% of these cases.[51]

Predisposing Factors: Bipolar disorder (25% risk), unwanted pregnancy, poor relationship with the partner,[15] hypothyroidism.[51]

m *Management*

1. Make a **referral** to a psychiatrist.[22]
2. **Anticipatory guidance:** The psychiatrist will **hospitalize** the woman for evaluation, suicidal precautions, and the beginning of therapy. **Treatment** may include electroshock therapy and administration of

tricyclic antidepressants, neuroleptic drugs, SSRIs, and lithium carbonate.[51]

3. The **spouse** will require support.[42]
4. **Complementary measures:** Some experts recommend **homeopathic** treatment for postpartum depression.[60]

• GENERAL POSTPARTUM HEALTH AND COMPLICATIONS

Postnatal Exercise

Indications: A return to exercise after pregnancy results in improved emotional status and decreased risk for PPH.[1]

Assessment of Readiness for Exercise: Consider the mother's fitness before delivery, mother-infant adjustment, and any birth injury sustained.

First 24 Hours: The woman may perform Kegel exercises, abdominal tightening, and leg stretches while breathing deeply to prevent thrombophlebitis.

After 3 Days: The woman may lie on her back with knees bent up and lift her head to look at her feet. When this maneuver causes no discomfort, abdominal strengthening exercises can be started slowly. Fatigue, pain, and numbness are signals to slow down or modify exercises. Beginning after 1 to 2 weeks, short walks can be taken.[69]

Readiness for a Regular Exercise Program: Gabbe et al[22] state that after an uncomplicated delivery, physical activity, walking up and down stairs, lifting heavy objects, driving a car, and doing muscle-toning exercises may be resumed for brief periods without delay and may be increased as the fatigue and lethargy of the postpartum period ease.

Exercise and Milk Production: Postnatal exercise does not decrease the volume or composition of breastmilk in lactating women, nor does it influence infant weight gain or maternal serum prolactin levels at 12 weeks after delivery.[18]

Postpartum Weight Loss

The weight gained during pregnancy is predictive of the weight that will be retained after delivery. A direct relationship has been noted between parity and increased weight. Most women are heavier 2 years after a pregnancy than women who have not been pregnant.[33]

Women who breastfeed tend to lose weight at the same rate as women who do not breastfeed according to Suitor,[63] but Lawrence[37] states that women who breastfeed return to their prepregnancy state sooner, and furthermore, have less risk of being obese in later life. Reifsnider and Gill[53] state that 80% of lactating women lose weight after delivery, some beginning as early as 15 days postpartum, and most lose 1 to 2 lb per month. Women who breastfeed for 1 year lose more weight during the second 6 months than they do during the first 6 months. The more frequently the woman breastfeeds, the greater her weight loss will be.[53]

Weight loss of up to 2 lb per month, achieved through a combination of diet and exercise, does not adversely affect lactation. Attempting to lose 4 lb per month through dieting alone, however, requires too great a reduction in caloric intake.[53] Women who increase their physical activity do not lose weight unless they also restrict their calories.[63] Aerobic exercise does not affect the quantity or composition of breastmilk. Returning to the prenatal weight is important to reduce the risks of obesity in later life,[53] including heart disease, diabetes, and some cancers.

Adynamic Colonic Ileus

Also called *pseudo-obstruction of the colon* (or Ogilvie syndrome), adynamic colonic ileus may occur over a 2- to 3-day period after vaginal or cesarean delivery.[40] Incidence varies from one in 1500 to 66,500 deliveries.[15] Symptoms include nausea, constipation, and abdominal distention. Perforation of the colon (associated with a 70% mortality rate) may occur at >12 cm diameter.[40]

Diagnosis: X-ray examination of the abdomen shows distention of the proximal colon.[40]

ⓜ Management

1. **Consult** with a physician when adynamic ileus is suspected.
2. **Anticipatory guidance:** Physician management will include fluid replacement and colonoscopy for diagnosis and treatment. If the colon reaches 10 to 12 cm in diameter, nasogastric suction and rectal tube are used for decompression to prevent rupture. Surgery may be necessary if medical and endoscopic treatment are unsuccessful, or if the bowel reaches the point of near perforation.[40]

Obstetric Paralysis

Pressure on the lumbosacral plexus or external popliteal, femoral, obturator, or sciatic nerves during labor may cause weakness of the flexors of the ankles and the extensors of the toes. Weakened ankle dorsiflexion, footdrop, and occasionally gluteal muscle weakness result. Neuralgia or cramplike pain may extend down the legs at delivery and persist afterward.[15] Complications of regional anesthesia, leg positioning, or a difficult forceps application may cause such an injury. Most of these injuries are minor and transient in nature.[22] See also symphysis pubis separation, p. 243.

ⓜ Management

1. **Consult** with the physician.
2. Obtain an **anesthesia** consultation if the woman received anesthesia during the birth process, as well as a **neurology** consultation.[22]

Management usually involves watchful waiting. Worsening may indicate a process that requires surgical intervention.
3. Consider a **physical therapy** consultation. **Equipment** such as a walker or wheelchair may be required.

Separated Symphysis Pubis

Relaxation of the pelvic girdle caused by hormonal (relaxin and progesterone) and biomechanical factors may result in separated symphysis pubis (SSP), although some degree of widening is normal and is present in 42% of women who are asymptomatic during the postpartum period. The condition occurs more often among Scandinavian women. Genetic predisposition may play a part. Previous SSP, SSP in a family member, multiparity, cephalopelvic disproportion (CPD), precipitous or difficult labor, excessive abduction of the legs at delivery, and operative deliveries predispose women to SSP. However, many cases of SSP occur during normal spontaneous vaginal deliveries without evidence of trauma or excessive forces.[17]

SSP manifests as localized pain in the symphysis pubis; difficulty walking, standing, or using the legs; sexual difficulties; low back pain; marked tenderness over the symphysis pubis; edema; ecchymosis; or a gaping joint defect palpable on physical examination. The pain may be exacerbated when the women ovulates after delivery. Onset may be abrupt, may be experienced by the woman as a bursting sensation, or may be heard as a crack at the time of delivery; or SSP may not be noticed until the woman tries to ambulate. Mild cases may resolve in 2 days to 8 weeks without intervention, while more serious cases may not resolve for 3 to 8 months.[17]

ⓜ Management

1. Manage mild cases with **pain medications** and close follow-up.[17]
2. **Advise bed rest with a tight binder** or a peritrochanteric belt wrapped tightly around the symphysis pubis to maintain alignment, **with a backboard** under the bed. **A trapeze bar** will facilitate movement. Ambulation is achieved with a **walker or crutches.**[17]
3. **Teach the woman** to shuffle, instead of picking feet up, to walk more comfortably. Advise her to avoid using stairs and to avoid abduction or adduction of the hip. Antiembolic stockings are worn. Isometric exercises will prevent thromboses caused by immobilization. A support person needs to be present with the woman at all times once she is discharged home.[17]
4. Provide **referrals** for physical therapy, an orthopedic surgeon, home health nursing, and a social worker if necessary. **Anticipatory guidance:** Lidocaine and/or hydrocortisone injections into the joint may provide relief.[17]
5. Surgical fixation of the joint is rarely required.[17]

Puerperal Fever: Differential Diagnoses

The standard definition of a postpartum fever is $\geq$38.0° C or 100.4° F on any 2 of the first 10 days after delivery, with the exception of the first 24 hours.[22]

Differential Diagnoses: Pelvic cellulitis, pelvic thrombophlebitis, or infection of a perineal injury. Nongenital causes of fever such as respiratory tract infection, pyelonephritis, breast engorgement, bacterial mastitis, thrombophlebitis, or cesarean wound infection[15]; other possibilities are cholecystitis, appendicitis, or a viral syndrome.[22]

Differential Diagnoses if the fever persists despite 48 hours of antibiotic therapy: Resistant organism, pelvic abscess, septic pelvic thrombophlebitis, relapse of connective tissue disease, or drug fever (eosinophilia due to antibiotic therapy).[22]

Septic Pelvic Thrombophlebitis

Septic pelvic thrombophlebitis occurs when an intrauterine infection seeds organisms into the venous circulation, the organisms damage the vascular endothelium, and thrombophlebitis is initiated.[22] Ovarian, renal, iliofemoral, and femoral veins and the vena cava may be affected by infection and thrombophlebitis.[15]

Two presentations are observed:

1. Lower abdominal or flank pain that may radiate into the groin occurs 2 to 3 days after delivery with chills and with or without fever. Nausea, vomiting, and abdominal bloating and guarding may be seen, as well as tachycardia, stridor, and dyspnea if a pulmonary embolism has occurred. Bowel sounds are decreased or absent. Fifty percent to 70% of women have a rope-like mass originating near one uterine cornu and extending laterally and toward the head.

2. An antibiotic course given for endometritis provides symptomatic relief, but temperature instability, chills, and tachycardia continue in this scenario, called *enigmatic fever.*[15]

Diagnosis: MRI and CT scan.[67] A trial course of heparin may be used by some physicians to make the diagnosis.[21]

Differential Diagnoses: Pyelonephritis, nephrolithiasis, appendicitis, broad ligament hematoma, adnexal torsion, and pelvic abscess.[22]

m *Management*

1. **Refer** the woman to the physician.
2. **Anticipatory guidance:** Physician management starts with administration of broad-spectrum **antibiotics:** Some physicians will administer anticoagulants.[21] Failure to improve with anticoagulation may require **surgical intervention** for ligation of the vessels or embolectomy by a vascular surgeon.[22]

• REFERENCES

1. American College of Obstetricians and Gynecologists (ACOG): *Exercise during pregnancy and the postpartum period,* Committee Opinion No. 267, Washington, DC, 2002, ACOG.
2. ACOG: *Antimicrobial therapy for obstetric patients,* Educational Bulletin No. 245, Washington, DC, 1998, ACOG.
3. Balch JF, Balch PA: *Prescription for nutritional healing,* ed 2, Garden City Park, NY, 1997, Avery.
4. Beck CT: A checklist to identify women at high risk for developing postpartum depression, *J Obstet Gynecol Neonatal Nurs* 27:39-45, 1998.
5. Bell KK, Rawlings NL: Promoting breastfeeding by managing common lactation problems, *Nurse Pract* 23:102-123, 1998.
6. Borrill J: Detecting and preventing postnatal depression, *Community Nurse* 4:19-20, 1998.
7. Budd S: Acupuncture. In Tiran D, Mack S, editors: *Complementary therapies for pregnancy and childbirth,* ed 2, Edinburgh, 2000, Baillière Tindall.
8. Buist A: Childhood abuse, parenting, and postpartum depression, *Aust N Z J Psychiatry* 32:479-487, 1998.
9. Buist A: Childhood abuse, postpartum depression and parenting difficulties: a literature review of associations, *Aust N Z J Psychiatry* 32:370-378, 1998.
10. Chaim W et al: Prevalence and clinical significance of postpartum endometritis, *Infect Dis Obstet Gynecol* 8:77-82, 2000.
11. Chamberlain G, Steer P: ABC of labour care: obstetric emergencies, *BMJ* 318:1342-1345, 1999.
12. Chaudron LH, Jefferson JW: Mood stabilizers during breastfeeding: a review, *J Clin Psychiatry* 61:79-90, 2000.
13. Cummings B, Tiran D: Homeopathy for pregnancy and childbirth. In Tiran D, Mack S, editors: *Complementary therapies for pregnancy and childbirth,* ed 2, Edinburgh, 2000, Baillière Tindall.
14. Cummings S, Ullman D: *Everybody's guide to homeopathic medicines,* New York, 1997, Jeremy P. Tarcher/Putnam.
15. Cunningham FG et al: *Williams obstetrics,* ed 20, Stamford, Conn, 1997, Appleton and Lange.
16. Dankner R et al: Cultural elements of postpartum depression: a study of 327 Jewish Jerusalem women, *J Reprod Med* 45:97-103, 2000.
17. Davidson MR: Examining separated symphysis pubis, *J Nurse Midwifery* 41:259-262, 1996.
18. Dewey KG et al: A randomized study of the effects of aerobic exercise by lactating women on breast-milk volume and composition, *N Engl J Med* 330:449-453, 1994.
19. Dombrowski MA et al: Kangaroo (skin-to-skin) care with a postpartum woman who felt depressed, *MCN Am J Matern Child Nurs* 26:214-216, 2001.
20. Epperson CN: Postpartum major depression: detection and treatment, *Am Fam Physician* 59:2247-2254, 2259-2260, 1999.
21. French RA, Cole C: An "enigmatic" case of back pain following regional anesthesia for caesarean section: septic pelvic thrombophlebitis, *Anaesth Intensive Care* 27:209-212, 1999.
22. Gabbe SG, Niebyl JR, Simpson JL, editors: *Obstetrics: normal & problem pregnancies,* ed 3, New York, 1996, Churchill Livingstone.
23. Gardner J: *Healing yourself,* ed 7 revised, Trumansburg, NY, 1982, The Crossing Press.
24. Griffith HW: *Healing herbs: the essential guide,* Tucson, Ariz, 2000, Fisher Books.
25. Hacker NF, Moore JG: *Essentials of obstetrics and gynecology,* ed 3, Philadelphia, 1998, WB Saunders.
26. Hendrick V, Altshuler LL, Suri R: Hormonal changes in the postpartum and implications for postpartum depression, *Psychosomatics* 39:93-101, 1998.
27. Hoffmann D: *The complete illustrated holistic herbal,* Boston, Mass, 1996, Element Books.

28. Hoffmann D: *The holistic herbal,* Findhorn, Scotland, 1985, Findhorn Press.

29. Idarius B: *The homeopathic childbirth manual,* Talmage, Calif, 1999, Idarius Press.

30. Jain KA, Olcott EW: Magnetic resonance imaging of postpartum pelvic hematomas: early experience in diagnosis and treatment planning, *Magn Reson Imaging* 17:973-977, 1999.

31. Johnson E: Shiatsu. In Tiran D, Mack S, editors: *Complementary therapies for pregnancy and childbirth,* ed 2, Edinburgh, 2000, Baillière Tindall.

32. Johnson TRB, Apgar B: Postpartum depression, *The Female Patient* Aug 1997. Available at: *http://www.obgyn.net/english/pubs /features/tfp/leopold.htm.*

33. Keppel KG, Taffel SM: Pregnancy-related weight gain and retention: implications of the 1990 Institute of Medicine Guidelines, *Am J Public Health* 83:1100-1103, 1993.

33a. Kloss J: *Back to Eden,* ed 2, Twin Lakes, Wis., 1999, Lotus Press.

34. Koehler N: *Artemis speaks: V.B.A.C. stories & natural childbirth information,* Occidental, Calif, 1985, Jerald R. Brown

35. Lamberg L: Safety of antidepressant use in pregnant and nursing women, *JAMA* 282: 222-223, 1999.

36. Lavender T, Walkinshaw SA: Can midwives reduce postpartum psychological morbidity? a randomized trial, *Birth* 25:215-219, 1998.

37. Lawrence RA: *A review of the medical benefits and contraindications to breastfeeding in the United States (Maternal and Child Health Technical Information Bulletin),* Arlington, Va, 1997, National Center for Education in Maternal and Child Health.

38. Mabey R et al, editors: *The new age herbalist,* New York, 1988, Collier Books.

39. Magiakou MA et al: Hypothalamic corticotropin-releasing hormone suppression during the postpartum period: implications for the increase of psychiatric manifestations at this time, *J Clin Endocrinol Metab* 81:1912-1917, 1996.

40. Mayer IE, Hussain H: Pregnancy and gastrointestinal disorders, *Gastroenterol Clin North Am* 27:1-36, 1998.

41. Medina IM: *Issues in women's health care: nutrition and herbs from menarche to menopause 3/28-29/98,* Brooklyn, NY, 1998, State University of New York Health Science Center at Brooklyn College of Health Related Professions Midwifery Education Program, course syllabus.

42. Meighan M et al: Living with postpartum depression: the father's experience, *MCN Am J Matern Child Nurs* 24:202-208, 1999.

43. Meyer S et al: The effects of birth on urinary continence mechanisms and other pelvic-floor characteristics, *Obstet Gynecol* 92:613-618, 1998.

44. Morrison EH: Common peripartum emergencies, *Am Fam Physician,* Nov 1, 1998. Published by The American Academy of Family Physicians. Available at: *http://www.aafp.org/afp/ 981101ap/morrison.html.*

45. Murata A et al: Prevalence and background factors of maternity blues, *Gynecol Obstet Invest* 46:99-104, 1998.

45a. Neifert MR: Clinical aspects of lactation: promoting breastfeeding success, *Clin Perinatol* 26: 281-306, 1999.

46. Nissim R: *Natural healing in gynecology,* San Francisco, 1996, Pandora (HarperCollins).

47. Ody P: *The complete medicinal herbal,* New York, 1993, Dorling Kindersley.

48. Page L: *Healthy healing,* ed 11, Carmel Valley, Calif, 2000, Healthy Healing Publications.

49. Parvati J: *Hygieia: a woman's herbal,* Berkeley, Calif, 1985, Bookpeople.

50. Parvati Baker J: Midwifery and herbs, *Midwifery Today* 26:29-31, Summer 1993.

51. Pedersen CA: Postpartum mood and anxiety disorders: a guide for the nonpsychiatric clinician with an aside on thyroid associations with postpartum mood; *Thyroid* 9(7): 691-697, 1999.

52. *Physician's desk reference (PDR) for herbal medicines,* Montvale, NJ, 1998, Medical Economics Co.

53. Reifsnider E, Gill SL: Nutrition for the childbearing years, *J Obstet Gynecol Neonatal Nurs* 29:43-55, 2000.

54. Righetti-Veltema M et al: Risk factors and predictive signs of postpartum depression, *J Affect Disord* 49:167-180, 1998.

55. Riordan J, Auerbach K: *Breastfeeding and human lactation,* ed 2, Sudbury, Mass, 1999, Jones and Bartlett.
56. Rose B, Scott-Moncrieff C: *Homeopathy for women,* London, 1998, Collins & Brown.
57. Schou M: Treating recurrent affective disorders during and after pregnancy: what can be taken safely? *Drug Saf* 18:143-152, 1998.
58. Seidman D: Postpartum psychiatric illness: the role of the pediatrician, *Pediatr Rev* 19:128-131, 1998.
59. Smith JW, Tully MR: Midwifery management of breastfeeding: using the evidence, *J Midwifery Womens Health* 46:423-438, 2001.
60. Smith T: *Homeopathy for pregnancy and nursing mothers,* Worthing, England, 1993, Insight Editions.
61. Spitz AM, Lee NC, Peterson HB: Treatment for lactation suppression: little progress in one hundred years, *Am J Obstet Gynecol* 179:1485-1490, 1998.
62. Stapleton H, Tiran D: Herbal medicine. In Tiran D, Mack S, editors: *Complementary therapies for pregnancy and childbirth,* ed 2, Edinburgh, 2000, Baillière Tindall.
63. Suitor CW: *Maternal weight gain: a report of an expert work group,* Arlington, Va, 1997, National Center for Education in Maternal and Child Health.
64. Suri RA et al: Managing psychiatric medications in the breast-feeding woman, *Medscape Womens Health* 3:1, 1998.
65. Tarr K: *Herbs, helps, and pressure points for pregnancy and childbirth,* ed 3, Provo, Utah, 1984, Sunbeam Publications.
66. Tiran D: Reflexology in midwifery practice. In Tiran D, Mack S, editors: *Complementary therapies for pregnancy and childbirth,* ed 2, Edinburgh, 2000, Baillière Tindall.
67. Twickler DM et al: Imaging of puerperal septic thrombophlebitis: prospective comparison of MR imaging, CT, and sonography, *AJR Am J Roentgenol* 169:1039-1043, 1997.
68. Ullman R, Reichenberg-Ullman J: *Homeopathic self-care,* Rocklin, Calif, 1997, Prima.
69. Varney H: *Varney's midwifery,* ed 3, Sudbury, Mass, 1997, Jones and Bartlett.
70. Weed S: *Menopausal years: the wise woman way,* Woodstock, NY, 1992, Ash Tree.
71. Weintraub TA, Paine LL, Weintraub DH: Primary care for women: comprehensive assessment and management of common mental health problems, *J Nurse Midwifery* 41: 125-138, 1996.
72. Yelland S: *Acupuncture in midwifery,* Cheshire, England, 1996, Books for Midwives Press.

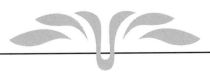

Chapter 5

The Newborn

History of the Newborn

A history of the newborn includes the following information.

Identifying Facts: Name, hospital number, date of birth, sex, feeding type

Family History: Diabetes, congenital anomalies, infectious diseases, cardiopulmonary abnormalities, health of father, siblings and other family members; medical conditions or traits that "run in the family"; consanguinity of parents.

Parental Demographics: Age, education, vocation, ethnic and racial backgrounds

Maternal History: Gravidity, parity, last menstrual period (LMP), estimated date of confinement (EDC), complications of previous pregnancies, medical/surgical and gynecologic histories, antepartum course (particularly substance abuse, gestational diabetes, preeclampsia, bleeding during pregnancy, size-dates discrepancy, polyhydramnios or oligohydramnios, infection or other illnesses, medications taken), extent and location of prenatal care, assessments of fetal well-being.

Maternal Laboratory Test Results: Blood type and Rh factor, antibody screen, rubella titer, serology, hepatitis panel, Hb and Hct values, tuberculosis (TB) testing.

Labor and Delivery: Date and time of delivery; weeks of gestation at delivery by dates and ultrasound examination; length of first and second stages of labor; fetal distress or acidosis; maternal fever; presence of meconium; length of rupture of membranes; presentation; complications; type of delivery; instrumentation; analgesia and time; anesthesia and complications; placental size, color, and odor; cord insertion; and appearance of the cord including number of vessels and size (stained? odor? abnormalities?)

Immediate Neonatal Period: Apgar scores, resuscitation, vital signs, temperature, vitamin K status; ability to suck, feed; alertness; whether infant has voided or passed meconium; jitteriness; unusual cry.

Neonatal Laboratory Test Results: Glucose level, blood type, Rh factor, Coombs' test, Hct.

Physical Assessment of the Newborn

Physical examination may be performed in any order, depending on the baby's state.

General Appearance

In the assessment of a neonate's general appearance check the following:

- General **muscle tone** and spontaneous **position.** Opisthotonos (an extended neck) may signal brain damage, birth asphyxia, or neurologic abnormalities. A premature infant may have a frog-legged appearance.
- Spontaneous **movement.** Lack of movement, asymmetry, or tremulousness may indicate birth asphyxia, respiratory difficulty, neurologic dysfunction, or prematurity.
- **State** or level of arousal. The infant may sleep lightly or deeply, may be awake making small or large peripheral movements, or may cry. Note ease of movement between states.
- **Overall motor movement.** Infant should move appropriately between states. Constant bicycling or swatting without stimulation; weak or asymmetric movements are abnormal. Jitteriness with sucking may be a sign of neurologic problems, hypocalcemia, hypoglycemia, or irritability associated with maternal drug use; while jitteriness that stops during sucking is most often a normal, physiologic activity.[13]
- **Moro reflex.** Lasts a maximum of 4 months.
- **Cry.** Consolable? Weak? High-pitched? A high-pitched shrill cry is associated with increased cranial pressure or drug addiction. A low-pitched, infrequent, hoarse cry may be associated with hypothyroidism or hypocalcemic tetany. The "cri du chat" sounds like a cat crying and may indicate chromosomal defects. Absence of crying suggests mental retardation or severe illness.
- **Weight, length, pulse, respirations, temperature.** Normal temperature is 37.6° to 37.8° C (99.7° to 100° F) rectally.

Skin

Skin **condition** may indicate several conditions. The **postmature baby** has paler, thicker skin, which may be peeling. The **premature infant** has thin, delicate skin, which tends to be dark red and to bleed and bruise easily.[53] Specific lesions are noted in Table 5-1.

- **Acrocyanosis** (cyanosis of the extremities) is normal for one day. Lobster-like mottling may be normal, occurring due to immature organ systems.[13]
- **Cyanosis.** Sometimes difficult to evaluate because of the polycythemia of the newborn; can be demonstrated by momentarily blanching the skin as is done for jaundice.

Table 5-1 / Miscellaneous Skin Conditions

Condition	Appearance	Timing	Course and Treatment
Acne neonatorum	Papules, occasionally pustules.	1-2 mo	Clears by 1-2 yr; medication is prescribed for extensive cases.[13]
Erythema toxicum	Like "flea bites," erythematous macules, papules, and pustules are present in 50% of newborns.[13]	Usually at 2-4 days, possibly at birth	R/O herpes simplex virus (HSV), *Staphylococcus* infection. Resolves within hours to 10 days.[53]
Hemangiomas	May be flat; commonly caused by dilated capillaries; or may be mass lesion, consisting of large, blood-filled cavities. Isolated or part of a syndrome.	Birth	Spontaneously involute in 5 to 10 yr. Steroids given if orifice affected.
Types of Hemangiomas			
Nevus flammeus (port wine stain)	Dilated capillaries, a macular lesion of variable size—pink/purple in white subjects, black in black subjects. May take up half body; common on face.	Birth	May fade but does not disappear. Laser treatment if skin becomes thick, nodular. May be associated with glaucoma or Sturge-Weber syndrome.[13]
Cavernosus hemangioma	Bluish, diffuse, cystic lesion with poorly defined borders	Birth	Grows—in 80% to no more than twice the original size, then spontaneously involutes. 50% gone by 5 yr. If nearby, may occlude trachea as it grows.[13] If large, may trap platelets and cause DIC or interfere with nearby organ function.[53]
Macular hemangioma (nevus simplex, stork bite)	Flat, salmon-colored patch, usually on face and neck; found in 50% of newborns.	Birth	Usually fades within the first year.[13]
Nevus vasculosus (strawberry mark)	Bright red, protuberant lesion, commonly found on face, scalp, back. May occur in multiples.	At birth, or may develop in early months	May expand rapidly to a stationary size, then spontaneously regress. By 5 yr, 50% are gone.[13]
Other Skin Manifestations			
Lanugo hair	Fine, soft hair present on premature infants on head, shoulders, and ears.	Birth	When located on lumbo-sacral spine may suggest occult spina bifida.
Milia	Tiny white papules on face; sebum blocking opening of follicles. On oral mucous membranes, called *Epstein's pearls*.	Birth	Rupture spontaneously and resolve usually within first weeks of life.[13]
Mongolian spots	Hyperpigmentation purple/black usually in sacral area, also abdomen, extremities.[41]	Birth	Fade in weeks to years.[53]

Table 5-1 / Miscellaneous Skin Conditions—cont'd

Condition	Appearance	Timing	Course and Treatment
	Present in 90% of African American and Asian American infants and 5% of white infants.		
Telangiectasia "stork bite" or "angel kisses"	Flat, irregularly shaped, salmon-colored patches on face, neck.	Birth	Usually fade within a year.

- **Jaundice.** Assessed by momentarily blanching the skin. Begins at head and moves down—note level (see p. 274).
- **Pallor.** May indicate edema, asphyxia, or shock.[53] An infant's head, right arm, and right chest may be pink, with the remainder of the body being pale or cyanotic, when the ductus has not closed. The line of demarcation vanishes as the ductus opens and peripheral vascular resistance drops.[13]
- **Plethora.** Ruddiness noted in the mucous membranes, less so on the soles and palms, may indicate polycythemia.[13]
- **Mottling.** May be due to transient skin temperature changes but may also be due to a serious illness, and the infant with mottled skin should be observed carefully.
- **Meconium staining.** Staining of vernix occurs within 15 hours of exposure to meconium. The fingernails stain within 6 hours.[30]
- **Texture and edema.** Edema may be differentiated from the state of being well-nourished by the presence of fine wrinkles at wrists and ankles.
- **Lesions, moisture, lanugo,** evidence of **birth trauma, pigmentation.**

Head

During examination of the head check the following:
- **Shape** and symmetry.
- **Proportion** to body and to face.
- **Circumference** (measured above ears). Changing as molding resolves[13] the head circumference is normally 32 to 38 cm in the average term infant. The head exceeds the abdominal circumference until 32 weeks of gestation, equals the abdomen in gestational weeks 32 to 36, and thereafter is smaller. An excessively large head may indicate hydrocephalus.[53]
- Sagittal, lambdoidal, and coronal **sutures.** Premature closure of suture lines is called *cranial synostosis*: sutures do not give when alternate

sides are pressed. Soft areas in the parietal bones along the sagittal suture are called *craniotabes* and are seen in premature infants and those who experienced uterine compression. Craniotabes are usually insignificant but must be investigated if they persist. Soft areas in the occiput are significant; and, when present, osteogenesis imperfecta, Down syndrome, cretinism, and other conditions must be ruled out.

- The diamond-shaped **anterior fontanel** is approximately 20 ± 10 mm,[53] but there is great variation, and the size of the fontanel is not significant.[13] It closes at 9 to 16 months. The **posterior fontanel**, which is triangular, may be closed at birth or is closed by about 4 months. The average size is 1 cm × 1 cm.[73] Fontanels should be flat: bulging indicates increased intracranial pressure, and depression indicates dehydration.[53]
- Presence of **molding** (overriding of the occipital and frontal bones by the parietal bones).
- Presence of a **cephalohematoma.** Sustained during labor and delivery, this subperiosteal hemorrhage is limited to one bone, usually the parietal, and does not overlie a suture. It may last about 8 weeks.[13]
- **Caput succedaneum** is swelling of the scalp where it presented through the cervix. Bruising may be seen. Caput may overlie suture lines.

Hair

- **Texture, direction** of growth.
- **Distribution.** Hair below the neck crease suggests syndromes associated with short and/or webbed necks.[13]
- Scalp **lesions.** Aplasia cutis congenita is a defect of the scalp.
- **Color.** Note concordance with race. Red hair in a black baby, for example, may indicate albinism. Note uniformity. A white forelock, for example, may be associated with deafness and mental retardation.

Face

- **Shape** and **expression.**
- **Eyelashes** and **eyebrows.**
- **Symmetry** at rest and during crying and sucking. Asymmetry may be due to hypoplasia or palsy of the seventh nerve.[53]

Eyes

Eyes may be most easily examined by holding the infant up and tilting gently forward and backward, when the baby will spontaneously reflexively open his or her eyes.[53]

- **Placement and symmetry.** Widely spaced eyes may be associated with congenital syndromes.
- **Size.** Normal size is 2.5 cm. Large eyes are called *hypertelorism;* small eyes are called *hypotelorism.* Both are associated with congenital

syndromes. Note the fit of the eyeballs in relation to the sockets. Note their depth.

- **Position.** Upward or downward slant may indicate congenital syndromes.
- **Corneal size and clarity.**[53]
- **Iris color.** Full pigmentation occurs at 10 to 12 months. A ventral cleft may be associated with defects in the lens and retina. Gold dots seen at the periphery of the iris, Brushfield's spots, may be normal or may be associated with Trisomy 21.
- **Sclera.** Normally clear but may be yellow with jaundice, hemorrhagic as a result of birth trauma, or blue with osteogenesis imperfecta.
- **Conjunctiva.** Small hemorrhages are common. Inflammation may be present as a result of erythromycin prophylaxis.[53]
- **Pupils.** Equal and reactive after 2 to 3 weeks.[13] The pupil is 1.8 to 5.4 mm in size.
- Symmetric **optical blink reflex.** Bright light causes blinking of both eyes and dorsiflexion of the head. Testing this reflex is done in lieu of visual acuity testing. The vision of a newborn is estimated to be about 20/600.
- **Dolls' eyes.** When the head is turned, eyes turn from midline to continue to look upward; considered normal for 10 days.
- **Red reflex.** Absent with cataracts.
- **Corneal light reflex** and **tracking of light** are noted.
- Transient **strabismus (cross-eyed).** Not a cause for concern if alternating eyes cross and if movements are convergent.
- Presence of **epicanthal folds.** May be associated with congenital defects.
- **Retina.** Should be clear on ophthalmoscopic examination.
- **Lacrimal duct.** Should be patent.
- **Eyelids.** Note edema or ptosis (drooping).[53]
- **Congenital glaucoma.** Evidenced by photophobia, excessive tearing, cloudy corneas, or large-appearing eyes.[13]

Ears

- **Symmetry and alignment.** Normal insertion is on an imagined line through the inner and outer canthus of the eye. Low-set ears may indicate a congenital syndrome, often with kidney defects.
- Extra **skin tags or pits.** Pedunculated skin tags may be ligated tightly at the base with suture.[53]
- **Shape. Cartilage** formation indicates maturity.
- **Hearing.** Infant turns toward whisper; startles in response to loud noise. Particularly important in cases of anomalies of the head and neck, family history of deafness, very low birthweight (VLBW), severe asphyxia, fetal infection, and other syndromes associated with deafness.[13]

- **Otoscopy** is done by pulling the pinna downward. Vernix caseosa may be present within the external canal or amniotic fluid may be seen behind the dull gray tympanic membrane.

Nose

- **Position and shape.** A position off midline or a flattened or beaked bridge may indicate congenital syndromes.
- **Nares.** Assessed for normal shape, symmetry, and **patency.** One nare is occluded at a time, and breathing is observed through the open nare, ruling out choanal atresia—occlusion of the posterior nares—which causes severe respiratory distress in the infant. Enlarged, bulbous, or absent nares may occur with congenital anomalies. Any **discharge** or **flaring** is noted.

Mouth

- **Size** and **shape.** A birdlike mouth is seen with fetal alcohol syndrome; a small mouth, microstomia, is seen with Down syndrome; and a wide mouth, macrostomia, is seen with metabolic disorders.
- **Symmetric grimace.**
- Intact arched **palate.**
- **Uvula** size and function. A bifid uvula may be associated with a submucous cleft palate. With normal neurologic function, the uvula will rise with crying.
- **Reflexes.** The **suck reflex** is present from 32 weeks' gestation to 3 to 4 months. The **rooting reflex** is present from 34 weeks' gestation to 3 to 4 months. The **gag reflex** should be present.
- **Lips.** Should be fully formed. A prolonged philtrum (groove from nose to upper lip) may indicate a congenital syndrome.[53]
- **Tongue** size. Macroglossia is associated with hypothyroidism.
- **Gums.** Precocious teeth are seen rarely in a normal newborn's mouth and will be shed before deciduous teeth erupt; teeth may also be present with some congenital syndromes.
- **Mucous membranes.** Note moisture. Excessive salivation may indicate a tracheoesophageal fistula or esophageal atresia. Thrush is identified by gray and white patches.
- **Chin.** Should be well proportioned. Micrognathia suggests Pierre-Robin syndrome.

Tongue

Note **size, proportion, color, coating, movement, tone,** length of **frenulum.**

Neck

- **Shape, lymph nodes,** presence of **masses.**
- **Movement.** The range of motion should enable the infant to rotate the chin to each shoulder. Congenital torticollis (head tilted to one

shoulder while the chin points to the other shoulder) occurs with a hematoma of the sternocleidomastoid muscle from a birth injury.[53]

- **Skin folds or webbing.** Webbing occurs with Turner's and other congenital syndromes.
- **Thyroid.** Normally found at midline without nodules.
- **Clavicle.** Fracture of the clavicle occurs in 1.7% to 2.9% of all term births, although many are not detected until a callous forms over the fracture at 2 to 3 weeks. A fracture usually occurs at the outer two thirds of the bone and may be palpated as crepitus, swelling, or tenderness along the shaft of the bone. Decreased motion in the affected hand or refusal to breastfeed while lying on the affected side may indicate discomfort.[13]

Arms

- **Length.** Proportionate (should reach upper thigh) and equal.
- **Movement** of arms and fingers.
- **Finger number and length.** The **grasp reflex** is present. Note syndactyly (fusion) or polydactyly (extra fingers). **Nails** should be normal in shape and extend beyond nail beds. Fingernails in premature infants may be rudimentary, whereas postmature infants' nails may extend past the fingertips.[53]
- **Capillary refill.** Normal ≤3 seconds.
- **Dermatoglyphics** of fingers and palms. The Simian crease, a single palmer crease from above the thumb to below the little finger, may be associated with a short stubby thumb and a short little finger and occurs with chromosomal anomalies such as Trisomy 21. Normal finger patterns are loops, arches, and whorls. Loops are the most common. The presence of more than four arches is considered abnormal. When the thumb is found under flexed fingers, it is called the cerebral thumb sign and may indicate a cerebral abnormality.
- **Gestational age markers.** The **square window** is done by estimating the angle between the palm and the forearm when the wrist is flexed forward. The **scarf sign** is performed by pulling one hand toward the opposite shoulder, like a scarf wrapped about the neck, noting the relationship of the elbow to the midline. A third test, the **arm recoil test,** is performed by flexing the forearm at the elbow for 2 to 5 seconds, fully extending it, and seeing how long it takes the infant to resume a flexed position. The latter two tests may be invalidated by birth injuries that alter the motor strength or integrity of the upper trunk or arms.

Chest

- **Shape** and symmetry.
- **Circumference** at nipples. The normal range is 30 to 36 cm, 1 to 2 cm less than head circumference (normal range, 30 to 36 cm).

- Development of **areolae.** Placement of **nipples.** Wide placement is seen in Turner's syndrome.[53] Supernumerary nipples are present with or without areolae in 1.2% to 1.6% of darkly pigmented infants, and less in lighter pigmented infants. In Caucasian infants, they may be associated with renal anomalies.

- Presence of **breast tissue.** Affected by nutritional status, fat deposition, and maturity. Milk production ("witches' milk") caused by maternal estrogen resolves at 1 to 2 weeks.[13]

- **Symmetry of expansion.** Lack of symmetry may signal diaphragmatic hernia, pneumothorax, or phrenic nerve damage.

- **Respirations.** Normally abdominal in the newborn; normal rate is 30 to 60 breaths/min, counted for a full minute. Rate >60 breaths/min indicates disease. Periodic breathing (Cheyne-Stokes respirations—up to 15 seconds of apnea without accompanying bradycardia) may be present. The infant displaying apnea longer than 15 seconds, with accompanying bradycardia, is at risk for sudden infant death syndrome (SIDS). Note seesaw respirations or paradoxical respirations. Signs of respiratory distress include **grunting, flaring** of the nostrils, **retraction** of intercostal muscles and the sternum, and the **use of accessory muscles.** Normal **breath sounds** are clear and equal, loud because of the thin chest wall, and almost all bronchovesicular. Rales are difficult to interpret in this period, but they should persist for only a few hours after birth.

- **Heart sounds.** Higher pitched than those of adults. **Sinus arrhythmia** (regular variance with respiration) is a normal finding. The **third heart sound** may be heard normally and is generally best heard at the apex. The **second heart sound** may normally split in infants. Both components of the S2 should be heard by 6 to 12 hours of age. The average **heart rate** is 110 to 160 BPM in healthy term infants, ranging from 90 to 180 BPM, depending on activity. In premature infants, the average heart rate is 140 to 150 BPM at rest.[53] A persistent rate >160 BPM may indicate central nervous system (CNS) irritability, congestive heart failure (CHF), fever, anemia, or another problem. Most premature beats are transient and benign.[13]

- **Murmurs.** Sixty percent of all newborns have murmurs. Most murmurs heard in the first days of life reflect the neonatal changes. Only occasionally does a murmur actually indicate a congenital defect.[13] A patent ductus arteriosus (PDA) is commonly heard at birth as a continuous machinery murmur but disappears in 2 to 3 days. A murmur heard at birth has a 1:12 risk of being due to congenital heart disease.[53]

When a murmur is heard and the practitioner is trying to determine whether it is transient or indicates a defect, the following factors favor the probability that a defect is present:

1. The patient has a first-degree relative with congenital heart disease.
2. The patient's mother had rubella or diabetes or used alcohol or a teratogenic drug during her pregnancy.

3. The patient was born prematurely or at a high altitude.
4. The patient has cyanosis, abnormal pulsations, or a physical appearance suggestive of a clinical syndrome.[46]

- The **point of maximal impulse (PMI).** Normally located on the left midclavicular line at the fourth intercostal space, variation may suggest cardiac anomaly. A pulsation in the suprasternal notch may be present with aortic insufficiency, PDA, or coarctation of the aorta. A **palpable thrill** in the suprasternal notch suggests aortic stenosis, valvular pulmonary stenosis, PDA, or coarctation of the aorta.
- **Pulses.** Narrow, thready pulses may indicate CHF or severe aortic stenosis; bounding may indicate PDA.[16] Note equality of intensity and timing between right and left brachial and femoral pulses.[53]
- **Blood pressure.** For the infant from birth to 7 days of age, a systolic BP ≥96 mm Hg is significant hypertension and BP ≥106 mm Hg is severe; for the infant 8 to 30 days old, a systolic BP ≥104 mm Hg is significant hypertension and BP ≥110 mm Hg is severe. NOTE: The appropriate-sized cuff, two thirds the length of the forearm, must be used, and the first Korotkoff sound heard is the systolic reading.[16]
- **Percussion.** Assessed with one finger, the newborn's lungs are normally hyperresonant throughout. Dullness may indicate an effusion or consolidation.[53]

Abdomen

- **Size and shape.** Normally protuberant. Flatness may be due to a diaphragmatic hernia with abdominal organs in the chest. Supraumbilical fullness may indicate duodenal atresia with gastric distention or hepatomegaly.[13] Abdominal distension suggests gastrointestinal (GI) disease. Note any masses.
- **Musculature.** Prune belly syndrome indicates hypoplastic kidneys and possibly other malformations.
- **Size.**
- **Bowel sounds.** Present 3 to 4 hours after birth with no visible peristalsis. Visible waves of peristalsis are present with intestinal obstruction.
- **Umbilicus** location (halfway between xiphoid and pubis) and condition. A mass may indicate a hernia; omphalocele (a hernia of the cord containing abdominal organs) or gastroschisis (a hernia lateral to the umbilicus that may contain abdominal contents). Omphalitis is an acute inflammation of the umbilical area.[53]
- Number of **umbilical vessels** (normally 2 arteries and 1 vein). A single artery is sometimes associated with kidney malformations.
- Palpation of abdominal organs.
- **Liver size and location.** Normally 1 to 3.5 cm below the costal margin at the midclavicular line and across the midline, with a soft, thin margin.[13] Assess by percussing the entire liver span—5.9 ± 0.8 cm in

the midclavicular line at term. A central or left-sided location suggests a cardiac anomaly.

- **Spleen.** Uncommonly, the tip may be felt.[53]
- **Kidneys.** Palpate lumbar or flank areas with infant's knees bent in fetal position. Normally 4 to 5 cm in size, right lower than left, moderately firm and lobulated.
- **Bladder.** Note distention.
- **Inguinal area.** Should be free of hernias. **Lymph nodes** are normally palpable in more than one third of all infants, most commonly in the inguinal region. Three to 12 mm in diameter, these nodes tend to persist.[13]

Genitals

- **Rectum** should be patent, as evidenced by passage of **meconium** within 12 hours of birth. Ninety-nine percent of term and 95% of preterm infants pass meconium within 48 hours. If no stool has been passed by 24 hours, suspect Hirschsprung's disease or cystic fibrosis.[53] **Anal wink** should be present.
  FEMALE GENITALS
- **Labia majora** should cover the **labia minora** and **clitoris** at term. Fullness in labia (usually unilateral, rarely bilateral) may indicate an inguinal hernia. Such a hernia enlarges with increased intraabdominal pressure such as crying. Maternal pregnancy hormones may cause protuberance of female genitalia.[53] Masculinization causes posterior fusion of the labioscrotal folds.[57]
- The normal **clitoris** is 1 cm or shorter.[57] Fully developed by 27 weeks, in the immature or undernourished infant it may falsely appear to be hypertrophied because surrounding structures are not full due to limited fat deposition.[13]
- **Vagina** should be patent; imperforate hymen may cause hydrometrocolpos and a lower abdominal mass.[53] Bloody discharge from vagina is caused by maternal estrogen. A fingertip space (at least 0.34 cm) should be present between the vagina and the rectum; a lesser measurement may indicate ambiguity.
- **Hymenal tags.** Virtually all females have redundant hymenal tissue. In 13%, hymenal tags extend 1 to 15 mm beyond the rim of the hymen. These tags disappear within the first few weeks of life.[13]
  MALE GENITALS
- Size and rugae of **scrotum** are noted. Scrotum may be enlarged as a result of the trauma of a breech delivery or due to a transitory hydrocele. Descent of **testes** should be confirmed; at least one testicle should be palpable in the canal or in the scrotum at term birth. Asymmetry reveals hydrocele or hernia of testicles.
- The midline fusion line of the scrotum should be present under the penis.

- The **penis** should stretch to a minimum length of 2 cm.[3] Chordee (curvature) is abnormal.
- The position of the **urethral opening** should be noted. Hypospadias is a ventral urethral opening; epispadias is a dorsal urethral opening. Either contraindicates circumcision; severe cases are investigated by sex chromosome analysis.[53]
- **Pigmentation** may reflect adrenal hormone exposure during pregnancy.[3]
- Character of **urine** is noted; in 95% of term and preterm infants, the first void occurs within 24 hours after birth.

Back

- **Spinal curve and integrity.** Any sinus openings, tufts of hair, protrusions, or overlying hemangiomas or pigmented nevi suggest meningomyelocele or pilonidal cyst.[53]
- **Trunk incurvation reflex.** Lasts 2 months.

Legs

- **Range of motion** and **movement of hips.**
- **Leg length.** Galeazzi sign is unequal length, suggesting dislocation of the shorter leg.
- Symmetric **location of knees.**
- Presence of a **hip click.** Perform Ortolani's test: with infant lying on back, place fingertips under hips and thumbs around bent knees; flex legs open 90 degrees. A click in a hip indicates congenital hip dysplasia.
- Symmetry of **gluteal folds.** Asymmetry suggests congenital hip dysplasia.
- **Foot alignment.** An imaginary line from the center of the heel through the center of the metatarsal-tarsal line should bisect the second toe or run between the second and third toes. A more lateral line indicates metatarsus adductus, the result of intrauterine positioning, which may resolve spontaneously within the first few years of life or may require casting and exercise. When the foot is deviated toward the midline, clubfoot, or talipes equinovarus is present and requires casting, splinting, or surgical correction.
- Number of **toes;** shape and formation of **toenails.**
- **Creases** on the soles of the feet. During gestation, crease formation progresses from toes to heel. Deep, absent, or vertical creases may be significant abnormalities.
- **Gestational age Markers.** The **popliteal angle** is determined by flexing the hips with thighs alongside the abdomen and then extending the knee, noting the popliteal angle, which diminishes with increasing age unless the child was in the frank breech position in utero. In the **heel-to-ear maneuver,** the legs are held together, hips are held down on the table, and feet are extended toward the ears.

Reflexes of the Newborn

The following reflexes are present in the normal newborn:

Anal Wink: Light stroking of anal area causes sphincter to constrict.

Babinski Sign: Firm stroke up the lateral aspect of the foot and over causes toes to fan and big toe to flex for a positive result. Present until 2 to 4 years of age.

Corneal Reflex: Touching cornea near outer canthus with dry wisp of cotton causes the eyelid to close (persists for life).

Crossed Extension: Hold one leg down; other leg will push hand.

Gag Reflex, Cough, Pupil Constriction: Persist for life.

Knee Jerk: Gently strike the knee; lower leg will jerk forward (persists for life). Because of the unfinished corticospinal tracts in infants, deep tendon reflexes (DTR) are variable and nonspecific.[67]

Magnet Reflex: With the infant's leg flexed, place a pen lightly under the toes; move the pen forward, and the foot will follow the pen forward.

Palatal Reflex: Also called *swallowing reflex.* Stimulating the palate should cause swallowing. Persists for life.

Trunk Incurvation: Holding the infant by the stomach, stroke the back along a line, 2 to 3 cm from the spine, from shoulders to buttocks. Normal response is lateral flexion in direction of stroke. Disappears after 2 to 3 months. Absent in infants with transverse spinal lesions.

Withdrawal: Legs draw up in response to painful stimulus.

Infantile Automatisms: Primitive reflexes that may be present at birth and disappear by approximately 4 to 6 months, when voluntary control begins. Absence of these reflexes at birth may indicate a severe CNS problem; persistence may be equally serious.

Blinking: Described under eyes, p. 253.

Moro Reflex (Startle Reflex): Produce a loud noise. The baby will abduct the arms symmetrically ("spreading"), form a C with open fingers, and then adduct the arms ("hugging").[13] Persists after 4 to 6 months only with cerebral disease.[67]

Palmar Grasp: Stroke palm; infant will grasp and hold (lasts 3 to 6 months). Absence suggests cerebral disease. Disappears by 3 months.[16]

Perez's Reflex: Place thumb at infant's sacrum and run upward toward head. Infant will extend head and spine while flexing knees and may urinate. Present for 2 to 3 months; absence indicates disease of the cerebrum or cervical spine, or a myopathy.

Placing: Brush front of tibia on table; infant steps up. Lasts 6 weeks. Best observed after 4 to 5 days of life; disappears by 2 to 5 months.

Plantar Grasp: Stroke sole of foot with a finger; toes will bend under, grasping and holding the finger. Lasts 8 to 15 months.[16]

Rooting Reflex: Stroke cheek; infant will turn, open-mouthed, in that direction.

Vestibular function reflex: Described under eyes above as "doll's eyes."

Sucking Reflex: Described under mouth above.

Tonic Neck or Fencing Reflex: With relaxed infant lying supine, turn head so that jaw is over one shoulder. The arm and leg toward which the head is turned should extend, and the opposite arm and leg should flex. Test both sides. Reflex diminishes at 3 to 4 months and resolves by 6 months, enabling infant to roll over.[16]

Walking or Stepping: When held so that feet rest on tabletop, infant will step (best seen at 4 to 5 days of age); lasts about 2 months.[67]

Gestational Age Determination

The New Ballard Scale (NBS) (see Figure 5-1) dates infants as young as 20 weeks.[15] The test, done while the infant is rested and quiet within 12 hours of birth, is accurate ±1 week on the infant <38 weeks' gestation and ±2 weeks on infants >38 weeks' gestation. Variables may affect testing. The compression of oligohydramnios, for example, causes misleading flexion. A condition that causes decreased fetal movement may make the infant appear less mature, with fewer sole creases. Fetal position, such as breech presentation, affects leg extension tests. Poor intrauterine nutrition and decreased fat may make an infant appear younger.[13] See descriptions of maneuvers earlier in text.

Classification by Birthweight and Gestational Age

Once the gestational age and the weight of the infant have been determined, the results are plotted on the graph of Battaglia and Lubchenco[17] (Figure 5-2), which indicates whether the infant is small for gestational age (SGA) (<10th percentile), appropriate for gestational age (AGA) (10th to 90th percentile), or large for gestational age (LGA) (>90th percentile). Any infant weighing <2500 g is classified as a low birthweight (LBW) baby despite age. The baby with a birthweight <1500 g is VLBW, and the baby weighing <1000 g is extremely LBW.[13]

Text continued on page 265

Neuromuscular Maturity

	−1	0	1	2	3	4	5
Posture							
Square Window (wrist)	>90°	90°	60°	45°	30°	0°	
Arm Recoil		180°	140°–180°	110°–140°	90°–110°	<90°	
Popliteal Angle	180°	160°	140°	120°	100°	90°	<90°
Scarf Sign							
Heel to Ear							

Physical Maturity

	-1	0	1	2	3	4	5
Skin	sticky friable transparent	gelatinous red translucent	smooth pink, visible veins	superficial peeling &/or rash, few veins	cracking pale areas rare veins	parchment deep cracking no vessels	leathery cracked wrinkled
Lanugo	none	sparse	abundant	thinning	bald areas	mostly bald	
Plantar Surface	heel-toe 40–50mm:–1 <40 mm:–2	>50mm no crease	faint red marks	anterior transverse crease only	creases ant. 2/3	creases over entire sole	
Breast	imperceptible	barely perceptible	flat areola no bud	stippled areola 1–2 mm bud	raised areola 3–4 mm bud	full areola 5–10 mm bud	
Eye/Ear	lids fused loosely:–1 tightly:–2	lids open pinna flat stays folded	sl. curved pinna; soft; slow recoil	well-curved pinna; soft but ready recoil	formed & firm instant recoil	thick cartilage ear stiff	
Genitals male	scrotum flat, smooth	scrotum empty faint rugae	testes in upper canal rare rugae	testes descending few rugae	testes down good rugae	testes pendulous deep rugae	
Genitals female	clitoris prominent labia flat	prominent clitoris small labia minora	prominent clitoris enlarging minora	majora & minora equally prominent	majora large minora small	majora cover clitoris & minora	

Maturity Rating

score	weeks
-10	20
-5	22
0	24
5	26
10	28
15	30
20	32
25	34
30	36
35	38
40	40
45	42
50	44

Figure 5-1 • The New Ballard Scale (NBS). (From Ballard J: New Ballard Scale, expanded to include extremely premature infants, *J Pediatr* 119:417-423, 1991.)

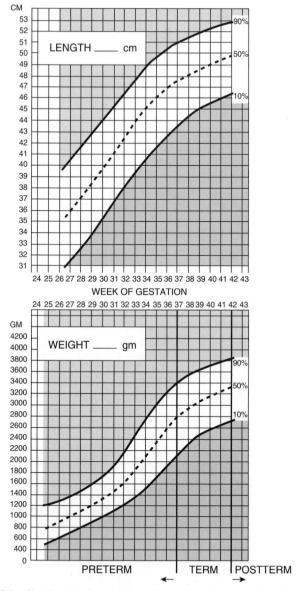

Figure 5-2 • Classification of newborns by birthweight and gestational age. (From Battaglia FC, Lubchenco LO: A practical classification of newborn infants by weight and gestational age, *J Pediatr* 71:159-163, 1967.)

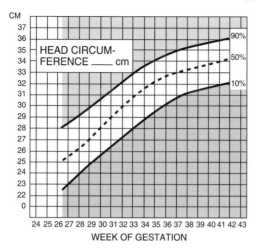

CM

HEAD CIRCUM-
FERENCE ____ cm

90%
50%
10%

WEEK OF GESTATION

Figure 5-2 • Cont'd. For legend, see previous page.

• HEALTH CARE OF THE NEONATE

Resuscitation of the Neonate

Preparation for Resuscitation

1. While awaiting a high-risk delivery, **assign roles:** determine who will manage the airway and ventilations; who will listen to the heart, place monitor leads, and provide cardiac massage; who will obtain vascular access; who will draw up medications; and who will record.
2. **Check and prepare the equipment:** turn on warmer and light; turn on the oxygen at 7 to 10 L/min; ensure the ability of the Ambu bag to create 20 to 35 cm H_2O pressure; test the laryngoscope light; choose the appropriate endotracheal (ET) tube and inset and with-

draw the stylet, bending it just shorter than the ET tube; turn on the suction and make sure that the suction creates 80 to 90 mm Hg negative pressure; turn on the cardiorespiratory, BP, and oxygen saturation monitors. Attach leads and probes.

3. Ascertain the need for **laboratory tests,** including cultures, cord blood gases, and pathologic examination of the placenta and arrange for these to be done.[68]

When the Baby Is Born

1. **Keep warm:** Place the infant under a preheated radiant warmer, stimulate by drying, remove wet linens, position with head slightly hyperextended. If thick or particulate meconium is present, perform tracheal suctioning before drying.

2. **Suction** mouth, then nose.

3. **Evaluate respirations.** If the baby is apneic or gasping, stimulate briefly. If the baby is not breathing, begin positive pressure ventilation with 100% oxygen at 40 to 60 breaths/min.[19] Thirty to 40 cm water pressure may be needed to inflate lungs initially, then follow with 15 to 20 cm. If pulmonary disease is present, 20 to 40 cm may be necessary. Bilateral breath sounds should be present, and modest chest movement should occur.[68] Give blow-by oxygen if the baby is breathing, or give several breaths with bag and mask, then evaluate the heart rate. For the infant with **central cyanosis** (cyanosis of the trunk), give free-flow oxygen at 80% to 100% and observe color. If color improves, withdraw the oxygen gradually. Otherwise, maintain the oxygenation. If the baby's color is good, observe the baby.[19]

4. **Check the heart rate** with a stethoscope or by palpating the umbilicus after about 30 seconds of positive pressure ventilation. For a heart rate <100 BPM, ventilate with an Ambu bag at a rate of 40 to 60 breaths/min with 100% oxygen. For a heart rate <80 BPM, begin cardiac compressions.[19]

5. If apnea continues, some practitioners perform **endotracheal intubation** immediately. Positive pressure ventilation can usually be achieved with bag and mask, however, and the inexperienced provider should not attempt intubation at this time. Exceptions to waiting include preterm infants who should be intubated because they will require intubation for stabilization and surfactant therapy; the infant suspected to have a diaphragmatic hernia who is intubated immediately to avoid distention of the stomach while it is located in the thoracic cavity; the infant who requires tracheal suctioning, who cannot be effectively ventilated with a bag and mask, and the infant for whom resuscitation is prolonged.[19] An ET tube the size of the infant's little finger is the correct size.[68]

6. The infant who requires positive pressure ventilation with a bag and mask for more than 2 minutes should have an **orogastric tube** placed. The stomach is then emptied, and the tube is left in place.[19]

7. Initiate **chest compressions** if 15 to 30 seconds of ventilation with 100% oxygen does not improve the heart rate >80 BPM. Use two fingertips on the lower third of the sternum. Alternately, use both thumbs, with hands encircling chest. Compress the chest against a firm surface $\frac{1}{2}$ to $\frac{3}{4}$ inch at a rate of 120, interspersing a respiration after every three compressions, for 90 compressions and 30 ventilations per minute. Reassess the heart rate every 30 seconds to determine whether compressions should be continued, unless resuscitation becomes prolonged.[19]

8. **Cannulate the umbilical vein** to allow administration of medications, volume expanders, and glucose[53] and withdrawal of blood for testing.[68] Clean the umbilical stump with Betadine (povidone-iodine), and advance a catheter 2 to 4 cm until blood returns.

9. Give **epinephrine 1:10,000** (0.1 to 0.3 mL/kg) rapidly IV or ET to increase cardiac rate and contractility; for peripheral vasoconstriction (increasing blood flow to vital organs); for asystole; or for failure to respond to 30 seconds of ventilations and compressions. Response should be seen in 30 seconds. Administration may be repeated every 3 to 5 minutes.[19] If there is no response, some authorities suggest giving 5 to 10 times the standard dose.[53]

10. The infant who has weak pulses with a good heart rate (hypotension), who responds poorly to resuscitation efforts, who has pallor despite oxygenation, or who has evidence of hemorrhage may be hypovolemic. Give a **volume expander,** 10 mL/kg, IV over 5 to 10 minutes. Four solutions are available: whole blood, 5% albumin–saline solution or other plasma substitute, normal saline solution, and lactated Ringer's solution. Administration may be repeated.[19]

11. Administer **4.2% sodium bicarbonate (NaHCO₃),** 2 mEq/kg—over at least 2 minutes—into the umbilical vein slowly if there is documented acidosis or if resuscitation is prolonged. Continue to support respirations, allowing carbon dioxide to blow off.[53] The heart rate should improve 30 seconds after administration.[19]

12. Give **Narcan** (naloxone), 0.1 mg/kg, rapidly ET, IV—or SQ or IM if necessary—if the mother received analgesia. Observe for a return of respiratory depression, signaling the need for further doses.[53] If the infant is addicted, Narcan may cause withdrawal seizures.[19]

13. Give **dopamine,** 50 mg in 250 mL,[53] at a IV rate of 5 to 20 µg/kg/min with volume expansion for poor peripheral perfusion, weak pulses, hypotension, tachycardia, and poor urine output.[19]

14. **Observe** the successfully resuscitated infant **for signs of encephalopathy,** including low Apgar scores, timing of extubation, feeding ability, tone, and the presence of seizures.[68]

Newborn Screening

Every state and U.S. territory now screens newborns for phenylketonuria (PKU) and congenital hypothyroidism.[6] These birth defects may result in serious illness, death, or severe retardation if they are not treated immediately. Many states and U.S. territories also screen newborns for the following conditions: galactosemia, sickle cell anemia, cystic fibrosis, congenital adrenal hyperplasia, biotinidase deficiency, and hearing loss.[49] The newborn screening program includes the screening tests themselves, education regarding the screening for providers and parents, retrieval of abnormal test results, confirmatory testing procedures to verify the diagnosis, genetic and psychosocial counseling for parents of affected newborns, medical management for the newborn, and outcome evaluation.[6]

Immunizations: Recommendations and Controversies

Figure 5-3 lists the immunizations recommended by the American Academy of Pediatrics. The **rotavirus vaccine,** RotaShield, was associated with intussusception and is no longer recommended.[2] The **oral polio vaccine** is no longer recommended because of the risk of contracting polio from the vaccine.[38] Demyelinating encephalopathy occurs once after administration of every million **measles vaccines** and occurs in 1 in 1000 actual cases of measles. Guillain-Barré syndrome occurs in one of every million **influenza vaccine** recipients.[1]

Immunization rates are falling because of concerns regarding side effects, dislike of giving infants multiple injections per visit, noncompliance and lack of access, lack of knowledge on the part of parents, and religious and philosophical objections. Proponents state that people who are currently parenting do not recall living with the serious threat of infectious diseases. Safer immunizations have been developed in response to parental concerns, and vaccines have been combined. They urge practitioners to educate and to take any office visit as an opportunity to immunize children if appropriate.[44] The risk that the unvaccinated person will contract a disease depends on the prevalence of the virus and contact with infected persons. Those unvaccinated individuals who do become infected may transmit the disease to a vaccinated person in whom immunity is not complete. A small increase in the percentage of an unvaccinated group significantly increases the risk of the disease to the whole group.[38]

Every year, 12,000 to 14,000 hospitalizations, injuries, and deaths associated with vaccination are reported to the Food and Drug Administration's (FDA's) Vaccine Adverse Events Reporting System (VAERS).[28] Between 1991 and 1994, 795 (2%) of the reported events were deaths; 72.4% of the deaths occurred within the first year of life, peaking at 1 to 3 months and declining until 9 months, after which death was relatively rare. (SIDS occurs in the same age pattern and has not been shown to be related to immunization.) Pediatric immunizations reported most often have been diphtheria, tetanus, and pertussis (DTP), oral polio, *Hemophilus influenzae* type B, and measles-mumps rubella (MMR) vaccines.[21]

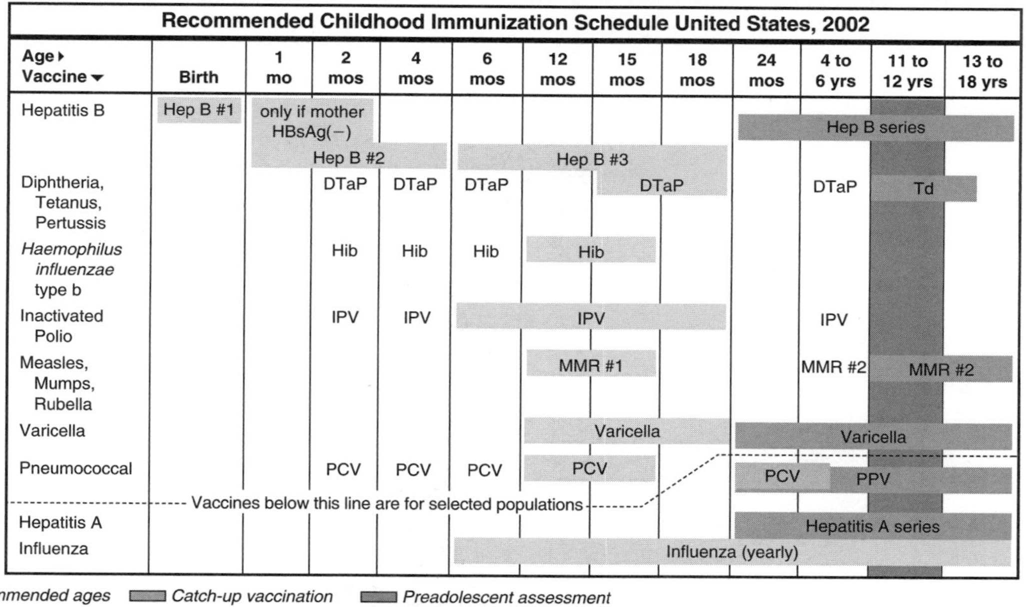
Recommended Childhood Immunization Schedule United States, 2002
Age ▸ Vaccine ▾
Birth
1 mo
2 mos
4 mos
6 mos
12 mos
15 mos
18 mos
24 mos
4 to 6 yrs
11 to 12 yrs
13 to 18 yrs
Hepatitis B
Hep B #1
only if mother HBsAg(−)
Hep B #2
Hep B #3
Hep B series
Diphtheria, Tetanus, Pertussis
DTaP
DTaP
DTaP
DTaP
DTaP
Td
Haemophilus influenzae type b
Hib
Hib
Hib
Hib
Inactivated Polio
IPV
IPV
IPV
IPV
Measles, Mumps, Rubella
MMR #1
MMR #2
MMR #2
Varicella
Varicella
Varicella
Pneumococcal
PCV
PCV
PCV
PCV
PCV
PPV
Vaccines below this line are for selected populations
Hepatitis A
Hepatitis A series
Influenza
Influenza (yearly)
Range of recommended ages
Catch-up vaccination
Preadolescent assessment

This schedule indicates the recommended ages for routine administration of currently licensed childhood vaccines, as of December 1, 2001, for children through age 18 years. Any dose not given at the recommended age should be given at any subsequent visit when indicated and feasible. ▭ Indicates age groups that warrant special effort to administer those vaccines not previously given. Additional vaccines may be licensed and recommended during the year. Licensed combination vaccines may be used whenever any components of the combination are indicated and the vaccine's other components are not contraindicated. Providers should consult the manufacturer's package inserts for detailed recommendations. Approved by the Advisory Committee on Immunization Practices (www.cdc.gov/nip/acip)*, the American Academy of Pediatrics* (www.aap.org)*, and the American Academy of Family Physicians* (www.aafp.org).

Figure 5-3 • Recommended childhood immunization schedule United States, January-December 2003. Approved by the Advisory Committee on Immunization Practices, the American Academy of Pediatrics, and the Animal Academy of Family Physicians.

The safety of immunizations is difficult to determine because some complications are relatively rare, because vaccines are given concurrently, because a vaccine may stimulate the infection itself and the complication may arise from the infection, and because the preservatives in vaccines may have side effects (e.g., thimerosal, which contains mercury with its potential for causing neurodevelopmental damage, or bovine products, which may carry bovine spongiform encephalopathy ["mad cow disease"]). The Institute of Medicine, in 1991 and 1994, reviewed 76 of the reported adverse events and found that 66% lacked sufficient evidence to determine causality.[38]

Vaccine opponents suggest that vaccines may be associated with diseases such as asthma and attention deficit disorder and that prospective studies that compare vaccinated and unvaccinated children in the development of these problems are needed. By kindergarten, children have been given 34 doses of vaccines against various illnesses. Some of these diseases, opponents would assert, are not serious. More research and informed consent of parents are urged.[28]

The National Vaccine Information Center (NVIC) can be reached for information at (800) 909-SHOT or http://www.909shot.com. The Centers for Disease Control and Prevention (CDC) can be reached at (800) 232-2522 or http://www.cdc.gov/nip. The telephone number for the Vaccine Adverse Event Reporting System is (800) 822-7967.

Circumcision

Circumcision is the removal of the foreskin of the penis. The only indication for circumcision in the newborn is parental choice. In the United States, about 70% of males are circumcised; in Canada, 48%; and in the United Kingdom, 24%. In Europe, Asia, and Central and South America, circumcision is uncommon. A national organization that has raised awareness regarding circumcision is the National Organization of Circumcision Information Resource Centers (NOCIRC), which can be contacted at (415) 488-9883, or http://www.nocirc.org. Contraindications to circumcision include hypospadias or any abnormality of the penis, prematurity, and illness.[35] Some providers delay the surgery for a baby with feeding problems because of the tendency of some infants to withdraw and sleep for 24 hours after the procedure.

An alternative provider is a mohel, a Jewish individual who has been certified to perform infant circumcision.[63]

Benefits

1. Decreased frequency of urinary tract infection (UTI)—from a risk of 1:100 in an uncircumcised male to 1:1000 in circumcised males.[5]
2. Prevention of penile cancer.[53] The risk of penile cancer is tripled for uncircumcised males, but the disease is so rare (9 to 10 cases per 1 million men) that the absolute risk remains very low.[5]

3. Prevention of phimosis (inability to retract foreskin) and paraphimosis (inability to replace a retracted foreskin over the glans).
4. Avoidance of a circumcision later in life, when the procedure is more expensive and causes more morbidity. Less than 25% of circumcisions done later in life are done for medical indications, however, and a significant number of infant circumcisions require revisions later in life.[53] Education about avoiding premature retraction of the foreskin might have prevented some of the medically indicated circumcisions.[35]

Complications[5,26]

Sepsis	Removal of excessive foreskin
Minor local infection	Scarring of the penile shaft
Urethrocutaneous fistulas	Complications from anesthesia
Meatal stenosis	Skin tags and skin bridges
Amputation of the distal glans	Curvature of the penis

The rate of complications is 0.2% to 0.6%.[5] (AAP, 1999).

Possible Psychological Ramifications

Immediate behavioral changes may include a long period of sleep, which makes the infant "unavailable for bonding and social interaction" for 24 hours. Long-term effects are unknown.

American Academy of Pediatrics Position Statement

In March 1999, the AAP[5] stated, "There is no absolute medical indication for routine circumcision." They determined that the absolute risks for UTI and for penile cancer are very low. The increased risk for sexually transmitted infections (STIs) is far less important, they concluded, than the behavioral risks for developing STIs. The risks of balanitis and irritation are equal in circumcised and uncircumcised boys. They urged parents to make an informed choice, weighing in religious, cultural, and ethnic traditions. They added that pain relief must be provided.

Pain Relief

Considerable new research shows that newborns circumcised without analgesia experience pain and stress. Choices include EMLA cream (topical mixtures of local anesthetics),[5] the injected dorsal penile block with 1% lidocaine (without epinephrine),[35] a subcutaneous ring block (injection into the midshaft of the penis),[5] and wine-soaked gauze for the baby to suck (used in ritual circumcision to reduce crying). Pacifiers reduce crying but **are not adequate analgesia.**[5]

Care of the Newly Circumcised Penis

Careful handwashing is used. A Vaseline gauze dressing is kept in place for 24 hours and changed with each diaper change. After circumcision, the glans is reddened; within 24 hours, it becomes edematous. A small amount of serosanguineous drainage is often present. At 24 hours, the Vaseline dressing is removed; the penis is washed with warm water and kept dry. Vaseline or A&D ointment may be applied. Healing begins within 2 days, when diaper changes become less painful, and is complete by about 1 week. Sponge baths are recommended until the circumcision and umbilical stump are healed. Avoid the use of soap and alcohol. If healing is slow or if excess drainage is seen, warm gauze soaks twice a day often promote healing. Observe for redness, swelling, a pustular drainage, fever, lethargy, or the inability to feed or void.[73]

Care of the Uncircumcised Penis

Wash external structures only. Do not forcibly retract foreskin or allow others to do so (including health care providers). The child can retract his own foreskin if he wants to. It does not need to be retracted regularly for cleaning until puberty. If irritation develops at the tip of the penis, apply A&D or antibiotic ointment. If a small amount of dirt lodges in the opening of the foreskin and is causing irritation, the foreskin can be slightly retracted and washed with warm water. If the dirt remains, apply a small amount of lubricant and remove.[59] Be aware that smegma is *not* a carcinogenic substance. It has a lubricating function and is rarely present before foreskin retraction.[73]

• TRANSITION TO LIFE

Heart of the Fetus and Newborn

Fetal Circulation

Oxygenated blood from the placenta enters the fetus through the umbilical vein where 50% enters the hepatic circulation and 50% enters the inferior vena cava via the ductus venosus, mixing with blood returning from the legs. The combined blood flows into the right atrium where it is directed across the foramen ovale to the left atrium. From there, the blood flows to the left ventricle and out into the aorta. The blood that has come into the heart from the superior vena cava flows primarily into the right ventricle and then into the pulmonary artery. Only 10% can flow into the constricted pulmonary capillary bed. The other 90% flows out the ductus arteriosus into the aorta.[53] See Figure 5-4 for a schematic illustration of fetal circulation.

Cardiac Events in the Transition to Life

At birth, expansion of the lungs and the increase in Po_2 cause the pulmonary vasculature to dilate. The right ventricle now empties entirely into the pulmonary vascular bed. Pulmonary vascular resistance is less than the systemic vascular resistance, and the shunt through the ductus arteriosus reverses. The high Po_2 causes constriction of the ductus arteriosus, which closes functionally by 10 to 15 hours, becoming the

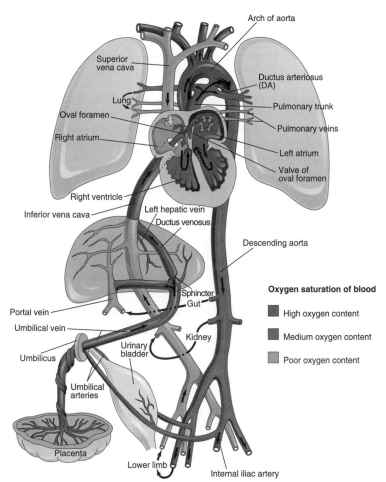

Figure 5-4 • A schematic illustration of fetal circulation. Arrows indicate the direction of blood flow. From Moore K, Persaud TVN: *Before we are born: essentials of embryology and birth defects,* ed 6, Philadelphia, 2003, Saunders.

ligamentum arteriosum. Blood returning from the pulmonary vessels to the left atrium increases left atrial pressure and gradually closes the foramen ovale; it is "functionally closed" by the end of the third month. The foramen ovale opens to a probe in 15% to 25% of adults. When the placenta is removed, the ductus venosus closes.[53]

In congenital heart disease, the ductus arteriosus and foramen ovale may remain open. Administration of prostaglandin E_1 will maintain the patency of these structures.[53] Indomethacin or ibuprofen hastens their closure.[72]

Persistent Fetal Circulation

Various congenital anomalies, meconium aspiration, or perinatal hypoxia can cause pulmonary bed vascular resistance to persist. The patent foramen ovale, patent ductus arteriosus (PDA), and right-to-left shunting of fetal life continue. The pulmonary vascular bed may develop increased muscularization, resulting in pulmonary hypertension.[53] Pulmonary blood flow is diminished, and the Po_2 may be very low. Infants who are older than 35 weeks' gestation and who are at low risk for retinopathy of prematurity are given oxygen sufficient to maintain an oxygen saturation of $\geq95\%$ to minimize pulmonary vasoconstriction secondary to hypoxia.[68]

Hyperbilirubinemia

The fetus, receiving oxygen from maternal blood, maintains a high RBC count with fetal Hb higher than is necessary for the neonate who is oxygenating blood in his or her own lungs. Those RBCs no longer needed when the infant begins breathing are broken down in the newborn's spleen; the liver, transiently limited in its ability to conjugate bilirubin, sometimes cannot adequately clear the bilirubin.[12] This results in hyperbilirubinemia, also called *physiologic jaundice* and *icterus neonatorum.*

Conjugated (direct) water-soluble bilirubin is excreted in the bile. Conjugated bilirubin is broken down in the liver and deposited in the intestines. In the adult, bilirubin passes into the small intestine and is reduced by the bacteria there to urobilinogen. Urobilinogen is excreted in the stool. Conjugated bilirubin cannot pass through intestinal lumen; remaining in the bowel, it is deconjugated and becomes available for resorption into the bloodstream. **Unconjugated (indirect) bilirubin,** a fat-soluble substance, has an affinity for extravascular tissue, where it is deposited when there is excess bilirubin in the blood. Bilirubin deposition in the skin and sclera cause jaundice. If the level of bilirubin deposited in the brain becomes high enough to cause lethargy, jaundice becomes pathologic. When the intestines are not moving (because the baby—now lethargic—is not eating well), the bilirubin is reabsorbed from the gut, thus beginning a vicious cycle.[61]

This **physiologic jaundice** usually begins at 2 to 3 days of life (3 to 5 days in breastfed babies).[12] It can be seen in the face at a serum level of approximately 5 mg/dL, moving downward as the bilirubin level climbs. It can be seen in the mid abdomen at approximately 15 mg/dL; and in the soles of the feet at approximately 20 mg/dL.[53] It decreases to approximately 2 mg/dL by 5 to 7 days.[12]

Kernicterus is the neurologic syndrome caused by the deposition of unconjugated bilirubin in the neonate's brain cells. Usually occurring with a serum bilirubin of >25 mg/dL, signs and symptoms include lethargy; poor feeding; loss of the Moro reflex; a rigid, arching back; bulging fontanels; shrill cry; and seizures. Seventy-five percent of infants who have kernicterus die; 80% of the survivors have severe neurologic damage.[53]

Incidence: Sixty percent of term infants and 80% of preterm infants have jaundice.[12]

Predisposing Factors for Indirect Hyperbilirubinemia[53,61]

Altitude	Delayed passage of stool
Maternal diabetes	Drugs (vitamin K, novobiocin, ASA,
Prematurity	sulfa)
A sibling who had	Trisomy 21
physiologic jaundice	Oxytocin induction
Polycythemia	Bruising or cephalhematoma
Breastfeeding	Weight loss
Chinese, Japanese, Korean,	LBW
and Native American race	First feeding >12 hours after birth
Male sex	<8 feedings in the first 24 hours

Pathologic Jaundice: Jaundice is pathologic when it can be seen within 24 hours, when the bilirubin increases by 5 mg/dL in 24 hours, when the bilirubin is >15 mg/dL, when the elevated level lasts more than a week in the term infant and more than 2 weeks in the premature infant, or when the infant becomes lethargic and feeds poorly.[53]

Laboratory Findings: In normal physiologic hyperbilirubinemia, the **indirect bilirubin** (total bilirubin minus direct bilirubin) of the cord blood is 1 to 3 mg/dL, rising at <5 mg/dL in 24 hours. The normal **conjugated** or **direct bilirubin** level is 0.0 to 0.4 mg/dL.[34]

Ⓜ Management

1. **Encourage early frequent feedings**, ≥8 feedings/24 hr, to help prevent jaundice. **Water supplementation is contraindicated.** (Water administration decreases thirst, the primary drive of infant appetite, thus actually serving to decrease the caloric intake and increase weight loss in the first week[61].) Some advocate supplementing breastmilk with formula to hasten the reduction of bilirubin concentrations.[12]

2. **Obtain** the following **lab work** on all patients with significant hyperbilirubinemia: direct and indirect bilirubin fractions, Hb, reticulocyte count, blood type, Coombs test, and a peripheral blood smear.[53]

3. **Teach** the mother of the slightly jaundiced baby who is discharged to **report lethargy, irritability, difficulty feeding, and infrequent passage of stool.**[61]

4. **Pediatric management: Phototherapy** converts the bilirubin in the skin to a form that is excreted in the bile. It is initiated at a serum bilirubin of 10 to 20 mg/dL.[53] The total bilirubin should decline 1 to 2 mg/dL within 4 to 6 hours of intensive phototherapy, and the level should continue to decline until discontinuance when the total serum bilirubin level falls to 14 to 15 mg/dL.[12] Should phototherapy fail, **exchange transfusions** are given to prevent neurologic damage.[53]

5. **Complementary measures:**
   a. Some experts recommend **homeopathic** remedies for jaundice.[76]
   b. To prevent jaundice or to treat slight physiologic jaundice in the first week, after the first 24 hours, a baby may be placed in natural light, undressed with skin exposed, for 5 to 10 minutes, morning and evening. On sunny days, the baby may be placed in a sunny window; on cloudy days it may be placed outside. Care is taken to protect the eyes, keep the baby warm, and prevent sunburn.[62,76]

Breastmilk Jaundice

Two percent of all mothers' breastmilk contains pregnanediol, which inhibits diglucuronide (the conjugated form of bilirubin) and also increases fatty acids, which inhibit albumin binding (keeping bilirubin in the plasma). In addition, some breastmilk contains substances that inhibit glucuronyl transferase conjugating activity, and some contains a glucuronidase that may cause jaundice. Genetic factors, inadequate early breastfeeding, supplementation with glucose water, and increased intestinal resorption of bilirubin caused by delayed passage of meconium may contribute to the development of jaundice.[52] Breastmilk jaundice occurs in 1 of every 200 breastfed babies. The unconjugated bilirubin becomes elevated between days 4 and 7, reaching maximum levels of 10 to 30 mg/dL during the second to third weeks. If breastfeeding is continued, the bilirubin will slowly decrease, possibly persisting at lower levels for 3 to 10 weeks. If breastfeeding is discontinued for 1 to 2 days with formula substitution, the serum bilirubin rapidly declines and does not increase thereafter. The infant may benefit from phototherapy. With breastmilk jaundice, there is no other sign of illness, and kernicterus does not develop.[53]

Ⓜ Management

1. After the diagnosis, the **breasts are pumped for 24 hours,** the baby is given formula, then breastfeeding is resumed, and the problem should be resolved.
2. **Complementary measures:** Romm[62] and Weed[76] note that the jaundice from breastfeeding is not harmful as long as the baby is vigorously feeding, and the decision to temporarily stop breastfeeding is optional.

Hypocalcemia in the Newborn

Hypocalcemia may occur as a result of hypoparathyroidism, abnormal vitamin D metabolism, a low calcium intake, or a high phosphate intake.[53]

Hypoglycemia in the Newborn

At delivery, the infant must make the transition from the continuous nutrient supply of the placenta to intermittent feedings. This is accomplished by breakdown of glycogen stores, gluconeogenesis, and fatty acid mobilization. Dietary carbohydrate intake provides 20% to 50% of the glucose metabolized by the newborn in the first few days of life. Immediately after birth, the blood glucose falls, with the nadir at 1 to 2 hours. It is promptly self-corrected by 3 hours and maintained thereafter.[39] The blood glucose should not drop below 40 mg/dL (serum or plasma levels are 10% to 15% higher). Severe, prolonged hypoglycemia may result in mental retardation, seizures, and/or subtle personality changes. Sequelae are more likely to occur when alternate fuel sources are inadequate, when hypoglycemic episodes are repetitive and prolonged, or when episodes are compounded by hypoxia.[53] Asymptomatic neonatal hypoglycemia is not, however, associated with neurodevelopmental sequelae.

Some researchers have suggested that blood glucose levels of 30 mg/dL for the first day and 40 mg/dL for the second day are more appropriate standards. The higher standard causes healthy infants to be misdiagnosed as hypoglycemic and to receive unnecessary supplementation.[61] According to Linder et al,[47] the sucking stimulation test can be performed on the newborn to determine whether a tremor is physiologic or an indicator of hypocalcemia or hypoglycemia. The examiner puts his or her finger into the mouth of the infant who is lying supine with head straight and hands free. The test result is positive if the tremor stops instantly and returns when the examiner's finger is removed. A positive test result together with an adequate glucose level determined with Dextrostix indicates a physiologic tremor requiring no further investigation.

Infants born to mothers with diabetes have transient hyperinsulinemia and diminished glucagon secretion. Infants with erythroblastosis fetalis are also prone to hyperinsulinemia, possibly because of the effects of hemolysis on insulin molecules. These infants are supported, if necessary, with IV glucose until the hyperinsulinemia abates.[53]

Signs and Symptoms of Hypoglycemia:

1. Signs of increased adrenaline secretion: tremor, jitteriness, pallor, sweating, and tachycardia.
2. Signs of low glucose in the CNS: irritability, bizarre behavior, lethargy, coma, convulsions.
3. Subtle signs: cyanosis, lethargy, apnea, hypothermia, hypotonia, poor feeding, or seizures.
4. Hypoglycemia may also be asymptomatic.[53]

The **incidence of symptomatic hypoglycemia** in newborns is 1.3 to 3.0 per 1000 live births.[53]

Predisposing Factors for Hypoglycemia:

Intrauterine growth restriction (IUGR)
Intrauterine hypoxia
Prematurity
Maternal diabetes
Respiratory distress
Polycythemia
Maternal receipt of excessive IV hypotonic glucose solutions during labor

Sepsis
Erythroblastosis fetalis
Cold stress

Maternal receipt of terbutaline or oral hypoglycemic agents[39]
Postmaturity[61]

(m) *Management*

1. **Do not routinely administer hypotonic glucose IV solutions** during labor.[61]

2. **Teach the mother** the following **practices to prevent infant hypoglycemia:** initiate breastfeeding as soon as possible, ideally about 20 minutes after birth, avoiding mother-infant separation until the latch-on has been accomplished. Breastfeed exclusively, at the first sign of hunger, and cuddle to discourage crying and perspiring.[39]

3. Some clinicians **test infants** at risk **for hypoglycemia** within the first hour after delivery.[61] Others suggest that the infant who exhibits symptoms of hypoglycemia or who is at risk for hypoglycemia have a heelstick done for determination of a blood glucose at 4 to 6 hours, before a feeding, by using a formal lab measurement. Maintain the level above 40 to 45 mg/dL. A lower value requires evaluation by pediatrics.[39] Pathologic neonatal hypoglycemia is confirmed with lab measurement of plasma glucose and diagnosis should not be made using glucose reagent strips and meter.[50]

4. The World Health Organization (WHO) and the AAP agree that **universal screening of newborns is inappropriate** and may result in misdiagnosis of hypoglycemia, impairment of breastfeeding initiation, delay of lactogenesis, insufficient milk supply, early termination of breastfeeding, and diminished maternal confidence in the ability to feed the baby.[39]

5. **Pediatric management:** For continued hypoglycemia and poor breastfeeding, **formula or IV glucose is preferable to oral glucose water,** which is low in calories and nutrients. Glucose water is stressful to the infant pancreas and may cause rebound hypoglycemia.[61]

Hypothermia in the Newborn

Heat loss occurs because of evaporative, convective, conductive, and radiant heat loss. Newborns, especially those ≤12 hours of age, have a limited ability to produce heat in a cold environment.[19] The premature infant with its thin epidermis, high surface to volume ratio, and reduced subcutaneous tissue is at particular risk, as are LBW infants and those who have hypoxemia, sepsis, or low body temperatures. Cold stress causes the infant to burn brown adipose tissue, releasing fatty acids and increasing oxygen consumption. Hypoglycemia, hyperkalemia, elevated BUN levels, metabolic acidosis, hypoxemia, and persistent fetal circulation may result.[29]

   Signs and Symptoms: Poor feeding; lethargy; cool skin; bright red color; edema; slow, shallow respirations; bradycardia.[29]

m *Management*

1. **Prevent hypothermia** by placing the baby directly onto the mother's skin (causing oxytocin release and enhancing bonding as well[51]) or onto a prewarmed radiant warmer, drying the baby with a prewarmed towel, removing the wet linen, covering the baby's head, and delaying the first bath.[19]
2. Core temperature should remain **>36.5° C.**[73]
3. A cold infant may be **warmed slowly** in an isolette 2° C higher than the infant's core temperature.[29]

Birth Injuries

Caput Succedaneum

Caput succedaneum is swelling of the soft scalp tissues in the area that was presenting through the cervix during labor. Caput succedaneum may overlie sutures, may be ecchymotic, and disappears within a few days without treatment.[53]

m *Management*

Complementary measures: Some experts suggest **homeopathic** measures to facilitate healing of caput succedaneum.[22]

Cephalhematoma

Cephalhematoma is a subperiosteal hematoma of a cranial bone (more than one cranial bone may be affected) that does not cross a suture line. No discoloration or swelling may be visible until hours after the delivery. A central depression with an organized osseous rim may be palpable. Most cephalhematomas resorb in 2 weeks to 3 months without treatment, but occasionally one is palpable for years as a bony prominence. A cephalhematoma may cause hyperbilirubinemia. Rarely, a massive cephalhematoma is associated with a skull fracture.[53]

m *Management*

Complementary measures: Some experts recommend a **homeopathic** remedy to facilitate healing.[22]

Clavicular Fracture

The most common fracture incurred by infants during birth,[58] clavicular fracture usually occurs during delivery of tight shoulders or in extraction of an arm during a breech delivery. The infant generally does not move the affected arm, the Moro reflex is absent, crepitus and bony irregularity may be palpated, and discoloration may be visible. The sternocleidomastoid muscle may spasm, hiding the supraclavicular depression where the fracture is located. In greenstick fractures, there may be movement and a Moro reflex.[53] There are no permanent sequelae.[58]

ⅲ Management

The affected arm and shoulder are immobilized. Within a week, a callous forms at the site of the fracture.[53]

Brachial Plexus Injury

A birth injury to the brachial plexus causes paralysis of the upper arm, which may or may not involve paralysis of the forearm and hand. Such an injury occurs with downward traction of the head during a shoulder dystocia or when arms are extended above the head during breech extraction.[53] Brachial plexus injuries are not necessarily prevented by cesarean delivery. Incidence is 0.15%; 4% to 9% of injuries persist.[32]

Injury Involving Upper Brachial Plexus Cranial Nerves C5 and 6 (Erb-Duchenne Paralysis)

When an injury involves the upper brachial plexus, the baby is unable to abduct the arm from the shoulder, rotate the arm externally, or supinate the forearm. The infant characteristically positions himself or herself with the affected arm adducted, internally rotated, the forearm bent into a prone position. Biceps and Moro reflexes are absent on the affected side. The outer aspect of the arm may have some sensory impairment. The forearm and the finger grasp remain strong unless the lower part of the plexus is also injured.[53]

Injury Involving Lower Brachial Plexus Cranial Nerves C7 and 8 (Klumpke's palsy)

An injury to the lower brachial plexus causes paralysis of the hand and is much less common than Erb-Duchenne paralysis.[75]

Phrenic Nerve Paralysis

Phrenic nerve paralysis, or diaphragmatic paralysis, is caused by injury of cranial nerves III, IV, and V and must be considered when irregular, labored respirations occur with cyanosis. Breathing is thoracic with breath sounds diminished on the affected side. Ultrasound or fluoroscopic examination reveals a flaccid diaphragm on the affected side and seesaw breathing. Supportive treatment includes IV feeding, positioning the infant on the affected side, and prevention of pulmonary infections until spontaneous recovery occurs in 1 to 3 months. Surgical intervention is rarely required.[53]

Facial Nerve Injury

Paralysis of the affected side of the face is caused by injury to the facial nerve in utero, during forceps delivery, or during the labor process. In this paralysis, the forehead is flat, the mouth is drawn to the unaffected side, the eye cannot be closed, the nasolabial fold is absent, and the corner of the mouth droops. Prognosis depends on whether the nerves were torn or compressed. Compression injury may improve within a few weeks[53] or may result in lifelong disability.[58] The exposed eye is protected, and neuroplasty is done if paralysis persists.[53]

Growth in the First Year of Life

An infant should regain his or her birthweight no later than 2 weeks after delivery, and after that, should gain at least 4 to 7 oz a week or a pound a month. A 7% weight loss should be carefully investigated; attempts should be made to identify the reason for the loss and to prevent more. If a 10% weight loss occurs, supplementation should be initiated to rehydrate the baby.[61]

• DEVELOPMENTAL AND MINOR HEALTH VARIATIONS

Colic

Defined by Nelson[53] as paroxysmal abdominal pain, presumably of intestinal origin, accompanied by severe crying, colic occurs in 15% to 35% of all term, healthy babies. It typically begins at 1 to 2 weeks of age and resolves abruptly or gradually by 3 to 4 months. It tends to have a diurnal pattern, increasing in intensity in the evening hours. The crying may begin suddenly and last for several hours. The baby may be pale around the mouth or flushed; legs are drawn up, hands are clenched, and feet are cold. The passage of feces or flatus may bring relief, or the baby may stop crying because of exhaustion.[53] Because of the excessive crying associated with colic, the risk for child abuse and neglect is increased.[43]

Some of the theories regarding the cause of colic include infant allergy to cow's milk or an allergen in the breastfeeding mother's diet; overfeeding; underfeeding; milk that is "too rich" or "too weak"; too much fat, sugar, or protein (especially for the infant who is bottlefed); holes in a bottle nipple that are too large or too small; swallowing of air caused by bottlefeeding; the position at the breast; prolonged pacifier use; the baby's temperament; smoke inhalation by the baby; or maternal anxiety.[61] Gas-producing foods have been blamed, but changing the diet rarely relieves colic.[53] Method of feeding is not associated with colic. Some have theorized that the CNS is immature, and stimuli that usually have no affect cause fussiness in these babies. Although stressful family relationships are associated with colic, these may be the result of, rather than the cause of, the colic. Rautava et al[60] found colic to be significantly associated with significant maternal stress, susceptibility to illness, self-confidence during pregnancy, and satisfaction with the birth and infant colic. These associations may indicate underlying maternal characteristics such as fearfulness or ambivalence that predispose the infant to colic.

Management

1. Frame **positive feedback** in terms of parents successfully learning how to deal with a high-needs baby.[73] Provide appropriate **referrals for the mother for support.**

2. **Suggestions for parents:**

   a. The breastfeeding mother should **try eliminating certain foods.** **Milk products** should be eliminated from the diet for a week to exclude milk allergy. Other allergens implicated in colic are beef, eggs, peanut butter, wheat, and high-acid fruits and vegetables.[61] Weed[76] suggests elimination of the cabbage family, onion, garlic, chocolate, butter, and sugar and restriction of prune juice to no more than one glass daily. Weed also notes two additional potential allergens, soy and pectin. Page[56] also suggests eliminating fried and fast foods, yeast breads, alcohol, and caffeine.

   b. **Try eliminating certain medications.** Maternal intake of laxatives[76] and iron supplements[61] may cause infant GI distress.

   c. Provide a **"stable emotional environment."**[62]

   d. **Improve feeding techniques** including adequate burping, holding the baby upright, and avoidance of overfeeding or underfeeding.[53] **Small, frequent feedings** may help.[76]

   e. **Infant comfort measures:**

      (1) Position the baby on his or her stomach on a **lambskin rug** while awake (removing lambskin for sleep because of SIDS risk).[71]

      (2) Hold the baby **astraddle the arm,** stomach down, with the head resting in the crook of the arm and the top of the legs in the hand for comfort.[76]

      (3) Place a **warm water bottle** on the infant's stomach.[53]

      (4) Before or during the fussy time, using warm hands and oil, **massage** the baby's abdomen clockwise; rub with little fingers, alternating hands, rubbing from under the ribs to the pubis for 15 minutes. "Bicycle" the legs up to the abdomen. Press each leg, then both legs, to the abdomen for 5 minutes.[62]

      (5) **Walk outside** with the baby in a sling.[62] Carrying, holding, or tight swaddling sometimes helps.[71]

3. Use **the REST model,** proposed by researchers who theorized that a disorganized sleep-wake cycle triggers excessive crying, with the infant becoming overstimulated and unable to self-soothe or fall asleep. The parents may unknowingly add stimulation in their efforts to soothe. The interventions are "REST" for infants and parents.

   a. **REST for infants** includes *regulation* of the environment to decrease stimulation until the infant can soothe himself or herself internally; *entrainment* that synchronizes the infant's behavior with outside signals such as light, noise, and activity; *structure* of the infant's routine with predictable outside clues about what is coming; and *touch* with chest-to-chest or skin-to-skin positioning and vertical ventral positioning that includes vestibular stimulation such as slow up-and-down movements to break through crying episodes and reduce arousal.

   b. **REST for parents** includes *reassurance* that the infant is not ill or in pain; *empathy* (listening and acknowledging the challenge); *support* when the midwife acts as an advocate for the mother, mobilizing resources; and *time-out,* which legitimizes the mother's need to take care of herself.

When this model was used, infant irritability resolved at 10 weeks rather than 12 weeks, mother-infant communication was improved, and parental stress was diminished.[43]

4. **Medical interventions** may be prescribed; however, babies with normal newborn irritability are often treated for organic disease when behavioral and/or feeding interventions would be more appropriate.[11] Medical interventions might include:
   a. Suppository or enema given to infant
   b. Sedative given to infant or parent
   c. Hospitalization of the infant for a change in routine and to allow the parents to rest if necessary for extreme cases[53]

5. **Complementary measures:**
   a. **Homeopathy** experts suggest their remedies for colic.[22,23,55,56,71]
   b. **Miscellaneous:** Apply cold, wet wool socks to the baby's feet; cover with dry cotton socks; the baby should fall asleep quickly.[76] Colic may be indicative of food allergies (especially if associated with constipation, frequent ear infections, dark circles under the eyes, restless sleeping, red cheeks, gas, spitting up a lot, and perspiring while feeding). The mother may want to eliminate foods that are most commonly associated with allergies. Reactions to a food occur in a breastfed baby 4 to 24 hours after the food is eaten by the mother.[69]
   c. **Nutritional suggestions:** The bottlefeeding mother may add 1 Tblsp or one capsule of **acidophilus** (or fresh yogurt) to every 8 oz of cow's milk. **Bottlefeeding mothers may try giving goat's milk**, which has the same amount of casein as human milk, very small fat globules, and high lactose levels, instead of formula. Ensure that the parent is providing skin-to-skin contact during feedings, as well as keeping the baby's head higher than the feet during feedings.[76]
   d. **Chinese medicine: Acupuncture** may be used in the treatment of colic.[78] Johnson[42] suggests incorporating stimulation of **acupressure** points into the clockwise abdominal massage: press the **Conception Vessel meridian** 3 times, then massage the descending colon; repeat 3 times. Then massage up the **Spleen meridian** (inner leg) and down the **Stomach meridian** (lateral thigh). Finally, press the point **Stomach 36** gently 3 times. **See charts and information on Chinese medicine, p. 559.**

e. **Herbs:** The following herbs are recommended for consumption by the **breastfeeding mother:**
   (1) **Catnip tea,** which relieves indigestion and is a remedy for colic.*
   (2) **Chamomile tea,** which is an antispasmodic, an antiinflammatory, and a mild sedative, making it useful for colic.[36,40,48,55,66] Steep 2 tsp dried herb in 1 cup of boiling water for 5 to 10 minutes.[55]
   (3) **Fennel tea,** which is antispasmodic and carminative, helps with dyspepsia, and is known to be useful for colic.† Drink 1 cup of infusion before breastfeeding.[40] **Fennel** is also recommended to be **given to the infant.** A carminative, fennel reduces colic pains.[40,48,55,56,76] Add 5 to 10 gtt tincture to a bottle or give 1 tsp of very dilute tea with a little maple syrup.[55] **See information on herbs, p. 563.**

Constipation

Constipation is diagnosed by the dry, hard character of the stool and not by frequency, because some infants pass stool only every 36 to 48 hours. Constipation is virtually nonexistent among breastfed babies who are receiving enough milk. The bottlefed infant may be receiving insufficient food, fluid, or bulk. A tight rectal sphincter may be present in the infant constipated since birth. Anal fissures or cracks may cause an infant to postpone painful bowel movements and become constipated.[53]

(m) *Management*

1. **Examine infant's anal area for fissures and cracks** and treat if they are present.[53]
2. **Dietary manipulation:** The bottlefed baby's formula may be adjusted by adding food, fluid, or bulk to ease constipation. The older child can have more cereal, fruits, and vegetables added to the diet. Prune juice (½ to 1 oz) is strictly a temporary measure.[53]
3. **Pediatric interventions:** When constipation is present from birth, a rectal **examination by the pediatrician** may dilate a tight sphincter sufficiently to resolve a stricture. **Suppositories** should be used strictly as a temporary measure, and **milk of magnesia** (1 to 2 tsp) is used only for severe constipation that has not responded to other interventions.[53]
4. **Complementary measures:**
   a. Some experts recommend **homeopathic** remedies for constipation.[71]
   b. **Acupuncture** may be used,[78] as may **shiatsu** massage.[42]

---

*References 36, 40, 48, 56, 69, 76.
†References 36, 40, 48, 55, 56, 76.

c. Herbalist Aviva Romm,[62] in her book regarding natural healing for babies and children, reminds us that constipation may occur as a result of **stress or a change in routine.** Other herbalists suggest that when a breastfed baby is constipated, the **mother is often also constipated,** and curing the mother cures the baby.[62,69]

d. **Nutritional suggestions: Blackstrap molasses,** ¼ to ½ tsp, has a laxative effect.[69]

e. The **reflexology** zone for the GI tract is in the arch of the foot. Clockwise massage of this area with the thumbs may effectively treat constipation in infants.[70] **See charts and information about reflexology, p. 567.**

Cradle Cap

Often beginning within the first year, cradle cap manifests as erythematous, papular, nonpruritic, crusty scaling of the infant scalp.[53]

m *Management*

1. If the scalp condition is associated with a generalized condition or becomes secondarily infected, **refer** to a pediatrician.[25]

2. **Advise parent:** Cradle cap may be controlled by use of a **mild shampoo** twice a week. Sesame, olive, or another **oil** may be massaged into the affected area a few hours before the shampoo; dilute castile soap, dilute witch hazel tea, or dry rolled oats in a small cloth sack may be used to **moisten, rub, and soften** the cradle cap; or hair may be combed with a **fine-tooth comb.**[62,69]

3. **Medical interventions** include the use of Selsun Blue or Sebutone shampoo or 2% ketoconazole cream rubbed into the scalp at bedtime, followed by a mild shampoo in the morning. Five to six courses, followed by weekly shampoos, may be required. Application of 1% hydrocortisone cream tid to inflamed areas may be helpful. Cradle cap usually clears in a few months.[53]

4. **Complementary measures:** Some herbalists mention **herbal** remedies for cradle cap.[55,76]

Dehydration

An infant loses water through diarrhea and evaporation from the skin and lungs. Having a large body surface area in proportion to the body mass increases evaporative loss. Excessive GI fluid loss also depletes the body of potassium and sodium, which must be replaced.[61] Signs and symptoms include decreased skin turgor, dry mucous membranes, depressed fontanels, tachycardia, tachypnea, decreased urine output (<6 to 8 wet diapers/24 hr), restlessness, apathy, weak peripheral pulses, mottled skin, cold and cyanotic extremities with capillary refill >2 to 3 seconds, hypotension, decreased motility or ileus, and compensated metabolic acidemia advancing to uncompensated acidemia when dehydration is more severe.[53] The child <2 years is unable to concentrate urine as efficiently as the older person, so concentrated urine (specific gravity >1.020) indicates more serious dehydration. The degree of dehydration is determined by weight loss: 10% weight loss is considered moderate and 15% is considered severe.[61]

(m) *Management*

1. **Advise the breastfeeding mother** that if the baby is able to take anything by mouth, it should be **breastmilk.** Even partial breastfeeding will reduce diarrhea. Additional rehydration fluids may be given by spoon or dropper to the breastfed baby. The **bottlefed** baby may have **milk products eliminated** for a period if diarrhea is severe.[61]
2. **Refer** the dehydrated infant for pediatric management. Treatment consists of hospitalization and IV fluid replacement when dehydration is moderate to severe.[61]

Diaper Rash

Friction and prolonged contact of the skin with urine, feces, diaper soap, or topical preparations may cause erythematous and scaly skin with papulovesicular or bullous lesions, fissures, or erosions. Secondary infection with bacteria or fungus is common. Intense inflammation may cause severe discomfort.[53] Disposable diapers, a cold, or teething may also cause diaper rash.[62]

(m) *Management*

1. Teach parents the following:
    a. **Diapering technique: Change diapers** often, gently washing the baby with mild soap and water and blotting skin dry. A hair dryer on the lowest setting may **dry the area** more thoroughly.[71] **Avoid the use of rubber pants.** Woolen soakers are an alternative.[76] Disposable diapers may create a drier environment.[53]
    b. **Eliminate possible irritants:** Disposable diapers may cause irritation, and cloth diapers or a different brand of disposable diapers may provide relief. Change the brand of detergent used. Try using soap flakes or Basic-H, rather than detergent, bleach, and ammonia to launder diapers. Add apple cider vinegar to the last rinse, and whenever possible, hang diapers in the sunlight to dry.[76]
    c. Exposing the buttocks to the **sun** for 10 minutes a day is healing.[62]
    d. Apply **protective topical agents,** such as zinc oxide or white petrolatum.[53]
2. **Medical intervention:** If the rash is red, painful, and raw with erythematous confluent lesions, skin-fold involvement, and multiple 1- to 2-mm pustules and papules at the periphery of the dermatitis, **refer** to the pediatrician to exclude yeast or bacterial infection. For yeast infection, an anticandidal agent will be helpful and may be used in conjunction with zinc oxide. When these measures are not effective or when candidiasis has been ruled out, application of 0.5% to

1.0% hydrocortisone cream for a limited time may be effective. Prolonged use can cause secondary complications, especially when fluorinated compounds are applied.[53]

3. **Complementary measures:**
   a. Some experts recommend **homeopathic** remedies for diaper rash.[71]
   b. **Nutritional suggestions: Identify the yeast sources** in the infant's or the breastfeeding mother's diet: wine, beer, and all spirits including vinegar[76]; bread; the skins of all fruits and vegetables; sugar; honey; and wheat.[62,71,76] Minimize yeast sources and **emphasize fish, grains, and beans** in the diet for 2 weeks to observe the baby's response.[62,76] The breastfeeding mother of an infected baby can take **niacinamide**, a B vitamin, 100 mg qd, to supplement the baby.[69]
   c. **Herbs:** A salve made from **calendula,**[14,36,62,71] **plantain,**[55,62,76] and **comfrey,**[36,54,62,76] applied externally, may be soothing and facilitate healing. **If candidiasis is present,** rinse the diaper area with **vinegar solution** after diaper changes and continue to use the salve.[27,69,76] **See information on herbs, p. 563.**

Bullous Impetigo

Infection of the skin with coagulase-positive *Staphylococcus aureus* most often occurs in the diaper area[18] but may also occur on the face, trunk, and extremities. Impetigo begins on intact skin, forming a rash of large blisters, or bullae. The bullae rupture easily, leaving a narrow rim around a moist eroded area. Regional adenopathy is generally absent. The skin may appear scalded. Constitutional symptoms are unusual but may be seen with widespread infection.[53] The infection is spread by direct contact with a person who has an infected, draining lesion or by a nonsymptomatic carrier of *S. aureus* in the nares. Incubation is usually 4 to 10 days.[18]

Laboratory Findings: Organism is identified by culture.[53]

ⓜ Management

1. **Report** the disease to the public health authorities.[18]
2. **Cleanse** the affected skin and treat with a **topical antimicrobial** (such as mupirocin tid to qid for 7 to 10 days).[53]
3. Advise parent to apply **warm dry compress,** which may localize the infection.
4. **Pediatric management:** The physician may incise abscesses to permit drainage. For severe cases, a **systemic antibiotic** may be prescribed.[18]
5. **Complementary measures:**
   a. Some experts recommend **homeopathic** remedies for impetigo.[23]
   b. **Herbs: Calendula** infusion salve or oil or dilute calendula tincture (1 Tblsp in 1 cup water) applied to sores a few times daily is an antiinflammatory antiseptic that will facilitate comfort, healing,

and prevent scarring.[36,48,62] **Goldenseal** acts as an antibiotic, may stimulate the immune system, and is effective when applied locally to impetigo, though it may stain the skin yellow.[36,45,48,62] **See information on herbs, p. 563.**

Diarrhea

Diarrhea may be caused by anatomic defects; malabsorption; endocrinopathies; food poisoning; neoplasms; milk allergies; immune deficiency disease; Crohn's disease; bacterial, parasitic, or viral infection; or ulcerative colitis. Infrequently, antibiotics are causative. Diarrhea is usually self-limiting, and the cause is not determined.[53]

(m) *Management*

1. **Assess nutrition:**
   a. **Breastfeeding** helps to prevent GI infections and diarrhea. Actual diarrhea in a breastfed infant is rare and should be considered infectious.[61]
   b. Although bottlefed babies' stools are usually firmer than those of breastfed babies, artificial feeding occasionally causes loose stools. **Overfeeding** in the first 2 weeks will cause loose stools. If overfeeding is suspected, the mother should withhold one or several formula feedings, substituting boiled water or an electrolyte solution. Most cases of diarrhea will quickly respond. Diarrhea in an artificially fed infant may also result from **formula contamination,** which is not serious and resolves easily.[53]
2. **Fluids with high osmolalities** as a result of excessive carbohydrate content and low sodium concentration (e.g., carbonated beverages, Kool-Aid, Jell-O, fruit juices) and tea **are inappropriate** for rehydration of infants, may cause hyponatremia, and may exacerbate diarrhea. Foods are reintroduced as soon as tolerated. The child should be **isolated,** and caregivers should use **good handwashing** technique.[53]
3. **Refer the infant with significant dehydration for pediatric treatment.** Fluids and electrolytes are replaced. Antibiotics are infrequently indicated.[53]
4. **Complementary measures:**
   a. **Acupuncture** may be used with success in the treatment of diarrhea,[78] as may **shiatsu.**[42]
   b. **Nutritional suggestions:** Never discontinue breastfeeding because doing so may worsen the diarrhea. If the child is old enough to eat solid food, the **pectin in applesauce** will help solidify the stool.[62] Consumption of **bananas, brown rice water, and carob** may help.[69]
   c. **Herbs:** A healing salve of **calendula, plantain, and comfrey may be applied to the anal area for comfort.**[36,54,62,76] **See information on herbs, p. 563.**

Remedies for Teething Pain

As the primary teeth erupt through the gums, irritation is noted and salivation increases. According to the *Nelson Textbook of Pediatrics*,[53] little evidence exists that teething can cause diarrhea, fever, facial rashes, or other systemic manifestations, although one contributor to the book mentions low-grade fever. Herbalist Romm,[62] on the other hand, states that teething is often accompanied by fever, diarrhea, irritability, earache, rhinorrhea, cough, and cold symptoms; but symptoms may be caused by the teething itself or by a virus contracted due to a lowered resistance to infection.

⑰ Management

1. **Comfort measures:** A pacifier or a teething ring that has been in the freezer may give temporary relief.[71]
2. **Complementary measures:**
   a. **Shiatsu** massage may comfort the teething baby.[42]
   b. **Homeopathy** experts recommend their remedies for the teething infant.[23,55,56,62,71]
   c. **Herbs: Catnip** tea[56,62,69] may be soothing when given to both mother and baby by cup, spoon, dropper, or bottle.[62] **Chamomile** is a mild sedative that may soothe a teething infant when given in small amounts.[48,55,56,62,71] Use tincture, 5 to 10 gtt up to tid, or put 1 to 2 gtt on a wet swab and apply to the gums.[55] **Clove oil** may be used as a topical anesthetic. Use in tiny amounts because more can be irritating.[56,62,69] **See information on herbs, p. 563.**

• NEONATAL DISORDERS

Erythroblastosis Fetalis (Hydrops Fetalis; Hemolytic Disease of the Newborn)

Maternal antibodies that cross the placenta cause hemolysis of fetal RBCs in the fetal syndrome resulting from maternal isoimmunization (see p. 94). Symptoms range in severity. Fifteen percent of infants have only mild laboratory evidence of hemolysis, while infants with severe anemia exhibit signs of hydrops. Liver, cardiac, and pulmonary complications may occur, as well as hyperbilirubinemia and hypoglycemia. The mortality rate of these infants has been dramatically reduced by the administration of prenatal RhoGAM at 28 weeks and by treatment with intraperitoneal or intravascular transfusion in utero.[24] Infants born with severe hemolytic anemia are treated by pediatrics with supportive therapy and receive exchange transfusions of type O Rh-negative blood, cross-matched to the mother.[53]

Failure to Thrive

Infants are generally diagnosed with failure to thrive (FTT) when their weight drops below the 3rd percentile or is two standard deviations below the mean standard weight for age. FTT may be due to organic factors (e.g., renal disease, congenital defects, or maternal starvation), nonorganic factors (insufficient caloric intake or disturbance in the mother-infant relationship), or both. Only about 18% of FTT cases are due to organic disease, regardless of whether the baby is breastfed or bottlefed. The baby with FTT may appear constantly fretful or may appear content and placid.[61] Children with nonorganic FTT remain shorter and lower in weight over the long term.[20]

Assessment of the breastfed baby and its mother includes a prenatal history; a history of the problem with descriptions of feeding including length, frequency, and infant behavior, as well as the mother's diet; physical examination of the baby; and observation of a feeding.[61] Health care providers need to be aware that breastfed babies grow at a different rate than do formula-fed babies after 4 months of age. The Fels Chart, used by many pediatric providers to determine normalcy of growth, was developed among a largely formula-fed group and is not representative for breastfed babies. When the breastfed baby's growth velocity drops off after 4 months, some babies are given a misdiagnosis of FTT.[37]

The mother of the calm, apparently contented baby with FTT may be waiting for hunger cues from the baby rather than initiating feedings. Alternately, the baby may not be actively suckling while at the breast. The mother should offer the breast more frequently and use a feeding tube device to increase the caloric intake, while pumping after feedings to increase the milk supply. The baby will often become increasingly alert and will awaken more often to be fed—including at night.[61]

A common cause of FFT is a rigid parenting style that structures parent-infant interactions, including feedings. Social pressure ("don't spoil the baby") may lead the mother to ignore hunger cues. Restrictions regarding the frequency of feedings or the length of time spent at each breast and inflexibility from day to day as the baby responds to its growth and caloric output are counterproductive. Awkward breastfeeding positioning may result in a baby's reluctance to nurse. Better positioning and coaching the mother to build up a milk supply should improve this baby's growth. A short frenulum (tongue-tie or ankyloglossia) in the baby may cause feeding difficulties. The mother who has been sexually abused, and for whom breastfeeding is linked in some way to that abuse, may not be feeding optimally. The mother who is dieting may have an inadequate milk supply (see p. 313).[61]

m *Management*

1. The **pediatrician** manages FTT.
2. With the benefit of a rapport developed during the pregnancy, the **midwife can offer** the mother **emotional and informational support.** Assess parenting style or concerns, support at home for breastfeeding, a history of sexual abuse, and nutritional or other contributory factors. Support the mother's breastfeeding frequently and on demand. Assist with positioning, working with the pediatrician to enhance the health of the breastfeeding couple.

3. **Complementary measures: Acupuncture** may be used in the treatment of FTT.[78]

Group B Streptococcal Sepsis of the Newborn

Colonization of the fetus with the gram-positive beta-hemolytic diplococcus, commonly found in the maternal lower intestinal and urinary tracts, occurs through ascending infection, across the placenta, or by contamination with passage through the birth canal. Two forms of this illness occur.

Early-Onset Neonatal Group B Streptococcal Infection

Early-onset Group B streptococcal (GBS) infection occurs within 7 days of delivery (usually within 6 to 12 hours) and is associated with a mortality rate of about 5% to 22%. Fifty percent of neonates are symptomatic at birth.[53] The infection is believed to be acquired in utero or during delivery. LBW infants are more often affected,[24] although 50% of the infants affected are full term. Initial symptoms may include cyanosis, apnea, hypotension, tachypnea, grunting, flaring, and retractions. Pulmonary effusion, infiltrates, and cardiomegaly are present. The disease ranges from asymptomatic bacteriuria to septic shock but generally manifests as pneumonia with bacteremia complicated by pulmonary hypertension. Persistent fetal circulation, generalized sepsis, and meningitis may occur. Neurologic sequelae are severe in 20% to 30% of cases and mild in 15% to 25% of cases.[53]

Late-Onset Neonatal Group B Streptococcal Infection

Late-onset GBS infection occurs 7 days to several months after delivery and involves sepsis and meningitis.[53] The mortality rate is 5% to 20%. Late-onset infection is the result of vertical transmission or nosocomial or community-acquired infection.[10] Sixty percent of cases manifest as meningitis, and survivors may have serious neurologic sequelae.[24]

Incidence

Twenty percent of pregnant women are colonized with GBS.[33] Only 1 in 100 colonized mothers have an affected baby,[18] but the rate is higher among at-risk infants (see Box 5-1). The more heavily a woman is colonized, the greater the risk that her infant will be colonized. With exposure to GBS, intact membranes may become inflamed, weaken, and rupture, causing premature labor.[53]

m *Management*

See screening and prophylactic treatment of the pregnant woman, p. 67. Pediatricians manage the neonatal infection.

Intrauterine Growth Restriction

IUGR is defined as a birthweight less than the 10th percentile for that population, although 70% of the infants identified by this definition are actually constitutionally small, incurring none of the IUGR risks.[29] On

• *Box 5-1 /* **Fetuses at Risk for Group B Streptococcal Sepsis** •

- Delivery at <37 weeks' gestation
- Prolonged rupture of membranes (>18 hr)
- A sibling with early-onset GBS disease
- Maternal intrapartum fever (temperature ≥38° C [100.4° F])
- Maternal GBS bacteriuria in current pregnancy
- Maternal vaginal/rectal GBS colonization identified by screening culture in current pregnancy[64]

examination, the infant with IUGR has little subcutaneous tissue, prominent eyes, dry skin, and an overly alert appearance. The infant is at risk for the following:

- Intrauterine fetal demise caused by hypoxia, acidosis, infection, or anomaly.
- Perinatal asphyxia as a result of placental insufficiency.
- Meconium aspiration syndrome.
- Hypoglycemia (due to decreased glycogen stores, increased usage of glycogen during hypoxia, and diminished gluconeogenesis).
- Polycythemia-hyperviscosity caused by fetal hypoxia-induced increased RBC production.
- Hypothermia (due to minimal fat stores, hypoxemia, hypoglycemia).
- Malformations caused by congenital syndromes, oligohydramnios-induced deformations, or TORCH infection.[53]
- Altered head size. IUGR that affects head size results in fewer and smaller brain cells. Verbal ability, visual recognition memory, and general neurodevelopmental outcome may be affected. IUGR also affects long-term growth.[31]

m *Management*

1. See p. 74 regarding antepartum management of IUGR.
2. The pediatrician manages the infant with IUGR. The newborn is observed closely for **hypothermia, hypoglycemia, polycythemia, and hyperviscosity.**[24] **Early feedings** are encouraged. The gestational age is estimated by using the New Ballard Scale (see p. 261), with the neurologic components being weighted more heavily because of the skin changes seen in babies with IUGR. The infant is examined for anomalies, infection, or any other cause of growth restriction.

Sudden Infant Death Syndrome

SIDS is the sudden death of an infant without known medical problems, except possibly a minor upper respiratory tract infection. SIDS usually occurs during sleep. The incidence peaks between 2 and 6 months of age.[61] The cause is unknown. SIDS results in more infant deaths than any other cause.[8]

Incidence: In 1998, 2529 babies died of SIDS in the United States (64 of every 100,000 live births). The SIDS rate has decreased by >40% since the launching of the 1992 Back to Sleep program.[8]

Predisposing Factors:

Maternal smoking (which doubles the risk with a dose-response relationship)
Bottlefeeding
Lower socioeconomic status
"Near-miss SIDS" incident[61]
Prone sleeping[65]
Maternal opiate use[77]
Use of soft bedding that traps exhaled gases causing rebreathing

LBW
Young maternal age
Multiparity
Male sex
Late or no prenatal care
Prematurity
Black or Native American race[8]

Prevention

1. Teach all parents the following:
    - **Place the baby to sleep on the back** to prevent rebreathing of expired gases. Side-lying is not recommended because it is unstable and infants will turn to the prone position.[8] Sleeping on the back was once discouraged because it was feared that aspirations might result. Since the Back to Sleep program began, there has been no increase in aspirations.
    - The **prone position is appropriate at times other than sleep** and is necessary for the baby to gain strength in the shoulders and to avoid flattening of the occiput.[8]
    - **Safe bedding:** A firm, tight-fitting mattresses should be used. Pillows, comforters, stuffed animals, and sheepskin—particularly dangerous when placed under the baby—should be removed from the crib. Use a warm sleeper instead of a blanket. If using a blanket, use a thin one and tuck it around the mattress so that it only reaches the baby's chest, making sure that the baby's head is uncovered.[8]
    - **Avoid overheating** the baby.[8]
    - **Sleeping with the mother** decreases the risk of SIDS.[61] The bed should only be shared by parents who do not smoke in bed and who do not use any drugs or substances that might alter their arousal.[8]
2. **Identify families at risk** and offer support services.[61]

Neonatal Withdrawal (Abstinence Syndrome)

Symptoms of neonatal withdrawal and interventions (when required) are listed in Table 5-2.

Table 5-2 / Neonatal Withdrawal Symptoms and Interventions

Symptom	Intervention
High-pitched cry	Swaddle
Inability to sleep	Decrease environmental stimuli; medication may be prescribed
Frantic sucking of fists, blistering hands	Dress in sewn-in mitts
Poor feeding	Feed small amounts at a time; observe for signs of dehydration; medication may be prescribed
Regurgitation, vomiting, diarrhea	Observe for triggering events and prevent; observe for dehydration; medication may be prescribed
Tachypnea, mottling	Observe for apnea, cyanosis, heart rate >180 BPM; place in semi-Fowler position.
Hyperactive Moro reflex and hypertonicity	Minimize handling
Increased activity may increase temperature	Exclude other causes of fever and maintain temperature through environmental measures
Tremors and seizures	Medications are prescribed for seizures; prevent pressure sores by turning
Risk for poor bonding	Room-in; minimize separation from mother; encourage skin-to-skin contact; involve social services
Yawning, sneezing, nasal stuffiness, perspiration	No intervention

Data from Nelson WE, senior editor: *Nelson textbook of pediatrics*, ed 15, Philadelphia, 1996, WB Saunders; Wagner CL et al: The impact of drug exposure on the neonate, *Obstet Gynecol Clin North Am* 25:169-194, 1998.

Toxicology Screening:

1. **Urine:** Amphetamines, marijuana, barbiturates, and opiates may be detected in fetal urine, as may cocaine for several days after maternal use. See Table 2-3, p. 110, for the timing of detection of drugs of abuse by urine toxicology.
2. **Meconium:** First developed at 18 weeks' gestation, a cumulative reservoir for cocaine and alcohol taken in the latter half of gestation.
3. **Hair:** Maternal hair (1.5 cm) can be analyzed to reveal the maternal use of narcotics, marijuana, cocaine, nicotine and cocaine in combination, and alcohol and cocaine in combination. Treated hair is less reliable. The infant's hair will reveal maternal drug use for 2 to 3 months after birth.[74]

• REFERENCES

1. Ada G: Vaccines and vaccination, *N Engl J Med* 345:1042-1053, 2001.
2. American Academy of Pediatrics (AAP): Immunization protects children, 2000 Immunization Schedule. Available at: *http://www.aap.org/family/parents/immunize.htm.*
3. AAP: Press release: AAP releases report on treatment of newborns with genital abnormalities. July 3, 2000. Available at: *http://www.aap.org/advocacy/releases/julgend.htm.*

4. Reference deleted in galleys.
5. AAP: Press release: New AAP circumcision policy released. March 1, 1999. Available at: *http://www.AAP.org/advocacy/releases/marcircum.htm.*
6. AAP: Issues in newborn screening, *Pediatrics* 89:345-349, 1992.
7. AAP Task Force on Circumcision: Circumcision policy statement (RE9850), March 1999. Available at: *http://www.aap.org/policy/re9850.html.*
8. AAP Task Force on Infant Sleep Position and Sudden Infant Death Syndrome: Changing concepts of sudden death syndrome: implications for infant sleeping environment and sleep position, *Pediatrics* 105:650-656, 2000.
9. Reference deleted in galleys.
10. ACOG: *Prevention of early-onset group B streptococcal disease in newborns,* Committee Opinion No. 173, Washington DC, 1996, ACOG.
11. Armstrong KL, Previtera N, McCallum RN: Medicalizing normality? management of irritability in infants, *J Paediatr Child Health* 36:301-305, 2000.
12. Augustine MC: Hyperbilirubinemia in the healthy term newborn, *Nurse Pract* 24:24-26, 29-32, 34-36, 42-43, 1999.
13. Avery GB, Fletcher MA, MacDonald MG: *Neonatology, pathophysiology and management of the newborn,* Philadelphia, 1994, JB Lippincott.
14. Balch JF, Balch PA: *Prescription for nutritional healing,* ed 2, Garden City Park, NY, 1997, Avery.
15. Ballard J: New Ballard Scale, expanded to include extremely premature infants, *J Pediatr* 119:417-423, 1991.
16. Barkauskas VH et al: *Health & physical assessment,* St Louis, 1994, Mosby–Year Book, Inc.
17. Battaglia FC, Lubchenco LO: A practical classification of newborn infants by weight and gestational age, *J Pediatr* 71:159-163, 1967.
18. Benenson AS, editor: *Control of communicable disease manual,* ed 16, Washington, DC, 1995, American Public Health Association.
19. Bloom R, Cropley C: *Textbook of neonatal resuscitation,* Elk Grove Village, Ill, 1996, American Heart Association and American Academy of Pediatrics.
20. Boddy J, Skuse D, Andrews B: The developmental sequelae of nonorganic failure to thrive, *J Child Psychol Psychiatry* 41:1003-1014, 2000.
21. Braun MM, Ellenberg SS: Descriptive epidemiology of adverse events after immunization: reports to the Vaccine Adverse Event Reporting System (VAERS), 1991-1994, *J Pediatr* 131:529-535, 1997.
22. Cummings B, Tiran D: Homeopathy for pregnancy and childbirth. In Tiran D, Mack S, editors: *Complementary therapies for pregnancy and childbirth,* ed 2, Edinburgh, 2000, Baillière Tindall.
23. Cummings S, Ullman D: *Everybody's guide to homeopathic medicines,* New York, 1997, Jeremy P. Tarcher/Putnam.
24. Cunningham FG et al: *Williams obstetrics,* ed 20, Stamford, Conn, 1997, Appleton and Lange.
25. Emmons L et al: Primary care management of common dermatologic disorders in women, *J Nurse Midwifery* 42:228-253, 1997.
26. Falk GT: Frequently asked questions about infant circumcision (1999). Available at: *http://www.parenthoodweb.com/Library/circfaq.htm.*
27. Feral C: Natural remedies, *Midwifery Today* 26:35-38, Summer 1993.
28. Fisher BL: Great debates: to immunize or not? (1999). Available at: *http://www.babycenter.com/debates/cons9.html.*
29. Gabbe SG, Niebyl JR, Simpson JL: *Obstetrics: normal & problem pregnancies,* ed 3, New York, 1996, Churchill Livingstone.
30. Galan H: Meconium-stained amniotic fluid: meaning and management, *OBG Manage* July 1999. Available at: *http://www.obgmanagement.com/799/cme799.html.*
31. Georgieff MK: Intrauterine growth retardation and subsequent somatic growth and neurodevelopment, *J Pediatr* 133:3-5, 1998.
32. Gilbert WM, Nesbitt TS, Danielson B: Associated factors in 1611 cases of brachial plexus injury, *Obstet Gynecol* 93:536-540, 1999.

33. Glantz JC, Kedley KE: Concepts and controversies in the management of group B streptococcus during pregnancy, *Birth* 25:45-53, 1998.

34. Gordon JD et al: *Obstetrics, gynecology & infertility*, Glen Cove, NY, 1998, Scrub Hill Press.

35. Greene A: What are the advantages and disadvantages of performing a circumcision on a newborn? 1999. Available at: *http://www.parenthoodweb.com/articles/phw720.htm.*

36. Griffith HW: *Healing herbs: the essential guide*, Tucson, Ariz, 2000, Fisher Books.

37. Guise JM, Freed G: Resident physicians' knowledge of breastfeeding and infant growth, *Birth* 27:49-53, 2000.

38. Hackley BK: Controversies in immunization practices: vaccine safety and implications for midwifery practice, *J Midwifery Womens Health* 47:16-27, 2002.

39. Haninger NC, Farley CL: Screening for hypoglycemia in healthy term neonates: effects on breastfeeding, *J Midwifery Womens Health* 46:292-301, 2001.

40. Hoffmann D: *The holistic herbal*, Findhorn, Scotland, 1985, Findhorn Press.

41. Jarvis C: *Physical assessment and health examination*, Philadelphia, 2000, WB Saunders.

42. Johnson E: Shiatsu. In Tiran D, Mack S, editors: *Complementary therapies for pregnancy and childbirth*, ed 2, Edinburgh, 2000, Baillière Tindall.

43. Keefe MR, Froese-Fretz A, Kotzer AM: The REST regimen: an individualized nursing intervention for infant irritability, *MCN Am J Matern Child Nurs* 22:16-20, 1997.

44. Kimmel SR et al: Breaking the barriers to childhood immunization, *Am Fam Physician* 53:1648-1656, 1996.

45. Kloss J: *Back to Eden*, New York, 1981, Benedict Lust.

46. Libman MD et al: Clues in diagnosing congenital heart disease, *West J Med* 13:392-398, 1992.

47. Linder N et al: Suckling stimulation test for neonatal tremor, *Arch Dis Child* 64:44-52, 1989.

48. Mabey R et al, editors: *The new age herbalist*, New York, 1988, Collier Books.

49. March of Dimes: *Core group of newborn screening tests recommended by the March of Dimes*, 2000. Available at: *http://www.modimes.org/HealthLibrary2/FactSheets/Newborn_Screening_Test.htm.*

50. Metzger BE, Coustan DR: Summary and recommendations of the Fourth International Workshop-Conference on Gestational Diabetes Mellitus, *Diabetes Care* 21(suppl 2):B161-B167, 1998.

51. Meyer K, Anderson GC: Using kangaroo care in a clinical setting with fullterm infants having breastfeeding difficulties, *MCN Am J Matern Child Nurs* 24:190-192, 1999.

52. Neifert MR: Clinical aspects of lactation, *Clin Perinatol* 26:281-306, 1999.

53. Nelson WE, senior editor: *Nelson textbook of pediatrics*, ed 15, Philadelphia, 1996, WB Saunders.

54. Nissim R: *Natural healing in gynecology*, San Francisco, 1996, Pandora (HarperCollins).

55. Ody P: *The complete medicinal herbal*, New York, 1993, Dorling Kindersley.

56. Page L: *Healthy healing*, ed 11, Carmel Valley, Calif, 2000, Healthy Healing Publications.

57. Parker LA: Ambiguous genitalia: etiology, treatment, and nursing implications, *J Obstet Gynecol Neonatal Nurs* 27:15-22, 1998.

58. Perlow JH et al: Birth trauma: a five-year review of incidence and associated perinatal factors, *J Reprod Med* 41:754-760, 1996.

59. Peron JE: Care of the intact penis, *Midwifery Today* 17:24, Nov 1991.

60. Rautava P, Helenius H, Lehtonen L: Psychosocial predisposing factors for infantile colic, *BMJH* 307:600-604, 1993.

61. Riordan J, Auerbach K: *Breastfeeding and human lactation*, ed 2, Sudbury, Mass, 1999, Jones and Bartlett.

62. Romm AJ: *Natural healing for babies and children*, Freedom, Calif, 1996, The Crossing Press.

63. Shechet J, Fried SM: Traditional Jewish circumcision of bris, *Am Fam Physician* 53:1070-1071, 1996.

64. Schrag SJ et al: Prevention of perinatal group B streptococcal disease: revised guidelines from CDC, *MMWR* 50:1-22, 2002.

65. Skadberg BT, Morild I, Markestad T: Abandoning prone sleeping: effect on the risk of sudden infant death syndrome, *J Pediatr* 132:340-343, 1998.
66. Stapleton H, Tiran D: Herbal medicine. In Tiran D, Mack S, editors: *Complementary therapies for pregnancy and childbirth*, Edinburgh, 2000, Baillière Tindall.
67. Swartz MH: *Textbook of physical diagnosis: history and examination*, ed 2, Philadelphia, 1994, WB Saunders.
68. Taeusch HW, Sniderman S: Neonatal resuscitation. In Taeusch HW, Christiansen RO, Buescher ES, editors: *Pediatric and neonatal tests and procedures*, Philadelphia, 1996, WB Saunders.
69. Tarr K: *Herbs, helps, and pressure points for pregnancy and childbirth*, ed 3, Provo, Utah, 1984, Sunbeam.
70. Tiran D: Reflexology in midwifery practice. In Tiran D, Mack S, editors: *Complementary therapies for pregnancy and childbirth*, Edinburgh, 2000, Baillière Tindall.
71. Ullman R, Reichenberg-Ullman J: *Homeopathic self-care*, Rocklin, Calif, 1997, Prima.
72. van Overmeire B et al: A comparison of ibuprofen and indomethacin for closure of patent ductus arteriosus, *N Engl J Med* 343:674-681, 2000.
73. Varney H: *Varney's midwifery*, ed 3, Sudbury, Mass, 1997, Jones and Bartlett Publishers.
74. Wagner CL et al: The impact of drug exposure on the neonate, *Obstet Gynecol Clin North Am* 25:169-194, 1998.
75. Wagner RK, Nielsen PE, Gonik B: Shoulder dystocia, *Obstet Gynecol Clin North Am* 26:371-383, 1999.
76. Weed S: *Wise woman herbal for the childbearing year*, Woodstock, NY, 1985, Ash Tree.
77. Willinger M, Hoffman HJ, Hartford RB: Infant sleep position and risk for sudden infant death syndrome: report of meeting held January 13 and 14, 1994, National Institutes of Health, Bethesda, Md, *Pediatrics* 92:814-820, 1994.
78. Yelland S: *Acupuncture in midwifery*, Cheshire, England, 1996, Books for Midwives Press.

Chapter 6

Infant Feeding

See care of the nonlactating breasts, p. 229.

• BOTTLEFEEDING

Indications: Maternal preference, substance abuse, human immunodeficiency virus (HIV) infection (in developed countries), human T-lymphocytic virus (HTLV-1) infection, or maternal use of certain medications.

Formula Composition: Most formula is made from cow's milk by processing the casein to smaller, digestible molecules and sterilizing to eliminate bacteria. The healthy formula-fed baby thrives by physiologically adjusting to wide ranges of protein, fat, carbohydrates, and minerals. Formula is made to simulate the mother's milk as closely as possible.[34] Formula may also be composed of soy products.

Method:

1. Good **handwashing** is essential.

2. **Utensils** and **bottles** are cleaned with a bottle brush in hot, soapy water or in a dishwasher and then boiled for 5 to 10 minutes **when the water supply is not contaminated.** Ideal bottles are widemouthed for easy cleaning, and the hole in the nipple should drip slowly.

3. The **formula** is mixed according to the directions. Failure to add sufficient water may result in dehydration. Bottles are filled with the average amount taken by the infant and refrigerated until used.

4. **Where the water supply is uncertain,** the formula can be sterilized by setting the bottles—filled with formula, nipples and caps loosely screwed on—into a large pot and boiling for 25 minutes. When cooled, caps are tightened and bottles are stored in a refrigerator.

5. **Temperature:** Traditionally, formula is warmed to liken it to breastmilk, although room temperature or cool milk is not harmful. The temperature is tested on the inside of the wrist. The microwave is not used for heating formula because uneven heating may burn the infant.

6. **The infant** should be **held for feedings** in much the same way as for breastfeeding. Propping of bottles deprives the infant of human

contact, may present the danger of aspiration for small infants, and increases the risk of milk entering the eustachian tube, causing otitis media. The infant should be allowed to drink at his or her own rate and should not be encouraged to take any more than he or she wants. The excess is discarded.

7. **Burp** the infant at regular intervals and after every feeding.

8. **Frequency:** Smaller infants may require feedings q2-3h, but most healthy infants want to be bottlefed q4h or so.[34]

9. **Quantity:** On the first day of life, the infant may take no more than 1 oz of formula at each feeding. During the following 2 weeks, most term infants take 1 to 2 oz q2-3h.[58] Thereafter, for about 6 months, the infant will usually take 7 to 8 oz.[34]

10. If a family cannot afford commercial formula, **an acceptable formula can be made** and should be recommended for use rather than cow's milk: To 15 oz water, add 1 Tblsp sugar and 10 oz evaporated milk (wiping the top of the can before opening). The result is 25 oz of formula at 20 kcal/oz. Evaporated milk has been heated and is more digestible than untreated cow's milk. This formula should be supplemented with a multivitamin with iron.[58]

• BREASTFEEDING

Anatomy and Physiology

The breast is made up of 15 to 20 lobes of milk-secreting glands, circularly arranged and surrounded by fat and connective tissue. The ligaments of Cooper are ligaments that attach these lobes to the chest wall. Each lobe is made up of alveoli and alveolar ducts that are surrounded by contractile myoepithelial cells. The alveoli drain into a lactiferous duct. Underneath the nipple, the lactiferous ducts become cone-shaped and form milk sinuses. The lactiferous ducts, surrounded by fibromuscular tissue, open onto the surface of the nipple (see Figure 6-1).[5]

Increased estrogen suppresses hypothalamic prolactin-inhibiting factor (dopamine) and stimulates pituitary prolactin secretion, which rises from the normal level of 10 to 25 ng/mL beginning at about 8 weeks' gestation to 200 to 400 ng/mL at term. Prolactin stimulates breast growth and colostrum production. During pregnancy, progesterone prevents lactation.[49]

When the placenta delivers at birth, estrogen and progesterone levels drop within 3 to 4 days. Prolactin stimulates the breast, causing breast engorgement and milk secretion before clearing from the circulation by about 7 days. Suckling stimulates nerve endings in the nipple and areola that send impulses to the hypothalamus, causing prolactin, oxytocin, and thyroid-stimulating hormone (TSH) to be released. Throughout lactation, prolactin levels are maintained at approximately 40 to 50 ng/mL. TSH plays a role in prolactin secretion. Prolactin maintains the casein,

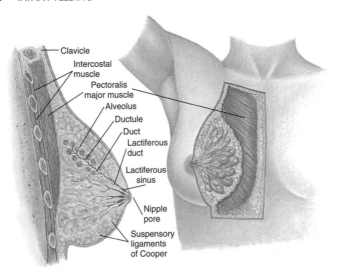

Figure 6-1 • Anatomy of the breast. (From Seidel H et al: *Mosby's guide to physical examination*, ed 5, St Louis, 2003, Mosby.)

fatty acids, lactose, and milk volume. Oxytocin contracts myoepithelial cells, empties the alveoli, and allows alveolar refilling. Milk ejection occurs not by mechanical negative pressure, but by the sensors in the areola stimulating the secretion of oxytocin, which causes contraction of alveoli into the lactiferous ducts underlying the areola, where it is removed by the infant. Oxytocin secretion may also occur as a conditioned response when the baby is present or cries. This release of milk is called "letdown." The milk that is available after the release of oxytocin is progressively higher in fat content ("hindmilk"). The amount of milk that is removed equals the amount of milk that is produced, both by the emptying of the ducts and by the release of prolactin stimulated by suckling. After the milk has come in, the most significant single determinant of milk volume is the frequency and efficiency of milk removal. The breast will store milk as long as 48 hours; milk production will then slow.[33]

Advantages of Breastfeeding for the Infant

The American Academy of Pediatrics (AAP) recommends exclusive breastfeeding for at least 4 to 6 months, with breastfeeding continuing for at least 1 year. The protective effect of breastfeeding increases the more the mother nurses the infant. Other advantages include:

1. The composition of the mother's milk changes to match the infant nutritional needs, with protein and mineral concentrations decreasing and lactose, water, and fat increasing in the first week of life.[2]
2. Breastmilk is free of contaminating bacteria.[34]

3. Breastmilk decreases allergy to and intolerance of cow's milk.
4. Breastmilk provides immunologic protection while the baby's immune system is developing. Infant secretory immunoglobulin A (IgA) is not established for 1 year; the full antibody repertoire is not established until 2 years.[46] Bacterial and viral antibodies and IgA antibodies make bacteria unable to adhere to the walls of the intestine. Breastmilk passes on protection for those diseases to which the mother is immune. It inhibits and kills harmful bacteria, decreasing gastrointestinal (GI) disturbances.[34] The child who is fully breastfed receives the most protection; a child being given formula for more than half of his or her feedings does not receive protection against illness.[39]
5. Breastmilk decreases the incidence of colic, otitis media, pneumonia, bacteremia, meningitis,[34] respiratory infections, asthma, urinary tract infections (UTIs), atopic eczema, necrotizing enterocolitis (in the preterm infant), Crohn's disease, insulin-dependent diabetes, and lymphoma.[46]
6. Breastfed babies have been noted to be more mature, secure, assertive, and more advanced developmentally and to develop visual acuity earlier.[26]

Advantages of Breastfeeding for the Mother

1. Breastfeeding causes quicker involution of the uterus.[34]
2. Breastfeeding is protective against ovarian cancer.[6]
3. The risk of premenopausal breast cancer is decreased, especially if the first lactation is before age 20 years and lasts for at least 6 months.[5]
4. The risk of osteoporosis is measurably less for women who have been pregnant and nursed their babies. Even though some bone loss occurs during lactation, it quickly returns to normal and sometimes exceeds baseline after lactation when calcium absorption, parathyroid hormone, and serum calcitriol markedly increase.[6]
5. The delay in ovulation favors spacing of children.
6. The secretion of prolactin increases relaxation and prolactin and oxytocin promote attachment.[31]
7. Ruth Lawrence,[26] physician breastfeeding expert, further states that breastfeeding "empowers a woman to do something special for her infant. The relationship of a mother with her suckling infant is considered to be the strongest of human bonds. Holding the infant to the mother's breast to provide total nutrition and nurturing creates an even more profound and psychological experience than carrying the fetus in utero."
8. Approximately $1000/yr is saved when the mother breastfeeds.[6]
9. Eliminating formula cans, bottles, and bottle liners is an ecologic advantage.[2]

Composition of Breastmilk

Colostrum may be expressed from the breasts from 12 weeks' gestation.[58] Deep lemon in color, its specific gravity is 1.040 to 1.060 as opposed to mature milk, which averages 1.030. The total amount of colostrum secreted a day is 10 to 40 mL. It contains valuable immunologic factors.[34] The mature milk comes in on the third or fourth postpartum day and is completely present at approximately 15 days. It is 90% water, and the baby does not require supplemental water for hydration.[58]

The baby is born with iron stores for 6 months. Human milk iron is well absorbed by the baby. Bioavailability of iron in human milk is 50% (7% in formula, 4% in infant cereals).[46] Iron-fortified cereals may be added when solids are begun.[34] Cholesterol is present in breastmilk regardless of the maternal dietary intake but has been removed from cow's milk formula.[26] Bioavailability of calcium from human milk is 75% (50% in formula). Zinc in human milk is 1% bioavailable (31% in cow's milk formula, 14% in soy-based formula).[46]

Human milk supplies all the water and nutrients necessary except the following:

- Vitamin K (given at birth) (0.5 to 1 mg IM at birth or 0.2 mg PO at birth; 0.2 mg PO at 1 to 2 weeks and 2 mg PO at 4 weeks).
- Vitamin D (if the baby is not exposed to the sun for at least 30 min/wk wearing only a diaper or 2 hours fully dressed).
- Fluoride after 6 months if the maternal water supply is not fluoridated.
- Vitamin B_{12} for babies whose mothers are strict vegetarians (requirement 0.3 to 0.5 µg/d).[46]

Initiation of Breastfeeding

When the unmedicated newborn is placed directly onto the mother's breast, it gives a birth cry that lasts from 30 seconds to 7 minutes, opens its eyes, and gradually (within the first hour) moves toward the mother's breast, massages the breast with its hands, finds the nipple, and sucks. The hand massage, skin-to-skin contact and sucking releases oxytocin in the mother, which enables attachment and milk production.[29,40] How the baby attaches to the areola may predict the success of subsequent feedings and the duration of breastfeeding.[23]

The baby should be allowed to empty the breast regularly during the time that colostrum is present. Regular emptying of the breast is the best stimulus for making milk. The infant should be allowed to nurse when hungry, whether or not there appears to be any milk.[34]

Signs of infant readiness to nurse include increased alertness, movements of the arms and legs, turning the head, hand-to-mouth movements and sucking fingers and hands, rooting, tonguing, smacking the lips, early sounds of discomfort, sometimes accompanied by faster breathing. Crying is the last cue, which may occur after the ideal time to begin nursing the baby. A crying baby may have to be comforted before he or she can nurse. The infant should grasp at least 1 inch of areola around the nipple to properly empty the sinuses of milk, holding the breast with the free hand so that the nipple is well back into the infant's mouth.[33]

Mothers' behaviors in the first 28 to 90 hours after birth are related to breastfeeding duration. Mothers who are more likely to be breastfeeding beyond 6 weeks after birth are far more likely to initiate a feeding when their baby is in a quiet alert state rather than crying or drowsy. Such cues should be pointed out to mothers in the first days to help them master awareness of their baby's needs.[9]

The infant empties each breast at every feeding,[34] and the beginning breast is rotated at every feeding. Neifert[33] suggests that some babies of women with large milk supplies may be more content to nurse on a single side per feeding. Infants should be fed at least q3h during the day and q4h during the night (counting from the beginning of one feeding to the beginning of the next),[34] or 8 to 12 times in a 24-hour period for 10 to 15 minutes per breast. An older baby may become efficient and require less time. Feedings may be clustered before a long stretch of sleep, and one 4- to 5-hour period of sleep per 24 hours is acceptable.[33] The mother replenishes 75% of the milk supply by 2 hours after the last feeding, and the baby should be nursed if he or she indicates the desire.[34] Frequent breastfeeding in the first days increases milk intake, promotes weight gain, lowers the incidence of hyperbilirubinemia, and promotes meconium passage.[33]

Early weight gain is overemphasized. Supplementing the baby to achieve a weight gain undermines breastfeeding. Babies are often sleepy for a few days and on the fourth day will "wake up" and nurse more vigorously. The mother should use both breasts at each feeding to stimulate the milk supply.[34] The AAP suggests that the couple experience two good feedings before being discharged from the hospital.[43]

Engorgement

Riordan and Auerbach[43] differentiate breast fullness from breast engorgement. Breast fullness is nearly universal among breastfeeding women. It occurs when the breastmilk comes in and does not preclude breastfeeding. Breast engorgement, however, occurs during the normally transient period of breast fullness when a delay or restriction of feedings, and possibly overhydration during labor, result in milk stasis. Engorgement is thought to be caused by venous and lymphatic stasis, increased congestion and vascularity, and milk accumulation and stasis. The woman feels heavy and full. The skin is taut, shiny, and red, and the breasts are warm, tender, hard, and vascular. Although some mothers experience only slight symptoms, other mothers experience multiple peaks of very firm, tender breasts for 2 to 14 days.[48] Engorgement may be accompanied by fever. The woman may experience brachial-plexus edema with numbness and tingling of the hands. In this circumstance, the baby may have difficulty latching. Engorgement and milk stasis are risk factors for mastitis. Further, back pressure on the alveoli causes a buildup of peptides that decrease milk production.[43]

m *Management*

Teach the mother:

1. Empty the breasts **early and frequently** (q2-3h).[48]
2. Use **massage** and **warm** showers, warm compresses, or immersion of the breasts in a basin of tepid water to reduce discomfort and stimulate milk flow at the next feeding.[43]
3. **Avoid supplementing,** which contributes to engorgement.[43]
4. Allow the **first breast to be completely emptied.**[43]
5. Be certain that the baby's **position** is correct for properly emptying the breast.[24]
6. **Express a small amount** of milk before latching to soften the area just behind the areola, enabling the baby to latch.[6] If a **nipple shield** helps a baby latch, hold, and effectively empty the breast, it may be helpful.[43] (See nipple shield discussion p. 310.)
7. Use **cold packs** for relief.[48]
8. Room temperature or cold, wet, or dry **cabbage leaves** have been found to give relief. Change when they become limp or wet.*
9. **Complementary measures for engorgement:**
   a. **Miscellaneous:** A grated **raw potato or carrot** poultice will draw heat out of the breast.[50] Although less dramatic than cabbage leaves, **geranium** leaves may also be used.[54] Maternal ingestion of **garlic** increases the infant's suckling, improves emptying of the breast, and reduces engorgement.[50]
   b. **Chinese medicine:** To relieve engorgement or to enhance relaxation enabling letdown, the following **acupressure** technique is suggested. The mother sits in a chair, and someone stands behind her and briskly rubs her back from the base of the neck to the bottom of her shoulder blades and along either side of the spine with the knuckles, stimulating the Bladder meridian.[43] **Acupuncture** may also be used to treat engorgement.[10] **See information on Chinese medicine, p. 559.**
   c. **Herbs:** Immerse the breast into a tea made of **marshmallow root;** apply on a poultice or use for massage.[36,37,50]

Promotion of Latching-on

- Suggest that the mother begin feedings with early signs of interest in the baby rather than waiting for crying when the baby is more frantic and less able to focus. The mother should soothe and **comfort the upset baby before attempting** latch-on.[33]

---

*References 6, 35, 40, 48, 50, 54.

- Encourage kangaroo-style **skin-to-skin contact** between feedings. A diaper-clad infant lies upright between or on one breast underneath the mother's clothes. Oxytocin is released, let-down is triggered, the milk supply is stabilized sooner; infants maintain their temperature, maternal anxiety is decreased, and mothers experience less engorgement and earlier mastery of breastfeeding. Maternal-infant attachment is also promoted.[31]
- **Express drops of colostrum** onto the nipple or drip glucose water or formula from a bottle onto the nipple to peak infant interest in latching-on.
- Use a breastpump to **draw out a flat nipple** and to initiate milk flow.
- Place a **silicone nipple** over the mother's nipple to get the resistant infant to begin sucking.[33] (See nipple shield discussion, p. 310.)

Signs that latch-on is correct include:
- Swallows are audible; sucks and swallows are rhythmic with short pauses
- Baby's extremities relax during feeding
- Baby's mouth is moist after feeding
- Mother is thirsty and drowsy and experiences uterine contractions during feeding
- After nursing, breasts are soft and nipples are elongated but not abraded.[48]

Letdown Reflex

The letdown reflex is generally well conditioned by 2 to 3 weeks, triggering the milk ejection reflex. The baby's suckling, or just the sight, sound, or smell of the baby may initiate letdown. The mother experiences letdown as a burning, pins-and-needles, stinging, and/or tingling sensation. It may be inhibited by alcohol, fear, anxiety, sore nipples, or embarrassment.[33]

Teach the mother the following measures to facilitate letdown:
- **Minimize stress**.[33]
- Allow breastfeeding to become **routine.** Do not hurry. Take a snack or drink with or before feedings. Nurse in the same place, play soothing music, lie down for a few minutes before and possibly during the feeding. Minimize distractions.[24]
- Perform **relaxation** exercises with deep breathing and visualizations of the milk flowing.[24]
- Use **warmth** to enhance letdown before feeding.[33]

Medical Interventions

Metoclopramide (Reglan) may be given to the mother for several days to facilitate the letdown reflex without adverse affects, although long-term administration may cause maternal depression.[43] **Oxytocin** nasal spray (Syntocinon, one spray in each nostril 2 minutes before nursing) may be used to stimulate the letdown. **Pregnancy is a contraindication.**

Headache is the major side effect. It may be used for several days and then discontinued.[5]

Sore Nipples

Transient soreness may occur during the first week after birth regardless of maternal hair color, skin color, or prenatal nipple preparation. Soreness lasting beyond the first week is abnormal and may be due to tongue-tie, impetigo, eczema, flat or retracted nipples, disorganized suckling, herpes simplex virus, improper infant positioning, breaking of the suction, excessive use of breastpump, nipple shields, moisture of the nipple, sensitivity to a substance used on the nipple, thrush, severe engorgement, the presence of *Staphylococcus aureus,* or unrelieved negative pressure.[43] Severe micrognathia, a high-arched palate, hypertonicity, tongue thrusting, and tongue sucking may also cause sore nipples.[33]

Restricting time at the breast is not indicated because it only delays the soreness, prevents the baby from getting the hindmilk, and may cause trauma by removing the infant from the breast.[43] Sore nipples can cause a reduction of the milk supply because an incorrect latch may not adequately stimulate the nerve endings under the areola that signal the central nervous system's hormone release, because incomplete emptying of the ducts causes decreased milk production, and because the woman with sore nipples may skip, postpone, or limit nursing.[33]

ⓜ Management

1. **Check positioning.** The mother should hold the baby close, with its chin pointing straight between its shoulders. The whole areola, or at least one inch of areola around the nipple, is in its mouth.[33] Supporting the breast with the other hand, even in small-breasted women, prevents the breast and nipple from slipping from gravity into a less desirable position.[6]
2. **Check the latch.** The tongue cradles the nipple, pressing it to the palate. Nothing is touching the tip of the nipple. If the mother feels the tongue thrusting or pressing on the end of the nipple, the mother or a helper can teach the baby to suck with a gloved finger pad side up. Turn the finger, then gently push the tongue down while moving the finger slowly out of the baby's mouth.[6]
3. **Teach the mother** the following measures:
   a. Stimulate the baby (by stroking the cheek or lips) to **open the mouth widely,** with the tongue extended over the lower gum line. At this time the mother inserts the breast, and the baby should latch on with 1 to 1.5 inches of areola around the nipple in the mouth.[6]
   b. Break the **suction** before removing the baby from the breast. Inserting the little finger (with a trimmed fingernail) into the gap at the back of the jaw, push the lower jaw down and break the suction.[34]

c. **Vary the position** for nursing (football hold, cradle position, and lying down stomach to stomach with the baby), rotating the spot on the nipple where the jaw takes hold.[34]

d. After nursing, **apply expressed milk** to the nipple—its bacteriostatic properties and oils are healing to the skin of the nipple.[6]

e. **Dry nipples** completely after feedings, using a hair dryer if desired.[34] Excessive dryness, however, may cause cracking.[33] Alternatively, keep nipples open to air for 15 to 30 minutes after each feeding. Avoid using plasticized breastpads, which keep moisture trapped next to the nipple. Change nonplasticized breastpads frequently to keep the nipples dry.[34] Tea strainers can be used inside the bra to keep moist fabrics off the nipples.

f. Before latching, apply an **ice cube** wrapped in a paper towel to the nipple for 5 seconds for its numbing affect and to bring out a flat nipple.[61]

g. Use **no soap** or other drying solutions on the nipples.

h. **Avoid plastic nipple shields if possible,** but they may be necessary as a transition tool.[34] (See discussion about nipple shields, p. 310.)

i. If the nipple is scabbing, **leave scabs alone.**

j. **Nurse more often** so that the baby isn't nursing as vigorously.[33]

k. **Enhance letdown** before feeding by starting feedings on the less sore nipple or by applying heat.

l. Apply **warm water compresses** after each feeding. The only means shown to improve nipple healing are warm water and pure lanolin in later weeks. Anything applied to the nipple must be safe for the infant or must be removed before feedings. Anything applied only to be removed may be worse than nothing at all.[43]

m. Apply pure **lanolin** to the nipples if desired,[33] although this remedy has not been proven useful in early weeks in clinical trials.[43]

n. Expose nipples to **fresh air and sunlight** for 20 minutes a day (sunshine through a window is adequate).[44]

o. A cool raw **cabbage leaf** worn inside the bra may help the nipples heal.[6]

p. **Breast shells** may be used to hold clothing away from sore nipples.[33]

q. A **milk blister** appears to be a blister on the tip of the nipple. It is a plugged nipple pore covered by epidermis. Treatment is a warm compress followed by immediately putting the baby to the breast. Sterile needle aspiration may be necessary if this does not work. Once open, ice packs, analgesics, breast shields, and a thin layer of antibiotic ointment will facilitate comfort and healing.[52]

r. **Consider time off:** If nursing is too painful or if bleeding and erosion are worsening, the mother may rest for 24 hours, expressing or pumping milk, and resuming slowly. Meanwhile, feed the baby by dropper, spoon, or cup.[43] Alternatively, Nelson[34] suggests pumping the breasts often, giving the colostrum or milk to the baby by bottle, and offering the breast 1 or 2 times a day when the mother is relaxed. Other authorities suggest that nipple confusion may result from this approach.[43]

4. The midwife may **consider antibiotics:** A thin layer of topical antibiotics and possibly low-dose steroid ointment for inflammation may be beneficial because *S. aureus* has been found to be present on sore nipples. The preparations are not harmful to the infant.[43] When moderate to severe discomfort, cracks, fissures, deep ulcers, or exudates are present, systemic antibiotics may speed healing as well as prevent mastitis.[33]

5. **Complementary measures for sore nipples:**
   a. Some experts recommend **homeopathic** measures for sore nipples.[12,45,47]
   b. **Herbs:** Herbalists suggest applying herbs and washing them off thoroughly before the next nursing. **Aloe vera gel,[44,50,61] calendula ointment,[44,54,61] and comfrey root ointment**[17,50,61] are suggested for use in this way. The thorough removal required when using an ointment or salve, however, may cause tissue damage. The use of infusions in a wash or a warm poultice, followed by exposure to the sun, followed by a bath or shower to cleanse the nipples before nursing may be more appropriate. **See information on herbs, p. 563.**

Candida Infection of the Nursing Couple

Candidiasis may be transmitted from mother to infant during childbirth, by care providers, or by equipment from infected infants. Candidiasis may follow antibiotic administration or may occur with immunosuppression.[34] Oral candidiasis, or **thrush,** is diagnosed when white, cheesy, curd-like plaques are identified on the buccal mucosa and the tongue. The patches can be scraped off, leaving the underlying skin raw and friable.[21] Discomfort may hinder feedings.[34] The infant may also have a *Candida* diaper rash (see p. 286).[6] The mother describes intense burning or shooting pains throughout the feeding, burning persisting between feedings for some, and itching for others. Nipples may appear normal, bright pink, or red and shiny. Small amounts of white material may accumulate in the folds. A yeasty odor may be noted on the breastpad. The mother may also have a vaginal monilial infection. There may be a recent history of antibiotics. No lab finding is reliable—the diagnosis is made on the basis of signs and symptoms.[6]

Ⓜ Management

1. Teach the mother to **keep the nipples dry.**[44]
2. The nipples may be bathed in 1 cup water containing 1 Tblsp **vinegar**, and then air dried q4h. The mixture may also be swabbed into the baby's mouth.[6]

3. **Hygienic measures:** Stress careful handwashing. Bras and all other clothing and fabric (e.g., washcloths, towels) are washed and thoroughly rinsed daily, as well as equipment, such as nipple shields, that contacts the breasts.[6] **Nipple shields may aggravate** a *Candida* infection.[44] A **pacifier** may also harbor *Monilia*.[3]

4. **Dietary measures:** Advise the woman to decrease dairy products, heavily sweetened foods, and artificial foods, which predispose her to *Candida* while she is healing from the infection.[52]

5. **Medical interventions:**
   a. **Antifungal medication:** Prescribe nystatin cream (Mycostatin, Nilstat, or Nystex) 1 million U qid applied locally.[34] Alternatives include Lotrimin or Mycelex bid-tid, miconazole 2% (Monistat-Derm or Micatin) bid-qid, or Nizoral cream 2% qd-bid. The creams are applied after rinsing nipples in warm water and allowing them to air dry. Oral Diflucan has been prescribed for recalcitrant cases without toxic effects noted in infants.[6]
   b. An **anti-inflammatory** cream combined with the anti-fungal treatment, such as Mycolog, may also provide comfort. A thin layer applied after nursing doesn't need to be washed off before the baby nurses again and has shown no ill effect on babies.[6]

6. Treat the **baby for thrush.** Prescribe Nystatin suspension 100,000 U/mL, 1mL to each side of mouth qid until 3 days after resolution of symptoms.[34] One to 2 weeks may be required for symptoms to disappear. A second course may be required.[6]

7. **Complementary measures:**
   a. Some experts recommend **homeopathy** measures for sore nipples.[13,45,57]
   b. A yeast infection of the nipples can be treated with unsweetened **yogurt** with active cultures applied to the nipples and nursed off the finger by the baby. The inside of the baby's mouth can also be "painted" with yogurt.[44,57]
   c. **Nutritional measures: Niacinamide**, a B vitamin, may help the baby with thrush. The mother takes 100 mg qd to supplement the baby.[53]

Inverted Nipples

The shape of the nipple "at rest" does not necessarily correspond with the shape of the nipple in the breastfeeding mouth. Inverted nipples may, however, make latching-on more difficult. Exercises and breast shells once prescribed have been shown to be ineffective.[43] Some inverted nipples spontaneously evert by the third trimester.[5] Exercising the nipple just before latching on seems to loosen nipple tissue and adhesions. A breastpump may be used, or the nipple may be manually stimulated and shaped. A cold cloth may be applied to cause an erectile response.[43] An ice cube wrapped in a paper towel may be applied to the nipple before the latch to help evert the nipple and provide comfort with the latch.[61]

The woman with an inverted nipple should place her thumb 1.5 to 2 inches behind the nipple while pushing back into the breast, assisting the baby to latch. This technique works best in a side-lying position. The infant's sucking also loosens adhesions.[43]

Nipple Shields

The nipple shield, a soft plastic disk shaped like a nipple and areola, can be placed over the nipple before the latch to assist the baby in latching or to protect tender nipple tissue. Use of the shield is associated with reduced milk transfer during feedings, but some lactation experts do use the device to bridge to effective breastfeeding. Indications include inverted nipples and very sore nipples. After nursing with a nipple shield, residual milk is pumped out, using the expressed milk for supplementation if necessary.[33]

Nipple Confusion

Sucking on an artificial nipple involves moving the tongue up to occlude the hole in the teat, releasing as much milk as the baby can swallow at a time. When latching onto the breast, the infant's tongue must be down, the nipple lying on top of it, and the baby must suck vigorously. The actions required of the baby are very different, and the breast requires more work on the part of the infant. Infants who have been given a bottle before breastfeeding is firmly established may develop a preference for the artificial nipple. Earlier supplementation with formula is associated with latching difficulties and shorter duration of breastfeeding.[33]

Pacifier Use and Breastfeeding

Pacifier use causes a faulty sucking technique and is frequently associated with breastfeeding problems.[42] The AAP[1] recommends that pacifiers not be used for breastfeeding babies. Auerbach[3] notes that using a pacifier to quiet a fussy baby does not provide fluids or calories to the baby, or stimulate the mother's breasts. Although pacifier use is associated with a shorter duration of breastfeeding, it is much less likely to affect infants whose mothers are confident about nursing.[59]

Adequacy of the Milk Supply

Most women are capable of producing more milk than their baby requires. Some infants will nurse for smaller amounts more frequently; others nurse for larger amounts less frequently, depending on infant preference and/or breast storage. Irregular or incomplete milk removal is the cause of most milk insufficiency problems. The position of the latch is important to the milk supply because the areola, when properly stimulated, causes release of the prolactin from the pituitary, which ensures an adequate milk supply.[33] In addition to a history of breast surgery (see p. 322), a major stress, postpartum hemorrhage (see Sheehan's syndrome, p. 485), anemia, or smoking cigarettes may reduce the milk supply.[43] Ergot preparations, pyridoxine, or diuretics will diminish the supply. Retained products of conception may inhibit pro-lactin secretion.[16] Box 6-1 lists the signs that the milk supply is adequate.

ⓜ Management

1. If the baby appears to be receiving adequate milk, **reassure** the mother, **educating** her about the expected frequency and length of feedings.
2. The infant who has a 7% weight loss should be carefully assessed. If a **10% weight loss** occurs, **supplementation** is used to rehydrate the baby.[43]
3. Infant milk consumption can best be measured by **weighing the infants before and after feedings.**[33] If the baby appears not to be receiving adequate milk, **increase the frequency** of feedings to q2-3h around the clock as well as on demand.[26] Neifert[33] suggests using a hospital-grade electric pump and pumping after every feeding to stimulate milk production. **See the baby again** in 2 days. The

---

• *Box 6-1 / Signs That the Milk Supply Is Adequate* •

- The baby is satisfied at the end of the feeding.[34]
- The baby is comfortable after a feeding for 2-4 hr, waking easily or awakening spontaneously after this period.[48]
- The baby gains weight appropriately.[34] An initial 10% weight loss is acceptable though unusual for the infant receiving adequate milk. Once the milk comes in, weight loss reverses and gain is seen by 4-5 days.[33] An infant regains its birth weight no later than 2 wk after birth, thereafter gaining at least 4-7 oz/wk or 1 lb/mo.[43] Breastfed infants grow as well as or faster than other babies for the first 2 mo, then less rapidly from 3-12 mo.[33] Nelson[34] stresses that the failure to gain must be measured over time and not measured daily or after feedings.
- In the first 2 days, infants may void only 1-2 times. After the milk is fully in (by day 4), most infants void colorless, dilute urine after most feedings a minimum of 6-8 times daily. Urate crystals ("brick dust") may be seen in the first 2-3 days but should not be seen once the milk is in.[48]
- The baby is having bowel movements.[43] By 5 days, when the milk comes in, infant stools are mustard in color, the consistency of yogurt with seedy curds. By 2-3 mo, it is not uncommon for a breastfed infant to go days or a week between stools.[33]
- The baby's mucous membranes are moist and skin turgor is good.[43]
- The milk progresses from scant, yellowish colostrum to copious, thin, bluish milk.[33]
- Breasts soften as the baby feeds.[48]
- Mother experiences hormonal signals such as drowsiness, thirst, and uterine contractions when the baby feeds.[48]

baby should have gained 2 oz in those 2 days and should catch up in its growth thereafter. If it doesn't, or if the baby appears dehydrated, initiate **supplementation** and involve a **lactation consultant.**[5]

4. The **LactAid system** in which a pliable plastic tube is taped next to the nipple and formula slowly dispensed as the baby sucks on the nipple, may be used.[5]

5. **Complementary measures for enhancement of the milk supply:**

   a. **Nutritional suggestions:** Foods that are said to increase the milk supply include oats,[44,50] beets, winter squash, almonds, avocados, brown rice, sea vegetables, thick grain-based soups and porridges,[44] leafy greens, barley, carrots (especially carrot juice),[44,61] apricots, asparagus, green beans, sweet potatoes, peas, and pecans.[61] Page[36] suggests Brewers' yeast intake (rich in B vitamins).

   b. **Reflexology:** Inadequate lactation may be enhanced by stimulation to the mammary gland regions on the top of the foot.[55] **See charts and information on reflexology, p. 567.**

   c. **Chinese medicine: Acupuncture** may be used to treat insufficient lactation.[10] A qualified **shiatsu** therapist will concentrate on the **stomach, spleen and kidney meridians** to increase the milk supply.[22] **See charts and information on Chinese medicine, p. 559.**

   d. **Herbs:** Riordan and Auerbach[43] suggest that all herbs be taken in small amounts. Avoid parsley and sage, which are recommended to decrease lactation. **Blessed thistle** leaves are the most widely suggested remedy to enhance lactation.* One hundred to 200 mg capsules can be taken qd-tid[30] or 200 to 400 mg of 70% silymarin (active component) tid.[56] **Fennel,**† **borage** leaves,[19,28,44,61] **red raspberry** leaves,[28,36,43,44,53] **marshmallow** root,[36,44,53] and **fenugreek**‡ are widely recommended. **Hops**[25,44,50,61] promotes the milk supply by relaxing the mother. Weed[61] suggests rotating through these herbs. **See information on herbs, p. 563.**

Growth Spurts

Many mothers will say that they gave up breastfeeding because they "did not have enough milk." Education about growth spurts may prevent some of these women from discontinuing nursing. At approximately 5 or 6 weeks, 3 months, and 6 months, growth spurts will occur. When the baby's weight has exceeded the threshold for the current milk supply, the baby will want to eat at more frequent intervals. Increased stimulation of the nerve centers under the areola stimulate more prolactin to be released from the anterior pituitary, and milk production increases over

---

*References 4, 17, 18, 25, 28, 30, 44, 50, 53, 56, 61.
†References 18, 25, 28, 35, 43, 44, 50, 54, 61.
‡References 17, 18, 25, 28, 35, 43, 50.

the next 24 to 48 hours. To meet the increased demand, the mother should nurse frequently and for as long as the baby desires. When the supply catches up, the baby will return approximately to its pre-growth spurt nursing frequency. If the problem persists longer than 3 to 4 days, evaluate breastfeeding adequacy.[33]

Nutrition During Lactation

Lawrence[26] states that a woman will produce adequate milk for her infant even if her diet is imperfect. Nutrition counseling is actually based on the need to replenish maternal stores. Caloric demand usually peaks at 6 months because most infants are eating additional foods after this time. The woman who is lactating should never eat less than 1800 kcal/d. Approximate breastmilk volume per day is 750 to 800 mL. Breastmilk volume does not vary with maternal weight, height, body mass index (BMI), dietary supplements, or additional fluids.[41]

Breastmilk contains approximately 20 kcal/oz regardless of maternal diet or other variables. Maternal stores are used if necessary. The fat content of the milk is similar from woman to woman and does not depend on the maternal diet, but it does vary from breast to breast, from the beginning to the end of a feeding, between feedings, and from one month to the next of lactation. Vitamin content of the milk varies with maternal diet, and fat-soluble vitamins may be taken from maternal stores. Calcium, zinc, and magnesium are maintained at a consistent level in the breastmilk at maternal expense, if necessary. The mother ideally takes in 1500 mg calcium/d. Fatty acid concentration is influenced by the maternal diet, and fatty acids are essential for brain and nerve development.[41] Vitamins A, B_{12}, and folic acid are also reduced in the breastmilk of women with poor dietary intake.[49]

The breastfeeding **vegan** mother (the vegetarian who does not eat milk or eggs) must take vitamin B_{12} to prevent methylmalonic acidemia in her infant. Vegetarian infants may not grow as quickly as their omnivore friends in their first 2 years.[34]

Dieting and Breastfeeding

Whether breastfeeding enhances postpartum weight loss is controversial.[51] Lawrence[26] states that breastfeeding women do return to their prepregnancy state sooner, and are, furthermore, at less risk to be obese in later life. Still other authors state that 80% of lactating women lose weight after birth, some beginning as early as 15 days after birth. Most lose 1 to 2 lb/mo. Women who breastfeed for 1 year lose more weight during the second 6 months than they do in the first 6 months. The woman who breastfeeds frequently will lose more weight.[41]

Women who want to lose weight should not attempt to lose more than 4 lb/mo through dieting alone because this requires the caloric intake to be too low. Up to 2 lb weight loss/mo through a combination of diet and exercise does not adversely affect lactation. Prolactin secretion increases when the energy spent exceeds the energy consumed to increase milk production.[41] The infants of women who lost 0.5 kg/wk through diet and exercise do not differ from the infants of nondieting, nonexercising mothers in weight and length.[27] Aerobic exercise does not affect the quantity or composition of breastmilk.[41] Women who increase their physical activity do not lose weight unless they also restrict their calories.[51]

Foods to Avoid During Lactation

Foods that may cause gastric distress and loose stools in the breastfeeding infant include cabbage, onions, tomatoes, some berries, chocolate, spices, and condiments. No food need be withheld, however, until the baby has had difficulty with it.[46] Foods that make the mother gassy will not necessarily make the baby gassy. Slusser and Powers[46] state that a breastfeeding mother is commonly advised to give up dairy products if the baby is fussy, when the problem is actually an inadequate latch, inadequate frequency and length of feedings, or a low milk supply. An offending food usually causes a reaction 4 to 24 hours after the mother has ingested it.[53]

Maternal Intake of Substances During Lactation

Cigarettes

Cigarette smoking should be discouraged in the nursing mother.[34] However, the infant who is exposed to secondhand smoke will experience upper respiratory infections and otitis more often, and breastfeeding provides some protection from these. Breastfeeding is also protective against the increased risk for sudden infant death syndrome among the infants exposed to secondhand smoke. Nicotine is absorbed in greater doses from the respiratory tract than from breastfeeding. Whether or not the mother stops smoking, therefore, it is beneficial for her to breastfeed. Smoking does lower the breastmilk volume because it depresses prolactin and oxytocin levels. Women who smoke tend to wean earlier.[60] Teach mothers not to smoke in the same room with the infant and to abstain from smoking for 2 hours before breastfeeding.[26] Nicotine is delivered in the breastmilk in a dose-related manner. Reports of irritability, restlessness, diarrhea, and tachycardia in breastfed babies of heavy smokers are rare.[11]

Alcohol

Alcohol use is discouraged.[34] Alcohol diminishes the ejection letdown reflex. It changes the flavor of the milk. Alcohol levels in the maternal serum and the breastmilk are equal. Up to one mixed drink, 8 oz wine, or two beers daily have not been shown to be detrimental to the infant.[41] The metabolite of alcohol that is believed to be the major cause of alcohol toxicity is acetaldehyde, and this substance does not appear in breastmilk. Infants whose breastfeeding mothers drink heavily have been shown to have gross motor delay at 1 year, although whether this reflects the alcohol intake during pregnancy or lactation is unknown.[26]

Caffeine

Caffeine is excreted into breastmilk in small amounts. Drinking 1 to 2 caffeine-containing beverages a day is not associated with a problem.[26] About 1% of the maternal dose goes to the baby.[46] Studies have shown that coffee does not alter the heart rate or sleep pattern of the term neonate. Preterm neonates, however, clear caffeine more slowly.[43]

Addition of Solid Foods

Withholding solid foods for the first 6 months of life diminishes the occurrence of atopic disease (allergic asthma, allergic rhinitis, atopic dermatitis, food allergies) in children who are at hereditary risk.[43] Solids can be swallowed when the extrusion reflex disappears at 4 to 5 months. When the mother decides to initiate solids, she may start with cereals and then add fruits. As less breastmilk is demanded, the milk supply will gradually diminish.[24] A common belief is that the addition of solids to an infant's diet will lengthen the night's sleep. This has never been shown in a study, and in fact an Australian study showed that 50% of infants 1 year of age did not sleep through the night.[46]

Breastfeeding "Strikes"

The infant may suddenly refuse to nurse rather than gradually so, as in self-weaning. Reasons that have been offered for such a "strike" include a change in the routine (such as mother leaving the house to work), leaving the baby with a bottle (even a bottle of breastmilk), a rebuke of the baby for having bitten the breast, or a separation from the baby for several days.[43] Alternately, the baby may be too hungry at the beginning of feedings and become impatient with the nursing; the mother may be eating a new food that the baby dislikes in the milk; the mother may be undergoing stress or tension; or the baby may be teething.

m *Management*

Offer the following suggestions to the mother[43]:
- Address the discomfort of **teething** (see p. 289).
- For the impatient baby, try **beginning feedings before the baby is very hungry.**
- During a strike, **do not give a bottle** if you do not wish to relinquish nursing. Breastmilk can be expressed and given from a cup, a feeding-tube device on the finger, or by allowing the baby to suck on a dropper, and solids can be increased.
- **Carry and hold the baby more** during this period.
- **Offering the breast when the baby is just falling to sleep or just waking up** may be successful.

Weaning

Ideally, weaning occurs when both mother and child are ready. Most infants in the United States are weaned within the first year of life. Child-led weaning usually occurs in the second or third years.[43] When the mother decides to initiate solids, less breastmilk is demanded and the milk supply will gradually diminish.[34] Page[36] suggests a rice drink to assist in weaning the infant from breastmilk. If weaning is sudden, see p. 229 for measures to decrease milk production in nonlactating breasts.

Variations in Breastfeeding Methods

Feeding on One Breast

Adequate nutrition can be given from one breast. Volume from one breast tends to be diminished; however, the milk tends to be creamier and will supply about 90% of the calories provided by a two-breast feeding.[43]

Working While Breastfeeding

Although returning to work is considered a barrier to breastfeeding by many, studies have shown that mothers who work continue to breastfeed as long as mothers who stay at home. Moreover, mothers who return to work and continue to breastfeed have 30% less absenteeism for infant illness than do mothers who are not breastfeeding.[46]

The following suggestions may facilitate breastfeeding for the working mother. Firmly establish breastfeeding in the first 4 to 6 weeks after delivery. If possible, extend the maternity leave. Once breastfeeding is established, begin to express milk and store it in the freezer to start a supply of frozen milk and to increase the maternal milk supply. When possible, work part-time or take the baby to work. When possible, use on-site childcare or childcare close to work, and feed the baby on breaks or have someone bring the baby to you for feedings. Express milk at work and leave it with the provider for the next day's feedings. Breastfeed full-time on days off. Feed more often at night and less frequently during the day. If pumping at work is impossible, pump at home after feedings. If expressing cannot be done, breastfeed when you can.[46]

Pumping the Breasts and Breastmilk Storage

After breastfeeding is established, the mother may wish to pump her breasts to store milk for use when she will be unavailable to feed the baby.[34] Cleanliness of the breast, hands, and equipment is important to prevent bacterial contamination. Hand pumps, battery-operated pumps, and electric pumps are available.[43] See Box 6-2 for those characteristics that are desirable in a breastpump.

FREQUENCY OF PUMPING. When the mother must pump full-time because of separation, illness, or prematurity of the baby, her regimen should include at least 8 pumpings in each 24-hour period.[43]

> • *Box 6-2 /* **Desirable Breastpump Characteristics** •
>
> - Flange that covers most of the areola.
> - Closely simulates a baby's suckling.
> - For the mother of an ill or premature baby, a pump that minimizes contamination by pathogens (all parts that contact the milk being dishwasher-safe with fewer, simpler parts that are easy to clean). Motorized pumps must have a trap to prevent milk from entering the motor. If milk enters the motor, the pump is returned to the manufacturer to be disassembled and sterilized. Sterilize parts for the compromised infant (immerse in boiling water for 10 min).
> - Cylinder and handle pumps are lightweight, portable, and inexpensive. They are ideal for occasional use. They are not the most ideal in simulating the baby's suckling and stimulating milk production, however; when this is a concern, an automated pump should be considered.
> - Automated pumps that give the greatest number of cycles per minute (>40 cycles/min) are the best at maintaining lactation, the most efficient at removing the hindmilk, high in fat, especially critical for LBW babies. Bilateral expression is more efficient in terms of time and volume and most effectively elevates prolactin. These pumps can be rented.
> - Medela's Pump-in-Style or Hollister's Purely Yours sell for less than $300, are lightweight, have car adaptors, include carrier cases with freezer packs for chilling and storing the milk, and run at >40 cycles/min. These pumps are for use for one infant only and are not for use with LBW babies where removing the hindmilk is especially important.
>
> Data from Biancuzzo M: Selecting pumps for breastfeeding mothers, *J Obstet Gynecol Neonatal* 28:416-426, 1997.

MEASURES TO TEACH THE MOTHER TO MINIMIZE SORE NIPPLES WHILE PUMPING

1. Use the smallest effective amount of suction. Use a well-fitting flange.
2. Begin letdown before beginning the vacuum of the pump. Facilitate letdown as discussed on p. 305. Timing may be helpful, such as pumping halfway between feedings instead of just after. What works early in the course of the pumping may not work after pumping for awhile.
3. Pause during pumping or pump for shorter periods more often.[43]

STORAGE OF BREASTMILK. Storage of milk must take into consideration bacterial growth and stability of the digestive enzymes. Guidelines for preterm babies are more stringent. Preterm milk is not as strongly antibacterial as is mature milk.[43]

- At 100° F, human milk is safely stored for <4 hours.
- Preterm milk is not stored at room temperature for >1 hour.
- At 77° F, the milk is safe for 4 hours.
- At 59° F (the temperature in a cooler with an ice pack), the milk is safe for 24 hours.

- Discard milk remaining unrefrigerated longer than 24 hours.[43]
- Breastmilk is stored safely in the refrigerator for 48 hours.[2]
- Breastmilk is stored safely in the deep freeze for up to 1 month.[34] Freeze as soon as possible after pumping, date, and use in chronologic order.
- Do not add fresh milk to already frozen milk.[43]
- Do not refreeze milk.[43]
- To thaw frozen milk, warm it slowly. Microwaving and other rapid warming adversely affects immunologic and nutritional properties of the milk.[43] Place it under running water or let it defrost in the refrigerator.[2] Any cream standing on the top is shaken into the milk.[43]
- Once thawed, milk can be kept in the refrigerator for 24 hours.[2]
- Giving fresh or refrigerated milk to the baby, as opposed to frozen milk, preserves its antibacterial properties.[43]

Breastfeeding in Special Circumstances

For breastfeeding and hyperbilirubinemia, see p. 276.

Breastfeeding and the Preterm Infant

Infants who are low birth weight (LBW) (<2000 g or 4½ lb) may have such fast growth rates that human milk alone is insufficient.[34] The World Health Organization (WHO) recommends fortification of human milk for the premature infant weighing <1500 g at birth or born before 32 weeks' gestation. Fortification supplies protein, calcium, phosphorus, and possibly zinc, copper, iron, and some vitamins that are not sufficient in breastmilk to meet the intrauterine requirement of these babies.[46]

The milk that a mother who has delivered prematurely produces is especially suited to the needs of the premature infant. The milk has higher concentrations of IgA, lactoferrin and other anti-infective properties; protein, fat, sodium, iron, and chloride; taurine for vitamin D absorption; and antioxidants such as beta-carotene and inositol (which decrease the incidence of bronchopulmonary dysplasia and retinopathy of prematurity). The lipids are more appropriate for the preterm infant, maximizing neurologic and visual development and reducing retinopathy. Preterm babies who are fed expressed breastmilk have higher scores on intelligence tests when measured at school age. According to numerous studies, advantages of breastfeeding preterm babies include greater tolerance of the feedings, resistance to infection, reduced risk of necrotizing enterocolitis, enhanced retinal development and visual acuity, enhanced developmental and neurocognitive outcome, and improved physiologic stability.[8]

Fewer preterm mothers breastfeed their infants; they also breastfeed for shorter durations. Maintenance of an adequate milk supply is challenging, and a mother may feel extreme pressure and vulnerability regarding the infant's intake. On the other hand, providing the baby's nurturance by giving breastmilk may be the only natural aspect of the baby's care that is preserved for this mother in the early months of the baby's life. She may feel validated by being the only one who can contribute breastmilk in a situation where her participation is otherwise limited.[43]

Pumping the breasts should begin as quickly as possible after birth. The frequency should equal the approximate frequency that a healthy term infant would nurse—ideally 8 to 12 times in a 24-hour period.[8] Skin-to-skin or kangaroo care improves physiologic stability and enhances breastfeeding in preterm infants. Ideally, at least one feeding a day is performed by pumping at the bedside and giving the fresh milk to the baby to preserve anti-infective qualities.[43]

Breastfeeding and Maternal Infection

Some infections are transferred to the baby in the breastmilk. The breastmilk also contains the mother's immunologic factors as she develops them. The baby may be exposed by routes other than breastmilk when the mother becomes ill. These factors are weighed in regard to the following maternal infections:

1. **Human immunodeficiency virus (HIV)** is present in breastmilk.[34] The longer the infant nurses after 28 days, the higher the risk of contracting HIV. In areas where the water is unsafe, however, the danger of HIV transmission is less than the danger of contracting serious illness from contaminated formula. In industrialized countries, therefore, breastfeeding is contraindicated when the mother is HIV positive. Breastfeeding is recommended, however, in third-world countries.[26]

2. **Cytomegalovirus (CMV)** is present in breastmilk.[43] Fifty percent to 80% of those exposed will become infected, but CMV is tolerated without sequelae by the newborn.[14] Antibodies to CMV are present in the breastmilk, minimizing illness in the newborn who is exposed to the disease anyway by droplet exposure.[26] CMV is not a contraindication to breastfeeding, except for preterm infants,[34] for whom expressed milk of the infected mother should be given only after it has been frozen at 20° C for 7 days.[26]

3. **Hepatitis A (HAV)** does not appear to cause serious illness in the newborn. Breastfeeding is not contraindicated when the mother has HAV. If the maternal infection occurs within 2 weeks of birth, the infant should receive gamma globulin[26] and vaccination.[2]

4. **Hepatitis B (HBV)** virus is present in breastmilk. Five percent to 15% of infants born to HBV-positive mothers are already infected prenatally,[43] and many more are infected during labor and birth.[34] Immunoprophylaxis and vaccination, however, are very protective when initiated at this time. When the baby has received immunoglobulin and vaccination, he or she can breastfeed with little risk unless the mother's nipples are cracked and bleeding.[43] If the

already lactating woman contracts HBV, the baby is given the vaccinations in an accelerated schedule (birth, 1 month, 2 months).[34]

5. **Hepatitis C (HCV)** spreads vertically in <10% of pregnancies, depending on the viral load of the mother. HCV is found in breastmilk, but in small quantities it is easily inactivated by stomach acids and not absorbed through the GI tract. Coinfection with HIV, however, increases the risk that the infant will contract both HCV and HIV. The benefits appear to outweigh the risks and breastfeeding is usually recommended unless the HCV-positive mother is coinfected with HIV.[43]

6. **Herpes (HSV)** may cause serious illness in the early months of life. If the neonate becomes seriously ill with HSV, nursing should cease and acyclovir administered for 1 week before resuming nursing.[43] Lawrence[26] suggests not resuming nursing until all lesions are healed. When the mother has an active lesion, she should practice careful handwashing technique, cover the lesions, and withhold nursing only for lesions near the breast.[43] For lesions on the mother's mouth, she should wear a mask and withhold kissing and nuzzling until they are healed.[26]

7. **Human T-lymphotropic virus (HTLV-1)** causes T-cell leukemia and lymphoma and is endemic in the Caribbean, Japan, and Africa. It is present in breastmilk, and HTLV-1 infection is a contraindication to breastfeeding.[43]

8. The **rubella** virus may be found in breastmilk after maternal immunization or with maternal infection but poses no risk for the infant.[34]

9. **Varicella-zoster (VZ; chicken pox)** does not cross in the breastmilk. Antibodies to the virus are present in the breastmilk, preventing or moderating the illness for the baby.[43] Transmission of VZ occurs by direct contact.[26] The mother who develops VZ while breastfeeding can continue nursing.[43] The mother who contacts VZ shortly before delivery and has not had time to produce antibodies is isolated from the baby. The mother pumps her milk, which is given to the baby. The baby should receive VZ immunoglobulin (VZIG). If the baby becomes ill (occurs within 16 days), he or she can rejoin the mother and breastfeed. Otherwise, the mother can commence breastfeeding the infant who remained well when lesions are crusted over.[2]

10. **Herpes zoster,** or shingles, does not preclude breastfeeding unless the lesions are on the breast. Careful handwashing technique is necessary. The infant should receive varicella zoster immune globulin.[2]

11. **Epstein-Barr virus** does not cause complications during lactation.[26]

12. **Tuberculosis bacilli (TB)** is spread by droplet and inhalation and not by breastmilk. In developed countries, once both mother and baby have begun treatment, breastfeeding can continue with the following precautions. INH, rifampin, and ethambutol may be taken by

the breastfeeding mother, but pyrazinamide and streptomycin should be avoided. The mother should take the drugs just after nursing and substitute a bottle for the next feeding to minimize drugs crossing to the baby. The already-lactating woman who contracts TB (has a positive PPD) is isolated from her baby until the diagnosis is made and treatment is begun. The mother pumps her breasts (giving the milk to the baby) and resumes breastfeeding 1 to 2 weeks into her medications. In underdeveloped countries, breastfeeding is not interrupted and the infant is treated.[26]

13. **Toxoplasmosis** does not contraindicate breastfeeding.[26]
14. **Lyme disease,** a tick-borne infection caused by a spirochete, has been identified in breastmilk. As soon as the diagnosis of Lyme disease is made, the mother should stop breastfeeding. If the infant is healthy, the mother can resume breastfeeding after beginning antibiotic treatment.[26]

Breastfeeding and Medications

PRINCIPLES

1. Most drugs pass into the breastmilk, but usually in small amounts, and the neonatal GI tract only absorbs some of the medication.
2. Very few drugs are contraindicated for breastfeeding women.[43]
3. Most breastmilk is actually produced during the feeding. The timing of a drug dose determines the quantity in the breastmilk. When the infant nurses at peak serum level, the maximum amount of drug will be ingested.[43] Medications relatively contraindicated may sometimes be taken with caution just after a feeding to minimize the baby's absorption.[2]
4. The blood pH, fat concentration of the milk, permeability of cellular and extracellular membranes in the breast, cellular transport mechanisms in the alveoli, drug metabolism by breast tissue, drug pH, molecular weight, half-life, and protein-binding and fat-solubility abilities affect the quantity of the drug in the breastmilk.[43]
5. The baby's age, maturity, personal sensitivity, and frequency and volume of breastfeeding affect the dosage received and its impact on the baby.[43]
6. Herbal products are not necessarily safe, and a poison control center or other information center should be consulted if the mother is using such substances.[26]

RESOURCES. The Physician's Desk Reference (PDR) is not a reliable source regarding the safety of drugs during lactation because the manufacturers are required to state that the drug is not recommended unless they have carried out extensive studies on that issue, although molecule size, pH, protein-binding, and other properties are supplied. Poison control centers may be able to provide information on the safety of drugs during lactation. The Breastfeeding and Human Lactation Study Center, which has a continuously updated computerized database available, can provide information to the health care professional.[26] The AAP Committee on Drugs uses a rating system to indicate the safety of drugs during lactation:

1. Contraindicated
2. Drugs of abuse: contraindicated
3. Radioactive drug requiring temporary cessation of lactation
4. Effect unknown; possibly of concern
5. Associated with significant effects on infants and should be used with caution
6. Usually compatible with lactation
7. Food and environmental agents that have an effect on lactation.[26]

Riordan and Auerbach,[43] ACOG,[2] and Lawrence[26] are resources regarding the safety of specific drugs.

Complications of Breastfeeding

True Lactation Failure

An inadequate milk supply may reflect a problem with milk synthesis, milk removal, or infant milk intake (infrequent or short episodes of nursing). Inadequate milk synthesis may be failure of mammogenesis (breast preparation during pregnancy), failure of lactogenesis (initiation of milk production), or failure of galactopoiesis (ongoing maintenance of milk supply).[62] Infants at risk for lactation failure include premature infants, twins and other multiples, jaundiced infants, intrauterine growth restriction (IUGR) babies, babies with latching-on difficulty, those with oral clefts or other oral anatomic abnormalities, and infants with respiratory, cardiac, or neurologic abnormalities or serious medical problems.[33]

BREAST REDUCTION AND AUGMENTATION. Breast reduction and augmentation may disrupt the ductal structure of the breast and innervation to the nipple. Infrasubmammary or axillary incisions are the least disruptive; periareolar incisions almost always damage milk ducts and innervation. Relocation of the nipples precludes breastfeeding unless the position has been partially altered while retaining ductal integrity. This technique results in a vertical scar from areola to the base of the breast. Initial engorgement may occur, then milk production will cease. Disruption of the innervation of the nipples interrupts prolactin and oxytocin stimulation, which stimulates milk production and ejection. This woman may not be able to produce milk or may only be able to establish a partial supply; but other women will be successful and some women will gain satisfaction from having tried.[6]

BREAST BIOPSY. Women with a periareolar incision may have impaired emptying of a part of the breast. Small biopsy sites away from the nipple are unlikely to affect lactation. Again, this woman may only be able to establish a partial milk supply, or no milk supply, but may be successful or may gain satisfaction from having tried.[6]

OTHER CONDITIONS ASSOCIATED WITH LACTATION FAILURE. **Conditions associated with lactation failure include tubular breast deformity, previous breast radiation, hypoplastic breasts, marked breast asymmetry,**[33] **widely spaced breasts,** or breasts that **failed to show pregnancy changes.**[48] Severe **PPH** may result in pituitary failure and failure of lactation. See Sheehan's syndrome, p. 485. **For mastitis, see p. 229.**

PSYCHOLOGICAL RAMIFICATIONS. Women may stop breastfeeding for a reason above or after a short trial because of nipple confusion from early supplementation, sore nipples, perceived inadequacy of breastmilk supply, or illness of mother or infant. The mother may have received inadequate or insensitive help or may have felt uncomfortable with the exposure and touching by others of their breasts. Many women perceive breastfeeding as a critical element of their maternal role, a symbol of their love and giving. The woman may feel a sense of failure, inadequacy, guilt, disappointment, and shame. She may be relieved to stop and then feel guilt for feeling relieved. Some women may have anticipated that breastfeeding would be "natural" and easy—an idealized image—not imagining the struggle that it can require. They may be angry at themselves or others. Self-doubts can linger for some time.[32] Resolution of these feelings may take a long time or may influence the breastfeeding of subsequent children. Support the woman in her decision to breastfeed with information, resources, and encouragement for as long as she wants to continue to try. Validate her efforts as well as her frustrations. Normalization of the challenge that breastfeeding can present may help the struggling mother. Encourage the mother to continue to try breastfeeding until she feels at peace with her decision to stop.

• FACILITY GUIDELINES FOR THE PROMOTION OF BREASTFEEDING

Birthing site policies and procedures regarding breastfeeding are known to affect the initiation and continuation of breastfeeding. The receipt of formula company gift packs at discharge, for example, decreases the likelihood of breastfeeding continuation for 2 months and increases the likelihood of the introduction of solid foods by 2 months.[7,15,20]

WHO and UNICEF issued the following facility guidelines in 1989. The first hospital to gain this status in the United States has a breastfeeding initiation rate of >90%.[38] Any birthing site may be designated as "Baby Friendly" if they meet the following criteria:

Ten Steps to Successful Breastfeeding

Every facility providing maternity services and care for newborns should:

1. Have a written breastfeeding policy that is communicated routinely to all health care staff.
2. Train all health care staff in the skills necessary to implement this policy.
3. Inform all pregnant women about the benefits and management of breastfeeding.
4. Help mothers initiate breastfeeding within 30 minutes of birth.
5. Show mothers how to breastfeed and how to maintain lactation even when separated from their infants.
6. Give newborns no food or drink other than human milk unless medically indicated.
7. Practice rooming-in, allowing mothers and infants to stay together 24 hr/d.
8. Encourage breastfeeding on demand.
9. Give no artificial teats or pacifiers to breastfeeding infants.
10. Foster the establishment of breastfeeding support groups and refer mothers to them on discharge from hospital or clinic.

The free formula and gift packs provided by formula companies have presented a major obstacle to this initiative in the United States. In other countries, a government agency implemented the Baby Friendly program. In the United States, a nongovernmental agency was awarded the task. An expert panel decided that the name and guidelines be revised, that birthing sites would assess themselves, and that provision and promotion of baby formula is not prohibited. Providers who work with women are urged to learn about breastfeeding, to become aware of public and facility policies regarding breastfeeding, to take an ethical stand and discharge patients without formula, to refuse gifts from the formula companies, and to take an active role in promoting positive standards in the birthing site, the prenatal care site, and in the community.[38]

• REFERENCES

1. American Academy of Pediatrics (AAP): Breastfeeding and the use of human milk, *Pediatrics* 100:1035-1039, 1997.
2. American College of Obstetricians and Gynecologists (ACOG): *Breastfeeding: maternal and infant aspects,* Educational Bulletin No. 258, Washington DC, 2000, ACOG.
3. Auerbach KG: Evidence-based care and the breastfeeding couple: key concerns, *J Midwifery Womens Health* 45:205-211, 2000.
4. Balch JF, Balch PA: *Prescription for nutritional healing,* ed 2, Garden City Park, NY, 1997, Avery Publishing Group.
5. Bedinghaus JM: Care of the breast and support of breastfeeding, *Womens Health* 24:147-160, 1997.
6. Bell KK, Rawlings NL: Promoting breastfeeding by managing common lactation problems, *Nurse Practitioner* 23:102-123, 1998.

7. Bergevin Y, Dougherty C, Kramer MS: Do infant formula samples shorten the duration of breast-feeding? *Lancet* 1:1148-1151, 1983.

8. Black KA, Hylander MA: Breastfeeding the high risk infant: implications for midwifery management, *J Midwifery Womens Health* 5:238-245, 2000.

9. Brandt KA, Andrews CM, Kvale J: Mother-infant interaction and breastfeeding outcome 6 weeks after birth, *J Obstet Gynecol Neonatal Nurs* 27:169-174, 1998.

10. Budd S: Acupuncture. In Tiran D, Mack S, editors: *Complementary therapies for pregnancy and childbirth,* ed 2, Edinburgh, 2000, Baillière Tindall.

11. Burrow GN, Ferris TF: *Medical complications during pregnancy,* 4 ed, Philadelphia, 1995, WB Saunders.

12. Cummings B, Tiran D: Homeopathy for pregnancy and childbirth. In Tiran D, Mack S, editors: *Complementary therapies for pregnancy and childbirth,* ed 2, Edinburgh, 2000, Baillière Tindall.

13. Cummings S, Ullman D: *Everybody's guide to homeopathic medicines,* New York, 1997, Jeremy P. Tarcher/Putnam.

14. Ely JW, Yankowitz J, Bowdler NC: Evaluation of pregnant women exposed to respiratory viruses, *Am Fam Physician* 61:3065-3072, 2000.

15. Frank DA et al: Commercial discharge packs and breast-feeding counseling: effects on infant-feeding practices in a randomized trial, *Pediatrics* 80:845-854, 1987.

16. Gabbe SG, Niebyl JR, Simpson JL: *Obstetrics: normal & problem pregnancies,* ed 3, New York, 1996, Churchill Livingstone.

17. Griffith HW: *Healing herbs: the essential guide,* Tucson, Ariz, 2000, Fisher Books.

18. Hoffmann D: *The complete illustrated holistic herbal,* Boston, 1996, Element Books.

19. Hoffmann D: *The holistic herbal,* Findhorn, Scotland, 1985, Findhorn Press.

20. Howard C et al: Office prenatal formula advertising and its effect on breast-feeding patterns, *Obstet Gynecol* 95:296-303, 2000.

21. Jarvis C: Physical assessment and health examination, Philadelphia, 2000, WB Saunders.

22. Johnson E: Shiatsu. In Tiran D, Mack S, editors: *Complementary therapies for pregnancy and childbirth,* ed 2, Edinburgh, 2000 Baillière Tindall.

23. Kennell J, McGrath S: Commentary: what babies teach us: the essential link between baby's behavior and mother's biology, *Birth* 28:20-21, 2001.

24. Kitzinger S: *Breastfeeding your baby,* New York, 1989, Alfred A. Knopf.

25. Koehler N: *Artemis speaks: V.B.A.C. stories & natural childbirth information,* Occidental, Calif, 1985, Jerald R. Brown.

26. Lawrence RA: *A review of the medical benefits and contraindications to breastfeeding in the United States (Maternal and Child Health Technical Information Bulletin),* Arlington, Va, 1997, National Center for Education in Maternal and Child Health.

27. Lovelady CA et al: The effect of weight loss in overweight, lactating women on the growth of their infants, *New Engl J Med* 342:449-453, 2000.

28. Mabey R et al: *The new age herbalist,* New York, 1988, Collier Books.

29. Matthiesen A et al: Postpartum maternal oxytocin release by newborns: effects of infant hand massage and sucking, *Birth* 28:13-19, 2001.

30. Medina IM: *Issues in women's health care: nutrition and herbs from menarche to menopause,* course syllabus 3/28-29/98, State University of New York Health Science Center at Brooklyn College of Health Related Professions Midwifery Education Program.

31. Meyer K, Anderson GC: Using kangaroo care in a clinical setting with fullterm infants having breastfeeding difficulties, *MCN Am J Matern Child Nurs* 24:190-192, 1999.

32. Mozingo JN et al: "It wasn't working": women's experiences with short-term breastfeeding, *MCN Am J Matern Child Nurs* 25:120-126, 2000.

33. Neifert MR: Clinical aspects of lactation, *Clin Perinatol* 26:281-306, 1999.

34. Nelson WE, editor: *Nelson textbook of pediatrics,* ed 15, Philadelphia, 1996, WB Saunders.

35. Ody P: *The complete medicinal herbal,* New York, 1993, Dorling Kindersley.

36. Page L: *Healthy healing,* ed 11, Carmel Valley, Calif, 2000, Healthy Healing Publications.

37. Parvati J: *Hygieia: a woman's herbal,* Berkeley, Calif, 1985, Bookpeople.

38. Philipp BL, Merewood A, O'Brien S: Physicians and breastfeeding promotion in the United States: a call for action, *Pediatrics* 107:584-588, 2001.

39. Raisler J, Alexander C, O'Campo P: Breastfeeding and infant illness: a dose-response relationship? *Am J Public Health* 89:25-30, 1999.

40. Ransjo-Arvidson A et al: Maternal analgesia during labor disturbs newborn behavior: effects on breastfeeding, temperature, and crying, *Birth* 28:5-12, 2001.

41. Reifsnider E, Gill SL: Nutrition for the childbearing years, *J Obstet Gynecol Neonatal Nurs* 29:43-55, 2000.

42. Righard L: Are breastfeeding problems related to incorrect breastfeeding technique and the use of pacifiers and bottles? *Birth* 25:40-44, 1998.

43. Riordan J, Auerbach K: *Breastfeeding and human lactation,* ed 2, Sudbury, Mass, 1999, Jones and Bartlett.

44. Romm AJ: *Natural healing for babies and children,* Freedom, Calif, 1996, The Crossing Press.

45. Rose B, Scott-Moncrieff C: *Homeopathy for women,* London, 1998, Collins & Brown.

46. Slusser W, Powers NG: Breastfeeding update 1: immunology, nutrition, and advocacy, *Pediatr Rev* 18:111-119, 1997.

47. Smith T: *Homeopathy for pregnancy and nursing mothers,* Worthing, England, 1993, Insight Editions.

48. Smith JW, Tully MR: Midwifery management of breastfeeding: using the evidence, *J Midwifery Womens Health* 46:423-438, 2001.

49. Speroff L, Glass RH, Kase NG: *Clinical gynecologic endocrinology and infertility,* ed 6, Philadelphia, 1999, Lippincott Williams & Wilkins.

50. Stapleton H, Tiran D: Herbal medicine. In Tiran D, Mack S, editors: *Complementary therapies for pregnancy and childbirth,* ed 2, Edinburgh, 2000, Baillière Tindall.

51. Suitor CW: *Maternal weight gain: a report of an expert work group,* Arlington, Va, 1997, National Center for Education in Maternal and Child Health.

52. Tait P: Nipple pain in breastfeeding women: causes, treatment, and prevention strategies, *J Midwifery Womens Health* 45:212-215, 2000.

53. Tarr K: *Herbs, helps, and pressure points for pregnancy and childbirth,* ed 3, Provo, Utah, 1984, Sunbeam Publications.

54. Tiran D: Massage and aromatherapy. In Tiran D, Mack S, editors: *Complementary therapies for pregnancy and childbirth,* ed 2, Edinburgh, 2000, Baillière Tindall.

55. Tiran D: Reflexology in midwifery practice. In Tiran D, Mack S, editors: *Complementary therapies for pregnancy and childbirth,* ed 2, Edinburgh, 2000, Baillière Tindall.

56. Tuso P: The herbal medicine pharmacy: what Kaiser Permanente providers need to know, *Permanente J* 3:33-37, 1999.

57. Ullman R, Reichenberg-Ullman J: *Homeopathic self-care,* Rocklin, Calif, 1997, Prima.

58. Varney H: *Varney's midwifery,* ed 3, Sudbury, Mass, 1997, Jones and Bartlett.

59. Victora CG et al: Pacifier use and short breastfeeding duration: cause, consequence, or coincidence? *Pediatrics* 99:445-453, 1997.

60. Ward S: Addressing nicotine addiction in women, *J Nurse Midwifery* 44:3-18, 1999.

61. Weed S: *Wise woman herbal for the childbearing year,* Woodstock, NY, 1985, Ash Tree Publishing.

62. Willis CE, Livingstone V: Infant insufficient milk syndrome associated with maternal postpartum hemorrhage, *J Hum Lac* 11:123-126, 1995.

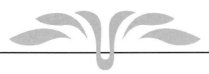

Chapter 7

Medical and Surgical Conditions and Considerations for Pregnancy

Preventive care of the essentially healthy woman includes the following screening:

Physical Examination: BP, body measurements (body mass index [BMI], weight), **breast** examination (annually), **oral cavity** examination, **pelvic** examination (annually, whether or not Pap test is indicated, as long as uterus is present), **rectal** examination (annually at 40 to 50 years), including **fecal occult blood** (annually at 50 years), **skin** examination, and **thyroid** examination.[74]

Screening Procedures:

• **Mammogram** (Recommended by American College of Obstetricians and Gynecologists [ACOG][13] every 1 to 2 years depending on history and risk factors for women aged 40 to 50 years; every year thereafter).

• **Sigmoidoscopy** (every 5 years after 50 years); **colonoscopy** for high-risk individuals—those with ulcerative colitis, those who have polyps detected after 40 years, and those who have a first-degree relative with colon cancer.[74]

Laboratory Studies: Cholesterol screening (nonfasting total cholesterol every 5 years; high-density lipoprotein [HDL] and low-density lipoprotein [LDL] at provider's discretion), **glucose, sexually transmitted infection (STI) and human immunodeficiency virus (HIV)** testing, **Pap** test (annually; after 3 normal results, every 3 years or at provider's discretion), **thyroid** function (routine screening is cost-effective for women older than 35 years[58]), **hepatitis** (surface antigen screening for at-risk populations), **urinalysis (UA).**[74]

Other Testing:

• **Tuberculosis (TB)** testing (for those at risk of exposure, see p. 387)

• **Hearing and vision** screening

Immunizations to Offer or Suggest:

• **Hepatitis B, tetanus/diphtheria** (every 10 years), **varicella, measles** (once if born after 1956), **rubella** (to women of childbearing age without immunity)

- **Influenza vaccine** (women who will be in the second or third trimester of pregnancy during Nov-Feb), annually after 65 years, at any age with a high-risk medical condition, health care providers for high-risk patients; household contacts of high-risk patients; residents of long-term care facilities)
- **Pneumococcus vaccine** (once after age 65 years; at any age with a high-risk condition as described for influenza vaccine).[74]

  Inquire Regarding:
- **Lifestyle practices** including tobacco use, alcohol and street drug use, physical activity, injury prevention such as seatbelt use, avoidance of environmental hazards, and exposure to violence
- **Nutrition** (including folic acid for preconception and calcium supplementation)
- **Sexual** history, activity, contraceptive needs, safe sex practices
- **Polypharmacy** practice
- **Depression** symptoms
- Use of **complementary healing practices**

• ABDOMINAL PAIN OF NONOBSTETRIC ORIGIN DURING PREGNANCY

Differential Diagnoses: Appendicitis, pancreatitis, gallbladder disease, bowel obstruction, liver disease, pyelonephritis (see p. 389), and inflammatory bowel disease are the most common sources of abdominal pain seen during pregnancy.[20] Ectopic pregnancy, ureteral colic, ruptured ovarian cyst, salpingitis, tubo-ovarian abscess, and infarcted uterine myoma should also be considered.[148]

Effect of Pregnancy on Diagnosis: The physical changes of pregnancy, changes in some serum enzyme levels, and alteration of the adrenocortical state make diagnosis more difficult in pregnancy. These factors are overcome by serial physical examinations and a heightened awareness of the potential for these conditions.[46] Delay in diagnosis and definitive treatment presents the greatest hazard for the pregnant woman with an acute abdomen.[162]

Table 7-1 describes the most common causes of nonobstetric pain during pregnancy, their presentation, diagnosis, management, how the condition affects pregnancy, and how pregnancy affects the condition.

• DERMATOLOGIC TERMINOLOGY

The midwife may encounter skin conditions and needs to be able to accurately describe them. Figure 7-1 illustrates common types of dermatologic lesions.

Text continued on page 336

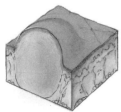

Nodule: Solid, elevated, >1 cm diameter
Tumor: As above, > few cm

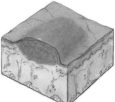

Wheal: Superficial, raised, transient, erythematous.
Urticaria (hives): Wheals coalesced extensively, intensely pruritic

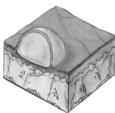

Cyst: Encapsulated, fluid-filled, in dermis or subcutaneous tissue

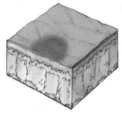

Macule: Nonpalpable, color changes; <1 cm diameter
Patch: As above; ≥1 cm diameter

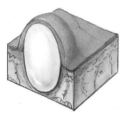

Vesicle: Clear, serum-filled, superficial, circumscribed, elevated, ≤1 cm diameter
Bulla: As above, >1 cm diameter

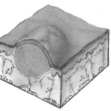

Papule: Solid, elevated, circumscribed, <1 cm diameter
Plaque: Papules coalesced to a lesion ≤1 cm diameter

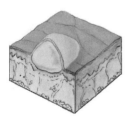

Pustule: Pus-filled, circumscribed, elevated

Figure 7-1 • Common skin lesions and their dermatologic names. (From Jarvis C: *Physical examination and health assessment*, ed 3, Philadelphia, 2000, WB Saunders.)

Table 7-1 / Nonobstetric Abdominal Pain during Pregnancy

	Appendicitis	Bowel Obstruction	Cholecystitis	Inflammatory Bowel Disease (Including Ulcerative Colitis and Crohn's Disease)	Pancreatitis	Liver Disease	Peritonitis
Clinical findings	Pain in RLQ radiating to R iliac crest at 4 mo; to upper R kidney at 8 mo; diffuse, colicky; may change with movement; uterine contractions may accompany. Leukocytosis is present; shift to left. Fever,[20] anorexia, N/V, rebound tenderness may be present.[162]	Triad: (1) Abd pain, possibly sudden in onset, colicky, periumbilical or poorly located; (2) persistent vomiting of odorous vomitus; (3) extreme constipation.[20] May come in waves, q4-5min in upper bowel; q10-15min in lower bowel obstruction.[46] A palpable bowel loop,[107] abd distention, abnormal bowel sounds, signs of peritonitis, fever, leukocytosis, dehydration,	Epigastric or RUQ abd pain, possibly sudden in onset, colicky, stabbing, or intermittent. May radiate to RUQ, R flank, shoulder or scapula. Anorexia, N/V, dyspepsia, low-grade fever, tachycardia, SOB, food intolerance (especially to fatty foods), tenderness with deep palpation of RUQ (Murphy's sign), and peritonitis may develop.[162]	Diarrhea is the most common SX during pregnancy.[20] Anorexia and wt loss also occur. Crohn's disease presents with N/V, colicky mid abd pain, or rectal bleeding. Ulcerative colitis affects the colon and rectum. Bloody diarrhea, rectal bleeding, urgency of defecation, and crampy low abdominal pain are present.[107]	Severe, often sudden, midepigastric pain radiating to back, or LUQ pain radiating to L flank, anorexia, N/V, diminished BS, fever (66%),[46] LUQ or diffuse tenderness to palpation.[20] In severe cases, guarding, rebound tenderness (peritonitis), ascites, flank ecchymosis present.[107]	Liver disease seen in pregnancy includes hepatitis (see p. 348), cirrhosis, HELLP syndrome (see p. 85), acute fatty liver of pregnancy (see p. 63), hepatic rupture (usually due to hypertension presenting with RUQ pain and shock); Budd-Chiari syndrome (hepatic venous outflow obstruction; rarely occurs in 3rd trimester and PP, with abd pain, ascites, and hepatomegaly	Abd and rebound tenderness, rigidity, guarding, severe pain, diminished BS, distention, thirst, restlessness, brown tongue, foul breath, projectile fecal vomiting, SOB, anxiety, pallor, and clamminess. Leukocytosis is present and clinical and lab findings specific to etiology.[55]

	altered electrolytes and renal function present.[20]				and AST, bilirubin, and alkaline phosphatase elevation); tumor; or acute porphyria (inherited metabolic disorder with "attacks" of ascites, abd pain, N/V, and psychiatric disorders,).[107]
Incidence during pregnancy	1 in 766-1500; more common in 1st or 2nd trimester.[46,162]	1 in 1500-66,431. Increasing due to higher incidence of PID and abd surgeries.[107,162]	0.05%-0.3% pregnant women have cholecystitis; 3.5%-10% have asymptomatic stones.[20]		1 in 3333 pregnant women are affected, most in late pregnancy or PP.[20]
Effect of pregnancy on the condition	Pain moves upward and toward the R flank with advancing gestation. Location delays peritonitis. Rebound tenderness and guarding less specific.[162]	When the uterus becomes an abd organ, when the head descends into the pelvis cavity, or when the uterus shrinks rapidly PP, intestinal volvulus occurs with sigmoid compression.[107,162]	Progesterone decreases the contractility of the gallbladder, causing increased volume and stasis. Elevated estrogen level causes cholesterol hypersaturation.[20]	Disease activity before pregnancy is usually sustained through the pregnancy.[107]	Pancreatitis during pregnancy is most often due to cholelithiasis. Hyperlipidemia of pregnancy is a predisposing factor.[20]

abd, Abdomen or abdominal; *BS,* bowel sounds; *bx,* biopsy; *EFM,* Fetal monitoring; *MD,* physician; *N/V,* nausea and vomiting; *OB,* obstetric; *PP,* postpartum; *pyelo,* pyelonephritis; *SOB,* shortness of breath; *sx,* symptom; *tx,* treatment; *wt,* weight.

Continued

Table 7-1 / Nonobstetric Abdominal Pain during Pregnancy—cont'd

	Appendicitis	Bowel Obstruction	Cholecystitis	Inflammatory Bowel Disease (Including Ulcerative Colitis and Crohn's Disease)	Pancreatitis	Liver Disease	Peritonitis
Effect of pregnancy on the condition—cont'd		Distention may be obscured by pregnancy. Leukocytosis is obscured by the normal leukocytosis of pregnancy.[20]					
Morbidity and mortality	3%-5% fetal mortality without perforation; up to 36% with perforation.[46]	Fetal mortality rises with advancing gestation: 36% in 2nd trimester; 64% in 3rd trimester. Maternal mortality 20%.[20,46]	5% fetal loss during abdominal cholecystectomy[20]; up to 60% in gallstone pancreatitis.[162]		Maternal outcome is favorable; fetal outcome is less so.[42]	Maternal and fetal outcomes worsen with the severity of the disease.[144a]	
Obstetric complications	Increased risk of 1st trimester SAB (33% in one study).[19] Risk of PTL in 2nd trimester (10%-43%).[20]		Increased risk of SAB with 1st-trimester surgery; PTL in the 3rd; less with laparoscopy.[20]	Chronic intestinal inflammation and disease flares are more harmful to pregnancy than	1st trimester SAB; PTL may occur in the 3rd trimester.[107]	SAB, PTL, IUGR,[2] fetal infection,[2] PP infection.[130]	

Diagnosis					
Ultrasound.[20] Differentiate from pyelo with cath UA.[162]	Upright and flat abd films, sometimes serial, with contrast.[20]	Ultrasound.[20]	Initial workup may include sigmoidoscopy or colonoscopy.[107] the drugs or surgery. Drugs are therefore continued in pregnancy. A perianal fistula in Crohn's may preclude episiotomy or vaginal delivery.[20]	Ultrasound may show dilated pancreatic ducts or cholelithiasis.[20] Elevated amylase (not specific), elevated lipase, or amylase: creatinine clearance ratio indicates acute pancreatitis in pregnancy.[107]	Hepatic hemorrhage may be detected with CT scan and ultrasound; paracentesis confirms intraabd bleeding.[107] Budd-Chiari diagnosed by liver bx, hepatic venography, or MRI. Abd film may show ascites, free air if a hollow organ ruptures, or the film may be normal.[160]

Continued

Table 7-1 / Nonobstetric Abdominal Pain during Pregnancy—cont'd

	Appendicitis	Bowel Obstruction	Cholecystitis	Inflammatory Bowel Disease (Including Ulcerative Colitis and Crohn's Disease)	Pancreatitis	Liver Disease	Peritonitis
Management	1. Prompt OB and surgical consultation.[20] MD evaluates the woman personally. 2. Aggressive surgical intervention is indicated.[162] Antibiotics indicated for perforation, abscess, or peritonitis.[107]	1. Prompt OB and surgical consultation. 2. In 1st and 3rd trimesters, conservative tx includes IV hydration, electrolyte correction, NG decompression, bowel rest, pain management and possibly antibiotics).[20]	1. Prompt OB and surgical consultation.[20] 2. IV fluid and electrolyte replacement; NG decompression, indwelling urinary catheter, and continuous EFM are indicated.[46] The earlier the surgical	An MD manages the GI disease. Sulfa drugs (pregnancy class C drugs) are used, and folate is supplemented. Steroids may be used.[20]	1. Prompt OB and surgical physician consultation.[20] 2. Management depends on severity, persistence of sx, and gestation.[20] 3. Mild disease without cholelithiasis is treated with IV hydration and	1. Midwife refers the patient with severe liver disease for MD management.[20] 2. Hepatic hemorrhage may require surgery. A stable hematoma may be conservatively managed with	1. Midwife refers the patient for MD management. 2. Identification of the cause is followed by specific tx, including IV hydration, correction of electrolytes, NG decompression, and observation for bowel obstruction.[55]

Prophylactic tocolytics cause fluid overload and ARDS; do not improve fetal outcome.[20]

resulting in nutrition problems, extended hospitalization, and the risk of recurrence (50%) and gallstone pancreatitis. 2nd-trimester surgery is often recommended.[162]

3. Surgery is indicated for failure of conservative tx, systemic toxicity recalcitrant pancreatitis.[46] Laparoscopy reduces OB complications.[23a]

intervention, the less risk of necrosis requiring bowel resection.[107]

correction of electrolytes, bland diet, or NG decompression and bowel rest.[20] IV alimentation may be indicated. With cholelithiasis, conservative tx, sx should improve within a wk.[107]

4. Surgery is indicated for abscess, ruptured pseudocyst, or hemorrhagic pancreatitis.[46]

careful BP control and C/S.[107]

3. Budd-Chiari tx may include thrombolytic therapy, surgical decompression, or liver transplantation.[107]

abd, Abdomen or abdominal; BS, bowel sounds; bx, biopsy; EFM, Fetal monitoring; MD, physician; N/V, nausea and vomiting; OB, obstetric; PP, postpartum; pyelo, pyelonephritis; SOB, shortness of breath; sx, symptom; tx, treatment; wt, weight.

• PREGNANCY IN THE WOMAN WITH CARDIOVASCULAR DISEASE

Effect of Pregnancy on the Maternal Heart

The pregnant woman's increased blood volume and decreased peripheral vascular resistance cause the heart to compensate by increasing rate and stroke volume, resulting in a 30% to 50% increased cardiac output, which is maximized by midpregnancy. S1 may be split; S3 may be heard. A systolic ejection murmur, caused by the increased blood volume crossing over the valves, is heard in 90% of pregnant women.[32] Chest x-ray examination shows minimal heart enlargement. The diaphragm displaces the heart upward and to the left, shifting the apex laterally. The electrocardiogram (ECG) during pregnancy shows a 15-degree left-axis deviation and mild ST changes in the inferior leads.[55]

At the beginning of labor, cardiac output increases about 13% over prelabor values. Uterine contractions increase this by another 34% by increasing the heart rate and extruding about 500 cc of blood into the central venous bed. Epidural anesthesia reduces this by 40%, and general anesthesia, by 25%. C/S before the onset of labor avoids the hemodynamic changes of labor but introduces the risks of apprehension, anesthesia, and surgical manipulation.[31] Cardiac output increases to almost 80% above prelabor values immediately after vaginal delivery, to 50% after C/S.[55]

Pregnancy and Maternal Heart Disease

In general, the higher the classification of the maternal heart disease, the more dangerous pregnancy is for the woman. Hemodynamic changes may worsen heart failure.[31] Artificial valve function may deteriorate during the pregnancy, requiring replacement after the pregnancy.[23] Postpartum changes may overwhelm a structurally damaged heart. Three to ten percent of mothers with a cardiac lesion give birth to an affected infant,[55] compared with 0.8% in the general U.S. population. The risk of giving birth to an affected infant is nearly 50% among women with some autosomal dominant defects.[31]

Cardiac signs and symptoms include chest pain related to effort or emotion, severe or progressive dyspnea, hemoptysis, and syncope with exertion. Findings on physical examination may include cyanosis, clubbing of fingers, grade 3 or greater systolic murmur, a diastolic murmur, a persistent split second heart sound during inspiration and expiration, persistent jugular venous distention, hepatomegaly, cardiomegaly, a sustained arrhythmia, or peripheral edema.[31]

Classifications of Cardiac Disease:

Class I: Uncompromised by heart disease
Class II: Activities slightly compromised by symptoms; comfortable at rest
Class III: Activities moderately or markedly compromised by symptoms; comfortable at rest
Class IV: Symptoms severe with activity and may occur at rest[55]

Preconceptional Counseling: For the patient with class III or IV cardiac disease, Cunningham et al[55] state that there is a significant risk of maternal death. Surgical correction of cardiac defects before conception may make a subsequent pregnancy safer. The woman with a prosthetic valve who takes warfarin—known to be teratogenic—is switched to heparin. The risk for heart disease in the infant is discussed.

Ⓜ Management During Pregnancy

1. The woman is **referred** to and managed by an obstetrician and is seen at least once during the pregnancy by a cardiologist.[31]
2. **Anticipatory guidance:** The woman with an artificial valve receives **anticoagulant therapy.**[23] Patients with class I and II disease are monitored closely throughout the reproductive year for signs of **congestive heart failure (CHF).** For the patient with class III or IV cardiac disease, prolonged hospitalization or **bed rest** is necessary. **Vaginal delivery** is preferable; C/S is performed for obstetric indications only.[55] Exhaustion or medications in the breastmilk may prevent the severely affected mother from **breastfeeding.**[31]

• ANTIBIOTIC PROPHYLAXIS FOR THE PREVENTION OF BACTERIAL ENDOCARDITIS

Box 7-1 gives the recommendation of the American Heart Association for antibiotic prophylaxis for the prevention of bacterial endocarditis.

Prophylactic antibiotics are given just before and 6 to 8 hours after a procedure. In cases of unanticipated bleeding, the antibiotics are probably effective if given within 2 hours. The patient already taking an antibiotic should receive an additional antibiotic from another class.[57]

• ENDOCRINE DISEASE

Diabetes Mellitus

Diabetes mellitus (DM) is characterized by hyperglycemia resulting from defects in insulin secretion, insulin action, or both. Autoimmune destruction of pancreatic β cells and/or peripheral insulin resistance are involved. Long-term chronic hyperglycemia is associated with damage, dysfunction, and failure of various organs including the eyes, kidneys, nerves, heart, and blood vessels.[65]

During pregnancy, the insulin requirement rises progressively because of the diabetogenic hormones of pregnancy and increased need.[88] β-Cell hyperplasia increases insulin secretion. Fasting glucose levels fall as a result of increased need. Women with gestational diabetes (GDM) cannot respond to the decreased peripheral sensitivity to insulin of pregnancy with an increase in the secretion of insulin as do other women. Fetal glucose levels equal maternal glucose levels, but insulin does not cross the placental barrier. Fetal hyperglycemia results in β-cell

• *Box 7-1* / Antibiotic Prophylaxis for Prevention of Bacterial Endocarditis as Recommended by the American Heart Association •

MEDICATION FOR CHILDBIRTH
- Ampicillin, 2.0 g IM or IV, plus gentamicin, 1.5 mg/kg (not to exceed 120 mg), within 30 min of delivery is followed by ampicillin, 1 g IM or PO, or amoxicillin, 1 g PO.
- **Penicillin-allergic:** Substitute vancomycin, 1 g, over 1 to 2 hr, plus gentamicin, 1.5 mg/kg (not to exceed 120 mg), completed within 30 min of delivery,[57] with no postpartum dose.[16]

PROPHYLAXIS ACCORDING TO CARDIAC CONDITION
IV prophylaxis is recommended for the following high-risk patients:
- Prosthetic cardiac valves
- History of bacterial endocarditis
- Cyanotic congenital heart disease
- Surgically constructed systemic pulmonary shunts or conduits

Oral prophylaxis is recommended for the following moderate-risk patients:
- Acquired valvular dysfunction
- Hypertrophic cardiomyopathy
- Mitral valve prolapse with valvular regurgitation and/or thickening of the leaflets

Prophylaxis is not recommended for the following conditions:
- Isolated secundum atrial septal defect
- Surgically repaired atrial septal defect
- Ventricular septal defect
- Patent ductus arteriosus (without residua beyond 6 mo)
- Previous coronary bypass graft surgery
- Mitral valve prolapse without valvular regurgitation
- Physiologic, functional, or innocent heart murmurs
- Kawasaki's heart disease without valvular dysfunction
- Rheumatic fever without valvular dysfunction
- Cardiac pacemaker or implanted defibrillators

PROPHYLAXIS ACCORDING TO THE PROCEDURE
Prophylaxis is recommended for patients undergoing the following procedures:
- Surgery or instrumentation of the GU tract
- Instrumentation of the urinary tract in the presence of a UTI
- Cystoscopy and urethral dilation
- Childbirth only when bacteremia is suspected [57]

Prophylaxis is not recommended for patients undergoing the following procedures:
- Cesarean section
- Vaginal hysterectomy (unless the patient is at high risk for endocarditis)
- Uterine D&C unless the tissue is infected
- TAB unless the tissue is infected
- Sterilization procedures
- Insertion or removal of IUDs unless the tissue is infected[57]

hyperplasia and hyperinsulinemia in the fetus. Insulin requirements change the most during weeks 20 to 32.[96]

Classification of Diabetes According to the Expert Committee on the Diagnosis and Classification of Diabetes Mellitus (ECDCDM), 1997

Type 1: Absolute deficiency of insulin secretion.[65] Onset usually occurs before 30 years of age. The acute complication is ketoacidosis; treatment is insulin therapy.[55]

Type 2: Insulin resistance and an inadequate compensatory insulin secretion response. May exist subclinically for some time; may be sufficient to cause pathologic changes. A fasting glucose level identifies type 2 diabetes.[65] Individuals tend to be >40 years old at onset, to be obese,[55] and to have a family history of DM. Native Americans and Mexican Americans are at increased risk.[133] The acute complication is hyperosmolar coma. This form of DM may or may not respond to insulin but does respond to sulfonylurea and exercise (decreases peripheral insulin resistance) and diet (obesity increases peripheral insulin resistance).[55]

Gestational diabetes: GDM is carbohydrate intolerance first recognized during pregnancy. DM may have predated the pregnancy without being identified and may persist afterward. Insulin may be required.[116] **Class A1** is diet-controlled GDM; **class A2** is insulin-dependent GDM.[55] **Impaired glucose tolerance (IGT)** and **impaired fasting tolerance (IFT)** are intermediate conditions in which glucose levels are above normal but are not high enough to be classified as DM.[65]

Criteria for the Diagnosis of Diabetes: If the patient is not pregnant, does not have unequivocal hyperglycemia, and is not in acute metabolic decompensation, any positive value is confirmed by repeat testing on a different day.

- A **random plasma glucose level** of ≥ 200 mg/dL with symptoms (polyuria, polydipsia, unexplained weight loss) is diagnostic of DM. *OR*
- A **fasting plasma glucose level** (≥ 8 hours without calories) of ≥ 126 mg/dL is diagnostic of DM; 110 to 125 mg/dL indicates IFT; <110 mg/dL is normal. *OR*
- In a **75-g glucose challenge**, a 2-hour plasma glucose level of ≥ 200 mg/dL is diagnostic for DM; 140 to 199 mg/dL indicates IGT; <140 mg/dL is normal (1997 ECDCDM recommendation for postpartum diagnosis of type 2 DM 4 to 6 weeks after delivery).[49]
- A **50-g glucose challenge** is recommended by ACOG[7] for screening pregnant women; (time and previous meals unimportant) a 1-hour plasma glucose level of ≥ 130 to 140 mg/dL indicates the need for an oral glucose tolerance test.[116]
- An **oral glucose tolerance test (OGTT)** is performed in the morning after an 8- to 14-hour fast. The woman remains seated and does not smoke. For a positive diagnosis, two or more of the values must be met or exceeded.[116]

Plasma glucose	50 g	100 g
Fasting	—	105 mg/dL
1 hr	140 mg/dL	190 mg/dL
2 hr	—	160 mg/dL
3 hr	—	145 mg/dL[65]

Type I DM and Pregnancy: Obstetricians manage these high-risk pregnancies. Maternal end-organ complications of diabetes may be accelerated. These women are at greater risk for spontaneous abortion (SAB), and their infants are at greater risk for anomalies (8% to 12% in the absence of preconceptional care),[31] intrauterine growth restriction (IUGR) (probably caused by uteroplacental vasculopathy),[118] macrosomia (tenfold risk),[69] and ketoacidotic episodes with a 20% fetal loss rate.[55] The perinatal mortality rate is 2% to 5%. With optimal obstetric care, the woman with diabetes can achieve a perinatal mortality rate equal to that of healthy women except for major malformations.[69]

Gestational Diabetes Mellitus

Risk Factors for GDM: (Fifty percent of the women with GDM have none of the following risk factors.[33])

DM in a first-degree relative
Obesity
History of abnormal glucose metabolism
Poor obstetric history

High-risk ethnicity
Advancing age
Prematurity, proteinuria, glycosuria, or hypertension in a previous pregnancy

Screening for GDM: In 1997, the ECDCDM recommended selective screening. However, because half of all women with GDM have no risk factors and because of the significant risks of GDM to mother and fetus, most prenatal care providers screen all women.[34] The pregnant woman is tested with the 50-g glucose challenge and the OGTT.

Glycosylated Proteins: Glycation reflects average glucose concentration over time. Glycosylated hemoglobin (HbA_{1c}) reflects glycemia over the last 2 to 3 months and is used to reflect glucose control and monitor treatment.[94] **Normal HbA_{1c}:** 2.9% to 6.9%. **Treatment goal:** <7%.

Risks for the Pregnant Woman With GDM: Greater risk of pyelonephritis,[31] preeclampsia,[116] polyhydramnios,[59] operative delivery,[135] lacerations, postpartum hemorrhage (PPH), postpartum endometritis,[76] GDM in subsequent pregnancies, and type 2 DM in later years.[91]

Risks to the Infant of the Pregnant Woman With GDM: Fetal malformations,[146] macrosomia,[33] shoulder dystocia and accompanying birth injuries,[76] neonatal hypoglycemia, hypocalcemia, hyperbilirubinemia, and polycythemia, permanent IGT,[116] altered neurobehavioral development as a result of altered metabolism, and obesity in childhood and adolescence.[153]

Ultrasonic Identification of Fetal Macrosomia: After 30 weeks' gestation, fetuses of mothers with GDM deposit extra fat in the abdominal and interscapular areas.[118] Sonographic fetal asymmetry (difference between abdominal diameter and biparietal diameter [BPD]) predicts the frequency and severity of shoulder dystocia.[44] For infants weighing 2500 to >4000 g, clinical estimated fetal weight (EFW) is significantly more accurate in identifying macrosomia than ultrasound.[84]

Exercise and the Woman With GDM: Exercise overcomes peripheral resistance to insulin.[88] Regular aerobic exercise lowers fasting and postprandial blood glucose levels and is suggested as an adjunct to dietary interventions during pregnancy.[116]

(m) *Management of Pregestational Diabetes or Insulin-Dependent Diabetes*

1. At the initial visit, **carefully date the pregnancy**, and order an **ultrasound examination to confirm** or establish dating. Order routine prenatal laboratory tests and an **HbA$_{1c}$** level.[116]
2. **Refer** woman to the obstetrician for management of a high-risk pregnancy.
3. **Anticipatory guidance:** The best pregnancy outcomes are brought about by **scrupulous glycemic control** through monitoring postprandial blood glucose levels[118] and administration of **insulin** for hyperglycemia.[88] **Glyburide,** the only oral hypoglycemic agent currently considered safe for use after organogenesis, may also be used. This sulfonylurea stimulates pancreatic β cells to secrete more insulin and crosses the placenta in minimal amounts.[51]

(m) *Management of the Woman With Gestational Diabetes*

1. Women with GDM are **managed by the midwife** with medical **consultation.**
2. Most women are managed with **dietary interventions.**[88] Box 7-2 describes the dietary guidelines.
3. Teach the woman to measure fasting and postprandial glucose levels (1 or 2 hours) by means of **fingerstick home glucose monitoring.**[96] Treatment goals are noted in Box 7-3.
4. **If the blood glucose level is not normalized by 2 weeks**, confirm compliance. Exclude infection. If these factors are absent, add insulin in **consultation** with an obstetrician.[96] Most practitioners begin with 20 to 30 U of insulin (two thirds long-acting and one third short-acting) in a daily dose before breakfast.[55]
5. Send periodic urine samples for **UA, culture and sensitivity** to exclude asymptomatic bacteriuria.
6. **Suggest regular aerobic exercise** 3 times/wk for ≥15 minutes.[116]
7. **Order an ultrasound examination** for detection of fetal anomalies for women with a fasting glucose level >120 mg/dL and those diagnosed as gestational diabetic during the first trimester.[116]
8. **Institute fetal movement counts** 8 to 10 weeks before term. **Initiate nonstress tests (NSTs)** from 32 weeks' gestation in cases

of class A2 GDM; near term in cases of class A1 GDM; intensify surveillance after 40 weeks.[116]

9. **Timing of delivery:** Amniocentesis to determine lung maturity is indicated when induction is considered before 38 weeks' gestation. Consider delivery at 38 weeks. Delay is associated with more macrosomic infants. Expectant management, however, allows for cervical ripening and increases the possibility of spontaneous labor, and it may be planned if fetal testing is reassuring and macrosomia is not suspected. Delivery after 40 weeks' gestation has not been associated with increased morbidity or mortality rates in mothers or infants when GDM is well controlled.[116]

10. **Route of delivery:** Moore[118] suggests that in making the decision regarding route of delivery, the following should be taken into account: the woman's history of macrosomia, shoulder dystocia,

• *Box 7-2 /* **Dietary Guidelines for the Woman With Gestational Diabetes** •

SIZE AND CALORIES

Woman's Body Size	Daily Calories
Normal weight	30 kcal/kg body weight
Overweight	24 kcal/kg body weight
Morbidly obese	12 kcal/kg body weight

NUTRIENT BALANCE
• 35%-45% supplied by carbohydrates
• 20%-25% by protein
• 35%-40% fat

GENERAL GUIDELINES
• Avoid sugar, concentrated sweets, and convenience foods.
• Eat about every 3 hr, including protein at every meal and snack.
• Eat a very small breakfast, no more than one starch/bread exchange.
• Eat high-fiber, low-fat meals.[88]

• *Box 7-3 /* **Capillary Blood Glucose Management Goals** •

• Fasting glucose level of ≤95 mg/dL
• 1 hr postprandial glucose level of ≤140 mg/dL *and/or*
• 2 hr postprandial glucose level of <120 mg/dL
• Avoid hypoglycemia, ketonemia, and ketonuria[116]

EFW of the present pregnancy, abdominal circumference/BPD ratio, clinical pelvimetry, and the mother's wishes. Prophylactic C/S may be considered for the woman with GDM whose baby's EFW is ≥4500 g. Induction for macrosomia is not indicated because it is associated with increased risk for C/S.[8]

11. **Breastfeeding,** associated with less obesity, and in some populations, with less diabetes in the offspring, is encouraged.[116]

ⓂIntrapartum Management

1. Maternal hyperglycemia during labor increases the risk of neonatal hyperglycemia, a rise in lactate and decline in pH that would occur during fetal hypoxic episodes. Treatment goals are stated in Box 7-4. **Test blood glucose levels every 1 to 4 hours.** Administration of exogenous insulin is infrequently required. Parenteral administration of glucose to meet basal energy requirements is suggested if the level is low; the recommended rate is 0.12 to 0.18 g/kg/h.[116]

2. Careful assessment of EFW, observance of labor progress, and **shoulder precautions** are paramount when macrosomia is suspected (see p. 184).[25]

3. **Pediatrics** is notified that the infant's mother had GDM. The baby is evaluated for hypoglycemia, hypocalcemia, polycythemia, hyperbilirubinemia, and anomalies.[116]

ⓂPostpartum Management and Evaluation of Women With Gestational Diabetes Mellitus

1. **Educate** the woman regarding the **prevention and symptoms of postpartum endometritis**—for which she is at increased risk.[41]

2. **Test with the 75-g glucose challenge at 6 weeks** postpartum and reclassify the diabetic status.[65]

3. **Teach the woman the signs and symptoms of DM**[116] and to notify the health care provider should they occur: polyuria, polydipsia, fatigue, weight loss, polyphagia, recurrent candidiasis, skin infections that will not heal, recurrent conjunctivitis, blurred vision, or susceptibility to infections.[65]

• *Box 7-4 /* Intrapartum Treatment Goal for Blood Glucose in the Woman With Gestational Diabetes •

- Plasma blood glucose level of 80 to 120 mg/dL *or*
- Capillary blood glucose level of 70 to 110 mg/dL[116]

4. **Discuss modifiable risk factors:** obesity, subsequent pregnancies, dietary fat intake, avoidance of drugs and nicotine, which adversely affect peripheral insulin resistance.[116]
5. Since all future pregnancies carry the risk of prepregnancy diabetes or GDM, **preconception planning** is important. Regulation of diabetes before conception decreases the risk for congenital anomalies. Folic acid supplementation (≥400 µg/d) is suggested.[116]
6. **Contraception for women with diabetes:** Low-dose oral contraceptives (OCs) may be safely used by women who have had GDM.[116] The woman should be normotensive, <35 years old, nonsmoking, and free of vascular disease. A subsequent pregnancy represents a greater risk for the woman's health than use of OCs. Careful follow-up (BP, weight, lipid profile, triannual glucose screening) is suggested.[11] The monthly combination contraceptive injection medroxy progesterone acetate and estradiol cypionate (MPA/E$_{2C}$; see p. 502) has no impact on carbohydrate metabolism and is acceptable for diabetic women without vascular complications.[122] Progestin-only contraception, however, may increase the short-term risk of developing DM.[116] Hispanic women who breastfeed and take progestin OCs experience a significantly increased risk of developing type 2 DM, and progestin OCs are not advised for these women.[92] Norplant is unavailable to diabetics because of the fear of litigation. Use of the intrauterine device (IUD) is avoided because of the risk of infection. Barrier methods and sterilization are suggested because they do not cause systemic side effects. Facilitate puerperal tubal ligation for these women if it is desired.[55]
7. **Complementary measures for diabetes: Osteopathy** may reduce the diabetic woman's insulin requirement. The woman with insulin-dependent diabetes who visits an osteopath should watch her glucose levels closely.[48]

Thyroid Disease

Normal Physiology

The hypothalamus produces thyrotropin-releasing hormone (TRH), which stimulates the anterior pituitary to release thyroid-stimulating hormone or thyrotropin (TSH). TSH stimulates the thyroid to release thyroxine (T_4) (a hormone produced with iodine).[133] One third of the T_4 is converted to T_3 (triiodothyronine), which is 4 times as potent as T_4, has one quarter the half-life, and is present in smaller amounts. About 99% of T_3 and T_4 circulate bound to proteins (mostly to thyroxine-binding globulin [TBG]). The molecules that are unbound are the biologically active ones.[145] The principle effect of the thyroid hormones is to alter or maintain the basal metabolic rate (BMR). The thyroid hormones inhibit the hypothalamus, as well as the anterior pituitary, in a feedback loop, diminishing TRH and TSH secretion.[133]

Effect of Pregnancy on Thyroid Function

TBG is approximately doubled by the end of the first trimester as a result of estrogen stimulation of hepatic production.[31] Total T_4 rises sharply in early pregnancy between 6 and 9 weeks, continuing to rise until it plateaus at 18 weeks. Free T_4 returns to normal after the first trimester. Total T_3 rises up to 18 weeks and then plateaus. During most of pregnancy, free T_3 and free T_4 stay within normal limits.[55] The normal pregnant woman's thyroid enlarges by about 13%.[69] The presence of a goiter or nodules is not normal and should be investigated.[55] The most accurate way to measure thyroid function during pregnancy is by determining free T_3 and T_4 levels. A low free T_4 level with an elevated TSH level reflects pituitary stimulation of a marginally responding thyroid gland and is the most sensitive measurement of hypothyroidism.[69]

Hypothyroidism and Hyperthyroidism

Table 7-2 describes the etiology, signs and symptoms, diagnosis, and management of hypo- and hyperthyroidism, as well as complications associated with these conditions in pregnancy.

Postpartum Thyroiditis

Thyroid disease, like other autoimmune diseases, may worsen after delivery. Five to ten percent of women develop thyrotoxicosis or hypothyroidism 3 to 8 months after delivery and are not diagnosed. This thyroiditis may cause hyperthyroidism, followed by transient hypothyroidism and then recovery. Presentation may mimic postpartum psychosis. A small painless goiter, palpitations, fatigue, depression, carelessness, and poor memory and concentration ability are seen. These women have microsomal autoantibodies that rise during pregnancy, peak 4 to 6 months after delivery, and return to normal 10 to 12 months after delivery. In 25%, permanent hypothyroidism eventually develops.[55]

ⓜ Management

1. **Refer** the woman to a physician for management.
2. **Anticipatory guidance:** Physician management includes β-blockade medications (propylthiouracil [PTU] is ineffective in this situation).[69]

• GASTROINTESTINAL DISEASE

Diarrhea

Diarrhea manifests as loose stools with abdominal cramps and is usually a self-limiting condition. Acute diarrhea is generally caused by food, drugs, or an infection. Chronic diarrhea is that lasting more than 2 weeks.[29]

Clostridium difficile is a spore-forming, gram-positive anaerobic organism; and *C. difficile*–associated disease is a gastrointestinal (GI)

Table 7-2 / Hypothyroidism and Hyperthyroidism

Hypothyroidism	Hyperthyroidism
Etiology	
Autoimmune destruction by antibodies (Hashimoto's disease), transient thyroiditis, pituitary or hypothalamic dysfunction, peripheral resistance to thyroid hormone; or medically induced by radioactive ablation, surgical removal, or antithyroid drugs.[133]	Graves' disease (most common) causes autoimmune stimulation by antibodies in exacerbations and remissions.[55] The initial stage of Hashimoto's disease may present as hyperthyroidism.[69] Toxic adenoma; toxic multinodular goiter; lymphocytic thyroiditis (painless and postpartum thyroiditis); trophoblastic tumors; and TSH-secreting pituitary tumors[133] may be etiologies. Half of the women with hyperemesis gravidarum have transient hyperthyroidism, but they are not thyrotoxic and do not require antithyroid measures.[133]
Signs and Symptoms	
Variable, may include lethargy, depression, reduced ability to concentrate, malaise, weakness, weight gain, cold sensitivity, hair loss and dryness, cool coarse skin, puffy hands and face, slow reflexes, muscle cramps, arthralgia, hoarse husky voice, bradycardia, menorrhagia, amenorrhea, infertility, anemia, cardiomyopathy, pericardial effusions, and a diffuse or nodular goiter. The goiter of Hashimoto's disease is symmetric and rubbery unless the woman is older and the gland is destroyed.[133]	Heat intolerance, nervousness, anxiety, tachycardia, diaphoresis, palpitations, atrial fibrillation, frequent bowel movements, oligomenorrhea, warm moist skin, weight loss, loosening of nails from nail beds, fatigue, weakness, exophthalmos, diplopia, lid lag, brisk DTRs, tremors, shortness of breath, thyroid bruit, diffuse or nodular goiter. In Graves' disease, the thyroid may be 2-3 times the normal size.[55]
Complications During Pregnancy	
IUGR, SAB, preeclampsia, placental abruption, and fetal developmental delays[5a] with lower IQ scores in fetuses whose mothers did not receive thyroid replacement during gestation.[83a]	Prematurity, low birthweight, and preeclampsia occur at greater rates.[55] In Graves' disease, the thyroid-stimulating antibodies are the IgG type, cross the placenta, and affect the fetal thyroid. Most often, Graves' disease remits during pregnancy and exacerbates immediately postpartum.[133]
Laboratory Findings	
Free T_4 and TSH levels are elevated. In Hashimoto's disease, antithyroglobin and antimicrosomal antibodies are elevated. Decreased TSH indicates pituitary malfunction; decreased TRH indicates hypothalamic dysfunction. During pregnancy, failure of total thyroxine to rise as expected is diagnostic.[133] An elevation in total cholesterol of approximately 4.3% occurs.[58]	Elevated thyroidal radioactive uptake (RAIU).[133]
Management	
The midwife consults with the physician. Thyroid supplementation is prescribed immediately on diagnosis.[5a] The TSH, T_3 and T_4 levels are monitored closely throughout pregnancy, the dosage being adjusted accordingly, as the requirement may increase 25%-50%.[5a] Women who have undergone surgical removal or radioactive ablation will require higher doses.[69] Screening women >35 yr of age during routine health examinations	The midwife consults with the physician. Radioactive ablation, surgical removal, or antithyroid drugs are medical interventions. During pregnancy, medical treatment is preferable. Propylthiouracil (PTU) or methimazole (Tapazole) is prescribed. PTU is used during pregnancy because it is protein-bound and thus less likely to cross the placenta or into the breastmilk; and Tapazole, inconsistently associated with aplasia cutis of the neonate, is

Table 7-2 / Hypothyroidism and Hyperthyroidism—cont'd

Hypothyroidism	Hyperthyroidism
compares favorably with other accepted health practices in cost-effectiveness.[58] ACNM[5a] recommends screening of women with a personal or family history of thyroid disease, as well as women who are symptomatic.	avoided. Side effects of PTU include agranulocytosis. The woman is directed to stop the medication and immediately report symptoms of sore throat and fever. The provider orders an immediate leukocyte count.[69] β-adrenergic antagonists may be ordered for women with acute adrenergic symptoms (tremor, tachycardia, diaphoresis).[133] One percent of women with Graves' disease have neonates with hyperthyroidism (most transient), and Pediatrics should be notified to carefully evaluate these infants.[69]

infection in the absence of the normal flora—usually after use of wide-spectrum antibiotics. Manifestations range from asymptomatic colonization to toxic megacolon and intestinal perforation. The primary symptom is diarrhea—watery; profuse; green, brown, or clear; foul-smelling; continuous or intermittent; often mucoid; rarely bloody. Cramping, fever, leukocytosis, abdominal tenderness and distention, nausea, vomiting, anorexia, malaise, and dehydration may be present. Enzyme-linked immunosorbent assays (ELISAs) or enzyme immunoassays (EIAs) detect *Clostridium* species.[3]

Ⓜ *Management of Diarrhea*

1. Advise oral **hydration.** Gatorade or Pedialyte may be helpful. Advise a bland carbohydrate diet called the ***BRAT diet***: bananas, rice, applesauce, and toast with the elimination of fats and/or milk products.
2. **Medical interventions:** Antiperistaltics include Imodium A-D (Food and Drug Administration [FDA] pregnancy risk category B), a synthetic opiate that temporarily slows intestinal transit time. The dosage is 4 mg initially, with 2 mg taken after each loose stool that follows. Drowsiness is a rare side effect. Opiates may be used. (Kaopectate is an adsorbent, which has not been proven to work clinically. Stools may become more formed, but losses of water, sodium, and potassium are increased. Pepto Bismol contains a salicylate product and is contraindicated during pregnancy.[29])
3. **Persistent diarrhea** requiring parenteral hydration mandates physician **consultation.**
4. **Management of *C. difficile*–associated disease:** Consists of isolation, hydration, electrolyte correction, and discontinuance of the antibiotic. For the moderate to severe case, metronidazole, 250 to 500 mg qid for 10 days, is the drug of choice.[3]

5. **Complementary measures for diarrhea:**
   a. Some experts recommend **homeopathic** treatment for diarrhea.[144]
   b. **Nutritional suggestions:** Soups, particularly **barley** soup with a dash of **cayenne**, may be soothing to the system. Add **cinnamon,** which relieves diarrhea, to **applesauce.**[52,77] **Garlic** is antibacterial and antifungal and is thought to replenish the intestines with the normal flora while killing pathogens. A capsule or a clove may be taken tid.[21,86,125,166] Odorless supplements are available.

Hepatitis

Hepatitis is inflammation of the liver caused by viral agents hepatitis A, B, C, D, E, and G[61]; by generalized infections; or by chemical irritation such as alcoholism or long-term use of medications such as acetylsalicylic acid (ASA), rifampin, Dilantin, or isonicotinic acid hydrazide (INH).[31] In the **prodromal phase** symptoms include malaise, myalgia, arthralgia, upper respiratory tract infection (URI) symptoms, headache, photophobia, anorexia, nausea, vomiting, diarrhea, constipation, and fever >39.5° C (103.1° F). In the **icteric phase** jaundice, right upper quadrant (RUQ)/epigastric pain, dark urine, and clay-colored stool are present. On physical examination, hepatomegaly with tenderness, splenomegaly, jaundice, palatial petechiae, and arthralgia are noted, and lymphadenopathy may be detected.[158]

Laboratory Findings: The WBC count is low to normal; aspartate aminotransferase (AST) and alanine aminotransferase (ALT) levels are elevated; bilirubin and alkaline phosphatase levels are elevated; mild proteinuria and bilirubinemia (preceding jaundice) are present; prothrombin time (PT) is prolonged in severe cases; and the serologic marker is detected. At diagnosis and again at 2 and 12 weeks, ALT and AST levels, CBC, PT, bilirubin level, and albumin/globulin ratio are determined and UA is performed.[158]

ⓜ *General Management*

1. **Refer** the acutely ill woman for physician management.
2. **Anticipatory guidance:** Physician management includes isolation, supportive therapy, avoidance of hepatotoxic agents such as alcohol or medications (OCs do not need to be discontinued), and control of nausea and vomiting and pruritus.[158]
3. Hepatitis is reported to the Public Health Department.
4. Contacts are treated with immunoglobulin (Ig) (0.2 mL/kg) and vaccines if necessary.[26]

Hepatitis A (Infectious Hepatitis)

Transmission of hepatitis A virus (HAV) is oral/fecal and rarely by blood.[37] No perinatal transmission occurs.[20] Incubation period is 15 to 50 days.[26] There is no chronic form. During pregnancy, it may cause preterm labor. See p. 319 regarding breastfeeding with HAV.

Laboratory Findings: HAV antibodies are present from the onset of symptoms for 4 to 6 months.[26] IgG anti-HAV indicates previous exposure, noninfectious state, and immunity.[158] ALT and AST levels rise.[82]

Hepatitis B (Serum Hepatitis)

The severity of hepatitis B virus (HBV) ranges from undetectable—except by elevated liver function tests—to fatal, fulminant disease. Incubation ranges from 45 to 180 days. Transmission is by skin or mucus membrane exposure to infective body fluids. Infected individuals are infectious for weeks before the acute illness phase and for the duration of the illness.[26] Perinatal transmission may occur as a result of an infected birth canal; hematogenous transplacental transmission may also occur.[87] Perinatal infection causes a 90% rate of chronic carriage.[26]

Chronic active HBV is manifested by varying degrees of jaundice in 20% of infected women, as well as by amenorrhea, multiple spider nevi, acne, hirsutism, multiple system involvement, and Coombs-positive hemolytic anemia, fatigue, malaise, and anorexia.[158] Infectiousness of chronically infected individuals varies greatly.[26] One to six percent of infected adults, 40% to 70% of children, and 90% of infants become chronic carriers.[36]

Laboratory Findings: See flowchart of laboratory values for hepatitis B (Figure 7-2).

HBsAg, the test usually performed to determine whether a person is infected, detects particles from the surface of the virus and is the first antigen to appear in the bloodstream. It is positive from weeks before the onset of symptoms to months after the onset of illness, persisting indefinitely in the chronically infected. The presence of this antigen indicates that the person is infectious.[82] The interval after **HBsAg** is cleared and before **anti-HBs** appears is an infective window.[158] **Anti-HBs (HBsAb)**

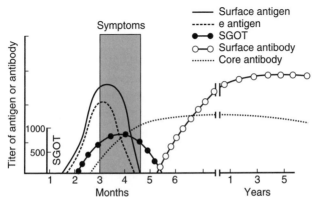

Figure 7-2 • Flowchart of laboratory values for hepatitis B. (From Stein JH, editor: *Internal medicine,* ed 4, St Louis, 1994, Mosby.)

is an antibody directed against the surface of the virus. Its presence marks complete resolution of the disease and it appears 4 to 6 weeks after exposure. A **positive HBsAg with a negative anti-HBs** indicates the chronic carrier state.[87] **Anti-HBc** (an IgG) appears at the onset of symptoms and persists indefinitely, indicating previous or chronic infection. **Anti-HBc** (an IgM) is present in high titers during acute infection. It persists in some cases of chronic hepatitis. **HBeAg** indicates ongoing viral replication, when the individual is highly contagious.[82] **Anti-HBe (HBeAb)** indicates slowed viral replication,[50] convalescence, or ongoing infection.[158]

Ⓜ Management During Pregnancy

1. **Routine prenatal labs include screening for HBsAg.**[26]
2. **Refer** the woman who is acutely ill to a physician; **consult** with the physician for a woman who has chronic hepatitis or is a carrier, depending on practice arrangement. All patients with HBV are tested for related diseases: hepatitis A, C, and HIV.[50] Interferon and antiretroviral agents may be given to shorten the duration of illness, lower the viral load, and decrease the frequency of chronic disease.[106] A hepatitis B vaccine is available, given in three doses. The woman **is monitored by means of liver function tests.**[82]

Ⓜ Management of HBSAG-Positive Mothers During Labor and Delivery

1. **Notify Pediatrics.**[82]
2. **Keep membranes intact** as long as possible.
3. **Avoid fetal skin breaks** such as that associated with fetal scalp electrode placement.
4. **Clamp the cord as soon as possible.**[50]
5. **Wait to give injections or to draw blood** until the baby has been washed.
6. Hepatitis B **immune globulin** (HBIG), 0.5 mL IM, is given to the neonate as soon as it is bathed (within 12 hours).[82] HBV **vaccine,** 0.5 mL IM, is given at the same time, in a different site, and repeated at 1 and 6 months.[26] Combined active and passive immunization prevents perinatal transmission in 85% to 95% of cases.[87]
7. **If the maternal HBsAg status is unknown,** treat the infant.
8. **Breastfeeding with HBV:** See p. 319.

Hepatitis C (Parenterally Transmitted Non-A, Non-B Hepatitis)

Hepatitis C virus (HCV) causes acute and chronic infection.[63] Sixty to seventy percent of infected individuals are asymptomatic; 20% to 30% have jaundice; and 10% to 20% have anorexia, vague abdominal discomfort, nausea, and vomiting. Rarely, the disease fulminates and is fatal. After ≥70% of adult cases, chronic hepatitis develops. Two or more decades usually go by with no symptoms. Fifteen percent of cases resolve, 26% to 50% develop chronic active hepatitis, and 8% to 62% develop cirrhosis.[120] Twenty percent develop hepatic carcinoma.[82]

Women at Risk Include: Blood transfusion recipients before 1990, hemodialysis patients, those with multiple sex partners or a history of STIs, those with a history of IV drug abuse in their lifetime, those who have sex with bisexual men, or those who have sex with hemophiliacs who received blood products before 1987.[63]

Transmission is largely parenteral.[120] Among steady sexual partners of people with HCV, 1.5% to 3% seroconvert.[63] Incubation ranges from 2 weeks to 6 months.[120] The infected person is contagious for 1 or more weeks before symptoms and remains so indefinitely.[26] **Perinatal transmission** occurs in 0% to 25% of pregnancies, depending on the maternal viral load, unless the mother is HIV-positive, when the rate is 14%.[63] Perinatal HCV infection is a chronic infection.[131] **See p. 320 regarding breastfeeding with HCV.**

Laboratory Findings: Ninety percent of patients are positive for anti-HCV within 12 weeks of onset. A quantitative HCV RNA assay (reverse-transcriptase polymerase chain reaction [RT-PCR] for HCV RNA) indicates treatment success. Infants are tested at 12 months. Earlier, maternal Ig is present.[120]

m Management

1. **Screen** at-risk women or those concerned that they have been exposed to HCV.
2. **Refer** the woman for physician management. **Anticipate guidance:** antiviral therapy (interferon alone or in combination with ribavirin, the latter contraindicated in pregnancy) may reduce viral load and prevent or slow disease progression. The woman is educated regarding transmission, safe sex practices, and maintaining liver health by receiving hepatitis A and B vaccinations and avoiding alcohol intake.[63]

Delta Hepatitis (Viral Hepatitis D)

Delta hepatitis is only present if HBV is present. It is found in the Mediterranean, North Africa, and South America and is rare in the United States except among IV drug users or patients who have received transfusions.[82]

Viral Hepatitis E (Enterically Epidemic or Fecal-Oral Transmitted Non-A, Non-B Hepatitis)

Viral hepatitis E (VHE) is rare in developed nations.[82] Transmission is oral/fecal or by contaminated water. Incubation period is 15 to 64 days. Clinical course is similar to that of HAV. No chronic or carrier form exists. Women in the third trimester of pregnancy are especially susceptible to the fulminant form, which has a death rate of 20%.[26] Mild infection increases the risk of SAB and stillbirth.[82] Sources vary regarding whether perinatal transmission occurs.

Hepatitis G ("Innocent Passenger" or "Accidental Tourist")

Discovered in 1995, two independent viral isolates, HGV and GBV-C, are present worldwide in many individuals infected with other hepatitis viruses. Transmission is by blood; the rate of perinatal transmission is 33%. Transmission may also occur as a result of organ transplantation and sexual contact.[22] It does not appear to affect the disease course of other viruses.[82]

• HEMATOLOGIC DISORDERS

Anemia

Deficiency in RBCs may be caused by hemolysis or by slow or defective production. Signs and symptoms include dizziness; headaches; weakness; shortness of breath with exertion; sore tongue; anorexia; nausea and vomiting; pica; depression; palpitations; jaundice; pallor of skin, mucus membranes, and nail beds; and spoon-shaped nails. At a hemoglobin (Hb) value ≤7.5, compensatory mechanisms may include increased stroke volume, tachycardia with or without a systolic murmur, and slight heart and liver enlargement.[134] See Figure 7-3 for a diagnostic decision tree for anemia.

The Effect of Pregnancy on Hematologic Parameters

Hemodilution or "physiologic anemia" occurs with a 50% expansion in plasma volume during pregnancy and a smaller increase in RBC mass. The increased plasma mass peaks at 24 to 28 weeks of pregnancy and then decreases, and the Hb and hematocrit (Hct) values are their lowest at 24 to 28 weeks, increasing toward term. Iron absorption increases as pregnancy advances: at 24 weeks, 36% of dietary iron is absorbed, and at 36 weeks, 66% is absorbed. The average diet (10 mg iron/d) will thus meet the demands of pregnancy.[75] Researchers have concluded that Hb values of 9g/dL for white women and 8 g/dL for black women are optimal.[70] Women with an Hb <8 g/dL have an increased risk for preterm birth and for having an infant with IUGR.[75] Box 7-5 details laboratory testing for anemia in pregnancy, testing for various types of anemia, and terms that are used to describe cells in the peripheral blood smear. See Appendix G, p. 588, for hematologic laboratory values.

Complications During Pregnancy[55]:

Increased perinatal mortality	Prematurity
Preeclampsia in the primigravida	High ratio of placental weight to
Low birthweight	infant weight (predictor of adult hypertension for the fetus)

Nutritional Deficiency Anemias

IRON DEFICIENCY ANEMIA. Occurs because of inadequate iron intake, malabsorption of iron, or excessive iron loss (genetic disorders, bone

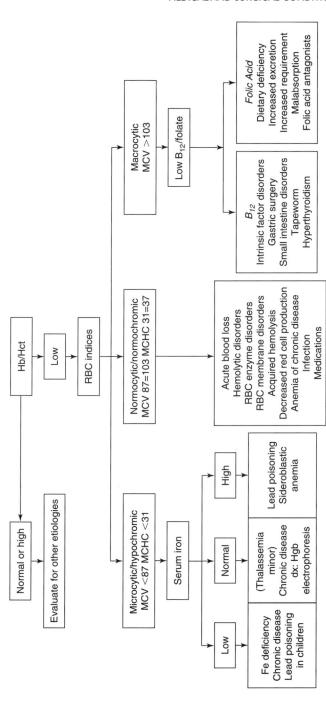

Figure 7-3 • Diagnostic decision tree for anemia. (From Payton RG, White PJ: Primary care for women: assessment of hematologic disorders, J Nurse Midwifery 40:120-136, 1995.)

• *Box 7-5 /* Laboratory Testing in Anemia—cont'd •

LABORATORY FINDINGS IN DEFICIENCY ANEMIAS

Iron Deficiency Anemia
Hb low; Hct Low; RBC indices: MCV <87; MCHC <31; RDW elevated. Presence of hemosiderin in bone marrow indicates no iron deficiency.[134] Serum ferritin reflects iron stores and is the first measure to fall with deficiency, but it also elevated with inflammation and infection, in which case a level < 60 to 100 μg is considered diagnostic of iron deficiency.[31] Serum iron falls when stores are depleted. Transferrin rises when stores are depleted, causing a low transferrin saturation level (<15%). When ferritin is <15 μg, RBCs are hypochromic and microcytic.

Folic Acid Deficiency
MCV >95 fl; serum folate ≤2.0; macrocytic hypochromic RBCs with ovalocytes; hypersegmented PMNs with lobes >3.27; vitamin B_{12} level is normal or slightly low. Leukopenia and thrombocytopenia are often present. LDH may be elevated as a result of ineffective hematopoiesis in the kidneys.[31]

Combined Iron and Folate Deficiencies
MCV normal; RBC size is measured to confirm.[31]

Vitamin B_{12} Deficiency Anemia
Early signs include low folic acid activity in plasma and neutrophil hyperseg-mentation. MCV may not reflect macrocytes if iron deficiency is present simul-taneously, but a peripheral smear may reveal some macrocytes. Nucleated erythrocytes are present; megaloblastic erythropoiesis is detected in the bone marrow. Thrombocytopenia and leukopenia develop as deficiency worsens.[55]

Pernicious Anemia
Macrocytic, hyperchromic RBCs; low RBC count; low Hb; elevated RBC indices; poikilocytosis is common.[31]

LABORATORY FINDINGS IN HEMOGLOBINOPATHIES

Sickle Cell Disease
Hb electrophoresis shows Hb S, a large quantity of fetal Hb, and the absence of Hb A.[111] Reticulocyte count and ESR are elevated. UA may show hematuria.[134]
- **Homozygous sickle cell (SS):** Almost entirely sickled Hb. Hct about 25%; reticulocyte count 20% to 40%.
- **Heterozygous sickle cell (AS):** 60% to 70% normal Hb; 30% to 40% sickled.[31]

α-Thalassemia
Hb electrophoresis at birth identifies small quantities of Bart's Hb; Hb H may be detected. Undetectable after 1 month of age. Intracellular inclusions indicat-ing Hb H may be detectable with supravital staining.[123] Microcytosis is present as a result of deficient synthesis of α-globin chains. Variations:
- **Bart's hemoglobin hydrops fetalis:** Complete absence of all α-globin chains including Hbs F, A, and A2
- **Alpha Thalassemia Minor:** RBC morphology shows microcytosis, hypochro-mia, abnormally shaped cells. Reticulocytes are present.
- **Hemoglobin H disease:** Microcytology. Intracellular inclusions in the RBCs after supravital staining. Moderate to marked anemia, decreased RBC indices, anisocytosis.[134]
- **"Silent carrier":** Microcytic anemia is present.

> • *Box 7-5* / **Laboratory Testing in Anemia—cont'd** •
>
> **β-Thalassemia**
> In β-thalassemia major, severe hypochromia and microcytosis (MCV <87; MCHC <37); fragmented poikilocytes, target cells, and large numbers of nucleated RBCs are present. Intraerythrocytic inclusions (excess α-chains, also called *basophilic stippling*) are present in the RBCs. Hb <5 g/dL. Hb electrophoresis: 75% is HbA; >3.5% is HbA2; fetal Hb is elevated in 50%. Individuals with lesser forms of the disease (β-thalassemia intermedia, minor, and minima) often have elevated levels of HbA as well. Unconjugated serum bilirubin and serum iron levels are elevated. TIBC is saturated.[123] Alternatively, diagnosis may be made by α- and β-chain synthesis or DNA probe.[31]
>
> **FINDINGS IN HEMOLYTIC ANEMIA**
> RBC, Hb, and Hct, levels are low. RBCs are normocytic and normochromic with normal indices. The reticulocyte count is elevated. Spherocytosis, elliptocytosis, or hemoglobinopathy is seen on the blood smear.
>
> **Hemoglobin C Anemia**
> 30% to 100% of RBCs are target cells. Spherocytes present.[134]
>
> **Hemoglobin E Anemia**
> Homozygous state (EE): Hb, Hct, and RBCs are slightly low; microcytosis with many target cells.[134]
>
> **G6PD Deficiency**
> RBC indices are normal. Spherocytes and poikilocytes are present. Haptoglobin level is low; LDH and bilirubin levels are elevated, and the reticulocyte count is high. Hemosiderin in the urine indicates hemolysis.[134] Gel electrophoresis confirms G6PD deficiency, and enzyme studies identify the exact deficiency.[145]
>
> ---
> NOTE: See Appendix G for normal hematology values and RBC smear terminology.

marrow damage, renal disease, neoplastic disease, chronic infection, hyperactive spleen, or bleeding from a tract or organ).[134] See Box 7-5 for laboratory findings.

Specific Complications: Pica, a symptom of nutritional deficiency, may exacerbate the deficiency by adding empty calories and binding iron in the gut.[31]

Ⓜ Management

1. **Nutritional counseling:** Teach the woman about **iron-rich foods** (Box 7-6). Advise her to add an ascorbic acid source **to enhance absorption** of nonheme iron supplements by as much as 30%. Adequate intake of vitamin A and vitamin B complex is also necessary for iron absorption.[21] Iron **absorption is inhibited** by fiber, oxalate, phytate (found in cereals, nuts, legumes, and greens), phosphates, excessive zinc and vitamin E, polyphenols (found in tea, coffee, and vegetables), and calcium.[75]

2. For the woman with a low ferritin level, **suggest oral iron supplementation** to achieve an optimal ferritin concentration for the

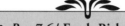

> ## • *Box 7-6 /* Foods Rich in Iron •
>
> | | |
> |---|---|
> | Dark green leafy vegetables | Egg yolks |
> | Dried fruits | Meat, including liver |
> | Legumes | Poultry |
> | Nuts | Fish, including shrimp, oysters |
> | Dark molasses | Fortified breads and cereals |

present pregnancy while maintaining stores for subsequent pregnancies. Recommended dosages vary by author, ranging from 27 to 60 mg/d[75,94a,141] to a daily dose of 200 mg of elemental iron.[55]

a. The 200-mg dose of elemental iron is reflected in these prescriptions:
   (1) Ferrous sulfate, 325 mg PO tid
   (2) Ferrous fumarate, 325 mg PO bid
   (3) Ferrous gluconate, 325 mg (two tablets tid)
   (4) Ferrous fumarate, 100 mg

b. Alternatives for women with difficulty with the above (a brand change may remedy a side effect):
   (1) Floridix iron (easily assimilated; take apart from vitamin A).[21]
   (2) Slow-Fe (sustained release preparation, reduces GI discomfort[94a]).
   (3) Ferrous sulfate in drop or elixir form.

c. **Client instructions:**
   (1) Side effects of iron supplementation may include nausea, constipation, gray or black stools, or diarrhea. Report troublesome side effects.
   (2) Ideally, take supplements with a vitamin C source, apart from meals and calcium sources, apart from the prenatal vitamin.
   (3) Keep the supplement out of the reach of children.

3. For the woman unable to tolerate oral iron, **IM Imferon is an alternative,**[55] but administration of this medication is painful, and it may stain buttocks. Imferon rarely causes rheumatologic and febrile reactions and anaphylaxis. It is contraindicated in women with autoimmune disorders.[31]

4. **Check reticulocyte count** after 4 weeks of supplementation. If no increase is seen despite patient compliance, discontinue iron supplementation and reevaluate.[55]

5. Once iron supplementation is begun, the body modifies its absorption and storage based on the new intake, and **supplementation should not be discontinued during pregnancy.**[75] After delivery, to replenish maternal supplies, **continue supplementation for 3 months** after anemia has been corrected.[55]

FOLIC ACID DEFICIENCY. Most women have folic acid deficiency but not anemia. It takes 20 weeks of a folic acid–free diet for signs and symptoms of anemia to appear.[134] Maternal stores are depleted before those of the fetus.[31] See Box 7-5 for laboratory findings.

Predisposing Factors for Folic Acid Deficiency[81,134]:

Enzyme deficiencies

Alcohol abuse

Low socioeconomic status

Adolescence

Use of folate antagonists
  (e.g., methotrexate)

Malabsorption syndromes

Anticonvulsant medications

Renal dialysis

Disorders of erythropoiesis

Malignancy

Multiple pregnancy

Multiparity

Hyperemesis gravidarum

Associated anemia

Cigarette smoking

Specific Complications: Fetal neural tube defects (NTDs) and cleft palate defects in pregnancy.[31]

m *Management*

1. **Consult** with a physician.
2. **Supplement folic acid.** Many women's diets are deficient in folate. Supplement a good diet with 400 μg and a poor diet with 800 μg to reduce NTDs by 72%.[81] If a hemolytic disorder such as sickle cell anemia or thalassemia is present, folate 5 mg PO qd may be prescribed.[31]
3. **Provide dietary counseling:** See Box 7-7 for dietary sources of folate.
4. **Complementary measures for folic acid deficiency:** Some experts recommend **homeopathic** remedies.[129]

VITAMIN B$_{12}$ DEFICIENCY. Specific symptoms of severe vitamin B$_{12}$ deficiency include paresthesia, weakness of the legs, coordination problems, visual disturbances, impairment of peripheral nerves, and permanent spinal damage. The cause may be gastric surgery, small intestine disorders, tapeworm, pregnancy, hyperthyroidism,[134] or a strict vegan diet.[172] **Pernicious anemia,** vitamin B$_{12}$ deficiency caused by a lack of

---

• *Box 7-7 / Foods Rich in Folic Acid* •

Dark green leafy vegetables	Yeast and enriched whole grains
Asparagus	Organ meats
Okra	Lean beef
Brussels sprouts	Fish
Artichokes	Legumes
Broccoli	Fresh fruit and vegetables
Chili peppers	Eggs
Orange juice	Cheese and milk

intrinsic factor, is more common in men and women older than 50 years.[134] See Box 7-5 for laboratory findings.

ⓜ *Management*

1. **Consult** a physician.
2. **Vitamin B$_{12}$** is given IM at monthly intervals.[55]

Hemoglobinopathies

SICKLE CELL ANEMIA. Sickle cell anemia is an autosomal dominant anemia in which the erythrocytes are brittle and sickle-shaped. They conform poorly to capillaries, particularly with dehydration, and hemolyze. The sickled cells sludge in the capillaries, causing tissue ischemia and infarction such as pulmonary emboli, stroke, and liver and kidney necrosis. Over time, altered perfusion through the organs affects their function. Compromise of the spleen's function results in increased incidence of infection, and women with sickle cell anemia are susceptible to pneumonia, parvovirus, and osteomyelitis. The kidneys lose their ability to concentrate urine, contributing to dehydration and acidosis, which exacerbates sludging with ischemia. Pulmonary infiltrates with fever, hypoxemia, and acidosis represent the greatest threat.[31] These episodes of increased sludging are called *crises*, and the affected individual may experience such a crisis rarely or frequently—averaging annually. See Box 7-5 for laboratory findings. The homozygous form of the disease, signs and symptoms, (almost exclusively sickled Hb) causes hemolytic anemia.[134] The heterozygous form, AS (partial sickled Hb), does not cause anemia but is associated with a kidney concentration defect. Scarring of the kidneys may increase the risk of pyelonephritis during pregnancy. Asymptomatic bacteriuria should be identified and treated aggressively in patients with the heterozygous form.[31] Sickle cell anemia occurs among 8% of American blacks. Hispanic, Mediterranean, Middle Eastern, and South Asian peoples are also at increased risk.[111]

Specific Complications in Pregnancy[31]:

SAB	Acute chest syndrome
12% stillbirth rate	IUGR caused by vascular occlusion
Preeclampsia (25%)	of the placental vascular bed
Thromboembolism	Compromised pelvic outlet
Infection (25% experience	caused by osteoporotic changes
urinary tract infections	
[UTIs])	

ⓜ *Management*

1. Offer all black patients **Hb electrophoresis** as part of their initial prenatal laboratory work.
2. The midwife may manage the woman with sickle cell trait (AS). **Refer** the patient with sickle cell anemia (SS) to an obstetrician who will probably co-manage her care with a hematologist.

3. Refer patients with sickle cell anemia (SS and AS) for **genetic counseling**. **Prenatal diagnosis** may be made by means of chorionic villus sampling (CVS) or amniocentesis.[31]

4. **Anticipatory guidance:** Physician management of the woman with sickle cell anemia (SS) includes frequent prenatal visits, iron and folic acid supplementation (5 mg daily), a high-protein, low-fat diet, lots of rest, and aggressive treatment of infections (especially asymptomatic bacteriuria).[31]

α-THALASSEMIA (INCLUDING HEMOGLOBIN H DISEASE AND BART'S HEMOGLOBIN HYDROPS FETALIS). Twenty-five percent of African Americans are α-thalassemia carriers or have the trait. Mediterranean and Asian peoples are also at increased risk.[123] Microcytosis occurs as a result of deficient synthesis of α-globin chains. See Box 7-5 for laboratory findings. α-Thalassemia occurs in four varieties of impaired Hb synthesis:

1. **"Silent carrier":** Mildest form; microcytic anemia but asymptomatic.
2. **Alpha Thalassemia Minor:** Essentially asymptomatic; splenomegaly present.
3. **Hemoglobin H disease:** More severe; unstable Hb H is formed to replace α-Hb. Hepatomegaly occurs; life expectancy is normal.
4. **Bart's hemoglobin hydrops fetalis**: Most severe form; fatal during intrauterine life or shortly after birth. Bart's Hb has such a high affinity for oxygen that it does not release the oxygen to the fetal tissues and anoxia occurs.[134]

ⓜ Management

1. **Screen** individuals of the mentioned ethnic groups.
2. **Consult** with the physician.
3. **Supplement folic acid** during pregnancy.
4. **Supplement iron for a** serum ferritin level <80 to 120 μg.[31]

β-THALASSEMIAS (COOLEY'S ANEMIA, THALASSEMIA MAJOR). β-thalassemias are seen in 40% of individuals from the Mediterranean, Africa, and some areas of Southeast Asia.[123] Hb synthesis damages the RBCs, resulting in chronic hemolysis, and ultimately, in iron overload. The iron damages the heart, liver, and endocrine organs. Transfusions, which are necessary to maintain the patient, add to iron overload. Splenomegaly occurs.[31] See Box 7-5 for laboratory findings. Many mutations exist. Four types are as follows:

1. **Thalassemia major:** Most severe form. Severe anemia manifests at 2 to 6 months of age. When untreated, erythropoietic tissues hypertrophy, causing thin bones and skeletal deformities, including a characteristic facies. Pallor, hemosiderosis, and jaundice cause a greenish brown cast to the skin. Hepatosplenomegaly, slow growth, delayed

puberty, diabetes caused by pancreatic effects, profound weakness, and CHF occur.[123] With regular transfusions and iron-chelating therapy, people with thalassemia major now live into their forties.[127]

2. **Thalassemia intermedia:** Normal growth and development with moderate anemia.
3. **Thalassemia minor:** Few if any symptoms.
4. **Thalassemia minima:** A silent carrier state.[134]

🅜 *Management*

1. **Screen** members of the mentioned ethnic groups.[31]
2. **Refer** women with thalassemia major to the physician and **consult** with the physician when managing any of the minor variations.
3. **Supplement folate** in women with thalassemia intermedia and minor. **Supplement iron** for a ferritin level of <80 to 120 µg.[31]
4. **Anticipatory management:** Physician management of the nonpregnant woman with thalassemia major includes transfusions and iron-chelating drugs, and eventually, splenectomy. Bone marrow transplants are curative.[123] The rare pregnancy in a woman with thalassemia major is managed by an obstetrician and requires close monitoring and maintenance of a Hb level of 10 g/dL.[31]

HEMOLYTIC ANEMIA. Possible etiologies include dietary deficiencies, malabsorption syndromes, metabolic disorders, hemorrhage, infection, malignancy, genetic predisposition, and immunologic defects or idiopathic etiologies.

Inherited hemolytic anemias include **spherocytosis,** a Northern European hereditary disorder characterized by hemolysis of spheroidal RBCs as they pass through the spleen; and **elliptocytosis,** an inherited disorder found in the Melanesian population. RBCs are oval or elliptical in shape, causing hemolysis with little or no anemia. Splenectomy may eventually be required for women with these conditions. **Hemoglobin C** anemia is inherited heterozygously by 2% to 3% of blacks and is usually asymptomatic in this form. Those homozygous for HbC are anemic with enlarged spleens and arthralgia. **Hemoglobin E** anemia is a mild anemia that occurs in 10% of Southeast Asian people.[134]

Chronic Renal Disease: Chronic renal disease causes a normocytic normochromic anemia because of decreased renal secretion of erythropoietin.[134] Recombinant erythropoietin may be given SQ in these cases, but hypertension is a side effect.[55]

Glucose-6-Phosphate Dehydrogenase Deficiency Anemia: G6PD deficiency anemia is an inherited RBC enzyme deficiency causing defective glucose-6-phosphatase activity that results in glycogen concentration in the liver, kidneys, and intestine. It is primarily seen among black males (10% affected); 25% of black women are carriers. Infections, surgery, and oxidant drugs are stressors that precipitate intravascular hemolysis, which varies from mild to fatal in severity. As patients grow older, the disease becomes less severe and more manageable.[123] See Box 7-5 for laboratory findings.

ⓜ Management of Hemolytic Anemia

1. **Consult** with the physician **or refer** the patient for management by a physician, depending on severity and practice arrangement. The **etiology** of the hemolysis is identified.
2. **Supplement iron and folic acid.**
3. **Provide patient education:** substances to avoid, symptoms to report, nutritional measures.
4. **Avoid administration of drugs that cause hemolysis and anemia.** See Box 7-8.
5. During pregnancy, **avoid OGTT** because it will cause severe lactic acidosis. **Treat infections** aggressively. These patients may be managed by **implementing dietary measures** including nighttime feedings by nasogastric (NG) or gastrostomy tube, frequent small feedings, or daily intake of uncooked cornstarch.[123]

Disseminated Intravascular Coagulation (Consumptive Coagulopathy)

In DIC, pathologic activation of procoagulants causes widespread activation of coagulation, resulting in platelet and coagulation factor consumption, a tendency for bleeding, fibrin buildup, and eventually, occlusion of small and midsize blood vessels causing multiorgan failure.[100] Renal failure, adult respiratory distress syndrome (ARDS), and microangiopathic hemolysis occurs. Thirty to fifty percent of DIC cases occur with gram-negative sepsis. Other common causes include cancer, trauma, vascular disorders (e.g., aortic aneurysm), reactions to toxins, and immunologic disorders (e.g., anaphylaxis). Obstetric etiologies include placental abruption, fetal death and delayed delivery, amniotic fluid embolism, septicemia,[55] saline-induced therapeutic abortion,[31] and preeclampsia.[100] See Box 7-9 for laboratory findings.

ⓜ Management

1. The midwife promptly **consults** the physician for management.
2. **Anticipatory guidance:** Physician management includes treatment of the underlying cause, often including facilitation of delivery. Vigorous volume expansion is used to treat persistent intravascular coagulation.[55] Heparin may be administered.[100] Fresh frozen plasma, cryoprecipitate, and/or platelet concentrate are administered to correct coagulation deficiencies.[69]

Idiopathic Thrombocytopenia Purpura

Idiopathic thrombocytopenia purpura (ITP) results from immune sensitization of platelets caused by drugs, viral infection, or a disturbed immune function disorder.[134] Antibodies target platelet membranes,

• *Box 7-8 / Drugs That Should Be Avoided Because They Precipitate Hemolysis in Women With G6PD Deficiency* •

Antimalarials

Primaquine
Parnaquine
Pentaquine
Plasmaquine

Sulfonamides

Kynex
Azulfidine
Sulfanilamide
sulfisoxazole
(Gantrisin)
sulfapyridine

Nitrofurans

Furadantin
Furoxone
Alta fur

Antipyretics and analgesics

Headache and cold remedies,
including phenacetin and
acetanilid (666, APC, Super
Ana Hist)
Anacin
Empirin
Aminopyrine
P-Amino salicylic acid
Bromo-seltzer
Aspirin in large doses
Stan back
Antipyrine

Miscellaneous Drugs and Chemicals

Methorexate (chemotherapy)
Acetylphenylhydrazine
Naphthalene mothballs (paradichlochlorobenzine
mothballs are safe)
Probenecid
Tolbutamide
Methylene blue
IV Berocca C
Black drought and other senna preparations
Vitamin K/H$_2$O solution analogue (Synkayvite
and Hykinone are safe)

removing platelets from the circulation in the spleen.[134] IgG also crosses the placenta during pregnancy and may destroy fetal platelets.[31]

• IMMUNOLOGIC DISORDERS

The Immunologic System

The body's immunologic system is composed of innate immunity (the protection provided by WBCs, the skin and stomach lining, and other compounds in the blood that destroy organisms and toxins) and acquired immunity (antibodies or humoral immunity, and sensitized lymphocytes or cellular immunity).

Immunoglobulins or Antibodies: "Humoral Immunity"

IgM: 10% of the body's Ig. Predominates in the early primary immune response. It carries ABO antibodies, is formed during blood transfusion reactions, and activates complement.

IgG: 75% of circulating Ig. The only Ig that crosses the placenta; fetal level equals mother's; protects the fetus from diseases to which mother is immune. Production escalates exponentially when a second exposure to an antigen occurs.

IgA: 10% to 15% of circulating Ig. Most abundant antibody. Present in high concentrations in colostrum. It lines and protects the baby's gut; may prevent allergies.

IgE: Called reagin. Activated when there is exposure to allergens and parasitic infection.

IgD: Function unknown; secreted in small amounts.[161]

T-Cells: "Cell-Mediated" Immunity

Human leukocyte antigen (HLA) binds to antigen cell surfaces and displays them to T cells. A T cell antigen receptor (TcR) on the T cell's surface then binds to a small antigenic fragment on the HLA molecule.[68] T cells protect against viruses, parasites, grafts, and slow-acting bacteria.

• *Box 7-9* / Laboratory Findings in Disseminated Intravascular Coagulation[100] •

Hypofibrinogenemia (approximately 100 mg/dL)	Schistocytosis
Presence of fibrin split products	Abnormal factors V and VIII
Lengthened PT, PTT, thrombin time	Thrombocytopenia
Leukocytosis	Abnormal thrombin time
Reticulocytosis	Low antithrombin III

Function begins in hours to days. Found in the thymus gland, T cells last a lifetime. Seventy-five percent of the T cells are called **helper T cells,** and they secrete **lymphokines,** which act on immune and bone marrow cells. It is helper T cells that are affected in acquired immunodeficiency syndrome (AIDS). Lymphokines stimulate growth and production of **killer T cells** and **suppressor T cells** (interleukins 2, 4, and 5) and stimulate **B-cell** growth and differentiation into plasma cells and Ig.[139]

Pregnancy and the Immune System

Nonspecific immunity is increased during pregnancy (more WBCs and enhanced phagocytosis). However, in the reproductive tract, phagocytosis is diminished by increase corticosteroid concentrations. This effect is especially true for gram-negative organisms and may explain the vulnerability of pregnancy women to disseminated gonococcal (GC) infection. Serum complement is elevated beginning at 11 weeks' gestation, enhancing chemotaxis and Ig stimulation of phagocytosis, but some of the proteins in the system are decreased, possibly delaying the role of complement in the immune response. This delay may be protective for the fetus.

To protect the fetus, the trophoblast presents minimal expression of the antigen major histocompatibility on its surface. Natural killer (NK) cells that respond to foreign cells without antigen recognition are suppressed, possibly explaining the vulnerability of pregnant women to *Listeria* and *Toxoplasma* infections. Locally, cytokines are secreted by the conceptus into the reproductive tract, protecting the fetus from NK cells while not endangering the overall immunity of the mother. All Ig levels are decreased by 15% to 32%, possibly by hemodilution. T-cell function is suppressed by alteration of the ratio of helper to suppressor T cells, improving arthritis in pregnant women but also resulting in increased vulnerability to viral infections.[139]

Human Immunodeficiency Virus (Acquired Immunodeficiency Syndrome)

HIV is a retrovirus that eliminates helper T cells. Two types have been identified, HIV-1 and HIV-2. HIV-2 appears to be less virulent.[26] HIV-1 is found worldwide and is most prevalent in the Americas and Europe; HIV-2 is prevalent in West Africa only.[168] Weeks to months after exposure to HIV, a self-limited 2-week-long mononucleosis-like syndrome called *the acute retroviral syndrome* occurs. During this time, the viral load is very high. Seroconversion begins the clinically latent period, occurring 8 days to 10 weeks after the initial illness. After 6 to 9 mo, the body stabilizes the viral load at an individualized level called the viral *set point*. A lower set point is a positive prognostic finding. Triple HIV drug therapy within the first 90 days lowers the set point. No symptoms may occur for months to years.[104] Box 7-10 lists the laboratory tests related to HIV and discusses their interpretation.

• *Box 7-10 /* **Laboratory Findings Related to Human Immunodeficiency Virus** •

FOR THE DIAGNOSIS OF HIV
- **Enzyme-Immunosorbent Assay (EIA):** Detects HIV at 3 to 4 wk. Approaches 99% in sensitivity and specificity. False-positive results are seen with laboratory errors, among multiparous women, after multiple blood transfusions, after recent influenza or hepatitis vaccines, with autoimmune disease, and others.
- **Western blot or an IFA:** Used to confirm the EIA. If inconclusive, repeat in 2 wk.
- **Referse transcriptase-polymerase chain reaction test RT-PCR test (HIV RNA RT-PCR):** Recommended if HIV-1 antibody test result is negative, yet the concern for HIV exposure remains high.
- **The Home Access HIV-1 Test System:** A home collection test is now available over the counter.

Diagnosis of HIV in Newborns
- **HIV RNA RT-PCR test:** Generally used within 24 hr of birth (sensitivity 93%).
- **HIV peripheral blood mononuclear cell (PBMC) culture:** Also recommended (McLaren & Imberg, 1998).

MONITORING OF HIV TREATMENT
- **CD4 or T4 helper cell count:** Immune cells depleted in HIV infection. <500 cells/mm^3 is abnormally low; <200 is diagnostic of AIDS in the HIV-positive individual. Highly variable, however, laboratory to laboratory, from concomitant illnesses, and time of day, varying from 50 to 300 cells/mm^3.
- **Percentage of lymphocytes that are CD4 cells:** More consistent marker. ≥0% is normal; ≤14% indicates severe immunologic suppression.
- **Viral load or burden:** Best indicator of disease progression. <10,000 copies/mL indicates low risk for disease progression; 10,000 to 100,000 indicates moderate risk; and >100,000 copies/mL indicates high risk for disease progression.[168]

In time, AIDS-related complex (ARC) appears with constitutional symptoms including lymphadenopathy, anorexia, chronic diarrhea, weight loss, fever, and fatigue. A diagnosis of AIDS is made when the CD4$^+$ cell count is <200/mm^3; when the CD4$^+$ T-lymphocyte percentage of total lymphocytes is <14%; or when an opportunistic infection, cancer, or another condition (wasting syndrome, HIV dementia, sensory neuropathy) occurs.[26] Women who are HIV-positive experience more genitourinary (GU) infections and have 5 times the risk of cervical neoplasia.[104]

Factors That Increase Transmission[26,79,104]:

High viral load	Uncircumcised male
More virulent HIV strain	Traumatic sex
STI in either partner (especially ulcerative)	Sex during menses
	Cervical ectopy

Factors That Increase Vertical Transmission[1,43,104,149]:

Virulent HIV strain	Disruption of fetal skin/mucus membrane
High maternal viral load	
Maternal drug use and cigarette smoking	AIDS diagnosis during pregnancy or up to 2 weeks after delivery

Severe prenatal anemia	Presence of other STIs
Rupture of membranes (ROM) >4 hours	Premature delivery
	Birthweight <2500 g
Chorioamnionitis and/or funisitis	Maternal vitamin A deficiency
Increased fetal "susceptibility"	

The Approximate Risk Per Episode of Exposure:

Receptive penile-anal sexual exposure	0.1%-0.2%
Receptive penile-vaginal intercourse	0.1%-0.2%
Contamination of intact skin	<0.1%
Mucous membrane exposure to infected saliva	<0.1%
Reception of a unit of HIV-contaminated blood	95%
IV needle or syringe exposure	0.67%
Percutaneous needlestick exposure	0.4%[37] (greater with deep injury, visible blood on the injuring device, and when the device had been in the infected person's blood vessel[168])

Risk of vertical transmission	
In the untreated woman	13%-30%
With AZT prophylaxis	5%-8%
With AZT prophylaxis and cesarean delivery	2%

NOTE: The risk of exposure to vaginal fluids or amniotic fluid is unknown.[104] The risk of receptive oral exposure is unknown, but transmission has been reported. Tears and urine are noninfectious.[37]

Pharmacologic Therapy

The HAART (Highly Active Antiretroviral Therapy) Regimen: Reduces viral load, maintains immune function, decreases risks of viral resistance and drug toxicity, and delays progression to AIDS. Side effects may reduce quality of life, drug regimen is inconvenient, drug resistance may limit future drug choices, long-term drug toxicity is unknown, and duration of effectiveness is unknown.[104]

Nucleoside Analogs (Nucleoside Reverse-Transcriptase Inhibitors): Inhibit reverse-transcriptase, an enzyme necessary for viral reproduction; prevent viral spread but do not eradicate virus.[159]

Protease Inhibitors: Act against HIV protease, making virus noninfectious.[159] Must be taken at specific times with dietary restrictions. Interact with many drugs.[104]

Non-Nucleoside Reverse-Transcriptase Inhibitors: Taken with nucleoside analogs and protease inhibitors. Alter the activity of reverse-transcriptase in a different way than nucleoside transcriptase inhibitors. Efavirenz is teratogenic and contraindicated in pregnancy.[159]

Interleukin-2: Bolsters immune response; regulates lymphocyte production.[168]

Hydroxyurea: Antineoplastic drug, teratogenic, contraindicated in pregnancy.[159]

m *Management of Well Women in Regard to HIV*

1. **Counsel all women regarding HIV risk factors** and risk reduction strategies, and then **offer testing with informed consent.**[6] The

woman at risk for recent exposure to HIV who **reports signs and symptoms of the acute retroviral syndrome** is again offered testing.

2. **Offer sexual postexposure prophylaxis** to the woman who has been exposed, making referrals as necessary.[104]

Care of the HIV-Positive Woman

1. Guard the woman's **confidentiality.**

2. **Consult** a physician and co-manage the early stages of HIV infection. As the disease advances, medical **referral** is necessary. Care is ideally **family-oriented** with social work support.[104]

3. **Report** HIV to the **health department.** Sexual contacts are notified.[104]

4. **Counsel regarding lifestyle measures:** Advise the woman to take precautions when caring for pets, handling food, and traveling to avoid contracting infections. Discuss the effects of smoking cigarettes, drinking alcohol, and using illicit drugs on one's immunity, general health, and judgment.[104] Review measures to protect contacts.

5. Solicit **symptom history** and observe for physical signs of disease progression or opportunistic infection. **Screen** regularly for **vaginal, cervical, and sexually transmitted infections (STIs).**[104]

6. When the HIV diagnosis is made, perform two **Pap tests,** 6 months apart. If findings are normal, repeat annually.[36]

7. **Refer** the woman with noncervical **genital ulcers** to a gynecologist.[104]

8. Perform a **purified protein derivative (PPD) test for TB and dual-anergy imaging annually.**[104]

9. **Vaccines: Pneumonia prophylaxis** every 3 years; the woman serology-negative for hepatitis B and at risk for exposure is given **hepatitis B vaccine**[104]**; influenza vaccine** (unless pregnant, see p. 369, number 10.)[159]

10. **Counsel regarding reproductive choices.**[6]

HIV and Pregnancy: In 1998 in New York State, 0.13% (1 in 769) women giving birth were HIV-positive; in New York City, this number was 0.71% (1 in 141).[159] Pregnancy does not exacerbate HIV progression, and pregnant women are medically managed in the same way as nonpregnancy women.[104] Perinatal transmission is increased with higher viral loads, but there is no safe lower level. The goal of treatment for the pregnant woman is to have <1000 copies/mL at delivery to minimize transmission.[159] Neonates who are infected vertically are more likely to be born prematurely, to be small for gestational age, and to have a smaller head circumference.[1] Failure to thrive, inherited immunodeficiencies, and other childhood health problems are seen.[26] In one study, 21% of infected neonates died at a median age of 27.6 months.[1]

ⓜ Management During Pregnancy

PRENATAL CARE

1. **Counsel and screen** all pregnant women as discussed above. **Co-manage** or **refer** to the physician, depending on severity of the disease.

2. The **initial laboratory workup** for the HIV-positive pregnant patient includes CD4$^+$ T-cell profile, quantitative HIV RNA, baseline liver and kidney studies (serum glutamate pyruvate transaminase [SGPT] and creatinine levels), hepatitis B and C panels, a PPD test, and urine toxicology.[104]

3. **Avoid invasive procedures** whenever possible to decrease perinatal transmission.[104] For the woman at risk for HIV, delay invasive procedures until HIV test results have been obtained.

4. Order an **early ultrasound examination for dating** to facilitate C/S at 38 weeks to reduce perinatal transmission.[159]

5. In the initial **assessment of** the HIV-positive pregnant patient, include questions regarding any **symptoms** of the disease **and any side effects or toxicity of treatments**. Observe for symptoms and physical **signs of disease progression** or the **presence of opportunistic infection**.[104]

6. The medical consultant offers **combination antiretroviral drug therapy** to treat the disease and reduce vertical transmission (long-term effects on the fetus are unknown).[159] The HIV-positive woman who declines combination drug therapy is evaluated and offered **azidothymidine (AZT) therapy** to prevent perinatal transmission.[6] She is counseled that AZT therapy reduces the risk of perinatal transmission from approximately 25% to 5% to 8% without known negative long-term effects for the baby.[53] Dosage: 100 mg zidovudine (ZDV) 5 times/d initiated at 14 to 34 weeks of gestation and continued through pregnancy.[38] The woman is confidentially registered with the CDC's registry for antiretroviral use during pregnancy at: Registrar, Antiretroviral Pregnancy Registry, PO Box 12700, Research Triangle Park, NC 27709-2700. Phone: (800)722-9292, ext 58465 or (919) 315-8465; Fax (919) 315-8981.

7. The woman who has a CD4$^+$ count of >500 cells/mm^3 is seen at **routine intervals for prenatal care.** Should signs of an opportunistic infection or advancing disease occur, she is seen biweekly or weekly.[104]

8. **Fetal surveillance:** A side effect of AZT therapy is bone marrow suppression with resultant fetal hydrops. Consider ordering an ultrasound examination each trimester. At 32 weeks' gestation, the woman with advanced disease begins fetal movement counting and biophysical profiles (BPPs).[104]

9. **Ongoing laboratory studies:**
   a. CD4$^+$ and HIV RNA every 2 to 3 months
   b. Women with CD4 >500 cells/mm^3: T-cell subsets and the viral load repeated each trimester
   c. Women receiving antiretroviral agents: monthly CBC with differential and platelets, SGPT, and creatinine to evaluate for toxicity.[104]

10. **Vaccines:** Give as above after the first trimester. The **influenza vaccine is contraindicated** in pregnant HIV-positive women because it may cause a transient rise in the viral load.[159]

11. **Counsel regarding good nutrition and fluid intake.** Deficiencies in protein and calories, zinc, calcium, magnesium, vitamins B_6, B_{12}, C, A, E, and β-carotene are seen in women with AIDS.[81] Vitamin A deficiency, which increases perinatal transmission, is addressed with supplementation and/or dietary measures.[149] Water intake is especially important for women taking indinavir (Crixivan) because nephrolithiasis is a side effect.[159]

12. Suggest **iron supplementation** because nucleoside analogues such as AZT cause bone marrow suppression.[159]

INTRAPARTUM CARE

1. **Scheduled C/S reduces the risk of perinatal transmission,** whether or not the mother is receiving AZT therapy. Once labor begins or the membranes rupture, it is unknown how long the benefit of C/S remains. The advantage is greatest for the mother with a high viral load; no benefit has been shown for women with a viral load of <1000 copies/mL of plasma. Perinatal transmission drops from the untreated 25%, to 5% to 8% with AZT, to approximately 2% with scheduled cesarean delivery. Maternal morbidity is, of course, greater with C/S. If the woman accepts C/S, it is scheduled at 38 weeks without amniocentesis for lung maturity testing.[17] **AZT** prophylaxis, when accepted by the mother, is administered 3 hours before surgery (dosage noted as follows).[159]

2. The physician may offer **Viramune** to reduce perinatal transmission.[159] Viramune is a non-nucleoside reverse-transcriptase inhibitor that has been used successfully in Africa; 200 mg is given to the mother at the onset of labor, and 2 mg/kg is given to the neonate within 72 hours of birth. Perinatal transmission is reduced by nearly 50% in a breastfeeding population.[80]

FOR THE WOMAN WHO CHOOSES TO DELIVER VAGINALLY

1. **Medications:** On admission to L&D, **continue administration of combination antiretrovirals** throughout labor. **AZT** is administered IV to the woman who accepts: 2 mg/kg over 1 hour, followed by 1 mg/kg/h throughout labor; administration is stopped when the cord is cut.[159]

2. **Maintain intact membranes** for as long as possible. Should spontaneous rupture of membranes occur, facilitate delivery to minimize fetal exposure. **Maintain the baby's skin integrity:** Avoid placement of fetal scalp electrodes, scalp sampling, and forceps or vacuum extraction delivery. After delivery, **handle the baby gently,** including while suctioning the nasopharynx. **Bathe** the baby to remove maternal body fluids as soon as the temperature is stable–before skin is punctured to obtain blood for glucose measurements or the vitamin K injection.[104]

POSTPARTUM CARE

1. See p. 319 regarding transmission of HIV by **breastfeeding** and related recommendations.
2. **Medications:** Combination antiretroviral therapy is continued until the 6-week examination when the CD4+ count and viral load are reevaluated. Stress the need for the woman to **continue her health care**.
3. In **reviewing newborn care**, teach the HIV-positive mother to avoid chewing the baby's fingernails or toenails, prechewing food, or sharing toothbrushes. Good handwashing is stressed. Any weeping lesion on the mother is covered. The mother can hold, kiss, and cuddle the baby and change the baby's diapers without gloves.[104]
4. The medical consultant will **address contraception.** Certain protease inhibitors—nelfinavir, ritonavir, rifabutin, and rifampin—diminish the effectiveness of OCs.
5. **Medication for the infant:** If the mother has accepted the therapy, Pediatrics will order AZT syrup for the first 6 weeks of life, beginning at 8 to 12 hours of life.[38]

m *Management of the Exposed Health Care Worker*

See the CDC's Internet home page at *http://www.cdc.gov* for up-to-date information on recommendations for post-exposure prophylaxis (PEP), or call the National Clinician's Postexposure Hotline at (888) 448-4911 and the HIV Postexposure Prophylaxis Registry at (888) 737-4448.

Systemic Lupus Erythematosus and Pregnancy

A chronic autoimmune disease, SLE does not affect fertility, although stillbirth, IUGR, and prematurity occur at an increased rate,[105] as do preeclampsia, hypertension, DM, and UTI.[99] Women may or may not have exacerbations of SLE during pregnancy and postpartum. The patient with well-controlled SLE is less likely to experience increased flares during pregnancy. A flare is manifested by hypertension and edema and must be differentiated from preeclampsia.[31] Pregnancy does not change the long-term prognosis of women with SLE.[69]

Diagnosis: The antinuclear antibody (ANA) reflects the presence of autoantibodies but is not specific for SLE.[112] Anticardiolipin antibodies, lupus anticoagulant antibodies, and a false-positive VDRL test result may be present.[69] A falling complement level or an elevated level of complement split products is diagnostic of an SLE flare.[99]

m *Management*

1. **Refer** the woman with SLE to an obstetrician who will co-manage her with an internist/rheumatologist to monitor for flares.
2. **Anticipatory management:** Management may include corticosteroids, nonsteroidal antiinflammatory drugs (NSAIDs), heparinization for treatment of antiphospholipid antibodies, early detection and

treatment of fetal cardiac complications, and fetal surveillance from 26 weeks' gestation on.[99] Route of delivery is determined according to obstetric indications. Whether the woman may breastfeed depends on maternal drug therapy.[31] Infants of women with SLE should be evaluated for heartblock that resolves spontaneously at 8 to 9 months.[99]

Antiphospholipid Antibody Syndrome

Thirty to forty percent of women with SLE have **antiphospholipid antibodies**, including anticardiolipin (ACA) and lupus anticoagulant antibodies (LA). Antiphospholipid antibodies may also appear as an isolated serologic finding. These antibodies cause recurrent venous or arterial thromboses and/or thrombocytopenia.[105]

ACA: High levels of this antibody against phospholipid are correlated with fetal distress or death.[31]

LA: Present in 5% to 18% of women with SLE, LA is an Ig inhibitor of coagulation that prolongs partial thromboplastin time (PTT), paradoxically causing thrombosis. In pregnancy, prostaglandin (PGI_2) production is inhibited, causing decreased invasion of the myometrium by the placental spiral arteries. It is associated with recurrent SAB, fetal death, and IUGR.[31]

ⓜ Management

1. **Screen** women with the following[55]:

   Recurrent SAB

   Unexplained second- or third-trimester loss

   Unexplained IUGR

   Early-onset severe preeclampsia

   False-positive VDRL test result

   History of deep venous thrombosis or pulmonary embolism

   Unexplained thrombocytopenia

   Prolonged coagulation studies

   Autoimmune or connective tissue disease

   Positive autoantibody test results

2. **Refer** the woman with ACA and/or LA to the obstetrician.

3. **Anticipatory guidance:** A combination of steroids, heparin, and/or low-dose aspirin may be used to treat affected women with variable success.[23]

• INFECTIOUS DISEASES

Cytomegalovirus

Infection with human (β) herpesvirus 5 (human cytomegalovirus [CMV]) causes no symptoms in many adults, though 15% exhibit a mononucleosis-like syndrome.[55] Transmission is by mucosal contact with body fluids. An infected person may shed CMV episodically for years. The incubation period is 3 to 12 weeks. There is no immunization or postinfection immunity.[26]

In the mother, a fourfold rise in the CMV-specific IgM antibody level confirms primary infection (single measurement is not meaningful, because 50% of adults carry the antibody). In primary infections, 4% of fetuses are affected; in recurrent cases, 0.19% to 1.5%.[62] In 5% to 10% of affected infants, cytomegalic inclusion disease develops. Intrauterine death may result; survivors may manifest microcephaly, mental retardation, motor disabilities, hearing loss, liver disease,[26] and learning disabilities.[62] Fetal infection is diagnosed sonographically[43] or by identification of the virus and IgM by amniocentesis or cordocentesis. Periodic ultrasound examination **monitors growth, calcifications, and other manifestations.**[62] The fetal heart rate tracing may show a true sinusoidal rhythm as a result of severe anemia.[121] Postnatal infection (less serious; no sequelae) may occur when the mother is shedding the virus in cervical secretions at delivery or when virus is present in breastmilk.[26] See p. 319 regarding breastfeeding by mothers with CMV.

Lyme Disease

Infection with *Borrelia burgdorferi* occurs through the bite of an infected tick.[66] In 50% to 70% of infected individuals, a lesion, called *erythema migrans* ("bulls-eye lesion"), is seen at the site 3 to 36 days later. The lesion begins as macules or papules and spreads to form red patches of erythema with a central papule of erythema, scales, or hyperpigmentation averaging 15 cm in diameter. A rash occurring in the first 2 days after a bite is an allergic reaction and not Lyme disease.[64] Fever, malaise, fatigue, headache, slightly stiff neck, jaw discomfort, chills, regional lymphadenopathy, and/or splenomegaly may also be experienced (stage 1). Without treatment, these symptoms may disappear or they may come and go for weeks. The infection disseminates in 2 to 12 weeks, causing arthralgia, myalgia, skin lesions, carditis, headache, stiff neck, photophobia, meningitis, and central nervous system changes (stage 2). Alternately, a patient may be asymptomatic during stage 2. The disease becomes chronic (stage 3) 6 weeks to 2 years after the bite. Some chronic carriers are asymptomatic; others have rheumatic, dermatologic, or neurologic manifestations. Although morbidity is extensive, the mortality rate is low.[112] Immunity is not conferred with infection.[66]

Lyme Disease During Pregnancy: There is no risk to the fetus of the woman who is seropositive but asymptomatic. Vertical transmission has been reported in the symptomatic patient,[64] but no syndrome of congenital anomalies is associated.[152]

Diagnosis: Laboratory diagnosis is made by indirect fluorescent assay (IFA) or ELISA for IgG and IgM anti-*B. burgdorferi* antibodies and confirmed by Western blot analysis, although the latter may not be positive for months. Seroconversion is prevented with early treatment. Lyme tick identification and analysis may also be done.[112]

🄜 *Management*

1. **Educate all women to** avoid tick exposure and observe bite sites for the bulls-eye lesion.[66]
2. **Refer to or consult** with the physician according to severity and practice arrangement.
3. **Advise removal of a tick** within 18 to 24 hours to prevent infection.[66] Use tweezers, and grasping the head, pull straight away until it releases its hold. Do not squeeze while pulling, or the spirochete may be injected into the patient. Complete removal of mouth parts is not necessary. Apply antiseptic to any remaining parts, and observe the site for rash.[117]
4. The woman who is **asymptomatic but serologically positive** requires no treatment.[64] For **early infection in the nonpregnant woman,** prescribe doxycycline (100 mg PO bid for 10 to 21 days) or ampicillin (500 mg PO tid for 10 to 21 days).[158] **During pregnancy,** give oral amoxicillin (500 mg PO for 21 days) or penicillin for 3 to 4 weeks. For penicillin-allergic women, give cefuroxime or erythromycin (250 mg PO qid for 10 to 21 days).[55,66]
5. See p. 321 regarding **breastfeeding** during maternal Lyme infection.

Mononucleosis

Mononucleosis is an acute infection with the Epstein-Barr virus (EBV), a herpes virus, and is common in young people 10 to 35 years of age. The disease is spread by oropharyngeal secretions from an infected person, and rarely, by blood transfusion. Viral shedding may continue for months after the acute illness. The woman may be asymptomatic or may develop a fatal infection manifested by fever, pharyngitis, malaise, headache, nausea and vomiting, myalgia, and jaundice. Chest pain or dyspnea accompany cardiac involvement; and photophobia, nuchal rigidity, or neuritis may signal CNS involvement. On examination, generalized lymphadenopathy (particularly the posterior cervical chain), erythematous pharynx and/or tonsils with or without exudate, palatial petechiae, palpebral edema, maculopapular or petechial rash, jaundice, hepatosplenomegaly, or nuchal rigidity may be seen.[158] An antibody to the EBV nuclear antigen may be detected 3 to 4 weeks after symptom onset. Pregnancy outcome is usually normal, although the risk of SAB and stillbirth is increased and there are unconfirmed reports of cardiac anomalies and cataracts.[31] The virus is not associated with complications during lactation.[97]

Toxoplasmosis

Toxoplasma gondii is an intracellular protozoan acquired by cats who have eaten infected birds or rodents or have contacted the feces of infected cats. The sexual stage of the life cycle of the protozoan occurs only in the feline intestine, and then the cat excretes the oocytes in the feces for 10 to 20 days. Feces are infectious after exposure to air for 1 to 5 days. In moist soil, feces remain infectious for about a year. Humans are infected by exposure to oocytes in dirty sandboxes or playgrounds where cats have defecated; by consumption of inadequately cooked meat, especially pork or mutton; by ingestion of water contaminated with cat feces; by consumption of milk from infected animals; by organ transplantation or transfusion; and hematogenously through the placenta. The incubation period is 5 to 23 days.[26] Immunity is conferred with infection. The presence of the specific IgM and/or rising IgG titers in infants identifies the disease. IgM antibody levels may persist for years.[55]

The infection may present without symptoms, as isolated lymphadenopathy, or with mononucleosis-like symptoms including fever, lymphadenopathy, and lymphocytosis that persist for days or weeks. During pregnancy, the infection crosses the placenta, causing congenital disease in about 50% of maternal cases. The likelihood of intrauterine infection increases with gestation: 10% of first-trimester fetuses are affected, though the manifestations are serious (CNS and liver affected; may cause death), whereas 60% of third-trimester fetuses are affected, though with milder disease.[43] A 1994 study, however, found that of 27 affected liveborn babies, all were symptom-free with normal neurologic development at 15 to 71 months of age.[27]

ⓜ Management

1. **Educate all pregnant women** to thoroughly cook meat and carefully cleanse hands and kitchen after handling raw meat. Frozen meat is still infective. Unless the pregnant woman is known to have antibodies to *T. gondii*, she should avoid changing cat litter boxes and contacting unfamiliar cats who may eat rodents. Litter boxes should be changed daily and disinfected, without shaking and dispersing oocytes. Cats are ideally well-fed inside cats. The pregnant woman should wear gloves when working in the garden and wash hands thoroughly afterward. Wash hands thoroughly before eating. Protect areas such as sandboxes from stray cats.[26]

2. **Refer to or consult** with the physician as appropriate, depending on the severity of the case and the practice arrangement.

3. **Anticipatory guidance:** When **fetal infection** is documented, the parents are referred for **genetic counseling.**[43] **Percutaneous umbilical sampling (PUBS)** may be used to **identify affected fetuses** and to direct management. Specific treatment is indicated for organ involvement.[26] Spiramycin decreases vertical infection but does not diminish the severity of fetal disease if it does occur.[55]

4. Toxoplasmosis is not a contraindication for **breastfeeding.**[97]

• MENTAL HEALTH AND SOCIAL ISSUES

Depression

A major depressive episode must be distinguished from "the blues," a time-limited normal life experience.[171] Depression may cause changes in appetite and body weight, sleep disorders, impaired self-care, failure to follow prenatal guidelines, and suicidality.[73] Lifetime incidence in women is 21%.[171] (See postpartum depression, p. 238.)

Predisposing Factors[95,171]:

Previous depression
Lack of social support
Stressful life events
Family history of depression
  or bipolar disorder

Personal or family history
  of suicide attempts
Medical illness or medications
Sleep deprivation

Diagnosis: Five or more of the following symptoms, including one of the first two, must be present for at least 2 weeks to make the diagnosis of depression: depressed mood for most of the day nearly every day, inability to sleep or excessive sleep, weight gain or loss, decreased appetite, fatigue, feelings of worthlessness or guilt, psychomotor agitation or retardation, inability to concentrate or make decisions, markedly diminished interest and pleasure in activities for most of the day nearly every day, or recurrent thoughts of death and/or suicide.[171]

ⓜ Management

1. **Rule out underlying medical illnesses.**[171]
2. **Refer** the woman who is depressed for psychological management.
3. **Anticipatory guidance: Nonpharmacologic therapies** include cognitive or interpersonal therapy, light therapy, sleep deprivation (for bipolar disorder), patient and family education. The **suicidal** woman may require hospitalization.[171] **Pharmacologic intervention** is made during pregnancy after the risks and benefits have been weighed. The mother's willingness to tolerate her depressive symptoms, vulnerability of other children in the home, and the possibility of worsening depression are taken into account.[73] Risks of pharmacologic treatment to the fetus include teratogenic risks, potential long-term neurobehavioral sequelae (long-term data are not currently available), and neonatal toxicity at birth. **Prozac** (a selective serotonin reuptake inhibitor) has been used extensively during pregnancy, and some tricyclic antidepressants may be used. Monoamine oxidase (MAO) inhibitors and other antidepressants are not recommended during pregnancy.[4]

Domestic Abuse

Domestic abuse occurs because there is an imbalance of power in a relationship resulting in coercion. It may involve hitting, pushing, throwing objects, forced sexual intercourse, verbal threats, depriving the woman of her reproductive and contraceptive choices, economic abuse, isolation, and intimidation.[151] During pregnancy the rate of domestic abuse is 0.9% to 65%.[56]

Signs of Domestic Abuse

Signs that a woman is the victim of domestic abuse include low self-esteem; trusting, passive, traditional behavior; social withdrawal; financial dependence; feeling of being trapped; fear of retaliation if located by perpetrator after leaving; depression; anxiety; suicidal ideation; insomnia; poor impulse control; substance abuse; multiple emergency department visits for minor burns, broken bones, or bruises; multiple injuries at various stages of healing[163]; chronic abdominal or pelvic pain; GI and GU problems; headaches; and chest pain.[14,137]

Effects on Pregnancy

The effects of domestic abuse on pregnancy include increased risk for late prenatal care,[71] unplanned and undesired pregnancy, closely spaced pregnancies, poor obstetric history, substance abuse, SAB, first- or second-trimester bleeding, anemia, poor weight gain, IUGR, cervicitis and vaginitis,[56] preterm labor, pyelonephritis, cesarean delivery, and trauma caused by falls and physical violence.[45]

Screening

Despite caregivers' discomfort with asking the questions for fear of offending the client, time constraints, or powerlessness to treat, women appreciate universal screening.[10] An abuse assessment screen is recommended for all women receiving prenatal care. One researcher suggests asking the following questions: (1) Within the last year, have you been hit, slapped, kicked, or otherwise physically hurt by someone? (2) Since you have been pregnant, have you been hit, slapped, kicked, or otherwise physically hurt by someone? and (3) Within the last year, has anyone forced you to have sexual contact?[56]

Sexual Abuse Survivors

Twelve to forty percent of women have experienced childhood sexual abuse. Women experience variable sequelae after childhood sexual abuse, depending in part on age at the time of abuse, frequency and duration of abuse, the use of force, the number of perpetrators, and whether the abuser was a biologic parent.[9] Sequelae of childhood sexual abuse may include diminished self-esteem, depression, eating disorders, substance abuse, suicidal behavior, dissociative disorder, anxiety, posttraumatic stress disorder,[150] lowered pain threshold, chronic headaches, GI, GU, musculoskeletal, and respiratory problems, addictions, and victimization as an adult (multiple sexual partners, STIs, unintended pregnancies).[9]

Pregnancy—being a physical, emotional, sexual, and spiritual experience—may bring up many related issues for a woman who has been sexually abused. Loss of control over her body, nakedness, exposure of the genitals, insertion of hands and/or instruments into the vagina, vaginal pain, lack of trust in her caregiver, the helplessness, pain, and lack of control and knowledge that may come with giving birth, and being the "patient" with health care providers who may be perceived as "authority figures" all simulate the abuse situation. A rekindling of the stress may occur, manifesting as intrusive reliving of the event, autonomic symptoms, or numbing and avoidance efforts (such as substance abuse, dissociation, or phobic reactions).[150] The woman may try desperately to be in control of the birthing situation, she may labor dysfunctionally—more often requiring epidural anesthesia and C/S. She may feel anger toward the infant who has "caused" vaginal trauma, bleeding, pain, and anxiety. Breastfeeding may be difficult because of bodily shame, discomfort in touching of the breasts, and fear of sexual arousal.[90]

Women who have been sexually abused want to be asked about it and about how the abuse is currently affecting them.[150] Failing to ask reinforces the survivor's belief that the abuse should not be talked about; that it is unimportant and should not be affecting her anymore. The question should be natural, the experience normalized by stating its frequency, and the woman should have control over the disclosure's timing and depth.[9]

Legal Responsibilities of the Health Care Provider

Health care providers may be held liable if they fail to ask whether a woman has been abused; if they accept an implausible explanation of injuries; if they report an abusive situation to the police without the woman's permission, endangering her; or if they fail to give appropriate referrals and information to women who have been identified as victims of domestic violence.[128]

🅜 Management

1. Provide **privacy and safety** in the office.[137] Privately **screen all women** for domestic and sexual abuse. Document denial.[113]
2. Offer nonjudgmental support. **Believe** the woman, **acknowledge** the trauma, and **affirm her and her courage in making the disclosure.** Be aware, and emphasize to her, that when the woman has revealed her story to you, the most important step—a courageous step—toward the end of the violent situation has been taken. **Destigmatize** the problem as one experienced by many others.[132]
3. **Safety** is the priority in caring for these women.[150] **Assess** danger; involvement of children; substance abuse by both partners; access to weapons; and threats that have been made.[137]
4. Assess **suicide** risk. Once the woman has a plan for the method of suicide, the situation is urgent.[137] Refer her to mental health specialists immediately and document.[113]

5. Provide **information and referrals and document.** The Legal Assistance Foundation will give her legal help regardless of whether she has funds or speaks English. Provide her with written literature with a list of local shelters. Suggest support groups.[56]

6. **Document** the history and physical examination, date and time of the examination, and time elapsed since the abuse.[5] Record all details of the abuse by using a body map and words to document current and past injuries and whether wound are consistent with injuries described. Document clinics, EDs, or physicians the woman reports having visited.[56] Document the woman's own words in quotes or use "pt states" as she names the abuser, describes the abuse, pain, and days taken off work because of abuse. Take pictures of current injuries if the woman signs a consent form.[113] Describe the woman's demeanor. Avoid using legal terms such as *alleged perpetrator* or phrases such as "patient claims" that imply doubt. Avoid charting conclusions such as "domestic violence" or "rape," which imply facts not in evidence and are inadmissible in court.[5]

7. Make a **follow-up** appointment in a few weeks, which is to be kept whether or not things are better.[56]

8. Care of the **sexually abused woman** during pregnancy:

   a. Develop an **egalitarian nonjudgmental relationship** with the client.[150] Give her control during procedures by discussing them ahead of time, encouraging her to make them easier by inviting a support person, allowing her to control the pace, increasing her visualization with a mirror, or having her place her hand over yours during an examination.[9]

   b. In preparing for birth, discuss previous health care experiences that may have an impact. **Normalize** her distress by discussing the likelihood of these issues surfacing during delivery. Discuss her **perceptions and fears** regarding birth and intrapartum procedures. Come to clear understandings and commitments regarding intrapartum care. Encourage her to bring any objects that will increase her sense of **control** (such as her own clothes). **Touch may be a boundary violation;** discuss her comfort with touch before labor. **Birth itself may be experienced as a violation** for this woman. Discuss differences between birth and the abuse experience.[150]

Women With Eating Disorders

Anorexia is the most common eating disorder in adolescent girls. Characteristics include avoidance of any fattening foods and other eating restrictions, interposed with binge eating and compulsive exercising. Psychologic factors may include a distorted body image, fear of maturity, control and independence issues, family obesity, and psychological issues. Treatment for anorexia includes nutritional, psychological, and medical support including hospitalization if the woman is in crisis.[115]

Bulimia is binge eating and induced vomiting.[119] Excessive use of laxatives—**purging**—may be part of the disorder. Eating disorders are very difficult to treat. Denial and minimization are experienced at a high level among these women.[101] In one study of 530 pregnant women, 4.9% reported an eating disorder.[165]

Physical Signs and Symptoms of Eating Disorders

General Appearance: Overweight or underweight; cachectic; easily fatigued; poor posture; muscle weakness, flaccidity, and tenderness

Affect: Listless, apathetic, inattentive, irritable

Skin: Rough, scaly, greasy, pale, pigmented, bruised with petechiae, darkness over cheeks and under eyes

Eyes: Pale conjunctiva, eyelids red or dry with redness or fissures at corners, dull cornea

Mouth: Lips dry and scaly with lesions at the corners; oral mucous membranes spongy and friable with receding gums; swollen scarlet tongue with hypertrophic or atrophic papillae; missing teeth

Hair: Dull, stringy, thin, brittle, easily plucked

Thyroid: Enlarged

Trunk: Tachycardia, cardiomegaly, hypertension, chest deformity at diaphragm, prominent scapulae

Abdomen: Hepatomegaly or splenomegaly with indigestion and diarrhea

Extremities: Paresthesia of hands; spoon-shaped, brittle, ridged nails; edema of legs; calf tenderness and tingling; decreased ankle and knee reflexes.[172]

Obstetric Complications

The woman with an eating disorder is at increased risk for the following obstetric complications[101]:

Low or excessive weight gain
SAB
Vaginal bleeding
Lower birthweights
Lower Apgar scores
Hypertension
Preeclampsia

Breech births
Instrumental and
  cesarean deliveries
Perinatal death
Fetal cleft palate
Developmental delays in offspring
Epilepsy in offspring

Management

1. **Screen** for the presence of eating disorders. Assess nonjudgmentally and with care and empathy.
2. **Display reading materials** in the office—introducing the subject as one of concern.
3. For the pregnant woman, as soon as possible attempt to **make the fetus "real"** for the woman to increase her bonding and motivation

to consider the needs of the fetus. Methods include sharing FHTs, fetal movement, and ultrasonic imaging.

4. **Refer** the woman **to a mental health care provider specializing in eating disorders**.
5. In the **postpartum period, screen the woman** for bonding with her infant, for infant feeding practices, and for depression.[101]
6. **Alert Pediatrics** to the mother's disorder, so that appropriate supervision and guidance can be provided to the woman in regard to feeding the child.

• NEUROLOGIC DISORDERS

Epilepsy and Pregnancy

Epilepsy causes decreased fertility in both men and women. Women with this seizure disorder are 85% as fertile as their healthy counterparts.[69] Fifty percent of women with epilepsy experience a change in the frequency of seizures during pregnancy.[55] Patients who experience more frequent seizures are generally the patients whose epilepsy will worsen with pregnancy. Changes in digestion and metabolism of medications, in other medications including dietary supplements, in compliance, and in sleep quantity make seizure control more difficult. Physician management includes close monitoring of drug levels.[69]

These mothers experience more preeclampsia, preterm and cesarean delivery and are more likely to have low birthweight (LBW) infants or infants with cerebral palsy, congenital anomalies, seizures, or mental retardation. The risk of perinatal death is increased. Epileptic drugs are teratogenic folate antagonists; and seizures cause hypoxia, which also causes anomalies (the latter being more dangerous). Dilantin (phenytoin), Tridione (trimethadione), and carbamazepine are associated with syndromes of growth deficiencies, a characteristic facies, and mental deficiencies.[55]

Headache

The International Headache Society has identified three classifications of headaches:

1. the tension headache due to tension in head and neck muscles;
2. the vascular headache (migraine and cluster); and
3. the organic headache (indicative of pathologic conditions such as tumors or intracranial bleeding).[24]

Headache Characteristics That Indicate Intracranial Pathology[78]:

"The worst headache of my life"
A change in a chronic headache pattern
Onset after trauma
Onset after age of 40 years

During exertion

Awakening the woman

Accompanying neurologic symptoms

Age >50 years with tenderness over temporal arteries

Any physical abnormality including neck stiffness, hypertension

Reassuring Signs That Indicate the Absence of Intracranial Pathology: Previous identical headaches, normal findings on neurologic examination, normal vital signs, supple neck, and improvement in the headache(s).[24]

Headaches and Pregnancy

Pregnancy tends to have a beneficial affect on headaches in 70% patients with migraine, particularly in the second and third trimesters for those women whose headaches are generally exacerbated by menses. Some women will experience migraines throughout pregnancy. Others have their first migraine during pregnancy. Tension headaches are likely to continue throughout pregnancy.[99]

m *Management*

1. **Refer or consult** with the physician as appropriate, depending on the headache's severity and the practice arrangement. Refer the patient who exhibits signs of a headache with intracranial pathology.
2. Advise the patient to begin by keeping a **"headache diary."** For 1 or 2 months, diet, menses, and any trigger events are recorded. Note patterns.[15,24,99]
3. Consider alternatives to any **medications** that may be causing the headaches. Advise the woman to make **lifestyle changes** that may prevent headaches: Avoid food triggers. Exercise to relieve stress, improve sleep, and release endorphins. Consider stressors and how they might be altered. Seek psychotherapy if necessary. Drink plenty of water. Stick to a routine with sleep and meals. Try relaxation techniques such as biofeedback, massage, meditation.[15] Hypnosis or acupuncture may prove helpful.[24]
4. **Tension headaches** may be treated with topical heat or cold; topical analgesic balms may be applied to affected muscles. Analgesics, muscle relaxants, anxiolytic medications, and trigger-point injection may ameliorate an acute episode. Antidepressants may be used with relief in the long-term.[24]
5. **Migraine headaches** may be improved by applying pressure to the affected side of the head or by taking aspirin or acetaminophen.[15] Sleep or rest in a dark room or application of cold may relieve a vascular headache.[24]
6. **A physician may prescribe pharmacologic interventions** that are prophylactic or abortive.
7. **See complementary measures, p. 33.**

• PULMONARY DISEASE

Asthma During Pregnancy

Asthma is airway hyperresponsiveness and inflammation[108] and may improve, worsen, or stay the same during pregnancy. Severe asthma is more likely to worsen with pregnancy than is mild asthma. Symptoms generally worsen between the twenty-ninth and thirty-sixth weeks of pregnancy. Labor and delivery are generally not associated with the worsening of asthma. Most women revert to their prepregnancy asthma baseline by 3 months postpartum.[147] Severe asthma is associated with prematurity and LBW.[31] During pregnancy, it is widely accepted that the risk to the fetus from untreated asthma is greater than the risk to a fetus from asthma medications.[31]

Ⓜ *Management During Pregnancy*

1. Patients with chronic asthma may not notice subtle respiratory compromise, although it is enough to affect the fetus. The **pregnant woman** with moderate to severe asthma may be asked to test and record her **peak flow every 12 hours.** These values are compared with her baseline values, and **medications need to be altered if the readings fall 20% to 30% below the baseline. Immediate medical attention is required if the readings fall 50% below the baseline.**[110]
2. **Carefully date** the pregnancy and obtain a baseline sonogram because of the **increased risk of IUGR.**
3. **When ordering commonly used drugs consider the following: Magnesium sulfate is indicated for preterm labor,** rather than terbutaline with its cardiorespiratory side effects. **Use fentanyl rather than morphine and meperidine** during labor, because the latter two can cause bronchospasm. **Avoid prostaglandin preparations** for induction and postpartum bleeding because they may cause bronchospasm. If administration of prostaglandin preparations is unavoidable, precede it with methylprednisolone 60 to 80 mg IV.[110]
4. **Complementary measures:** Some experts recommend **homeopathic** remedies for asthma.[129]

Fifth Disease (Erythema Infectiosum or Human Parvovirus B19 infection)

The fifth childhood rash to be described in the medical literature, fifth disease is a mild, usually nonfebrile disease. About 50% of U.S. adults have serologic evidence of past infection. It is characterized by an erythema that gives a slapped-face appearance. A lace-like rash may also appear on the trunk and extremities; it fades and then may reappear for 1 to 3 weeks more after exposure to the sun or a warm bath.[26] Malaise, lymphadenopathy, pruritus, and URI may occur.[121] In adults, arthralgias and arthritis may persist for months after the infection. The disease is communicable 5 to 10 days before the rash develops and is probably not communicable once the rash is present. It is spread by respiratory droplets, hand-to-mouth transfer, vertically from mother to fetus, and rarely, through blood products.[62] The transplacental transmission rate is 33%.[55] Infection does confer immunity. The incubation period is 4 to 14 days.[62] Infection during the first half of pregnancy is associated with a 10% risk of fetal anemia with hydrops and a 10% risk of fetal death.[26] Midpregnancy infection is associated with an approximate 12% fetal loss.[55] Fewer than 1% of the fetuses infected in the latter half of pregnancy are affected. Those who survive do not have sequelae. Parvovirus-specific IgM antibodies are present in serum on the third day of the infection and persist for 30 to 60 days. IgG antibodies are detectable on the seventh day of illness. If they are present in the absence of IgM, they indicate immunity.[62] The maternal α-fetoprotein (AFP) level usually rises with infection.[140]

Respiratory Tract Infection

Viral rhinitis, the "common cold," is caused by more than 200 viruses. Symptoms include inflammation of the nasal mucosa with rhinorrhea, nasal congestion, sneezing, sore throat, nonproductive cough, headache, fever, malaise, myalgia, hoarseness, and lymphadenopathy.[158] Transmission is by airborne droplets. Colds are contagious for the first 2 to 3 days; 38% of household contacts will become infected. The incubation period is 1 to 3 days.[62]

Pharyngitis causes the symptoms of viral rhinitis, as well as mild erythema of the pharyngeal mucosa; tonsillar exudate; and vesicles on tonsils, uvula, and palate (also on palms and soles of feet with Coxsackie virus). Bacterial pharyngitis, usually caused by **Group A β-hemolytic streptococci** (GABHS), presents with the same symptoms but with a sudden onset, enlarged cervical nodes, malaise, edema of tonsils and pharyngeal mucosa, palatial petechiae, abdominal pain, and a generalized scarlatiniform rash. A throat culture is positive for bacteria (negative for viral pharyngitis). Pharyngitis is transmitted by respiratory secretions. GABHS pharyngitis is additionally transmitted by contaminated foods. The person with GABHS pharyngitis is infectious for 2 to 3 weeks and noninfectious after 24 hours of treatment with penicillin. Incubation is 1 to 3 days. GABHS pharyngitis is reportable, and isolation is required for the 24 hours of treatment. **Gonorrheal** pharyngitis manifests with symptoms similar to those of GABHS pharyngitis.[26,158]

Acute bronchitis is the presence of a cough without pneumonia, sinusitis, or other respiratory disease. **Pneumonia** is infection of the pulmonary alveoli. **Atypical pneumonia** is infectious and has an insidious onset, with the symptoms of viral rhinitis and pharyngitis, as well as cough and fever. **Pyogenic pneumonia** is noncommunicable and has a rapid onset. The findings on lung examination may be normal, or may show diffuse adventitious sounds, focal rales, or dullness to percussion if consolidation is present. If the patient has hypoxemia, tachypnea and retractions may occur. If fever and abnormal breath sounds are present, a chest x-ray film should be obtained to rule out pneumonia.[98] Sputum may be sent for Gram staining and culture, but in 50% of cases the organism is not identified.[109]

Influenza is a systemic viral infection that may exacerbate preexisting bronchitis or asthma.[89] It is infectious from respiratory secretions 24 hours before to 7 days after onset, and incubation is 1 to 5 days. Ten to twenty percent of individuals become infected after exposure.[62] CBC shows leukopenia; nasal secretions may be cultured or tested for antigen within 72 hours of onset; chest x-ray film may show bronchitis or pneumonia.[158] Influenza is particularly dangerous for pregnant women in the second and third trimesters, and immunization is recommended (in Oct and Nov) for all those who will be in those trimesters during influenza season (Dec-Mar). The HIV-positive pregnant woman is the exception, because the influenza vaccine transiently increases the viral load.[159] Transplacental infection is rare.[62]

m *Management*

1. Recommend **influenza immunization** as suggested above.
2. For **mild disease,** advise rest; increased intake of fluids; use of a steam vaporizer; warm saline gargles tid; and cough suppression with over-the-counter (OTC) preparations containing dextromethorphan, diphenhydramine, or codeine (with proper precautions). Encourage the woman to stop smoking and support cessation. Educate her regarding preventing transmission by covering mouth, handwashing, etc. Acetaminophen is advised for fever, *not* ASA (contraindicated in pregnancy and predisposing to Reye's syndrome). Topical nasal sprays are suggested for *no more* than 3 to 5 days to prevent rebound nasal edema.[158] The woman with influenza or GABHS pharyngitis is isolated. Antibiotics are not prescribed unless pneumonia is suspected.[98]

   Regarding the use of antihistamines in pregnancy: Avoid antihistamines during the first trimester. Chlor-Trimeton (chlorpheniramine maleate) and Benadryl (diphenhydramine hydrochloride) are generally safe during pregnancy when used sparingly. Zyrtec (cetirizine), Claritin (loratadine), and Allegra (fexofenadine) have not been adequately tested for safety during pregnancy and must definitely be avoided in the first trimester. In rare cases, routine use of Benadryl and hydroxyzine during pregnancy has resulted in neonatal withdrawal. Benadryl taken with Restoril may cause stillbirth. Retrolental fibroplasia occurs more frequently in premature infants whose mothers were using first-generation antihistamines during the last 2 weeks of pregnancy; this has not been observed in term infants.[28]
3. When **gonorrheal pharyngitis** is diagnosed, see p. 430 for treatment, report the disease, and advise treatment of contacts.

4. **Consult with or refer** to the physician, depending on the severity of the illness and the practice arrangement. Consult for recurrent infections, for peritonsillar abscess, for the patient who is unable to swallow, and patients with comorbidities—including smoking.[109]
5. **Complementary measures**:
   a. The experts suggest many **homeopathic** remedies for URI.[54,129,144,155,167]
   b. **Acupuncture** may be used to relieve cough and chest congestion.[30]
   c. **Herbs: Chamomile,** used in a facial steam, will relieve rhinitis, or as a gargle relieves a sore throat.* **Echinacea** is an immune system stimulant that prevents colds. Because it is antimicrobial and antiviral, this herb is especially effective for URIs.[†] Echinacea may be given in the form of tea (1 to 2 tsp root simmered in 1 cup water for 10 to 15 minutes) tid or as tincture 1 to 4 mL tid.[86] **Garlic** is antiviral, antibacterial, antifungal, and diaphoretic; and it is a pulmonary antiseptic. It is secreted largely through the lungs and so is particularly effective for infections of the lungs, colds, and flu.[‡] A clove or a garlic capsule (to eliminate odor) may be taken tid as a preventative or once an infection is present.[86] **Ginger** is antiinflammatory and antipyretic and can be used for URI.[86,94a,103,115,125] See notes regarding the safety of ginger during pregnancy on p. 40. **See information on herbs, p. 563.**

Rubella (German Measles)

Infection with the rubella virus causes a mild, febrile viral disease with a diffuse punctate and maculopapular rash in 50% of individuals. Children often have few constitutional symptoms; adults usually have 1 to 5 days of low-grade fever, headache, malaise, rhinitis, conjunctivitis, and arthralgia. Rubella is infectious for a week before and at least 4 days after the rash appears. Transmission is by droplet.[26] The incubation period is 16 to 18 days. Twenty percent of pregnant women are susceptible to rubella.[62] Laboratory findings are a fourfold rise in the specific antibody titer between acute and convalescent phases or the presence of a rubella-specific IgM indicating recent infection. Serum is tested 7 to 10 days after the onset of illness and repeated 2 to 3 weeks later.[26]

Congenital rubella syndrome occurs in 85% of those fetuses infected before 9 weeks' gestation and 52% of those infected during weeks 9 to 12; it rarely occurs in those infected after week 16.[62] Infection during the first trimester may result in SAB; intrauterine death; or major malformations of the eyes, ears, brain, and heart.[55]

---

*References 86, 93, 103, 125, 136.
[†]References 21, 77, 86, 93, 103, 115, 125, 126, 129, 136, 166.
[‡]References 21, 86, 103, 125, 126, 136, 166.

ⓜ Management

1. **Report** the infection to the local health authority.[26]
2. **Immunoglobulin,** given after exposure in pregnancy, may modify the severity of the infection. Immunoglobulin has been given in large doses (20 mL) to women who have been exposed and would not consider an abortion, but the value of this practice has not been confirmed.[26]
3. **Refer** the woman who has contracted rubella in early pregnancy to a genetic counselor **regarding the risk to her fetus.**
4. **Rubella vaccine:** If they are not immune, women planning to marry, postpartum women, and health care workers should all receive the vaccine. Pregnant women are screened for the presence of rubella antibodies. Women known to be pregnant are not vaccinated because of theoretical concerns, and women are urged not to conceive for 3 months after receiving the vaccine. In one study, however, the infants of 200 women inadvertently immunized shortly before conception or during the first trimester showed no congenital defects.[26] Breastfeeding is not contraindicated after vaccination.

Tuberculosis

TB is infection with *Mycobacterium tuberculosis* complex. Mycobacteria enter the respiratory system via airborne droplets and implant in a respiratory bronchiole or alveolus. The bacilli divide slowly; their lack of toxins fails to stimulate an immediate response in the host. The organisms grow for 4 to 12 weeks, until they reach a number sufficient to elicit a cellular immune response. Granulomas form that limit multiplication and spread of the organism but do not eradicate it. This primary complex is usually not visible on a chest x-ray film. It is usually detected by the PPD skin test. At this point, the individual has **latent TB** and is not contagious. No symptoms are present.[18]

TB becomes active when bacilli multiply and the resulting immune response destroys host tissue.[109] Symptoms of active TB include fever (in 37% to 80%), anorexia, weight loss, night sweats, malaise, fatigue, chills, cough persisting ≥3 weeks (initially nonproductive and then productive of sputum), and, rarely, hemoptysis. Rales may be heard in the involved area. Approximately 10% of all healthy untreated persons with latent infection will develop active disease, usually within 2 years. HIV-positive people have an annual 10% or greater risk of the disease becoming active. In rare cases the disease disseminates throughout the body. Acid-fast bacilli in stained sputum or other body fluid smears, confirmed by identification of the organism by culture though negative acid-fast smears, do not exclude TB. Chest x-ray findings include pulmonary infiltrates, cavitation, and fibrosis.[26]

TB During Pregnancy: Pregnancy does not alter the course of TB. Congenital TB occurs rarely when transmission occurs by fetal aspiration of infected amniotic fluid or by hematogenous spread.[154]

High-risk Groups:
- Country of origin: Asia, Africa, the Caribbean, and Latin America
- Institutional risk: Correctional institutions, nursing homes, homeless shelters, drug treatment centers
- Substance abuse risk: Drug-injecting persons; alcoholics
- Illness-related risk: HIV seropositivity, diabetes, cancers, severe kidney disease, other medical illnesses
- Other risks: Contact with of an infected person; elderly persons, or children <4 years[18,40]

Skin Testing: Mantoux test or purified protein derivative (PPD) test: The **PPD test** is the injection of 0.1 cc Mantoux PPD just below the surface of the skin of the inner forearm, creating a wheal 6 to 10 mm in diameter. The result is read 48 to 72 hours later. Results are interpreted according to the risk of the population.[35] **Pregnancy** does not alter the PPD result, as was once thought, and the fetus is not affected by the PPD.[154]

ⓜ Management

1. **Screen all pregnant women** for TB with the **PPD** test.[35]
2. **Consult with or refer** to the physician when a woman has a positive PPD test result or when TB is suspected, depending on severity and practice arrangement.
3. **Anticipatory guidance:** Active TB is ruled out by **chest x-ray** and **sputum smear and culture for acid-fast bacillus (AFB)**. The **pregnant woman with a positive PPD** test result has a chest x-ray with the abdomen shielded in the second trimester.[35]
4. Report TB to the **local health authority** and give further care in consultation with these experts.[18] Care may include **isolation,** treatment of **contacts,** and **preventive treatment** to prevent progression to active disease (isoniazid and rifampin). The likelihood of disease progression before delivery determines whether INH administration is begun during pregnancy. In general, it is delayed until after delivery.[35] If a woman receiving medication becomes pregnant, she should continue use of the medications, but when possible, streptomycin, pyrazinamide, or ethionamide should be discontinued. INH, rifampin, and ethambutol can be used during pregnancy without concern regarding teratogenicity.[154] Women who have been treated for latent TB are educated regarding the symptoms of active disease in the unlikely event that the disease progresses.[109]

For information on **TB and its treatment during breastfeeding,** see p. 320.

Varicella (Chickenpox)

Varicella is infection with human α-herpesvirus 3 (varicella-zoster virus).[26] Symptoms are fever, chills, arthralgia, and myalgia, followed in a few days by the outbreak of macules that change to fluid-filled pruritic vesicles within hours. The rash begins on the head and neck and spreads to the trunk and extremities; vesicles break open and then crust over. The vesicles occur in successive crops, so that there are lesions of varying maturity at any given time. Vesicles are monocular and collapse on puncture. They are more abundant on covered areas of the body but may be so few in number that they are unnoticed. Potential complications include pneumonia, encephalitis, and postherpetic neuralgia.[124] The virus may become latent in the skin ganglia and later reactivate as shingles (herpes zoster).[26]

Varicella is transmitted by droplet spread of secretions or vertically. It is communicable from 2 days before the vesicles appear until all lesions have crusted over.[62] The incubation period is commonly 3 to 17 days. Infection confers immunity,[26] and about 80% of adults unaware of having had varicella are immune when tested.[156] Laboratory studies include visualization of the virus by electron microscope (EM), isolation of the virus in cell cultures, detection of viral antigen in smears with fluorescent antibody, identification of viral DNA by PCR, and measurement of serum antibodies.[26]

Varicella Infection During Pregnancy

Approximately 10% of pregnant women are nonimmune. In early pregnancy, varicella infection is associated with a 2% risk of a congenital varicella syndrome[62] manifested by brain, eye, and bone deformities; hydronephrosis; and cutaneous scars.[169] Varicella infection is also associated with a 50% fatality rate.[156] Near term, preterm labor may occur.[26] Maternal infection in the 5 days before and 3 days after delivery results in neonatal varicella infection in 20% of cases, with a 30% to 50% neonatal mortality rate.[156]

Ⓜ Management

1. **Consult with or refer to** a physician as appropriate, depending on severity and practice arrangement.
2. Varicella infection is a **reportable** disease in some states.[26]
3. Women who are **exposed during the first 20 weeks of pregnancy** and are uncertain of their varicella status are given varicella-zoster immune globulin (VZIG) and are tested for immunity. Within 96 hours, give **VZIG,** which modifies or prevents disease.[43] Treat the **woman in whom varicella infection develops** with mild analgesics and antipyretics. **Refer** her to the physician for acyclovir if she has a high fever, extensive rash, or pulmonary symptoms. **Anticipatory guidance:** The physician may use ultrasound examination and PUBS to identify fetal infection. Identification of the viral genome in the amniotic fluid does not mean that the infant has been affected.[43]
4. For the **woman at 20 weeks or more gestation but not expected to give birth within 10 days,** treat as described previously, except that the ultrasound examination and PUBS are unnecessary. The fetus receives passive immunity from the mother. Tocolysis may be necessary.[169]

5. For the **woman at term who may deliver within 6 days, notify Pediatrics.** Give VZIG to the mother. The infant receives VZIG at birth. The mother in whom varicella infection develops just before delivery is isolated from her infant. She should pump her breasts, and the milk may be given to the baby; transmission does not occur through the milk.[97] Fifty percent of these infants will not develop varicella infection. The mother can commence breastfeeding when her lesions are crusted over. The other 50% of infants develop varicella infection within 16 days. They can move into the room with their mothers, and infant and mother are isolated together.[142] Thirty percent of infants die from pneumonia and disseminated disease in this circumstance.[26]

6. For **maternal varicella infection within 72 hours postpartum,** mother and baby should receive VZIG.[142]

7. For the **mother and/or baby exposed after 72 hours postpartum,** test mother for serologic immunity. As the breastfeeding mother develops antibodies, she passes them to the infant, preventing infection or at least ensuring a mild course for the infant.[97] Treat the infant of the nonimmune mother, or the bottlefed infant, with VZIG.[169]

8. **Varicella immunization** is 97% effective.[123] Offer the vaccine during preconception counseling or postpartum. Advise the woman to avoid pregnancy for 3 months after receiving the vaccine.[169]

• URINARY TRACT DISORDERS

Effect of Pregnancy on Normal Renal Function

Kidney volume increases by 30% as a result of hypertrophy during pregnancy. The physiologic hydronephrosis of pregnancy (dilation of the renal collecting system) is probably hormonally mediated. Mechanical blockage of the ureter at the pelvic brim increases pressure in tubules above the pelvic brim. Smooth muscle relaxation contributes to increased vesicoureteral reflux. Because of the increased cardiac output and decreased peripheral (and thus renal) vascular resistance that occurs in pregnancy, the glomerular filtration rate (GFR) increases by 50% in normal pregnancy, beginning as early as the fifth week of gestation. Blood urea nitrogen (BUN), serum creatinine, and serum uric acid levels are lower in early pregnancy and rise toward the end of gestation. Glucosuria occurs commonly as the glucose load is increased, and the tubules are inefficient in reabsorbing glucose.[31]

Urinary Tract Infection

UTI is infection of one or more parts of the urinary tract and includes asymptomatic bacteriuria, cystitis, and pyelonephritis. Bacteria may ascend through the urethra to the bladder or through the ureters to the kidneys, enter by the hematogenous route (rare), or by the lymphatic channels that connect the bowel and the urinary tract.[83] Box 7-11 lists the laboratory findings related to UTI.

Predisposing Factors for UTI[138]:

Previous UTI	Frequent intercourse
Pregnancy	Decreased urethral resistance
Vulvovaginitis	of the postmenopausal urethra
Urethral diverticula	Mechanical obstruction (renal
Poor hygiene	calculi, urethral stricture)
Urethral catheterization	Systemic factors such as DM,
Infrequent or incomplete	sickle cell trait, or cystic
emptying of bladder	renal disease

Signs and Symptoms:

- **Asymptomatic bacteriuria:** Bacteria in the urine in the absence of symptoms.
- **Cystitis:** Infection of the bladder characterized by dysuria, urgency, frequency, voiding in small amounts, nocturia, suprapubic abdominal pain with or without hematuria, and incontinence.[83]
- **Pyelonephritis:** This infection of the upper urinary tract occurs more commonly in the second half of gestation and is often abrupt in onset. The patient may have a fever (as high as 42° C) or hypothermia (as low as 34° C). Fifteen percent of women with acute pyelonephritis also have bacteremia.[55] Fever, chills, flank pain and tenderness, nausea and vomiting, dehydration, tachycardia, and cystitis symptoms are present. Unilateral or bilateral costovertebral angle tenderness is present. In the pregnant woman, preterm labor[138] and fetal tachycardia may occur.[20]

UTI and Pregnancy: Pregnancy enhances the progression of asymptomatic bacteriuria to symptomatic UTI.[47] Maternal UTI during pregnancy is associated with preterm birth, premature rupture of membranes (PROM), fetal death, low Apgar scores, mental retardation, IUGR, and—when the UTI results in endotoxemia—cerebral palsy.[72]

ⓜ *Management*

IN THE NONPREGNANT WOMAN
1. **Prescribe antibiotics:**
   a. Macrodantin (nitrofurantoin), 100 mg qid PO for 7 days (if not G6PD-deficient) *OR*
   b. Azogantrisin (sulfisoxazole), 2 g stat then 1 g qid for 10 to 14 days[83] *OR*
   c. Ampicillin, 500 mg PO q6h, for 7 to 10 days if sensitive by culture only (many organisms are resistant)[60]
   d. Gabbe et al[69] suggest a 3-day course of antibiotics, saving longer courses for persistent cases: Keflex (cephalexin), 250 mg PO qid for 3 days; Macrobid (nitrofurantoin macrocrystals) 100 mg PO bid for 3 days; Gantrisin, 2 g for 1 dose then 1 g qid PO for 3 days;

• *Box 7-11 /* Urinary Laboratory Studies •

URINALYSIS

- **Appearance:** Color reflects concentration; turbidity in acidic urine indicates crystallization or precipitation of urates; in alkaline urine, phosphates. Although this precipitation may occur in the bladder, it more often forms as the specimen cools after voiding.
- **Specific gravity** or osmolality: Higher value indicates greater concentration.
- **Urobilinogen:** Not present in normal urine. Bilirubin is converted by colonic bacteria to urobilinogen, which is then excreted in the feces or urine.
- **Glucose:** Not present in normal urine. During pregnancy, mild glucosuria is seen with normal blood sugar levels as a result of decreased renal threshold.
- **Protein:** Not present in normal urine.
- **Hemoglobin:** Not present in normal urine.
- **Ketones:** End products of fatty acid metabolism; make urine acidic.
- **Leukocyte esterase:** Detects neutrophil granulocytes. Positive value indicates >10 leukocytes/mm^3.
- **Urinary nitrate:** Reflects bacterial reduction of urinary nitrate to nitrite, best tested in first morning void. Certain bacteria will not be reflected by this test.
- **Microscopy:** Examination for WBCs (indicating inflammation), RBCs, epithelial cells, casts, and bacteria.
- **Casts** (cylindrically shaped protein masses that form in renal tubules, reflecting high protein, low flow in tubules, and acidic pH): Red, white, and tubular epithelial cells may be trapped in a cast, as well as Hb, myoglobin, hemosiderin, or other substances. As the cells disintegrate, they may be described as simply "granular." WBC casts indicate inflammation of tubules; RBC casts reflect glomerular damage; mixed or granular casts may reflect a combination. Clear casts may be present in small numbers in normal specimens.[145]

CYSTITIS LABORATORY FINDINGS: Bacteriuria, pyuria, RBCs, nitrites.[169]

PYURIA: Five or more WBCs in a high-power field. Pyuria with RBCs and bacteriuria suggests an infection. Pyuria without bacteriuria suggests inflammation, possibly caused by a foreign body, tumor, or urinary TB.

PYELONEPHRITIS LABORATORY FINDINGS: Casts are present with renal parenchymal disease.

GRAM STAIN is almost always positive with a positive urine culture.[83]

URINE CULTURE:

<10,000 colonies	No infection[145]
20,000 colonies	One pathogenic organism with pyuria and a symptomatic patient; some clinicians will treat[55]
25,000-100,000 colony-forming units per milliliter of a single pathogenic organism	Asymptomatic bacteriuria, requires treatment[16]
>100,000 colonies pathogenic bacteria[55]	UTI; requires treatment
>100,000 **mixed bacteria**	Represents contamination

PATHOGENIC ORGANISMS: *Escherichia coli; Neisseria gonorrhea; Proteus* species; *Klebsiella* species; *Pseudomonas aeruginosa; Corynebacterium* species; *Staphylococcus aureus;* β-hemolytic streptococci; *Enterococcus* species,[169] *Citrobacter freundii,*[72] TB,[143] group D streptococci. In the immunosuppressed or diabetic patient, yeast can cause a UTI.[83]

NONPATHOGENIC ORGANISMS: α-Hemolytic streptococci; *Staphylococcus epidermidis; Lactobacillus* species.[169]

or in the midtrimester, Bactrim or Septra (trimethoprim-sulfamethoxazole), 800 mg or 160 mg PO bid for 3 days; amoxicillin, 250 mg PO tid for 3 days; Augmentin (amoxicillin and clavulanate potassium), 250 mg PO qid for 3 days, or ampicillin, 250 to 500 mg PO qid for 3 days if sensitive by culture only.[20]

2. For **discomfort,** a urinary analgesic such as Pyridium (phenazopyridine hydrochloride), 100 mg PO bid, for 2 to 3 days may be prescribed: Pyridium is **contraindicated during pregnancy.**[83]

3. **Advise rest,**[83] **hydration** by drinking as much water as possible during treatment, and **avoidance of alcohol and caffeine.**[12]

4. Consider suggesting **a preventative antifungal** medication when prescribing antibiotics that disrupt vaginal flora.

5. **To prevent recurrence:**

   a. Evaluate for **risk factors.** In the nonpregnant woman, evaluate the size and type of **diaphragm** as a possible cause of the UTI. **Spermicide-coated male condoms** have been associated with *Escherichia coli* UTIs in young women.[36] Screen black women for **sickle cell trait,** if not screened previously.

   b. **Educate** the woman:

      (1) Maintain good personal **hygiene,** including wiping from front to back after urinating, washing daily, and washing before and after intercourse. Drink more **fluids,** particularly water. **Urinate frequently**, at least every 2 to 3 hours. **Avoid douching** and use of vaginal deodorants and **perfumed or dyed** toilet paper or feminine hygiene products. Wear panties with a **cotton crotch.**[12]

      (2) **Vitamin C,** 500 mg PO bid, keeps the urine acidic. Grapefruit juice and carbonated drinks make the urine basic and should be avoided.[83]

      (3) Drink **cranberry juice** (also available in tablets) to decrease UTIs.[129]

6. Obtain a **follow-up urine culture** 2 weeks after a course of antibiotics has been completed. Advise the woman that symptoms should be gone within 48 to 96 hours of treatment, or she should call.[69]

7. **Relapse** of the UTI may occur within 2 to 3 weeks. After 3 weeks, another infection is generally due to reinfection with another organism.[83] **Consult with physician for recurrent infections.** Take a careful history regarding compliance with drug regimen and counsel accordingly. Prescribe a second course with a new drug to which the bacteria are sensitive. Reculture 2 weeks after that course is complete.

8. For more than three episodes of **"honeymoon cystitis"** in 6 mo, consider prophylaxis: Bactrim or Septra, 1 tablet, to be taken PO after intercourse or nitrofurantoin, 50 mg, to be taken after intercourse.[138] Follow up every 3 months, then annually if asymptomatic.

9. **Consult** with a physician for **pyelonephritis.**[20]

DURING PREGNANCY

1. **Screen** all pregnant women for bacteriuria at registration for prenatal care and treat as indicated.[47] Screen women at risk for UTI again at 28 weeks' gestation.[138]
2. For **asymptomatic bacteriuria, prescribe antibiotics:** Treat as described previously, using Azogantrisin, Bactrim, or Septra **only in the second trimester.**[83]
3. Recommend **rest** and **hydration.**[83]
4. **Consult** with a physician when **pyelonephritis** is suspected or when there are signs of **preterm labor.**[20]
5. **Anticipatory guidance: Mild pyelonephritis symptoms** without signs of preterm labor are treated on an outpatient basis with trimethoprim-sulfamethoxazole-DS (double strength), one tablet PO bid for 7 to 10 days (in the second trimester) or Augmentin, 500 mg PO tid, if culture-sensitive.[69] The patient who is **moderately ill with pyelonephritis or who has signs of preterm labor is hospitalized for** IV hydration and close monitoring of urinary output and signs of pulmonary involvement, sepsis, preterm labor, anemia, thrombocytopenia, and adult respiratory distress syndrome (ARDS).[20] IV antibiotics are given empirically until culture sensitivities are received.[69]
6. The woman who has β-*Streptococcus* **organisms** in her urine must be treated and should also receive intrapartum prophylactic antibiotics.[60] See p. 67.
7. For the woman who has UTI symptoms but no bacteriuria, consider *Chlamydia* urethritis, vulvovaginitis (see pp. 428 and 476), and interstitial cystitis. The latter is chronic, sterile inflammation of the bladder and is treated by a urologist or a urogynecologist. Warm sitz baths and Pyridium may give temporary relief.
8. **Complementary measures for UTI:**
   a. **Acupuncture** has been used with success in the treatment of cystitis and other urinary maladies.[30,129]
   b. **Homeopathy** experts have many suggestions for UTI.[54,129,144,155,167]
   c. **Nutritional suggestions:** Two **cranberry capsules** are recommended, to be taken q3h, at the first hint of a bladder infection.[129] A clove of **raw garlic** taken daily is a urinary tract antiseptic and will ward off cystitis and other infections.[85,157,164] **Vitamin C** (1000 mg) may be taken with cranberry juice bid. Vitamin B supplementation, taken in the morning and evening, and small frequent meals with plenty of roughage are also recommended.[67] Drinking the remaining liquid from pearl **barley** cooked with double the required water and strained, with a little lemon juice, is healing for cystitis.[157]
   d. **Reflexology:** Cystitis may be treated with reflexology, but **during pregnancy great caution should be used** to prevent the infection

from moving upward. Work only in the direction of the zones for the kidneys to the ureters and then the bladder. In a woman in whom calculi are suspected, caution must be exercised because treatment may dislodge a stone, moving it to an area where it can cause a blockage.[164] **See charts and information on reflexology, p. 567.**

e. **Herbs: Agrimony** is used for cystitis and for hematuria.[86,103,157] **Buchu** is a urinary tract antiseptic[85,103,126]; it is used to treat bladder and urethral irritation and may be a diuretic.[77,126,129] But Mabey et al[103] warn that **buchu should be avoided in the presence of kidney disease; buchu is also contraindicated in pregnancy. Burdock** aids kidney function and heals cystitis.[77,86,103] **Corn silk** tincture or tea is a urinary demulcent, reducing pain and discomfort.* **Couch grass** is a diuretic and a mild antibiotic that soothes mucous membranes,[77,85,103,126,157] but it is often contaminated with an ergot-containing fungus and **should be used with caution during pregnancy.**[77] **Dandelion root** is effective against UTI.[115,129,136] **Echinacea** is antimicrobial; it works to heal infections by stimulating the immune system. It is also a urinary tract antiseptic, and its use will help curb pain and inflammation.[77,85,115,125,129] Echinacea may be given as 1 to 4 mL of tincture tid or as tea (1 to 2 tsp root simmered in 1 cup water for 10 to 15 minutes) tid.[86] Echinacea tea may be used as a rinse after having sex if the infections routinely follow intercourse.[129] **Goldenseal** is a soothing urinary demulcent that acts as an antibiotic and stimulates the immune system.[77,85,115,129] **Goldenseal** tea may also be used as a rinse after having sex if the infections routinely follow intercourse.[129] **Goldenseal is contraindicated in pregnancy. Horsetail** is used to treat infections of the urinary tract, as well as kidney and bladder stones; as an astringent it reduces bleeding† and incontinence.[86] Horsetail may be applied in a warm compress or consumed as tea (1 cup daily).[170] **Marshmallow** is soothing to the urinary tract mucous membranes and is useful in the treatment of UTI and for hematuria.[85,103,115,129,157] One oz marshmallow root steeped in 1 pint hot milk may be consumed q30min.[129] **Stinging nettle** eases cystitis.[115,129,157,170] It may be consumed as a tea (1 cup infusion tid) or applied in a warm compress.[170] **Uva ursi** or **bearberry** is a urinary demulcent and disinfectant that relieves urinary pain and is a diuretic. It was used extensively for UTI before other drugs were developed. It turns the urine green.‡ Bearberry may be given as tincture, 1/2 dropper bid[115]; consumed as 2 to 3 cups of tea daily for no more than 7 days[85]; or taken in capsules for 14 days.[129] It

---

*References 67, 85, 103, 115, 126, 129, 157.
†References 77, 85, 103, 115, 126, 129, 136, 157.
‡References 77, 85, 103, 115, 126, 129, 157.

is toxic when used long-term, but safe when used medicinally.[126] **Yarrow** is a urinary antiseptic and is indicated in UTI.[85,93,103,126,157] Yarrow may consumed as tea (1 to 2 tsp dried herb steeped for 10 to 15 minutes in 1 cup boiling water) tid or as tincture, 2 to 4 mL tid.[86] **Yarrow is contraindicated in pregnancy. See information on herbs, p. 563.**

Urolithiasis

Stones in the urinary tract complicate 1 in 90 to 3800 pregnancies. Signs and symptoms include severe flank pain, often radiating to the lower abdomen, nausea, vomiting, urinary frequency or urgency, and hematuria. UTI and preterm labor may accompany lithiasis. Diagnosis is made by ultrasound examination.

ⓜ Management

1. **Consult** with a physician.
2. **Anticipatory guidance:** Conservative management (bed rest, analgesia, and hydration) allows 75% of stones to pass spontaneously. Management may involve cystoscopy with ureteral stent placement, ureteroscopy with stone manipulation, percutaneous nephrostomy, or surgery. Extracorporeal shock wave lithotripsy is contraindicated during pregnancy.[107]
3. **Complementary measures:**
   a. **Nutritional measures:** A low-acid diet is indicated. Avoid oxalic acid, present in rhubarb and spinach.[85]
   b. **Herbs: Corn silk** is useful for urinary lithiasis. A diuretic, it soothes the mucous membranes. **Couch grass** is also a diuretic and urinary demulcent and is useful for urinary lithiasis. **Gravel root** is antilithic.[85,103,126] **Hydrangea** is used to treat bladder stones.[77,85,103,126] **Marshmallow** is used to treat kidney stones and soothes the mucous membranes.[77,85,103] **Parsley piert** is an antilithic and a soothing diuretic[85,103,126,136] and is taken as tincture, 2 to 4 mL tid, or tea made with 1 to 2 tsp dried herb.[86] **Bearberry (uva ursi)** is an antiseptic specific for urinary lithiasis, to be added if infection is present[85,103,126]; but may be toxic when used long-term.[103] **See information on herbs, p. 563.**

• REFERENCES

1. Abrams EJ et al: Neonatal predictors of infection status and early death among 332 infants at risk of HIV-1 infection monitored prospectively from birth, *Pediatrics* 96: 451-458, 1995.
2. Aggarwal N et al: Pregnancy and cirrhosis of the liver, *Aust N Z J Obstet Gynecol* 39: 503-506, 1999.
3. Alef K: *Clostridium difficile*-associated disease, *J Nurse Midwifery* 4:19-29, 1999.
4. American Academy of Pediatrics Committee on Drugs: Use of psychoactive medication during pregnancy and possible effects on the fetus and newborn, *Pediatrics* 105:880-887, 2000.

5. American College of Nurse-Midwives (ACNM): How do you document domestic violence? *Quickening* 33:24, 2002.

5a. ACNM: Society releases position statement on hypothyroidism, *Quickening* 30:20, 1999.

6. ACNM: Statement on HIV/AIDS, *Quickening* 29:19, 1998.

7. American College of Obstetricians and Gynecologists (ACOG): *Gestational diabetes*, Practice Bulletin No. 30, Washington, DC, December 2001, ACOG.

8. ACOG: *Fetal macrosomia*, Practice Bulletin No. 22, Washington, DC, November 2000, ACOG.

9. ACOG: *Adult manifestations of childhood sexual abuse*, Educational Bulletin No. 259, Washington, DC, July 2000, ACOG.

10. ACOG: *Domestic violence*, Educational Bulletin No. 209, Washington, DC, July 2000, ACOG.

11. ACOG: *The use of hormonal contraception in women with coexisting medical conditions*, Practice Bulletin No. 18, Washington, DC, July 2000, ACOG.

12. ACOG: *Decreasing your chance of a urinary tract infection*, ACOG Woman's Health column, 1999. Available at: *http://www.acog.com/from_home/publications/womans_health/wh8-25-7.htm.*

13. ACOG: *When should you get a mammogram?* ACOG Woman's Health column, 1999. Available at: *http://www.acog.com/from_home/publications/womans_health/wh 10-13-7.htm.*

14. ACOG: *Getting help for domestic abuse*, ACOG Woman's Health column, October 1999. Available at: *http://acog.com/from_home/publications/womans_health/wh10-20-7.htm.*

15. ACOG: *Headache*, Education Pamphlet AP124, December 1998. Available at: *http://www.acog.com/from_home/wellness/featured-pep.htm.*

16. ACOG: *Antimicrobial therapy for obstetric patients*, Educational Bulletin No. 245, Washington, DC, March 1998, ACOG.

17. ACOG Committee on Obstetric Practice: *Scheduled cesarean delivery and the prevention of vertical transmission of HIV infection*, Committee Opinion No. 219, Washington, DC, August 1999, ACOG.

18. American Thoracic Society and the Centers for Disease Control and Prevention (AST and CDC): Diagnostic standards and classification of tuberculosis in adults and children, *Am J Respir Crit Care Med* 161:1376-1395, 2000.

19. Anderson B, Neilsen TF: Appendicitis in pregnancy: diagnosis, management, and complications, *Acta Obstet Gynecol Scand* 78:758-762, 1999.

20. Angelini DJ: Obstetric triage: management of acute nonobstetric abdominal pain in pregnancy, *J Nurse Midwifery* 44:572-584, 1999.

21. Balch JF, Balch PA: *Prescription for nutritional healing*, ed 2, Garden City Park, NY, 1997, Avery.

22. Balistreri WF: "G"—another form of viral hepatitis? *J Pediatr* 131:503-506, 1997 (editorial).

23. Barbour LA, Pickard J: Controversies in thromboembolic disease during pregnancy: a critical review, *Obstet Gynecol* 86:621-633, 1995.

23a. Barone JE et al: Outcome study of cholecystectomy during pregnancy, *Am J Surg* 177: 232-236, 1999.

24. Barrett E: Primary care for women: assessment and management of headache, *J Nurse Midwifery* 41:117-124, 1996.

25. Ben Shachar I, Weinstein D: High risk pregnancy outcome by route of delivery, *Curr Opin Obstet Gynecol* 10:447-452, 1998.

26. Benenson AS, editor: *Control of communicable diseases manual*, ed 16, Washington, DC, 1995, American Public Health Association.

27. Berrebi A et al: Termination of pregnancy for maternal toxoplasmosis, *Lancet* 344:36-39, 1994.

28. Briggs GG: Antihistamines. Drugs, pregnancy, and lactation, *OB GYN News* 36:24, 2001.

29. Brucker MC, Faucher MA: Pharmacologic management of common gastrointestinal health problems in women, *J Nurse Midwifery* 42:145-162, 1997.
30. Budd S: Acupuncture. In Tiran D, Mack S, editors: *Complementary therapies for pregnancy and childbirth*, Edinburgh, 2000, Baillière Tindall.
31. Burrow GN, Ferris TF: *Medical complications during pregnancy*, ed 4, Philadelphia, 1995, WB Saunders.
32. Campbell C: Primary care for women: comprehensive cardiovascular assessment, *J Nurse Midwifery* 40:137-149, 1995.
33. Carr CA: Evidence-based diabetes screening during pregnancy, *J Midwifery Womens Health* 46:152-158, 2001.
34. Carr SR: Screening for gestational diabetes mellitus, *Diabetes Care* 21(suppl 2):B14-B18, 1998.
35. Centers for Disease Control and Prevention (CDC): Fact sheets. Tuberculosis information. Diagnosis of latent TB infection and TB disease. Updated June 23, 2000. Available at: *http://www.cdc.gov/nchstp/tb/pubs/tbfactsheets/250102.htm.*
36. CDC: 1998 guidelines for treatment of sexually transmitted diseases, *MMWR Recomm Rep* 47(RR-1): 1-111, 1998.
37. CDC: Public Health Service statement: Management of possible sexual, injecting-drug-use, or other nonoccupational exposure to HIV, including considerations related to antiretroviral therapy, *MMWR Recomm Rep* 47(RR-17):1-14, 1998.
38. CDC: Public Health Service Task Force recommendations for the use of antiretroviral drugs in pregnant women infected with HIV-1 for maternal health and for reducing perinatal HIV-1 transmission in the United States, *MMWR Recomm Rep* 47(RR-2):1-30, 1998.
39. Reference deleted in galleys.
40. CDC: Guidelines for preventing the transmission of *Mycobacterium tuberculosis* in health-care facilities, 1994, *MMWR Recomm Rep* 43(RR-13)1-132, 1994.
41. Chaim W et al: Prevalence and clinical significance of postpartum endometritis, *Infect Dis Obstet Gynecol* 8:77-82, 2000.
42. Chang CC et al: Acute pancreatitis in pregnancy, *Chung Hua I Hsueh Tsa Chih (Taipei)* 61:85-92, 1998.
43. Chescheir NC, Hansen WF: New in perinatology, *Pediatr Rev* 20:57-63, 1999.
44. Cohen BF et al: The incidence and severity of shoulder dystocia correlates with a sonographic measurement of asymmetry in patients with diabetes, *Am J Perinatol* 16:197-201, 1999.
45. Cokkinides VE et al: Physical violence during pregnancy: maternal complications and birth outcomes, *Obstet Gynecol* 93:661-666, 1999.
46. Coleman MT, Trianfo VA, Rund DA: Nonobstetric emergencies in pregnancy: trauma and surgical conditions, *Am J Obstet Gynecol* 177:497-502, 1997.
47. Connolly A, Thorp JM Jr: Urinary tract infections in pregnancy, *Urol Clin North Am* 26:779-787, 1999.
48. Conway PL: Osteopathy during pregnancy. In Tiran D, Mack S, editors: *Complementary therapies for pregnancy and childbirth*, Edinburgh, 2000, Baillière Tindall.
49. Conway DL, Langer O: Effects of new criteria for type 2 diabetes on the rate of postpartum glucose intolerance in women with gestational diabetes, *Am J Obstet Gynecol* 181:610-614, 1999.
50. Corrarino JE: Perinatal hepatitis B: update & recommendations, *MCN Am J Matern Child Nurs* 23:246-253, 1998.
51. Coustan DR: Oral hypoglycemic agents for the ob/gyn, *Contemp OB/GYN* 46:45-63, 2001.
52. Crawford AM: *Herbal remedies for women*, Rocklin, Calif, 1997, Prima.
53. Culnane M et al: Lack of long-term effects of in utero exposure to zidovudine among uninfected children born to HIV-infected women. Pediatric AIDS Clinical Trials Group Protocol 219/076 Teams, *JAMA* 281:151-157, 1999.
54. Cummings S, Ullman D: *Everybody's guide to homeopathic medicines*, New York, 1997, Jeremy P. Tarcher/Putnam.

55. Cunningham FG et al: *Williams obstetrics,* ed 20, Stamford, Conn, 1997, Appleton and Lange.
56. Curry MA, Perrin N, Wall E: Effects of abuse on maternal complications and birth weight in adults and adolescent women, *Obstet Gynecol* 92:530-534, 1998.
57. Dajani AS et al: Prevention of bacterial endocarditis, *JAMA* 277:1794-1801, 1997.
58. Danese MD et al: Screening for mild thyroid failure at the periodic health examination: a decision and cost-effectiveness analysis, *JAMA* 276:285-292, 1996.
59. Dashe JS et al: Correlation between amniotic fluid glucose concentration and amniotic fluid volume in pregnancy complicated by diabetes, *Am J Obstet Gynecol* 182:901-904, 2000.
60. Delzell JE Jr, LeFevre ML: Urinary tract infections during pregnancy, *Am Fam Physician* 61:713-721, 2000.
61. Ellett ML: Hepatitis A, B, and D, *Gastroenterol Nurs* 22:236-244, 1999.
62. Ely JW, Yankowitz J, Bowdler NC: Evaluation of pregnant women exposed to respiratory viruses, *Am Fam Physician* 61:3065-3072, 2000.
63. Emmett P: Hepatitis C: the silent epidemic, *Nurse Week* 12:14-16, 1999.
64. Emmons L et al: Primary care management of common dermatologic disorders in women, *J Nurse Midwifery* 42:228-253, 1997.
65. The Expert Committee on the Diagnosis and Classification of Diabetes Mellitus: Report of The Expert Committee on the Diagnosis and Classification of Diabetes Mellitus, *Diabetes Care* 20:1183-1197, 1997.
66. Feder HM: Lyme disease vaccine: good for dogs, adults, and children? *Pediatrics* 105:1333-1334, 2000.
67. Feral C: Natural remedies, *Midwifery Today* 26:35-38, 1993.
68. Fleisher TA: Back to basics: immune function, *Pediatr Rev* 18:351-356, 1997.
69. Gabbe SG, Niebyl JR, Simpson JL: *Obstetrics: normal & problem pregnancies,* ed 3, New York, 1996, Churchill Livingstone.
70. Garn SM et al: Maternal hematologic levels and pregnancy outcome, *Semin Perinatol* 5:155-162, 1981.
71. Gazmararian JA et al: Prenatal care for low-income women enrolled in a managed-care organization, *Obstet Gynecol* 94:177-184, 1999.
72. Gebre-Selassie S: Asymptomatic bacteriuria in pregnancy: epidemiological, clinical, and microbial approach, *Ethiop Med J* 36:185-192, 1998.
73. Gold LH: Treatment of depression during pregnancy, *J Womens Health Gend Based Med* 8:601-607, 1999.
74. Gordon JD et al: *Obstetrics gynecology & infertility,* Glen Cove, NY, 1998, Scrub Hill Press.
75. Graves BW, Barger MK: A "conservative" approach to iron supplementation during pregnancy, *J Midwifery Womens Health* 46:156-166, 2001.
76. Gregory KD et al: Maternal and infant complications in high and normal weight infants by method of delivery, *Obstet Gynecol* 92:507-513, 1998.
77. Griffith HW: *Healing herbs: the essential guide,* Tucson, Ariz, 2000, Fisher Books.
78. Grimes DA, editor: Headache, migraine, and oral contraceptives, *Contracept Rep* 8:12-14, 1998.
79. Grimes DA, editor: STDs as cofactors for HIV infection: taking a sexual history, *Contracept Rep* 17:3-11, 1996.
80. Guay LA et al: Intrapartum and neonatal single-dose nevirapine compared with zidovudine for prevention of mother-to-child transmission of HIV-1 in Kampala, Uganda: HIVNET 012 randomised trial, *Lancet* 354:795-802, 1999.
81. Hally SS: Nutrition in reproductive health, *J Nurse Midwifery* 43:459-470, 1998.
82. Hayes C: *The alphabet soup of viral hepatitis: A-G.* Handout for lecture at the American College of Nurse-Midwives' Annual Convention, May 25, 1998, San Francisco, Calif.
83. Hacker NF, Moore JG: *Essentials of obstetrics and gynecology,* ed 3, Philadelphia, 1998, WB Saunders Company.
83a. Haddow JE et al: Maternal thyroid deficiency during pregnancy and subsequent neuropsychological development of the child, *N Engl J Med* 341:549-555, 1999.

84. Hendrix NW et al: Clinical and sonographic estimates of birth weight among diabetic parturients, *J Matern Fetal Investig* 8:17-20, 1998.

85. Hoffmann D: *The complete illustrated holistic herbal*, Boston, 1996, Element Books Limited.

86. Hoffmann D: *The holistic herbal*, Findhorn, Scotland, 1985, Findhorn Press.

87. Jackson SL, Soper DE: Sexually transmitted diseases in pregnancy, *Obstet Gynecol Clin North Am* 24:631-644, 1997.

88. Jovanovic L: American Diabetes Association's Fourth International Workshop-Conference on Gestational Diabetes Mellitus: summary and discussion. Therapeutic interventions, *Diabetes Care* 21(suppl 2): B131-B137, 1998.

89. Kennedy MM: Influenza viral infections: presentation, prevention, and treatment, *Nurse Pract* 23:17-37, 1998.

90. King MC, Ryan J: Woman abuse: the role of nurse-midwives in assessment, *J Nurse Midwifery* 41:436-441, 1996.

91. Kjos SL et al: Contraception and the risk of type 2 diabetes in Latina women with prior gestational diabetes, *JAMA* 280:533-538, 1998.

92. Kjos SL et al: Hormonal choices after gestational diabetes, *Diabetes Care* 21(suppl 2):B50-B57, 1998.

93. Kloss J: *Back to Eden*, New York, 1981, Benedict Lust Publications.

94. Ko GTC et al: Combined use of a fasting plasma glucose combination and HbA1c or fructosamine predicts the likelihood of having diabetes in high-risk subjects, *Diabetes Care* 21:1221-1225, 1998.

94a. Kolasa KM, Weismiller DG: Nutrition during pregnancy, *Am Fam Physician* 56: 1205-1212, 1995.

95. Lamberg L: Safety of antidepressant use in pregnant and lactating women, *JAMA* 282:222-223, 1999.

96. Langer O: Maternal glycemic criteria for insulin therapy in gestational diabetes mellitus, *Diabetes Care* 21(suppl 2): B91-B98, 1998.

97. Lawrence RA: *A review of the medical benefits and contraindications to breastfeeding in the United States*, Maternal and Child Health Technical Information Bulletin, Arlington, Va, 1997, National Center for Education in Maternal and Child Health.

98. Leiner S: Acute bronchitis in adults: commonly diagnosed but poorly defined, *Nurse Pract* 22:104-117, 1997.

99. Leppert PC, Howard FM: *Primary care for women*, Philadelphia, 1997, Lippincott-Raven.

100. Levi M, Cate HT: Disseminated intravascular coagulation, *N Engl J Med* 341:586-592, 1999.

101. Little L, Lowkes E: Critical issue in the care of pregnant women with eating disorders and the impact on their children, *J Midwifery Womens Health* 45:301-307, 2000.

102. Reference deleted in galleys.

103. Mabey R et al, editors: *The new age herbalist*, New York, 1988, Collier Books.

104. MacLaren A, Imberg W: Current issues in the midwifery management of women living with HIV/AIDS, *J Nurse Midwifery* 43:502-525, 1998.

105. Magid MS et al: Placental pathology in systemic lupus erythematosus: a prospective study, *Am J Obstet Gynecol* 179:226-234, 1998.

106. Malik AH, Lee WM: Chronic hepatitis B virus infection: treatment strategies for the next millennium, *Ann Intern Med* 132:723-731, 2000.

107. Mayer IE, Hussain H: Abdominal pain during pregnancy, *Gastroenterol Clin North Am* 27:1-36, 1998.

108. Mays M, Leiner S: Pharmacologic management of common lower respiratory tract disorders in women, *J Nurse Midwifery* 42:163-175, 1997.

109. Mays M, Leiner S: Primary care for women: management of common respiratory problems, *J Nurse Midwifery* 41:139-154, 1996.

110. Mays M, Leiner S: Asthma: a comprehensive review, *J Nurse Midwifery* 40:256-268, 1995.

111. March of Dimes Birth Defects Foundation: Newborn screening tests, 1998. Available at: *http://www.modimes.org/HealthLibrary2/FactSheets/Newborn_Screening-Test.htm*

112. McCowan CB: Systemic lupus erythematosus, *J Am Acad Nurse Pract* 10:225-231, 1998.

113. McFarlane J, Parker B: Physical abuse, smoking, and substance use during pregnancy: prevalence, interrelationships, and effects on birth weight, *J Obstet Gynecol Neonatal Nurs* 25:313-320, 1996.

114. Reference deleted in galleys.

115. Medina IM: *Issues in women's health care: nutrition and herbs from menarche to menopause: 3/28-29/98*, course syllabus, Brooklyn, NY, 1998, State University of New York Health Science Center at Brooklyn College of Health Related Professions Midwifery Education Program.

116. Metzger BE, Coustan DR: Summary and recommendations of the Fourth International Workshop-Conference on Gestational Diabetes Mellitus. The Organizing Committee, *Diabetes Care* 21(suppl 2):B161-B167, 1998.

117. Meyers J: Lyme disease: a challenge and an opportunity for nurse practitioners, *J Am Acad Nurse Pract* 10:315-319, 1998.

118. Moore TR: Fetal growth in diabetic pregnancy, *Clin Obstet Gynecol* 40:771-786, 1997.

119. Morgan JF, Lacey JH, Sedgwick PM: Impact of pregnancy on bulimia nervosa, *Br J Psychiatry* 174:135-140, 1999.

120. Moyer LA, Mast EE, Alter MJ: Hepatitis C: routine serologic testing and diagnosis, *Am Fam Physician* 59:79-88, 1999.

121. Murray M: *Antepartal and intrapartal fetal monitoring*, ed 2, Albuquerque, NM, 1997, Learning Resources International, Inc.

122. National Association of Nurse Practitioners in Women's Health (NPWH): *New option in hormonal contraception: monthly combination contraceptive injection*, Washington, DC, 2001, NP Communications, NPWH (suppl for continuing ed, pp 4-17).

123. Nelson WE et al, editors: *Nelson's textbook of pediatrics*, ed 15, Philadelphia, 1996, WB Saunders.

124. Niederhauser VP: Varicella: the vaccine and the public health debate, *Nurse Pract* 24: 74-76, 79, 83-84, 1999.

125. Nissim R: *Natural healing in gynecology*, San Francisco, 1996, Pandora (HarperCollins).

126. Ody P: *The complete medicinal herbal*, New York, 1993, Dorling Kindersley.

127. Olivieri N: Thalassemia: clinical management, *Baillieres Clin Haematol* 11:147-162, 1998.

128. Orloff LE: Effective advocacy for domestic violence victims, *J Nurse Midwifery* 41: 473-494, 1996.

129. Page L: *Healthy healing*, ed 11, Carmel Valley, Calif, 2000, Healthy Healing Publications.

130. Pajor A, Lehoczky D: Pregnancy in liver cirrhosis: assessment of maternal and fetal risks in eleven patients and review of the management, *Gynecol Obstet Invest* 38:45-50, 1994.

131. Palomba E et al: Natural history of perinatal hepatitis C virus infection, *Clin Infect Dis* 23:47-50, 1996.

132. Paluzzi PA, Houde-Quimby C: Domestic violence: implications for the American College of Nurse-Midwives and its members, *J Nurse Midwifery* 41:430-435, 1996.

133. Payton RG, Gardner R, Reynolds D: Pharmacologic considerations and management of common endocrine disorders in women, *J Nurse Midwifery* 42:186-206, 1997.

134. Payton RG, White PJ: Primary care for women: assessment of hematologic disorders, *J Nurse Midwifery* 40:120-136, 1995.

135. Persson B, Hanson U: Neonatal morbidities in gestational diabetes mellitus, *Diabetes Care* 21(suppl 2):B79-B84, 1998.

136. *Physician's desk reference (PDR) for herbal medicines*, Montvale, NJ, 1998, Medical Economics Co.

137. Poirier L: The importance of screening for domestic violence in all women, *Nurse Pract* 22:105-122, 1997.

138. Polivka BJ, Nickel JT, Wilkins JR III: Urinary tract infection during pregnancy: a risk factor for cerebral palsy? *J Obstet Gynecol Neonatal Nurs* 26:405-413, 1997.

139. Priddy KD: Immunologic adaptations during pregnancy, *J Obstet Gynecol Neonatal Nurs* 26:388-394, 1997.

140. Pustilnik TB, Cohen AW: Parvovirus B19 infection in a twin pregnancy, *Obstet Gynecol* 83:834-836, 1994.

141. Reifsnider E, Gill SL: Nutrition for the childbearing years, *J Gynecol Neonatal Nurs* 29:43-55, 2000.

142. Riordan J, Auerbach K: *Breastfeeding and human lactation*, ed 2, Sudbury, Mass, 1999, Jones and Bartlett.

143. Roberts JA: Management of pyelonephritis and upper urinary tract infections, *Urol Clin North Am* 26:753-763, 1999.

144. Rose B, Scott-Moncrieff C: *Homeopathy for women*, London, 1998, Collins & Brown.

144a. Russell MA, Craig SD: Cirrhosis and portal hypertension in pregnancy, *Semin Perinat* 22:156-165, 1998.

145. Sacher RA, McPherson RA: *Widmann's clinical interpretation of laboratory tests*, ed 10, Philadelphia, 1991, FA Davis.

146. Schaefer-Graf UM et al: Patterns of congenital anomalies and relationship to initial maternal fasting glucose levels in pregnancies complicated by type 2 gestational diabetes, *Am J Obstet Gynecol* 182:313-320, 2000.

147. Schatz M, Zeiger RS: Asthma during pregnancy: what to do, *J Respir Dis* 19:731-738, 1998.

148. Scroggins KM, Smucker WD, Krishen AE: Spontaneous pregnancy loss: evaluation, management, and follow-up counseling, *Prim Care* 27:153-167, 2000.

149. Semba RD et al: Maternal vitamin A deficiency and mother-to-child transmission of HIV-1, *Lancet* 343:1593-1597, 1994.

150. Seng JS, Hassinger JA: Relationship strategies and interdisciplinary collaboration. Improving maternity care with survivors of childhood sexual abuse, *J Nurse Midwifery* 43:287-295, 1998.

151. Shank SL: *Domestic family violence: confronting the monster*, Roseville, Calif, 1999, National Center of Continuing Education.

152. Shapiro ED: Lyme disease, *Pediatr Rev* 19:147-154, 1998.

153. Silverman BL et al: Long-term effects of the intrauterine environment. The Northwestern University Diabetes in Pregnancy Center, *Diabetes Care* 21(suppl 2):B142-B149, 1998.

154. Simpkins SM, Hench CP, Bhatia G: Management of the obstetric patient with tuberculosis, *J Obstet Gynecol Neonatal Nurs* 25:305-312, 1996.

155. Smith T: *Homeopathy for pregnancy and nursing mothers*, Worthing, England, 1993, Insight Editions.

156. Smith WJ et al: Prevention of chickenpox in reproductive-age women: cost-effectiveness of routine prenatal screening with postpartum vaccination of susceptibles, *Obstet Gynecol* 92:535-545, 1998.

157. Stapleton H, Tiran D: Herbal medicine. In Tiran D, Mack S, editors: *Complementary therapies for pregnancy and childbirth*, Edinburgh, 2000, Baillière Tindall.

158. Star W, Lommel LL, Shannon MT, editors: *Women's primary health care: protocols for practice*, Washington, DC, 1995, American Nurses.

159. Stein E, Handelsman E, Matthews R: Reducing perinatal transmission of HIV: early diagnosis and interventions during pregnancy, *J Midwifery Womens Health* 45:122-129, 2000.

160. Stein JH, editor: *Internal medicine*, ed 4, St Louis, 1994, Mosby–Year Book.

161. Stites DP, Terr AI, Parslow TG: *Basic & clinical immunology*, Norwalk, Conn, 1994, Appleton & Lange.

162. Tarraza HM, Moore RD: Gynecologic causes of the acute abdomen and the acute abdomen in pregnancy, *Surg Clin North Am* 77:1371-1394, 1997.

163. Tillett J, Hanson L: Midwifery triage and management of trauma and second/third trimester bleeding, *J Nurse Midwifery* 44:439-448, 1999.

164. Tiran D: Massage and aromatherapy. In Tiran D, Mack S, editors: *Complementary therapies for pregnancy and childbirth*, Edinburgh, 2000, Baillière Tindall.

165. Turton P et al: Incidence and demographic correlates of eating disorder symptoms in a pregnant population, *Int J Eat Disord* 26:448-452, 1999.

166. Tuso P: The herbal medicine pharmacy: what Kaiser Permanente providers need to know, *The Permanente J* 3:33-37, 1999.

167. Ullman R, Reichenberg-Ullman J: *Homeopathic self-care*, Rocklin, Calif, 1997, Prima.

168. Ungvarski P: Update on HIV Infection, *Am J Nurs* 97:44-52, 1997.

169. Varney H: *Varney's midwifery*, ed 3, Sudbury, Mass, 1997, Jones and Bartlett.

170. Weed S: *Menopausal years: the wise woman way*, Woodstock, NY, 1992, Ash Tree.

171. Weintraub TA, Paine LL, Weintraub DH: Primary care for women: comprehensive assessment and management of common mental health problems, *J Nurse Midwifery* 41:125-138, 1996.

172. Worthington-Roberts BS, Williams SR: *Nutrition and lactation*, ed 6, Madison, Wis, 1997, Brown & Benchmark.

Chapter 8

Gynecologic Conditions and Considerations for Pregnancy and Contraception

1. **Introductions** and woman's reason for the visit.
2. **Data collection:** Age, menstrual history, medical/surgical history, family history, gynecologic history, obstetric history, contraception history, and any relevant sexual and social history.
   a. **Menstrual history:**
      (1) Age at **menarche,** frequency of menses, and number of days of menses (often noted by practitioners as age at menarche X number of days in the usual cycle X number of days of menses), and whether the flow is heavy or light
      (2) Premenstrual and **menstrual-associated symptoms** or disorders
      (3) First day of the **last menstrual period** and whether it was normal in timing, number of days, menstrual-associated symptoms, and amount of flow
      (4) **Menopausal history** if appropriate, including symptomatology, whether the quality of life is impacted, and interventions used (see Chapter 10)
   b. **Family history:** Include diabetes, cardiac disease, cerebrovascular disease, hypertension, thrombophlebitis, and cancer (particularly breast and ovarian cancers).
   c. **Medical/surgical history:**
      (1) Include inquiries regarding headaches, thyroid disease, cardiac disease, hypertension, diabetes, gastrointestinal (GI) or urinary tract disease, vascular disease, anemia or other hematologic disease
      (2) History of surgery or serious injury

       (3) Current medications, including over-the-counter (OTC) drugs; drugs of abuse; and herbs, supplements, and complementary remedies

  d. **Obstetric history:** Year each pregnancy ended, number of weeks gestation, route of delivery, length of labor, sex and weight of infant, whether living now, perineal injury, any complications

  e. **Gynecologic history:**
       (1) History of gynecologic surgery or conditions (including tumors, cysts, fibroids)
       (2) History of an abnormal Pap smear, treatment, and follow-up
       (3) History of intermenstrual spotting or bleeding
       (4) Last mammogram and results
       (5) History of vaginal, cervical, or uterine infection
       (6) History of incontinence of feces or urine
       (7) Presence of abdominal, back, or pelvic discomfort

  f. **Contraception history:** See p. 495.

  g. **Sexual history:**
       (1) Whether currently sexually active, sexual preference, number of partners and whether mutually monogamous
       (2) Whether any condition affects the woman's sexuality

  h. **Social history:**
       (1) Whether she smokes cigarettes or uses other substances
       (2) Whether she is a victim of domestic violence

3. Conduct a **physical examination** (PE), including BP, breast examination (including BSE instruction), and abdominal and pelvic examinations (see p. 5). During the pelvic examination, collect a **Pap smear and cultures** if indicated and perform a rectovaginal examination if indicated.
4. See p. 327 for health care **screening** that is recommended for all women through the life cycle.
5. See Chapter 9 regarding **contraceptive** planning if required.
6. Determine **diagnoses,** share them with the woman, and together with the woman develop a **plan** for her presenting concern, including any referrals and the return visit.

• ADOLESCENT GYNECOLOGY VISIT

Teenagers face many risks. Twenty-one percent of high school girls report being physically or sexually abused. Seventy-five percent of all adolescent deaths are caused by accident or violence. Sixty-six percent of teenage girls have had sex by the twelfth grade, and 1 in 8 women aged 15 to 19 years becomes pregnant each year.[5,15] Females aged 15 to 19 years have the highest rates of sexually transmitted infections (STIs), especially chlamydia and human papillomavirus (HPV), because they are biologically at increased risk for infection, they frequently have unprotected intercourse, and because they experience barriers to health care.[31]

In 2000, 24% of a group of girls in the United States in fifth through twelfth grades were overweight; 45% reported dieting and 13% reported eating behaviors such as binge eating and self-induced vomiting.[15]

ACOG[15] recommends that a teenage girl have her first gynecologic visit at 13 to 15 years and her first pelvic exam and Pap smear by the age of 18 years or younger if she is sexually active. Health care providers should strive to remove the health care barriers faced by adolescents, including uninsured or underinsured status, lack of funds for copayments, limited access to appropriate services, lack of transportation, lack of culturally appropriate care, and confidentiality issues.[5] Teens fear the PE. They fear birth control and are ambivalent about using it. Providers should be prepared to talk to them about sexual risk-taking behavior, substance abuse, smoking, domestic violence, sexual abuse, STIs, contraception, depression, suicide, accidental trauma, and eating disorders. Lifestyle counseling should include the fact that they need to be consuming 1200 to 1500 mg calcium and exercising at least 3 times/week for 20 minutes.[15]

The provider should inform the adolescent and her parent, separately and together, that the adolescent has a right to confidentiality unless the young woman discloses any risk of bodily harm to herself or others. All states require parental consent for medical care of a minor. However, all states also have statutes (with limited exceptions according to the CDC) allowing minors to consent to certain health care services, including STI treatment, HIV testing and treatment, mental health treatment, prenatal care and delivery services, and treatment for drug and alcohol abuse. The further exception is the emancipated minor who can consent for her own care, including married minors, those who live on their own and are self-supportive, those in the Armed Forces, and those who parents.[13]

• BREAST DISEASE

History of the Woman Presenting With a Breast Lump:

Menstrual history

Menopausal history if appropriate

Obstetric history, including lactation

Gynecologic history, including exogenous hormones and mammograms

Personal and family history of breast disease

Alcohol and cigarette use

Irradiation history

Regarding the lump: tenderness, cyclic changes, whether enlarging, any discharge

Breast Examination: See the PE section regarding breast examination on p. 5. Normal structures sometimes mistaken for a breast lump include a prominent rib or costochondral junction, a firm margin at the edge of the breast, the edge of a defect from a biopsy, a lobulated circular terminus of firm breast tissue at the border of the areola, or the firm ridges of tissue near the inframammary fold. Generally, when the finding is present symmetrically (also in the other breast), it is a normal variation. When findings are equivocal and a mammogram is normal, the examination may be repeated in 1 month.[44] Careful examination of the lymphatic system of the breast is necessary (see Figure 8-1).

The breast is illustrated in Figure 6-1, p. 300.

Breast Cancer

Incidence: In the United States, 1 in every 8 women who lives to age 90 years will develop breast cancer.[63] Women have a 1 in 231 chance of developing invasive breast cancer from birth to age 39 years, a 1 in 25 chance from age 40 to 59 years, and a 1 in 15 chance from age 60 to 79 years. In 1999, 175,000 women and 1300 men were expected to develop breast cancer.[36]

Risk Factors for Breast Cancer (cumulative)[38]:

Early menarche with late menopause

Nulliparity or first term pregnancy when >34 years

Benign breast disease

Increasing age and postmenopausal status

Heavy body weight after menopause

Personal history of breast cancer

History of endometrial cancer (slight increase)

Obesity

Affluence

Alcohol consumption (dose-dependent)

Cigarette smoke exposure in adolescence

Irradiation

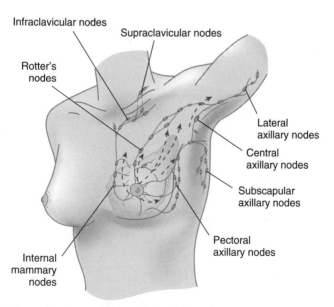

Figure 8-1 • Lymphatic drainage of the breast. (From Matteson PS: *Women's health during the childbearing years: a community-based approach,* St Louis, 2001, Mosby.)

- Race: In the United States, Caucasians and African Americans have twice the risk for breast cancer as Asians.[141]
- Family history: A first-degree relative increases risk 2 to 3 times; high-dose oral contraceptive (OC) use by a woman whose first-degree relative had breast cancer increases the woman's risk 3.3 times. Relatives with bilateral disease and a family history of ataxia-telangiectasia increase the risk.[61]

NOTE: Eighty percent of all breast cancers occur in women with no risk factors.[96] The associations once theorized between dietary fat and fiber intake and breast cancer have not been established by clinical studies.[72,103]

Risk Reduction:

- Lactation slightly decreases the risk of premenopausal breast cancer (reduction proportional to the amount of time lactating).
- Younger age at first lactation.[106]
- Physical activity at work and during leisure time.[146]

Hereditary Early Onset Breast Cancer Syndrome: Accounting for only 10% of all breast cancer cases, women who inherit mutant alleles of the breast cancer susceptibility genes BRCA1 or BRCA2 have an elevated risk of breast and ovarian cancer. The syndrome is suspected when 3 or more closely related individuals develop breast and/or ovarian cancer by age 45 years. One in 800 Caucasian women and 1 in 40 Ashkenazi Jewish women carry the mutation.[95]

Screening for Breast Cancer

Table 8-1 lists historic and physical examination findings and whether the finding indicates that a mass is likely to be benign or malignant.

- Breast **self-examination** monthly from the age of 20 years is recommended. Women themselves discover 70% to 90% of lumps. Sensitivity of this exam is 20% to 30%.[141] Examination should be done after menses, comparing breasts. The woman should first observe her breasts in the mirror in 3 positions: arms down, overhead, and on the waist with body bent slightly forward, looking for skin changes, puckering, and distortion of tissue or nipples. Next, she places one arm behind the head; using the other hand, she palpates the breast using pads of fingers from top to bottom, from under the arm to the lower bra line, then across the breast continuing in a vertical strip pattern from the collar bone down, parallel to the breast bone. Light, medium, and firm pressure is used. The axillary area is checked carefully. The woman with large breasts lies supine, supporting the breast with one hand while palpating with the other.[105]
- **Mammography** every 1 to 2 years from age 40 to 49 years and an annual mammography after age 50 years are recommended.[8] The mammogram's sensitivity is 91%; approximately 10% of palpable tumors cannot be seen on mammogram. Specificity is 98%.[141] The

Table 8-1 / Evaluation of History and Physical Findings of a Breast Mass and Likelihood of Breast Cancer

Findings Likely Benign	Findings Likely Malignant
History	
Prior trauma may indicate fat necrosis[105]	Concurrent bone pain, weight loss; history of breast cancer, new lump, opposite side
Pain and tenderness[18]	No pain and tenderness[105] in 85%; present in 15% cancers[141]; possibly lymphatic blockage[105]
Varies with menstrual cycle[18]	No variation with cycle[18]
No discharge	Watery (33%), sanguinous (27.5%), sero-sanguineous (12.9%), or serous (5.9%) nipple discharge is present[96]; present with 2% breast cancers— spontaneous, unilateral, confined to one duct most worrisome[141]
Physical Findings	
Multiple, indistinct lumps; rubbery or cystic consistency with smooth borders & mobility within breast tissue[19]	Single, firm, definite mass on exam; most commonly found in upper outer quadrant[141]
Bilateral venous engorgement	Unilateral venous engorgement
No axillary or supraclavicular mass	Axillary or supraclavicular mass rarely present, but may indicate metastasis[141]
Any nipple deviation is bilateral, symmetrical	Unilateral nipple retraction or deviation[141]
Any nipple excoriation is bilateral	Unilateral nipple excoriation[105]
Skin dimpling or peau d'orange is absent	Peau d'orange present; skin dimpling present[141]
No fixation to chest wall[18]	Fixation to chest wall[18]
Inflamed, hot may indicate abscess if postpartum or lactating	Inflamed, hot may be ominous in a nonlactating woman[141]
Firm, palpable radial ducts indicate cystic disease	Abnormal contour of breast as woman moves; asymmetric with other breast[105]
Freely movable, slippery mass may be fibroadenoma[105]	Ulceration and edema may be late signs seen with lymphatic blockage[105]
Distinct borders	Indistinct borders[44]

death rate from cancer among women age 40 to 49 shows no improvements in women who underwent mammography until 12 to 14 years later. At that time, screened women are 16% less likely to die from breast cancer. This delayed benefit led the National Institutes of Health (NIH) Consensus Development Conference to conclude "each woman must decide for herself" whether to undergo mammography. The risk of a false-positive result requiring a biopsy is 47.3% to 56.2% after 10 mammograms. Among women age 50 to 74 years, mammography reduces the risk of dying from breast cancer by 26%. Most physicians recommend informed, routine screening in this group. False-positive mammograms do not adversely affect most women's decisions for follow-up screening.[27]

- **Clinician breast examination** is recommended triennially until age 39 years, then annually.[36] Sensitivity of the clinician exam is 57% to 70%, depending on technique and time spent.[141]

- **Genetic screening** may identify the risk of a woman having familial breast cancer. Testing is suggested for the woman with a strong family history, as discussed. Genetic testing may affect health insurance status. Even if the mutation is present, at this time there is not enough evidence to recommend prophylactic surgery.[96] Screening suggested for female BRCA1 carriers would be conducted by a gynecologist and includes physical breast examination every 6 months from the age of 20 years, annual mammogram from the age of 25 years and every 6 months after the age of 50 years, pelvic examination every 6 months beginning at age 30 years, and annual transvaginal ultrasound and CA-125 testing after age 30 years. Advise the patient about experimental breast cancer prevention trials (tamoxifen), and discuss prophylactic mastectomy (although this does not completely remove the risk) and prophylactic oophorectomy at age 35 years or when childbearing is complete.[95]

Diagnostic Procedures

1. **Cytology of nipple discharge.** This procedure has a high false-negative rate and is unreliable (nipple is washed; fluid is expressed and placed on slide, then sprayed with fixative).[105]
2. **Mammography.** A low-dose x-ray is taken of the breasts. This procedure is not useful in young women or during pregnancy because of the density of breast tissue.[105] Sensitivity is 76% to 94%. Approximately 10% of tumors that are palpable and carcinogenic cannot be seen on mammograms. Specificity is >90%. A dose of 40 mrad per view is delivered during the mammogram (compared with 1000 mrad for a computed tomographic [CT] scan).[141]
3. **Ultrasonography.** This procedure has a sensitivity of 88% and a specificity of 97%. It is usually performed on women <30 years.[141] It determines whether a mass is solid or cystic.[105]
4. **Ductography or galactography.** A tube is threaded into a duct and dye is injected. This procedure is indicated for patients with persistent bloody nipple discharge. An intraductal papilloma may be outlined, but it has limited ability to distinguish benign from malignant lesions.[105]
5. **Biopsy.** Ninety percent of women referred for biopsy do not have cancer.[96]
   a. **Fine-needle biopsy** or aspiration (FNA) has 98% sensitivity and up to 100% specificity. Local anesthesia and sometimes light sedation are used.[141] Normal cystic fluid is straw colored or greenish and is discarded. Bloody or cloudy fluid is suspicious and is sent for cytology. A cyst may collapse with aspiration, requiring no further treatment.[105]
   b. **Stereotactic needle biopsy** is a 1-hour outpatient procedure for which light sedation may be given. The woman lies prone on a special table with the breast hanging down. Under a local anesthetic,

a radiologist guides an automated large-bore needle radiologically or ultrasonographically to the area and multiple cores of tissue are taken. There is a minor risk of hematoma or infection. Specialized equipment is necessary. The stereotactic needle biopsy has 89% sensitivity and up to 94% specificity.[141]

c. **Core-cutting needle biopsy** is a biopsy with a large-bore cutting needle; it has 90% sensitivity and up to 100% specificity. The procedure is conducted under local anesthesia, sometimes with light sedation.[141] Several needle passes may be required with minor discomfort. There is a small risk of hematoma and infection. A pressure dressing is applied and acetaminophen or ibuprofen is advised for discomfort afterward.

d. **Open surgical biopsy** has 91% sensitivity and up to 100% specificity.[141] Excisional biopsy is surgical removal of the lesion or lumpectomy; incisional biopsy is partial removal of a mass. A pressure dressing is left in place for 24 to 48 hours. Complications include bleeding, hematoma, and infection.[105]

e. **Wire-guided or needle localization biopsy** has 89% sensitivity and up to 100% specificity.[141] Nonpalpable lesions that can be seen on mammography are marked by the radiologist under local anesthesia with a needle or a wire as indicators for the surgeon to follow with excisional biopsy.[36]

6. **Magnetic resonance imaging (MRI)** may be used in women with dense breasts to examine nonpalpable breast masses, but it is expensive.[105]

7. **Lymphatic mapping** is a new, somewhat controversial technique. The sentinel node (determined by dye or a nuclear medicine scan to primarily drain the affected part of the breast) is removed and others are spared. Women with small tumors (<1 cm) and clinically negative lymph nodes may benefit from this approach.[36]

Types of Breast Cancer

Breast cancer is designated as either ductal (arising from the ductal epithelium) or lobular (arising from the epithelium of the terminal ducts of the lobules) and is further designated by its degree of metastasis:

1. In-situ (noninvasive)
2. Locally invasive
3. Regional metastasis (metastasis to the lymph nodes)
4. Distant metastasis (5% of breast cancer cases are diagnosed at this point)[141]

LOBULAR CARCINOMA IN SITU. Lobular carcinoma in situ (LCIS) is solid, extensive atypical lobular hyperplasia. It is clinically undetectable and diagnosed microscopically only when incidentally found on tissue submitted for another reason. LCIS is precancerous, indicating a 7 to 10 times greater risk of developing invasive carcinoma in either breast. The finding is considered a high-risk marker and the woman is followed as high risk.[141] LCIS is seen in 3% to 5% of breast cancers, occurring more often in premenopausal women.[105]

DUCTAL CARCINOMA IN SITU. Ductal carcinoma in situ (DCIS) is a proliferation of malignant cells within the ductal-lobular system without invasion of the surrounding breast parenchyma. It is usually diagnosed when microcalcifications are seen on mammography. It is precancerous alone but also occurs with 28% of all breast cancers, frequently with invasive cancer.[105]

INVASIVE DUCTAL CARCINOMA. Sixty-five percent to 80% of all invasive breast cancers are invasive ductal carcinomas.[141] The tumor is stony hard on palpation and is diagnosed histologically.

INVASIVE LOBULAR CARCINOMA. Five percent to 10% of all breast cancers are invasive lobular carcinomas. This carcinoma is diagnosed histologically.

MEDULLARY, MUCINOUS, PAPILLARY, OR SARCOMA CANCERS. These cancers coexist in <10% of all breast cancers. Medullary cancer is fast growing but is associated with a good prognosis.[105]

INFLAMMATORY BREAST CANCER. Inflammatory breast cancer is a local response to any type of carcinoma[141]; it occurs in 1% to 4% of all breast cancers.

PAGET'S DISEASE. Paget's disease involves infiltration of the epidermis of the nipple and the duct system by breast carcinoma cells without direct invasion of breast tissue. It presents as excoriation of the nipple or as a subareolar mass[139] and is usually associated with invasive intra-ductal or invasive carcinoma. It is present in 2% of breast cancers.[105]

m *Management*

1. The midwife who identifies a breast mass orders a **mammogram and refers** the woman for surgical evaluation.
2. **Anticipatory guidance: Tissue sampling** may be done as described above. The diagnosis is made and confirmed histologically.[38] The aggressiveness and estrogen sensitivity of the tumor are deter-mined.[105] Estrogen sensitivity allows for tamoxifen treatment. **Staging** is conducted and treatment decisions made.[90] X-rays, bone scans, lab work, and/or CT scans may be required to detect metasta-sis.[105] The type of **surgery** depends on tumor size and location and breast size. Options include lumpectomy, partial mastectomy, axil-lary node dissection, simple mastectomy, modified radical mastec-tomy, and radical mastectomy. Breast-conservation surgery can

usually be done with early detection.[90] Breast reconstruction may be part of the initial surgery or may be done after radiation and chemotherapy.[96]

Adjuvant therapies after surgical intervention, including radiation, chemotherapy, tamoxifen, and ovarian ablation, have improved the survival rate.[111] Premenopausal or postmenopausal status, tumor size and type, and nodal involvement are factors.[90]

3. **Management during pregnancy:** The breast changes of pregnancy and lactation may obscure the diagnosis of breast cancer, delaying treatment and worsening the prognosis. A suspicious breast mass is pursued as vigorously during pregnancy as at other time.[41] When the tumor is estrogen receptor negative, a therapeutic abortion (TAB) does not improve the chance for a cure. Surgical intervention is usually well tolerated by mother and fetus. Ovariectomy is acceptable after 8 weeks' gestation, when the placenta has assumed progesterone production. Breastfeeding is discouraged among women receiving chemotherapy. Some researchers have suggested that the origin of cancer is a virus that might be transmitted by breastfeeding. If a neoplasm is present in the remaining breast, bottlefeeding is usually recommended to avoid increased bloodflow to the breast.[38]

Pregnancy After Breast Cancer

There is little evidence that pregnancy or lactation after breast cancer changes the prognosis for cancer-free survival. A 2- or 3-year delay before conception is considered prudent.[41] A thorough evaluation ideally precedes conception, including scans, chest x-ray, and mammography. Pregnancy probably does not cause, but may accelerate, a recurrence.

Prognosis

As the number of reported breast cancer cases rises, a continuous 1% to 2% improvement in mortality rate has been noted in countries with a high incidence, such as the United States and Canada, possibly due to early detection and high quality of treatment.[141] In 1995, a 95% 10-year survival rate was reported for stage 0 breast cancer and an 88% 10-year survival rate for stage I. Stage II patients had a 66% 10-year survival rate; stage III had a 36% rate and stage IV had a 7% rate. Axillary dissection improved 10-year survival in stage I patients, from 66% to 85%.[56] In 2000, *Lancet* published a report by the Early Breast Cancer Trialists' Collaborative Group reporting that the death rate from breast cancer had fallen nearly one third among British women and about 25% among American women in the previous decade, due in part to earlier diagnosis, better surgery, chemotherapy, and radiotherapy—but most importantly because of the widespread, prolonged use of tamoxifen.[48]

Fluid Cysts

Fluid cysts exist alone or with fibrocystic changes. They are identified and well defined by ultrasonography and are found in women aged 35 to 50 years. Fluid cysts regress with menopause and do not increase the risk of cancer.

Differential Diagnoses: Fibroadenoma, fat necrosis, breast cancer.

ⓜ *Management*

1. **Order a mammogram** for women older than 30 years.
2. **Order ultrasonography,** recommended for women <25 to 30 years.[19]
3. **Refer** the patient to a surgeon.
4. **Anticipatory guidance: Fine-needle aspiration** is performed for diagnosis of a mass in a woman older than 25 years. A cyst that contains bloody fluid, does not drain completely, or recurs must be excised.[19] **Danazol** may be prescribed.[139]

Fat Necrosis

An injury, such as surgery or blunt trauma, even minor, causes a hematoma. The hematoma turns into fat, and fibrous tissue fixes the lump to the skin, sometimes causing nipple retraction. The mass is dominant, tender, irregular,[129] often mobile, and firm. Induration may be present. The mass may be cystic filled with an oily substance or may be a solid calcified mass.[19] Fat necrosis occurs most frequently in overweight, perimenopausal, large-breasted women. The mass does not change cyclically, but over time may increase in size, regress, or remain unchanged for years. It may be caused by breast surgery, radiotherapy, or malignant neoplasm.[139]

Differential Diagnosis: Cancer.

ⓜ *Management*

1. The midwife **refers** the patient to an obstetrician or surgeon.
2. **Anticipatory guidance: Mammography, fine-needle aspiration**, or **open biopsy** may be used. **Expectant management** is the treatment if the trauma is recent.[129]

Fibrocystic Changes

Fibrocystic changes, the most common breast condition, are benign and self-limiting. These round lumps in the breast may be firm or soft, are freely movable, and are tender, especially before menses.[96] Representing a change from the normal response and regression to cyclic hormonal stimulation,[105] "fibrocystic changes" is an umbrella term for bilateral changes due to calcification, mild hyperplasia, or fibrosis. Before the early 1980s, this group of conditions was called "fibrocystic breast disease" until studies showed that such changes were present in at least 50% women of reproductive age and 58% to 89% of women at autopsy. The significance is unknown.[19]

Complications: Women who have benign breast disease with epithelial hyperplasia with or without atypia are at increased risk for breast cancer.[6]

ⓜ Management

1. Order **mammography** to exclude malignancy and **refer** the woman to a surgeon.
2. **Anticipatory guidance:** If a **single solid mass** is palpated, excisional **biopsy** is indicated. A palpable mass may be aspirated. Conservative follow-up is indicated if the aspirant is not bloody, if the cyst resolves after aspiration, and if there are no other signs of malignancy. Excisional biopsy is performed if the cyst recurs after several aspirations.[105] **Fibrocystic changes** are treated if breast pain interferes with sleep or activity or when recurrent cyst or mass formation causes repeated surgical interventions.[19]
3. **Recommend lifestyle changes when the diagnosis has been made:** A well-fitting **supportive bra** promotes comfort.[19] **Eliminating caffeine** and **cigarette smoking** reduces discomfort for many women. **Over-the-counter (OTC) analgesics** are recommended for discomfort.[105]
4. **Pharmacologic interventions:** OCs or supplementary progestins during the secretory phase of the cycle may reduce pain. If the breast discomfort is a **side effect of OCs**, wait 3 cycles for spontaneous improvement; if there is none, switch to a lower estrogen and higher progesterone OC.[105] (Vitamin E supplementation, diuretics, and avoidance of caffeine and chocolate have not been shown to be useful in alleviating pain in fibrocystic breasts.[19])
5. If these measures do not improve the pain, the midwife **refers** the woman for further medical intervention.
6. **Anticipatory guidance: Bromocriptine**, **danazol**, and **tamoxifen** may be prescribed to control symptoms. **Bilateral simple mastectomy** is rarely indicated for pain but may be considered after multiple biopsies or after a biopsy that reveals precancerous cells.[105]
7. **Complementary measures:**
   a. **Homeopathy** is recommended by some authors for relief.[75]
   b. **Herbs: Evening primrose oil** 1500 mg qd may control cyclic pain. Side effects may include bloating and nausea.* **See information about herbs, p. 563**.

Fibroadenoma

Fibroadenoma is a solid, smooth, encapsulated, moveable lump, usually painless, most often located in the upper outer quadrant.[96] It may be single or multiple, unilateral or bilateral and may grow, remain unchanged, or regress. Most grow to about 1 to 2 cm, uncommonly reaching

---

*References 18, 19, 37, 97, 105, 107.

4 cm.[139] These lumps enlarge during pregnancy and lactation, and regress at menopause.[19] This benign proliferation of ductal epithelium, connective tissue, and fibrous stroma grows slowly with unopposed estrogen stimulation. Fibroadenoma is the most common breast tumor in women <25 years, and its presence, together with a family history of breast cancer, increases the risk for cancer.[96]

Differential Diagnoses: Cyst, cancer.

m *Management*

1. The midwife **refers** the patient to a surgeon.
2. **Anticipatory guidance: Aspiration or ultrasound** rules out a cyst.[139] The woman <25 years, because of the low risk of cancer, may choose not to have the fibroadenoma excised. **Excision** is the definitive treatment, however, for the woman >35 to 40 years, for a large fibroadenoma, when there are other risk factors for breast cancer, if the fibroadenoma enlarges, or if the woman prefers.[96]
3. **Fibroadenoma and the use of OCs:** The woman who has a history of fibroadenoma has a small but significant risk of breast cancer if she has currently uses OCs or has used them within the previous 9 years. The increase is restricted to women with localized disease and the risk of metastatic disease is reduced, suggesting that the difference actually reflects earlier diagnosis of existing disease. A history of fibroadenoma is not considered a contraindication to OCs.[6]

Galactocele

A firm, nontender, milk-filled mass caused by a blocked lactiferous duct. It usually develops with the cessation of breastfeeding but may also occur with OCs or galactorrhea.[105]

Differential Diagnoses: Fluid-filled cyst, fibroadenoma, breast cancer.

m *Management*

1. **Order mammography and/or ultrasound.**
2. The midwife **refers** the woman to a surgeon.
3. **Anticipatory guidance:** The surgeon will do an **FNA.** A milky substance with fat globules microscopically is diagnostic. The FNA may be curative, the galactocele may need multiple aspirations, or it may resolve spontaneously.[139] If the mass does not resolve after aspiration, excisional biopsy is conducted to exclude cancer.[105]

Interductal Papilloma

Epithelial tumors within the ductal system are common among perimenopausal and postmenopausal women. Trauma to the duct causes bloody or serous discharge from the nipple. The duct is tender, and pressure carefully applied to areas of the areola identifies the source of the discharge. A single affected duct does not predispose the woman to cancer, but when multiple ducts are affected, it can become cancerous. The latter usually affect younger women and present as a mass. The condition is usually, but not always, unilateral.[139]

Differential Diagnosis: Single vs. multiple interductal papilloma, duct ectasia, physiologic nipple discharge, breast cancer.[139]

ⓜ *Management*

1. **Order a mammogram** for women >30 years to exclude cancer.
2. The midwife **refers** the patient to a surgeon.
3. **Anticipatory guidance:** Cytology of discharge may (or may not) be reliable. **Aspiration fluid** is more reliable **for cytology** findings. **Ductogram** is done to locate the affected duct. **Excision** of the involved duct is the treatment. Alternately, with a normal mammogram, **expectant management** may be chosen, and the discharge sometimes ceases over time if the papilloma necroses.[96]

Mammary Duct Ectasia

Mammary duct ectasia, also called periductal mastitis, plasma cell mastitis, or comedomastitis, is the distension of terminal collecting ducts resulting in inflammation, fibrosis, and dilation as the secretions extravasate.[60] The condition causes a sticky, multicolored discharge from the nipples (red discharge is distinguished from blood by a dipstick or a Hemoccult card).[96] It occurs most often in women aged 45 to 55 years. On exam, a fixed, deep, soft, poorly delineated or firm mass is located centrally below the areola. Breast pain and tenderness, pain, itching, and redness around the nipple and areola, nipple retraction due to shortening ducts, and peau d'orange may be seen. The condition is noncyclical and may become infected and abscess, be bilateral, appear and subside within a week, or become chronic.[139] May occur with obstruction, atrophy, inverted nipples, or lactation.[60]

ⓜ *Management*

1. Order a **mammogram** to exclude cancer.
2. If discharge resembles galactorrhea, order a **serum prolactin** level to exclude prolactinemia.[139]
3. **Refer** the patient to a surgeon.
4. **Anticipatory guidance:** The **surgeon may not intervene** in early stages of inflammation. Hygiene and a lack of further stimulation during this time is important.[96] If inflammation becomes moderate to severe, the physician will prescribe **antibiotics** and do an **incision and drainage.** Local **excision** of ducts may be performed.[139]

Mastitis (Nonlactational)

Mastitis is an inflammatory reaction to fluid extravasated from a dilated alveoli and is often bilateral.[60] Mastitis is a rare cause of a multicolored nipple discharge. It may originate from squamous metaplasia of the ducts, periareolar abscesses, or cellulitis with bacteremia and usually occurs in immunocompromised patients.[96] (See p. 229 regarding puerperal lactational mastitis.)

ⓜ Management

1. **Refer** the patient to a surgeon.
2. **Anticipatory guidance:** Treatment includes **antibiotics and incision and drainage** if necessary.[96]

Nipple Discharge

For galactorrhea, see next section.

Physiologic Discharge: Bilateral, serous, arising from multiple ducts, secreted by the breasts into the ductal system, and usually absorbed into the blood and lymphatic systems. It may be expressed during breast examination or sexual activity. Nipple discharge is generally benign in nature.[96]

Pathologic Discharge: Discharge involving a diseased breast usually comes from one duct and is expressed spontaneously, not on manipulation. The discharge is persistent, intermittent, and the color is variable (clear, yellow, green-gray, pink, bloody). Etiologies include mastitis, intraductal papilloma (44%), duct ectasia (23%), and cancer (11%). Only when the fluid is bloody is cytology of the fluid useful.[19]

ⓜ Management

1. The midwife orders a **mammogram** and **refers** the woman for surgical evaluation. For **anticipatory guidance,** see breast cancer management, p. 411.

Galactorrhea

Galactorrhea is milk production in the absence of pregnancy or lactation,[19] is usually bilateral, and arises from multiple ducts. It is usually caused by hyperprolactinemia from pituitary action or inadequate hypothalamic inhibition of the pituitary.[139]

Etiologies:

1. Physiologic (e.g., chest wall stimulation such as breast manipulation, stress, surgery), possibly related to the stimulation of the areola causing prolactin release.[19]
2. Pathologic (e.g., primary hypothyroidism, hypothalamic disease, pituitary disease, production of prolactin by a neoplasm, chronic renal failure).
3. Anovulatory conditions in which prolactin levels are elevated or "functional" (idiopathic).[96]
4. The following drugs may induce galactorrhea[19,139]:

Reserpine	Dibenzoxepine antidepressants
H$_2$ blockers	(Asendin)
Thioxanthenes (Taractan)	Papaverine derivatives

Butyrophenones (Haldol)
Benzamines (Reglan, sulpiride)
Narcotics
α-Methyldopa
Calcium channel
   blockers (Verapamil)

Chronic opiate use (methadone
   or morphine)
Tricyclic antidepressants
Cimetidine (Tagamet)
Phenothiazines
Combination OCs (administration
   or discontinuation)

Ⓜ Management

1. The midwife **refers** the woman to a physician.
2. **Anticipatory guidance:** Galactorrhea is **confirmed by microscopic visualization of fat globules** in the fluid. Lab work includes measurement of human chorionic gonadotropin **(hCG)** (exclude pregnancy) and **serum prolactin. A prolactin value** >20 ng/mL connotes hyperprolactinemia and suggests hypothyroidism. A **thyroid-stimulating hormone (TSH)** level will exclude thyroid disease. A level >200 to 300 ng/mL indicates a pituitary tumor. Levels between are probably caused by medication, local stimulation, an exaggerated physiologic response, or microadenoma.[19,96] **Imaging studies of the pituitary** may include a lateral x-ray of the sella turcica, CT, or MRI.[134]

   Physiologic causes are treated by **removing the precipitating event.** Other causes of hyperprolactinemia may be treated with **bromocriptine** (Parlodel).[139] **Surgical resection of an adenoma** has high complication and recurrence rates and is usually only considered if the woman cannot tolerate bromocriptine.[19]

• CERVICAL CONDITIONS

Cervical Cancer

When columnar cells are exposed to the pH and hormones of the pubertal woman's vagina, they are replaced by squamous cells of the ectocervical epithelium. The area undergoing this squamous metaplasia, called the transformation zone, is particularly vulnerable to carcinogens. Cervical eversion is increased when the woman is taking OCs; during pregnancy the transformation zone increases, and at menopause the area shrinks.

If cellular alterations occur during this process, they result in an atypical transformation zone that initiates cervical intraepithelial neoplasia (CIN). Mild dysplasia, CIN I (affects the inner third of the cervical epithelium) may regress, remain at this stage, or may progress to moderate dysplasia, CIN II. CIN II affects the inner half to two thirds of the cervical epithelium. Ten percent to 15% of patients with CIN II progress to severe dysplasia, with full-thickness epithelial involvement, and carcinoma in situ (CIN III). Thirty-five percent of patients with carcinoma in situ progress to frankly invasive carcinoma, a 3- to 20-year process.[67]

Predisposing Factors:

Initial sexual intercourse at age <20 years

Increased parity

Young age at marriage

Young age at first pregnancy

Women who have sex with nonmonogamous men

Divorce

Lower socioeconomic status[67]

Multiple sexual partners

HIV infection

Approximately 20 HPV genotypes[137]

Cigarette smoking (dose-related: risk for CIN III increased by 5.85 times with >1 pack/d[42])

Signs and Symptoms: Abnormal bleeding (postcoital, intermenstrual, postmenopausal) and discharge (serous, mucoid, or purulent) with a foul odor may be present. No other symptoms are present until the disease has advanced. On speculum examination, a cancerous lesion may appear as a small, hardened, granular area—ulcerative, necrotic, or bulging and friable. Surrounding tissue may be normal or may show chronic cervicitis. Bloody, serous, or purulent discharge may be present. Alternately, an endocervical lesion may not be visible.[67]

Screening: See cervical cytology, p. 422.

Cervical Cancer and Pregnancy

The diagnosis of cervical cancer may be missed during pregnancy because the vaginal bleeding may be mistaken for a threatened abortion or another pregnancy complication. Colposcopy is easy because the transformation zone is exposed because of physiologic eversion. The prognosis is similar to the nonpregnant woman.[41]

ⓜ Management of Cervical Carcinoma

1. **Refer** the woman with cervical cancer to a gynecologist.
2. **Anticipatory guidance:** See Figure 8-2, the decision tree for the management of cervical cytology results. **Staging** of cervical cancer involves biopsies, cystoscopy, sigmoidoscopy, chest and skeletal x-rays, IV pyelogram, and liver function tests. **Hysterectomy** may be suggested followed by **adjuvant treatment** (radiation and/or chemotherapy).[56]
3. **Management during pregnancy:** Biopsies can still be taken. Endocervical curettage and cone biopsy are undesirable because of the danger of bleeding, rupture of membranes, and preterm delivery. MRI may be used as a staging tool.[41] Carcinoma in situ may be managed conservatively, with therapy initiated 6 weeks postpartum. Microinvasive carcinoma diagnosed during pregnancy may also be managed conservatively, with colposcopic examination every 8 weeks and hysterectomy taking place with cesarean delivery. Frankly invasive carcinoma is more urgent, and the pregnancy <22 to 26 weeks' gestation may be interrupted to pursue treatment.[67]

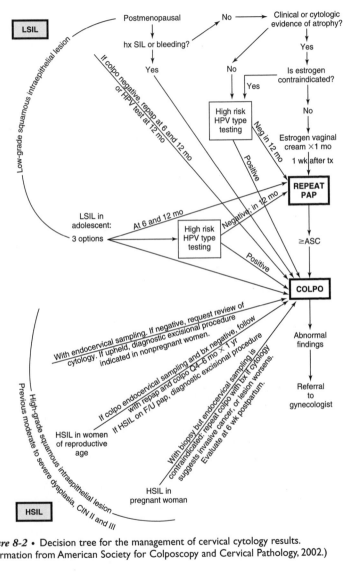

Figure 8-2 • Decision tree for the management of cervical cytology results. (Information from American Society for Colposcopy and Cervical Pathology, 2002.)

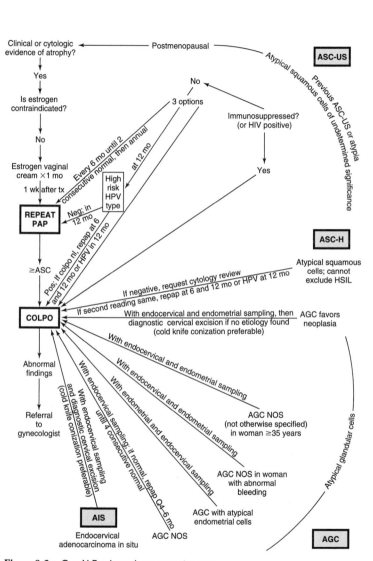

Figure 8-2 • Cont'd For legend, see opposite page.

Cervical Cytology: The Papanicolaou Smear

Cervical cancer is the second most frequent cause of death in women across the world.[108] Screening with the Pap smear has dramatically reduced this number in industrialized countries, where cervical cancer is only the tenth leading cause of all cancer deaths,[137] one tenth of what it was 50 years ago.[25] Five percent to 19% of the 50 million Pap smears performed annually require follow-up.[108]

Technique:
1. Have the woman **avoid lubricants and douches** for 24 hours before the examination.[137]
2. Treat vaginitis before taking the Pap.[137] **Vaginal spotting** does not preclude taking a Pap smear.[17]
3. Take the Pap smear **before** doing **cultures** and the **bimanual** exam. Without disturbing the epithelium, **remove copious vaginal discharge.** Take an **ectocervical scrape** with a moistened Ayres spatula, and take an **endocervical smear** by gently rotating the moistened brush in the os.
4. **Two techniques are available:**
   a. For the **traditional Pap slide technique,** gently smear the sample onto a slide, avoiding clumping. Immediately spray fixative onto the slide from 10 inches or more away to avoid specimen disruption.[137] Much of the sample is discarded with the sampling devices in this technique. Air drying and irregular cell distribution and matter may prevent visualization of cells.[88] A single Pap smear collected in this manner has a 50% false-negative rate.[9]
   b. For the **liquid-based** cytology or **Thin** Prep technique, rinse the sampling device in a vial containing a preservative solution where a slide is prepared from the cells. With this method, the number of satisfactory specimens is increased and more pathology (especially low-grade disease) is identified than with the traditional slide technique.[88] Liquid-based cytology is more expensive than the traditional Pap slide test, and some express concern that its use may result in high-risk women being screened less frequently.[126] It results in more false-positive results, increasing the number of biopsies and colposcopies for healthy women. ACOG concluded in 1999 that liquid-based cytology is not the standard of care as long as Pap tests are conducted annually, but some researchers have concluded that its increased sensitivity make it the superior screening device.

Screening Recommendations: Annual Pap smears are recommended by the American Cancer Society, ACOG, and the National Cancer Institute for women 18 years and older or for younger, sexually active women. After 3 consecutive normal smears, testing is done every 3 years, at the discretion of the woman and her care provider, depending on her risk factors for cervical cancer. Risk factors include multiple sexual partners, cigarette smoking, HPV, or HIV infection.[17] The woman should still receive annual breast and pelvic examinations. Some providers prefer to repeat the Pap smear annually to compensate for the error that may occur in the sampling technique or in the Pap interpretation.[25]

Screening Alternatives: Some researchers suggest HPV DNA testing for triage of atypia. Sensitivity compares to cytology but specificity is lower.[21]

Ⓜ Management of Results

1. **Consult or refer** for abnormal Pap results. See Figure 8-2 for the management of abnormal cervical cytology results.
2. **Anticipatory guidance:** Management of cervical lesions includes **surgical excision** (by excision or punch biopsy), a **loop electrosurgical excisional procedure (LEEP), cryotherapy**, and **laser ablation therapy.** A 1998 study found these three approaches to be equal in complications and in persistence of squamous intraepithelial lesion.[101] **Diagnostic cone biopsy** removes tissue higher in the endocervical canal than other techniques, has a higher cure rate, and is recommended for noncompliant patients who might not come back for examinations for recurrence.[101] **Endocervical curettage (ECC)** is done routinely after colposcopy, except during pregnancy, or under colposcopic visualization after conization.[17]

Cervicitis

Infection of the endocervical canal is evidenced by yellow, mucopurulent discharge, spotting, pressure, dyspareunia, dysmenorrhea, backache, and/or urinary urgency and frequency. On exam, the cervix appears eroded, granular, irritated, friable, and ulcerated. Pain is present with cervical motion. Nabothian cysts may be seen. The wet mount shows many WBCs. Inadequate treatment of gonococcal or chlamydial cervicitis may result in pelvic inflammatory disease (PID)[67] (see p. 425).

Differential Diagnoses: Gonorrhea (GC), chlamydia (CT), cervical cancer, salpingitis, syphilis, chancroid, granuloma venereum.

Laboratory Studies: Pap smear, GC and CT cultures, aerobic culture, CBC, and erythrocyte sedimentation rate (ESR). The WBC will show a shift to the left. The ESR will show whether the infection is chronic.

Ⓜ Management

1. Collect **Pap smear, wet mount, and cultures.**
2. **Treat the specific organism** according to CDC guidelines.
3. **Consult or refer** for the woman with chronic cervicitis, an abnormal Pap smear, or PID for further evaluation.

Polyps (Cervical or Endocervical)

Polyps originate from the ectocervix, endocervix, endometrium, or vagina when local inflammation results in cellular hyperplasia and proliferation.

Growth may be stimulated by OCs. Premenopausal women most often have endocervical polyps; ectocervical polyps occur more often after menopause.[139] Endometrial polyps may arise from uninterrupted estrogen stimulation.[79] Most occur among women in their fourth and fifth decades. Polyps may ulcerate or may become secondarily infected, causing spotting. One percent or less become malignant.[67] A polyp may keep the cervical os open, causing cervicitis and low-grade endometritis (which will spread after a dilation and curettage [D&C]). Polyps commonly recur. Symptoms may include leukorrhea or spotting, or the woman may be asymptomatic. On exam, endocervical polyps appear purple to cherry-red on a long, thin pedicle. Ectocervical polyps are light gray with a short, broad base. Smooth on palpation, friable, single or multiple, a polyp may be millimeters to a few centimeters in diameter.[139]

Differential Diagnoses: Small prolapsed myoma, retained products of conception, sarcoid, cervical cancer, squamous papilloma,[139] squamous cell carcinoma, or adenocarcinoma.[67]

m *Management*

1. **Exclude concurrent infections** by performing cultures, wet mount, **CBC** to evaluate bleeding, and **Pap smear** (should be normal with polyps).[67]
2. The midwife may **remove the polyp** with a punch biopsy or by grasping the polyp at the stalk with a twisting motion, curetting the base, then sending the specimen for histologic evaluation. Control the bleeding with pressure, Monsel's solution, or cautery.[67]
3. If the source of bleeding is uncertain, such as an endometrial polyp that cannot be seen on examination; if the polyp does not easily avulse; if the procedure is excessively painful; or if abnormal bleeding continues after polyp removal; **refer** the woman to a gynecologist.[139]
4. **Anticipatory guidance:** Hysteroscopy or D&C may be used to diagnose endometrial polyps. Tissue is submitted to pathology.[79]

• INFECTIOUS PROCESSES

Bartholin's Cyst or Abscess

The Bartholin's gland is a mucus-secreting nonpalpable 0.5 to 1.0 cm structure with ducts 1.5 to 2 cm long opening just lateral to the vaginal orifice. Duct occlusion results in a nontender mass, usually 1 to 4 cm (up to 10 cm) in size, noted at the entrance of the vagina. Occlusion may occur secondary to congenital stenosis or atresia, thickened mucous at the outlet, mechanical trauma, or neoplasm. When the cystic fluid becomes infected, an abscess forms. Many organisms may cause this infection. Bilateral Bartholin's cysts suggests GC.[139]

A simple cyst may be asymptomatic. An abscess usually develops over a 2- to 3-day period and may spontaneously rupture within 72 hours.

It appears swollen, hot, and fluctuant. The labia may be distorted. "Pointing" occurs at the site of impending rupture. It may cause dyspareunia or painful walking or sitting. Extensive inflammation may cause systemic symptoms.[139]

Differential Diagnoses: Cyst vs. abscess, neoplasm, STI, or sebaceous cyst.

ⓜ *Management*

1. **Small, asymptomatic cysts require no treatment.**
2. **Culture** a draining cyst and **exclude other STIs.**
3. Do a **CBC** for extensive inflammation.
4. For an **uninfected** Bartholin's cyst during pregnancy, **postpone treatment until after pregnancy** because of the hyperemia of pregnancy. In the rare event that it interferes with delivery, perform needle aspiration. A Bartholin's **abscess,** however, **must be drained and cultured** during pregnancy.[41]
5. Indications for **referral** to a gynecologist for treatment include rapid enlargement, increasing pain, abscess formation, or hemorrhage into the cyst. Sitz baths may cause the Bartholin's cyst to spontaneously rupture within 72 hours, but it will likely recur. Broad-spectrum antibiotics will delay ripening of the abscess.[139]

   Anticipatory guidance: Surgical options include **"fistulization"** (catheter placed for drainage is left in place for body to epithelialize a new opening); **"marsupialization"** (a 2 cm incision is made between the gland and the vagina, and the lining of the gland is sewn to the vaginal wall, creating a new opening); **"window procedure"** (a small, oval piece of skin is excised, including the cyst wall, and sutures are placed along the newly excised margin); or **excision** of Bartholin's gland (may result in cellulitis, hemorrhage, hematoma, incomplete removal, subsequent recurrence, and painful scarring; is only recommended if the abscess is huge, multiocular, or recurrent).[139]

Pelvic Inflammatory Disease

Pelvic inflammatory disease (PID) is infection of the uterus, fallopian tubes, and adjacent pelvic structures not associated with pregnancy or surgery.[112] Microorganisms spread from the vagina and/or endocervix to the endometrium (causing endometritis), fallopian tubes (causing salpingitis or tubo-ovarian abscess [TOA]), or contiguous structures (with pelvic peritonitis).[77] Inflammation of the upper genital tract usually follows infection with CT or GC, although other organisms may be present, including *G. vaginalis, Haemophilus influenzae*, enteric gram-negative rods, and *Streptococcus agalactiae*, as well as cytomegalovirus, *M. hominis*, and *U. urealyticum*.[30] Signs and symptoms are highly variable and may include lower abdominal pain, adnexal tenderness, cervical motion tenderness (chandelier's sign), fever, purulent vaginal and cervical discharge. A palpable abdominal mass may be present.[77] Delay in diagnosis allows further inflammation in the upper reproductive tract.[30]

Complications:

Hydrosalpinx	Infertility (20%)
TOA[145]	Chronic pelvic pain (9%)
Adverse pregnancy	Ectopic pregnancy
outcome	Increased risk for
Infant pneumonia	reproductive tract cancer
Neonatal death (20%)	Vulnerability to HIV[64]

Tubo-Ovarian Abscess

TOA occurs in 1% to 4% of PID cases and is the most serious complication. Rupture of a TOA carries an 8.6% mortality rate.[145] TOA is usually present with a polybacterial infection that includes aerobes and anaerobes. The woman (50% have a PID history) experiences pelvic or abdominal pain, fever (80%), and leukocytosis (80%). ESR and C-reactive protein levels are elevated. Pelvic examination shows cervical pain on motion and extreme pelvic tenderness, and a mass may be palpable. Once ruptured, peritonitis and shock may ensue.[131]

Hydrosalpinx

Hydrosalpinx is the accumulation of oviductal fluid in the ampullar lumen due to occlusion of the infundibulum. Women with this condition have a low conception rate (10% after in vitro fertilization [IVF]), have a 50% first trimester spontaneous abortion (SAB) rate,[1] have an increased rate of ectopic pregnancy,[142] and may experience chronic pelvic pain.[29]

Predisposing Factors for PID:

Trichomonas infection[145]	Intrauterine device (IUD) use
Douching (dose-related risk[28])	Cigarette smoking
STI exposure	Sexual activity at a young age
Lower socioeconomic group	Invasive medical procedures
Failure to use contraception	in the genital tract
Multiple sexual partners	Adolescence[77]
PID history	

Diagnosis: Diagnosis is made according to clinical symptoms and cultures, confirmed by rapid improvement (48 to 72 hours) with treatment. A clinical diagnosis of PID is correct 65% to 90% of the time, as confirmed by laparoscopic findings. Additional evidence includes wet mount with >30 WBCs in a high-power field, elevated ESR, and elevated C-reactive protein. Definitive criteria include histopathologic evidence of endometritis on endometrial biopsy or sonography or another imaging technique showing fluid-filled thickened tubes, TOA, free pelvic fluid, or laparoscopic evidence of PID.[30,31]

Ultrasound is instrumental in the diagnosis of TOA and in conservative management. A complex or cystic adnexal mass with multiple echoes and septations describes a TOA ultrasonographically. Laparoscopy is the gold standard for diagnosis.[145]

Differential Diagnosis: Ectopic pregnancy, endometriosis, ovarian cysts, cancer, myoma, appendicitis, pancreatitis, septic abortion, acute cholecystitis, GC vs. nongonorrheal PID, mesenteric lymphadenitis.

PID During Pregnancy: Rarely, salpingitis may occur during the first 12 weeks of pregnancy, before the fusion of the chorion and the decidua, while organisms may still ascend from the cervix.[78] The pregnant woman with PID is at high risk for maternal morbidity, fetal wastage, and preterm delivery.[31]

HIV and PID: The HIV-positive woman will respond to the same antibiotic coverage but may have a more severe course of PID and more often requires surgical intervention.[31]

ⓜ Management

1. **Educate** all women regarding safe sex, STIs, and high-risk behaviors.
2. Obtain **history** including last menstrual period (LMP) and determine whether the woman is pregnant.
3. Collect **cultures** and **wet mount;** when PID is suspected, **consult** the physician.[77]
4. **Anticipatory guidance:** When **laparoscopy** is conducted by the physician for diagnosis, other procedures that may be done include pelvic irrigation, lysis of adhesions, drainage and irrigation of unilateral or bilateral pyosalpinx, and drainage and irrigation of TOA.[102] **Outpatient treatment** is indicated for the woman with mild symptoms. **Hospitalization** for parenteral antibiotics is indicated when the woman is severely ill, has a TOA, does not respond to oral antibiotics, or when a surgical emergency cannot be excluded. **Pregnant women** are hospitalized and given parenteral medications.[30]
5. Sexual **partners** are treated if they had sexual contact with the woman within 60 days of the onset of symptoms.[30]
6. **Instruct** the woman regarding the importance of completing the full medication course, and the need to keep follow-up appointments.

Sexually Transmitted Infections

Chancroid (Ulcus Molle, Soft Chancre)

A chancroid is an ulcerative bacterial genital infection caused by the organism *Haemophilus ducreyi*. More commonly seen in tropical and subtropical locations,[31] *H. ducreyi* is becoming more prevalent in some U.S. cities. In 1997, 32% of genital ulcer cases in New York City were *H. ducreyi*.[46] The diagnosis may be made if one or more painful genital ulcers are present, regional lymphadenopathy is present, and *T. pallidum* and herpes simplex virus (HSV) are excluded. Suppurative inguinal adenopathy is very strong evidence of chancroid.[30] Minimally symptomatic lesions may appear on the cervix or vaginal wall. Alternately, women may carry the organism asymptomatically. Transmission is sexual, and autoinoculation may occur in infected persons to nongenital areas. The woman is infectious as long as the organism is present in the lesion or nodes, possibly months without treatment, and 1 to 2 weeks with treatment.[20] Infection does not confer immunity.[2] Incubation period is 3 to 14 days.[20] The presence of chancroid increases HIV transmission. In the United States, it often coexists with *T. pallidum* or HSV.[30]

Effect on Pregnancy: No known hazard for the fetus.[31]

Differential Diagnoses: Syphilis and HSV.[31]

Laboratory Findings: Definitive diagnosis is made by culturing *H. ducreyi*; however, many laboratories do not have the special culture medium required. The sensitivity of the culture even on the special media is <80%.[30]

⑩ Management According to the CDC's 2002 Recommendations

1. Screen for **concurrent STIs,** including HIV. If negative, retesting in 3 months is suggested. Exclude syphilis and HSV. **Diagnosis is made by exclusion** due to the poor laboratory sensitivity. In areas where chancroid is frequently seen, many health care providers treat for both syphilis and chancroid before they get culture results.[30]
2. **Reporting** the disease is required in many states.[20]
3. **Pharmacologic treatment:**
   a. Azithromycin 1 g PO in a single dose (safety in pregnancy/lactation not established) *or*
   b. Ceftriaxone 250 mg IM in a single dose *or*
   c. Ciprofloxacin 500 mg bid PO for 3 days (contraindicated in pregnant/lactating women and women <18 yr) *or*
   d. Erythromycin base 500 mg PO tid for 7 days.[30]
4. **Improvement should be seen** symptomatically within 3 days and objectively by 7 days, or reevaluate diagnosis. Large ulcers may take >2 weeks to heal. Fluctuant lymphadenopathy heals more slowly than the ulcers and may require incision and drainage.[30]
5. **Treat partners** with whom there was sexual contact within 10 days of symptom onset even if symptom free.[30]

Chlamydia

Chlamydia trachomatis (CT), an obligate intracellular gram-negative parasite,[78] is the most prevalent STI in the United States. CT causes trachoma, genital infection, and lymphogranuloma venereum in adults (see p. 442). Symptoms are similar to GC, with a mucopurulent cervical discharge (clear, white, or amber), erythema, edema, friability of the cervix, bartholinitis, and urethral syndrome. Sixty-seven percent to 74% of women with genital infections, however, are asymptomatic.[3] Reiter's syndrome, a syndrome of urethritis, conjunctivitis, and arthritis, may occur.[28]

Transmission may be perinatal or by vaginal, oral, and anal sex.[28] The period of communicability is unknown. Incubation is probably 1 to 2 weeks or longer.[20] PID, ectopic pregnancy, and infertility may result from the infection.[31] Endocervical CT is associated with an increased risk of acquiring HIV infection. GC coexists in >40% of pregnant women who have CT.[78]

Effect on Pregnancy: SAB, fetal death, preterm premature rupture of membranes (PPROM), preterm delivery, and postpartum endometritis and salpingitis occur with increased frequency. Two thirds of the neonates born through an infected genital tract become infected.[78] Infections of the newborn include ophthalmia neonatorum that may result in blindness (occurring in 35% to 50% of infants born to untreated women) and chlamydial neonatal pneumonia (affecting 11% to 20% of infants born to untreated women).[28]

ⓜ Management According to the CDC's 2002 Recommendations

1. **Educate** all women regarding safe sex, STIs, and high-risk behaviors.
2. **Screen.** During pregnancy, screen at the first prenatal visit. For high-risk women (young age, multiple or new sexual partners, lack of barrier contraception, history of STIs), screen again in the third trimester.[78] Evaluate for **concurrent STIs.** Clinically, GC and CT are difficult to differentiate, and treatment is recommended for both when one is suspected.[30] Gather **history of sexual contacts** within last 10 days and LMP. **Determine whether pregnant.** (If the woman is pregnant and delivery is imminent, **notify pediatric staff.**)
3. **Culture endocervix** (may be done during menses). Exclude concurrent STIs including GC, syphilis, and HIV. Culture or treat presumptively for GC.[30]
4. **Pharmacologic treatment:**
   a. **Recommended regimens for nonpregnant women** (including HIV-positive women):
      (1) Azithromycin 1 g PO in a single dose (safety in pregnancy/lactation not established) *or*
      (2) Doxycycline 100 mg PO bid for 7 days (contraindicated during pregnancy)[30]
   b. **Alternative regimens for nonpregnant women:**
      (1) Erythromycin base 500 mg PO qid for 7 days *or*
      (2) Erythromycin ethylsuccinate 800 mg PO qid for 7 days *or*
      (3) Ofloxacin 300 mg PO bid for 7 days (contraindicated during pregnancy/lactation) *or*
      (4) Levofloxacin 500 mg PO qd for 7 days[30]
   c. **Recommended regimens for pregnant women:**
      (1) Erythromycin base 500 mg PO qid for 7 days *or*
      (2) Amoxicillin 500 mg tid for 7 days[30]
   d. **Alternate regimens for pregnant women:**
      (1) Erythromycin base 250 mg PO qid for 14 days *or*

   (2) Erythromycin ethylsuccinate 800 mg PO qid for 7 days *or*
   (3) Erythromycin ethylsuccinate 400 mg PO qid for 14 days *or*
   (4) Azithromycin 1 g PO in a single dose[30]
5. **Treat presumptively for GC (p. 431).**[30]
6. **Advise the woman** to abstain from sexual intercourse for 7 days, until asymptomatic, and until partners have been treated and 7 days have passed.[30]
7. **Test of cure** is required for all pregnant women because their regimens may be less efficacious. It is not necessary for nonpregnant women if there are no symptoms and if reinfection is not suspected. Rescreening 3 to 4 months later, however, has demonstrated high rates of reinfection, which is associated with a higher risk of PID.[30]
8. **Refer partner(s)** for treatment: all those with whom the patient had sexual contact within 60 days, or the most recent partner whenever contact occurred.[30]
9. The disease is **reportable** in most states.

Gonorrhea *(Neisseria gonorrhoeae)*

GC is a gram-negative anaerobic intracellular diplococcus that infects columnar and transitional epithelium. The woman is most commonly asymptomatic.[78] She may have a yellow vaginal discharge that itches and burns or discharge from the urethra, Bartholin's glands, or Skene's glands. Twenty percent experience endometritis after two or more menstrual cycles. The infection spreads during the menses because of the open os and the presence of nutrients. Timing of infection during the first week of the cycle indicates salpingitis. Rectal infection causes pruritus, tenesmus, and discharge. Symptoms range from mild cervicitis to cystitis, menstrual changes (increased cramping and flow), and pharyngitis to septicemia with arthritis, skin lesions, and rarely endocarditis and meningitis.[20] Complications include the pelvic pain, infertility, and ectopic pregnancy that may follow PID. Disseminated GC infection is manifested by petechial or pustular skin lesions, arthralgia, or septic arthritis. Perihepatitis, endocarditis, or meningitis may occur.[30]

Infection is transmitted by contact with mucous membrane exudate of infected individuals, almost always as a result of vaginal, anal, or oral sexual activity or vertical mother-to-infant transmission. The risk of contracting GC from a single act of intercourse is 60% to 90% for the woman and 20% to 30% for the man.[28] The incubation period is 2 to 7 days or longer. Untreated individuals are infectious for months. The individual is noncommunicable 24 hours after treatment.[20] Other STIs often coexist with GC, including CT in 40%.[3]

Laboratory Findings: Gram stain of the discharge (60% sensitivity), or bacteriologic culture on medium such as Thayer Martin media is diagnostic.[78] In systemic cases, blood cultures are positive for GC.[3]

Effect on Pregnancy: Salpingitis rarely occurs during the first 12 weeks of pregnancy before the fusion of the chorion and the decidua while organisms may still ascend from the cervix. Disseminated GC infection occurs more often during pregnancy. Untreated GC is associated with premature birth, low birthweight (LBW), PPROM, chorioamnionitis, postpartum endometritis, and neonatal transmission causing ophthalmia neonatorum, sepsis, genital infection, and abscess at the site of the scalp electrode.[78]

ⓜ Management According to the CDC's 2002 Recommendations

1. **Educate** all women regarding safe sex, STIs, and high-risk behaviors.
2. **Screen.** During pregnancy, screen at the first prenatal visit. For high-risk pregnant women (young age, multiple or new sexual partners, lack of barrier contraception, history of STIs), screen again in the third trimester.
3. Gather the **history** of sexual contacts within last 10 days and LMP. **Determine whether pregnant.** (If the woman is pregnant and delivery is imminent, **notify pediatric staff.**)
4. Evaluate for **concurrent STIs.** Clinically, GC and CT are difficult to differentiate, and treatment is recommended for both when one is suspected.[30]
5. **Culture endocervix** (may be done during menses), the pharynx, and rectum if appropriate. Obtain a **Gram stain** for a presumptive diagnosis. Exclude concurrent STIs including GC, syphilis, and HIV. **Culture or treat presumptively for CT.**[30]
6. **Pharmacologic treatment** of uncomplicated GC infection (including HIV-positive women):
   a. **Recommended regimens for nonpregnant women**[30]:
      (1) Cefixime 400 mg PO in a single dose *or*
      (2) Ceftriaxone 125 mg IM in a single dose *or*
      (3) Ciprofloxacin 500 mg PO in a single dose *or*
      (4) Ofloxacin 400 mg PO in a single dose *or*
      (5) Levofloxacin 250 mg PO in a single dose
   In addition, if CT has not been excluded:
      (1) Azithromycin 1g PO in a single dose *or*
      (2) Doxycycline 100 mg PO bid for 7 days
   b. **Alternative regimens for nonpregnant women**[30]:
      (1) Spectinomycin 2 g IM in a single dose for patients who cannot take a cephalosporin or a quinolone *or*
      (2) Ceftizoxime 500 mg IM in a single dose *or*
      (3) Cefotaxime 500 mg IM in a single dose *or*
      (4) Cefoxitin 2 g IM in a single dose with probenecid 1 g PO *or*
      (5) Single-dose quinolones (contraindicated for treatment of GC acquired in Hawaii, Asia, the Pacific, and California, where there are high rates [up to 14.3%] of quinolone-resistant GC):
         (a) Gatifloxacin 400 mg PO in a single dose *or*
         (b) Lomefloxacin 400 mg PO in a single dose *or*
         (c) Norfloxacin 800 mg PO in a single dose

c. **Recommended regimens for pregnant women (quinolones and tetracycline are contraindicated in pregnancy; treat with a recommended or alternate cephalosporin)**[30]:
   (1) Cefixime 400 mg PO in a single dose *or*
   (2) Ceftriaxone 125 mg IM in a single dose *or*
   (3) Ceftizoxime 500 mg IM in a single dose *or*
   (4) Cefotaxime 500 mg IM in a single dose *or*
   (5) If cephalosporins are not tolerated, spectinomycin 2 g IM in a single dose

In addition, if CT has not been excluded:
   (1) Erythromycin base 250 mg PO qid for 14 days *or*
   (2) Amoxicillin 500 mg PO tid for 7 days

d. **Recommended regimens for treatment of pharyngeal GC**[30]:
   (1) Ceftriaxone 125 mg IM in a single dose *or*
   (2) Ciprofloxacin 500 mg PO in a single dose (contraindicated in pregnancy)

In addition, if CT has not been excluded:
   (1) Azithromycin 1 PO in a single dose (safety in pregnancy/lactation not established) *or*
   (2) Doxycycline 100 mg PO bid for 7 days (contraindicated in pregnancy)[30]

e. **Recommended regimen for treatment of infection of the conjunctiva**[30]: Lavage the infected eye with saline solution once. Administer ceftriaxone 1 g IM in a single dose.

f. **Prophylaxis for gonococcal ophthalmia neonatorum** (the efficacy in preventing chlamydial ophthalmia is unclear)[30]:
   (1) Silver nitrate 1% aqueous solution in a single application *or*
   (2) Erythromycin 0.5% ophthalmic ointment in a single application *or*
   (3) Tetracycline 1% ophthalmic ointment in a single application

7. **Refer** the woman with **disseminated GC** to the physician. **Anticipatory management:** Hospitalization and parenteral antibiotics are required.[30]

8. Individuals who are "not cured" with the above regimen have probably actually been cured and reinfected because **treatment failure** with these regimens is rare. Follow-up cultures are not necessary unless the woman remains symptomatic, in which case order culture with sensitivities and exclude other STIs.[30]

9. Treat sexual **partners** of infected individuals who had sexual contact within the last 60 days or the most recent contact, regardless of timing.[30]

10. **Counsel** regarding safe sex. Other safety measures include urinating before and after sex and daily perineal hygiene. The woman should avoid sexual intercourse until her treatment is complete and she and her partners are asymptomatic.[31]

11. GC is **reportable** to the public health department.

Granuloma Inguinale (Donovanosis)

The intracellular gram-negative bacillus *Calymmatobacterium granulomatis* is rarely seen in the United States but is seen more often in tropical and developing regions, specifically southern Africa, India, Papua New Guinea, and central Australia. A bacterial disease of the skin and mucous membranes of the genitalia, this disease is progressive and chronic. Beginning as a painless indurated papule or nodule, the disease spreads slowly in nontender, friable, beefy-red granulomatous, ulcerative, fibrotic scarring lesions. There is no lymphadenopathy. Secondary bacterial infection or infection with another STI may occur.[30] Untreated, the process may destroy the external genitalia and spread to other parts of the body. Transmission is presumably by direct contact with lesions during sexual activity. In studies, only 20% to 65% of the sexual partners of infected persons have been infected. The condition is probably infectious as long as there are open lesions present. The incubation period is probably 1 to 16 weeks.[20]

Laboratory Findings: Intracytoplasmic rod-shaped organisms (Donovan bodies) are diagnosed in Wright or Giemsa-stained smears of granulation tissue or by histologic examination of biopsy specimens. Exclude *Haemophilus ducreyi* (chancroid) by culture in appropriate media.[20] Donovan bodies cannot be grown on culture media.[31]

🅜 *Management According to the CDC's 2002 Recommendations*

1. **Educate** all women regarding safe sex, STIs, and high-risk behaviors.
2. Gather history of sexual contacts within last 10 days and LMP. Determine whether pregnant.
3. **Pharmacologic regimens:** Drug-resistant strains have occurred. Continue therapy for 3 weeks or until all lesions have completely resolved.[30]
   a. **Recommended regimens for the nonpregnant woman**[30]:
      (1) Doxycycline 100 mg PO bid for at least 3 weeks *or*
      (2) Trimethoprim-sulfamethoxazole 1 double-strength tablet (800 mg/160 mg) PO bid for at least 3 weeks.
   b. **Alternate regimens for the nonpregnant woman**[30]:
      (1) Ciprofloxacin 750 mg PO bid for at least 3 weeks *or*
      (2) Erythromycin base 500 mg PO qid for at least 3 weeks *or*
      (3) Azithromycin 1 g PO once a week for at least 3 weeks
   c. **Recommended regimens for the pregnant woman:** Erythromycin base 500 mg PO qid for at least 3 weeks. Consider adding an IV aminoglycoside (e.g., gentamycin). Doxycycline and ciprofloxacin are contraindicated during pregnancy.
4. **Sexual partners** who had sexual contact with the infected woman within 60 days preceding symptoms or those with symptoms are referred for evaluation and treatment.[30]

5. **Report** the disease to the public health department.[20]

Herpes Simplex Virus

HSV is seen in two forms, types 1 and 2. HSV2 causes the majority of genital infections. Beginning as a localized primary lesion, both HSV1 and 2 are characterized by latency and recurrences. A primary case of HSV occurs when the woman acquires HSV but carries no antibodies to HSV1 or HSV2. A nonprimary, first-episode case is one in which the woman has antibodies to HSV1 and she acquires HSV2, or vice versa. These cases are difficult to distinguish clinically from recurrent or reactivation cases in which the woman carries the antibody to the virus that is causing an outbreak.[78] Many are infected with the virus and are unaware of it.[31]

Primary Infection with HSV1: May be mild or unnoticed or may have occurred in childhood. Ten percent will have fever and malaise lasting a week or more. Gingivostomatitis, vesicular lesions in the oropharynx, severe keratoconjunctivitis, a generalized cutaneous eruption, meningoencephalitis, acute pharyngotonsillitis, or sometimes fatal congenital HSV may occur (see below).[20] In a primary case, lesions are larger in size and number. Initial vesicles rupture and leave a shallow ulcer. Inguinal lymphadenopathy is present. Lesions spontaneously resolve in approximately 3 weeks.[11] **Recurrences** of HSV1 usually causes clear vesicles on an erythematous base located on the face or lips that crust and heal within a few days (herpes labialis, fever blisters, or cold sores). Reactivation may be triggered by fever, trauma, or a concurrent disease. Circulating antibodies are not affected by reactivations.[20] Recurrences of genital HSV1 infection are much less frequent than those of HSV2 infection.[30]

Primary Infection with HSV2: Usually sexually transmitted, involving a primary lesion—the appearance of small, painful, superficial blisters—usually on the cervix or vulva in women, with accompanying flulike symptoms. Lesions spontaneously resolve at approximately 3 weeks.

Increased shedding of the virus in the lower genital tract occurs for 3 months after the initial lesions have healed.[11] The virus then becomes latent in the nerve-cell bodies of sensory ganglia.[78] **Recurrences** occur in 50% of infected women—with viral shedding, with or without symptoms—on vulva, perineal skin, buttocks, and legs, depending on sexual practices.[20] Triggering stimuli may include ultraviolet light, immunosuppression, and trauma. Recurrent infections are typically less severe and of shorter duration.[78]

Laboratory Findings: Multinucleated giant cells with intranuclear inclusions are seen in tissue scrapings. Diagnosis is confirmed by direct fluorescent antibody (FA) tests or isolation of the virus from oral or genital lesions, biopsy, or by demonstration of HSV-DNA in lesion or spinal fluid. HSV-specific IgM suggests, though not conclusively, a primary infection.[20] Cytologic tests only have a 60% to 70% sensitivity. Viral cultures of the ulcers (obtained by unroofing a lesion and testing the fluid) are 80% sensitive in early primary and nonprimary first-episode cases and 40% sensitive in recurrent cases.[11]

Serologic testing for HSV may be performed to distinguish a primary from a nonprimary first-episode case; a second test is indicated in 2 to 3 weeks.[11] Routine weekly cultures in the absence of a lesion are not recommended in pregnancy because these cultures are not predictive of infants at risk.[78]

Transmission: HSV1 is spread by contact with an infected person's saliva. The virus may be present in the saliva for 7 weeks after stomatitis. Contact with the hands may cause herpetic whitlow (HSV infection of the hand). HSV2 is usually spread through sexual contact. Primary genital lesions are infectious for 7 to 12 days; recurrent lesions are infectious for 4 to 7 days. HSV1 and 2 may be found at various sites, depending on oral, genital, and anal contact. The incubation period is 2 to 14 days.[20] The annual risk of acquiring HSV infection from a sexual partner is 31.9% for a woman with no HSV antibodies. Women who are HSV1 positive run a 9.1% risk of acquiring HSV2 during a year of sexual contact with an infected partner. Asymptomatic shedding (in both saliva and genital secretions) causes more than half of the cases of transmission.[11]

Complications During Pregnancy: Vertical transmission is more likely to occur during a primary case of HSV1. HSV2 is as likely to be transmitted in either primary or recurrent outbreaks.[11] Vertical hematogenous dissemination is uncommon but may occur. Alternately, infection may ascend through the cervix with or without ruptured membranes.[78] Primary HSV infection during the first trimester increases the risk of SAB, stillbirth and, rarely since the introduction of acyclovir, microcephaly, microphthalmia, intracranial calcifications, and chorioretinitis. Late primary infection may cause preterm labor. Vertical transmission by vaginal deliver occurs in 50% of primary HSV cases, in 33% of nonprimary first-episode cases, and in 1% to 3% of recurrent cases.[11] Infection is occasionally spread by internal fetal monitoring.[78] Neonatal disease may remain localized to skin, eye, and mouth (no mortality risk but it may progress); it may affect the central nervous system (CNS; 15% mortality); or it may become disseminated (57% mortality).[11]

Transmission During Breastfeeding: See p. 320.

ⓜ Management of the Nonpregnant Woman According to the CDC's 2002 Recommendations

1. **Educate** all women regarding safe sex, STIs, and high-risk behaviors.
2. Gather **history** of sexual contacts within last 10 days and LMP. Determine whether pregnant.
3. The clinical diagnosis of genital HSV is insensitive and nonspecific, and the classic lesions are absent in some patients. The HSV serotypes

differ in their course, requiring different counseling. The clinical diagnosis of HSV is therefore confirmed by laboratory testing. Cytologic testing (Tzanck preparation and Pap smear) are unreliable. Perform a **viral culture.** False-negative viral cultures are common, so confirm the diagnosis with **type-specific serologic testing** in cases with healing lesions (making specimen poor) or recurrences.[30]

4. **Pharmacologic treatment:** Systemic antiviral drugs ameliorate primary and recurrent episodes or may be used as a daily repressive treatment. They do not eradicate the virus or decrease asymptomatic viral shedding. Once medications are discontinued, the disease reverts to its former severity and frequency of recurrences.[30]

   a. **For the first outbreak**[30]:
      (1) Acyclovir 400 mg PO tid for 7 to 10 days *or*
      (2) Acyclovir 200 mg PO 5 times/d for 7 to 10 days *or*
      (3) Famciclovir 250 mg PO tid for 7 to 10 days *or*
      (4) Valacyclovir 1 g PO bid for 7 to 10 days

   NOTE: Treatment is extended if healing is incomplete after 10 days.[30]

   b. **For recurrences** (The woman is provided with a prescription to self-initiate treatment immediately when symptoms or the prodrome begin.)[30]:
      (1) Acyclovir 200 mg PO 5 times/d for 5 days *or*
      (2) Acyclovir 400 mg PO tid for 5 days *or*
      (3) Acyclovir 800 mg PO bid for 5 days *or*
      (4) Famciclovir 125 mg PO bid for 5 days *or*
      (5) Valacyclovir 500 mg PO bid for 3 to 5 days *or*
      (6) Valacyclovir 1 g PO qd for 5 days

   c. **Daily suppressive therapy** (Does not entirely eliminate asymptomatic viral shedding and transmissibility but reduces frequency of recurrences by 70% to 80%. Discontinue after 1 year of therapy to reassess changes in the frequency of outbreaks due to the natural disease course. Not prescribed to those who are serologically positive but clinically asymptomatic.)[30]:
      (1) Acyclovir 400 mg PO bid *or*
      (2) Famciclovir 250 mg PO bid *or*
      (3) Valacyclovir 500 mg PO qd *or*
      (4) Valacyclovir 1 g PO qd

   NOTE: Valacyclovir 500 mg PO qd may be less effective than other regimens for the woman with frequent outbreaks.[30]

5. **Educate** the woman regarding the natural course of the disease, the potential for recurrences, asymptomatic viral shedding, sexual transmission (need to abstain from sexual activity during prodromal symptoms and while a lesion is present, to inform partners that she has HSV, and to use condoms during all sexual encounters), the risk of neonatal infection, and benefits and limitations of antiviral therapy. Dispel the concern that HSV causes cancer (HSV2 is at most a

cofactor in cervical cancer). Further information is available for clients at the CDC National STD/HIV Hotline: (800) 227-8922 and at http://www.ashastd.org.[30]

6. **Complementary measures for HSV:**
   a. **Homeopathy** experts suggest homeopathy remedies for HSV outbreaks.[41,113,121,149]
   b. **Ice** applied locally or **baking soda** baths may be comforting.[85,113] Local application of cornstarch, rubbing alcohol, and **cold milk** compresses applied for 5 to 10 minutes 5 to 6 times/d help dry lesions and enhance comfort.[85]
   c. **Nutritional suggestions:** L-Lysine 500 to 1000 mg is suggested daily[18,85,149] as well as **vitamin C** 5000 to 10,000 mg.[18,85,149] **Garlic** is an antiviral.[62,85,110] Other supplementary suggestions include **vitamin A** 50,000 U daily (no more than 10,000 U if pregnant), **vitamin B complex** ≥50 mg tid,[18,85] **vitamin B$_6$** 250 mg tid,[113] **vitamin E** 600 IU daily,[18,85] and **zinc** 30 to 100 mg qd in divided doses.[18,149]

      Minimize the following foods that contain L-arginine: coffee, grains, chicken, chocolate, corn, dairy, meat, peanut butter, nuts and seeds. Avoid citrus.[18,113]
   d. **Herbs: Burdock**, **contraindicated in pregnancy,** 15 to 60 g/L of liquid for local use as a compress or taken orally 6 to 25 drops of tincture tid is helpful.[62,107,113,138] **Calendula** ointment or infused oil, **contraindicated in pregnancy,** can be applied locally; a sitz bath with calendula tea is healing. Calendula tincture may also be diluted with three parts water applied locally with a cotton swab tid.* **Echinacea** extract, **contraindicated in pregnancy,** is antiviral, stimulates the body's immune system, and is useful in treating HSV. It may be taken orally or used locally to treat inflammation and pain.[18,62,10,113,117] At the first sign of a HSV recurrence, Nissim[107] suggests taking 25 drops of Echinacea tincture in a little water, repeating q2h for 6 to 8 hours. Continue the tincture qid during the outbreak. It shortens the outbreak and decreases recurrences. **Goldenseal, contraindicated in pregnancy,** can be taken internally by capsule, tea, or extract or used locally to treat inflammation and pain.[18,62,85,113,117] **Myrrh, also contraindicated in pregnancy,** applied locally as a diluted tincture or as a poultice, treats inflammation and pain. Diluted tincture of myrrh applied to lesions helps them dry faster, though it will sting.[18,85,113,138] **Tea tree oil,** an antibiotic, stimulates the immune system. It can be applied locally or added to the sitz bath.[85,110,113,138] **See information about herbs, p. 563.**
   e. Authors encourage getting a lot of rest and reducing stress.[18,113]

---

*References 40, 62, 85, 113, 130, 138, 149.

ⓜ Management of the Pregnant Woman According to the CDC's 2002 Recommendations

1. As in the nonpregnant woman, **confirm the diagnosis** with viral culture and type-specific HSV serologic testing.[30] Gather the history of recent sexual contacts.

2. **Counsel** the HSV-negative woman with an HSV-positive partner to avoid acquisition of HSV in the third trimester by avoiding oral or genital contact. Educate the woman as described for the nonpregnant client.

3. **Pharmacologic management:** Although **acyclovir** is a category C medication during pregnancy, numerous studies and a registry maintained since 1984 have failed to identify a risk to the fetus. Use in primary, severe disease appears to be safe.[78] Acyclovir hastens healing of the lesion, reduces lesion pain, reduces viral shedding, and decreases recurrences—possibly reducing the number of cesarean sections required.[30] It may diminish vertical transmission to the fetus in utero.[11] Newer antivirals, **valacyclovir** and **famciclovir,** are class B medications. They require less frequent dosing than acyclovir, and they are approved by the FDA to treat primary cases and recurrences and for suppression during pregnancy. Medications are prescribed at the same dosage as for the nonpregnant woman.

4. **Delay invasive transcervical procedures** until active lesions have resolved.

5. In the case of the woman with **PPROM remote from term** who has active HSV, the physician weighs the risk of HSV against the risks of prematurity. Delivery may be delayed for glucocorticoid therapy while treating with an antiviral agent.[11]

6. Cesarean section is advised before the membranes rupture when a **primary genital HSV lesion is present in late pregnancy or when a recurrent lesion is present when labor begins.** When the membranes have spontaneously ruptured, cesarean section is performed as soon as possible. A maximum period after rupture of the membranes has not been determined beyond which cesarean delivery does not benefit the fetus.[11]

7. For the woman with a **recurrent lesion distant from the vulva**, such as the buttock, the risk of vertical transmission is approximately 3%. Cervical shedding occurs in 2% of these women. Cesarean section is not recommended for these women. Apply an occlusive dressing to the lesion and proceed with vaginal delivery.[11]

8. Local infection may result from the use of scalp electrodes, even with no lesion present. **Scalp electrodes are contraindicated** when genital lesions are present and are used only when indicated when there are no lesions present.[11]

9. See the complementary measures noted for the nonpregnant woman, some of which may be suggested during pregnancy.

Human Papillomavirus (Condyloma Acuminata)

HPV is an STI that usually affects the lower genital tract. More than 80 genotypes exist, and more than 20 affect the cervix.[137] Box 8-1 lists common HPV genotypes that confer risk. Several strains may coexist in one individual. Left untreated, warts may regress spontaneously, may remain unchanged, or may grown and multiply.[30] Many young women are transiently infected with HPV for 12 to 24 months.[137] Cauliflower-like growths, known as condyloma acuminata, are seen mostly in moist areas of the genitalia and rectum. They may be painful, friable, and/or pruritic. Papillomas of the cervix are flat. When a cervical infection with certain high-risk HPV genotypes persists, there is an increased risk for cervical cancer. Smoking, the presence of other infections, and the immunocompetence of the woman determine whether HPV will progress to cancer.[104] Removal of visible HPV lesions does not change the course of the disease or alter the risk for cervical cancer. Recurrence of the warts within several months of treatment is common and probably represents recurrence rather than reinfection.[30]

Transmission is by direct contact, autoinoculation, fomites, vertical transmission, and sexual contact.[20] Removal of the visible warts may or may not reduce infectivity. The period of communicability is unknown and the incubation period is variable. The communicability of subclinical warts is unknown. The duration of infectivity is uncertain and whether future sexual partners should be told about past HPV infection is unclear.[30] Laryngeal papillomas rarely develop on the vocal cords and epiglottis of children who have been born through a birth canal infected with those warts.[20]

Complications During Pregnancy: Elevated estrogen levels of pregnancy may accelerate growth of condylomata acuminata, causing obstruction of the birth canal. These warts may be friable, and their presence may increase the risk of hemorrhage with childbirth.[78]

The risk of vertical transmission increases with increased maternal viral load. Transmission may occur during fetal passage through the birth canal and may be transmitted hematogenously by crossing the placental

• *Box 8-1 / HPV Genotypes* •

- HPV types 16, 18, 31, 33, and 35 are strongly associated with cervical neoplasia. They may be found in visible genital warts and may be associated with external genital squamous intraepithelial neoplasia. These types are also associated with vaginal, anal, and cervical intraepithelial dysplasia and squamous cell carcinoma.[30]
- HPV types 6 and 11 are the usual causes of the cauliflower-type growths on external genitalia. These types are rarely associated with invasive squamous cell carcinoma of the external genitalia.[30]

barrier.[144] Risk of transmission to the infant is <1 in 1000. Neonatal infection may manifest itself as laryngeal papillomatosis or genital tract or rectal disease.[78] The time between rupture of membranes and delivery may influence transmission. Rupture of less than 2 hours resulted in no vertical transmission in the 1999 study of Tenti et al. Thirty percent of the infants of infected mothers had positive initial nasopharyngeal samples, but all were clear by 5 weeks and remained so for 18 months.

Vaccination: A controlled trial was recently conducted on a three-part vaccination that has been developed for women who are HPV16 negative. The presence of this genotype puts women at high risk for cervical cancer. The vaccine, when recipients were followed for 17 months, appeared to be 100% effective in preventing HPV16 infection; a placebo group reported a 3.8% incidence of persistent HPV16 infection per 100 woman-years. No serious adverse reactions were reported. No cross-protection with other HPV genotypes occurs.[87]

Diagnosis: To identify cervical HPV infection, a cervical swab is taken of the transformation zone and put into transport medium. HPV DNA is identified in the laboratory.[137] Biopsy of visible lesions may be performed. HPV may also be identified on the Pap smear, although this report is not reliable.[78]

ⓜ Management of Lesions of the External Genitalia According to the CDC's 2002 Recommendations

1. **Educate** all women to avoid direct contact with lesions on another person. Using a condom probably reduces transmission.[20] A website is available for client education: *http://www.ashastd.org.*
2. **R/O neoplasm** with colposcopy and/or biopsy. An external HPV lesion is not an indication for colposcopy or to perform Pap smears more frequently than annually.[30]
3. **R/O concurrent STIs.**[31]
4. **R/O pregnancy.** Podophyllin, podofilox, interferons, and 5-fluorouracil are contraindicated during pregnancy.[78]
5. **Treatment:** NOTE: Treatment of external warts is guided by client preference, available resources, and the clinician's experience. No one treatment is superior and whether infectivity is reduced is unclear. Recurrence may occur. Genital warts are not associated with cervical cancer. A woman may choose to forego treatment and await spontaneous regression of external warts. Warts located on moist surfaces tend to respond better to topical treatment than warts on dry surfaces. Change treatment modality if there is not substantial improvement after 3 treatments or complete resolution after 6 treatments. Persistent hypopigmentation or hyperpigmentation may be seen after ablative treatment. Depressed or hypertrophic scars may occur rarely, especially if there was insufficient healing between treatments. Treatment may rarely result in chronic pain (vulvodynia) of the vulvar region (see p. 467).[30]

a. **Patient-administered treatments** (the first treatment is ideally applied by the clinician to demonstrate proper technique; patients must be able to reach and identify warts):

(1) **Podofilox** 0.5% solution or gel (an antimitotic drug **contraindicated during pregnancy**): Using a cotton swab for solution or a finger for gel, the woman applies the treatment to the visible wart(s) bid for 3 days, followed by 4 days of no therapy. Repeat as necessary 4 times. Total wart area should not exceed 10 cm^2, and the daily total dose of podofilox should not exceed 0.5 mL. Most patients feel mild to moderate local irritation with application.[30] *or*

(2) **Imiquimod** 5% cream (Aldara) **(contraindicated during pregnancy):** Apply with a finger at hs 3 times/wk for as long as 16 weeks. Wash the area with mild soap and water 6 to 10 hours after application. May clear warts by 8 to 10 weeks. Imiquimod stimulates the body's own immune system to fight the virus by stimulating the production of interferon and cytokines. Local inflammatory reactions, usually mild to moderate, are common.[30]

b. **Provider-administered treatments:**

(1) **Podophyllin resin** 10% to 25% in compound tincture of benzoin is an antimitotic **(contraindicated during pregnancy).** Petroleum jelly may be applied to the skin around the lesion with a gloved finger. Apply a small amount of podophyllin to each wart and allow to air dry. Use <0.5 mL/session, applying to <10 cm^2. Some experts suggest washing off after 1 to 4 hours to reduce local inflammation. Repeat weekly if necessary.[31] Never apply to raw or open tissue. Be sure the lesions are dry before clothing is replaced. A sanitary napkin prevents the staining of clothing.[28]

(2) **Trichloroacetic acid (TCA) or bichloroacetic acid (BCA)** 80% to 90% are caustic agents that chemically coagulate proteins. Apply petroleum jelly to the skin around the lesion with a gloved finger. Apply a small amount of the acid to warts. TCA is thin and spreads easily. Allow to air dry, forming a white, frosty appearance, before the woman sits up. Powder with talc or baking soda to remove unreacted acid if excess is applied or to counteract burning. Repeat weekly if necessary.[30]

6. If the above are unsuccessful, **refer** to a physician.

7. **Anticipatory guidance:** A physician may use cryotherapy, surgical removal of warts (most benefits the woman with a large number or area of warts), laser surgery (for extensive warts nonresponsive to other treatments or for intraurethral warts), or intralesion recombinant interferon (requires frequent office visits and has frequent systemic adverse effects).[30]

8. **Follow-up:** With self-administered treatments, a return appointment a few weeks into therapy to assess success may be helpful. Women concerned about recurrences may return in about 3 months.[30]

9. Treatment of sexual **partners** is not necessarily recommended due to the lack of data regarding whether reinfection causes recurrences or whether treatment reduces infectivity. Referral may be beneficial for education and counseling, however.[30]

10. **Complementary measures: Herbs: Thuja (contraindicated in pregnancy)** may be used externally in tincture form painted on the warts tid.[40,107,121] **See information on herbs, p. 563.**

ⓜ *Management of Lesions of Cervix, Vagina, Urethral Meatus, Mouth, or Anus According to the CDC's 2002 Recommendations*

1. After education and exclusion of concurrent STIs and pregnancy, **refer** the woman to a physician.

2. **Anticipatory guidance:** Vaginal warts may be treated with podophyllin, TCA, or BCA by some clinicians, but absorption is increased from this area and other clinicians question its safety. Cryotherapy or surgical removal may be used.[30]

ⓜ *Management During Pregnancy*

1. After education and exclusion of concurrent STIs, the midwife **refers** the woman to the obstetrician for management of HPV.

2. **Anticipatory guidance:** The physician will exclude neoplasm. Removal is recommended by many experts.[30] Recommended treatments include carbon dioxide laser ablation, cryotherapy with liquid nitrogen or cryoprobe, or surgical excision. Treatment in the third trimester decreases the risk of recurrence before labor, decreasing the risk of transmission to the infant. Whether cesarean delivery is protective is unknown. HPV is, therefore, not an indication for abdominal delivery unless warts are large and obstructive.[30,78]

ⓜ *Management of Subclinical Human Papillomavirus Infection*

May be diagnosed by Pap smear, colposcopy, or after application of acetic acid. Neither acetic acid nor a pap smear is specific for HPV, however. A Pap diagnosis of HPV does not always correlate with HPV testing. Manage according to the degree of dysplasia. No treatment is effective for subclinical HPV. Most sexual partners of women infected with subclinical HPV are already infected. Whether subclinical HPV is as infective as warts is unknown.[30]

Lymphogranuloma Venereum (Lymphogranuloma Inguinale, Climatic, or Tropical Bubo)

Lymphogranuloma venereum (LGV) is a genital infection usually seen in tropical climates and rare in the United States. It is caused by chlamydia trachomatis.[30] Beginning as a small, painless ulcer at the inoculation site on the vulva, the initial lesion may go unnoticed. Lymphadenopathy, often unilateral, is the usual presenting symptom. Enlarged glands (buboes) may adhere to the skin, creating sinuses. The infection may progress to the rectum and the rectovaginal septum. Elephantiasis of the genitalia may occur. Fever, chills, headache, anorexia, and joint pain may be present. Disease course is long. Transmission is by contact with an open lesion, probably through sexual contact. Infectiousness lasts while active lesions are present, from weeks to years. Twenty percent to 65% of partners become infected. The incubation period is variable, ranging from 3 to 30 days for a primary lesion, up to several months if a bubo is the first manifestation.[20]

Diagnosis: Exclude other causes of inguinal adenopathy and genital ulcers and test serologically.[30]

Laboratory Findings: Complement fixation titers ≥1:64 are diagnostic of LGV.[30]

ⓜ Management According to the CDC's 2002 Recommendations

1. **Educate** all women regarding safe sex, STIs, and high-risk behaviors.
2. Evaluate and treat for **concurrent STIs.** Offer HIV counseling and testing.
3. Collect **history** regarding recent sexual partners and LMP. **Determine whether pregnant.**
4. **Pharmacologic treatment for the nonpregnant woman (including HIV-positive women):**
   a. Doxycycline 100 mg PO bid for 21 days is the preferred treatment (contraindicated during pregnancy).
   b. **Alternative regimen:** Erythromycin base 500 mg PO qid for 21 days is an alternative treatment, and the one recommended during pregnancy and lactation.
5. **Buboes may require drainage** by aspiration through healthy tissue or incision and drainage to avoid inguinal/femoral ulcerations.[30]
6. **Instruct the woman to refrain from sexual contact** until all lesions are healed and until her partner is cured.
7. Refer sexual **partners** during the 30 days preceding diagnosis for treatment.[30]

Molluscum Contagiosum

Molluscum contagiosum is a viral disease of the skin caused by the Molluscipoxvirus. It manifests as a smooth, firm, rounded papule with a depression at the head.[50] Pale-colored and 2 to 5 mm in diameter (rarely >15 mm), lesions may occur on the lower abdominal wall, pubis, genitalia, and thighs. Children may have lesions on the face, trunk, and extremities. Fifty to 100 lesions may become confluent and form a single plaque. Individual lesions last 2 to 3 months; untreated, the condition lasts 6 months to 2 years. Mechanical removal may shorten the disease course. The disease is communicable as long as lesions are present;

incubation period is 7 days to 6 months.[20] Transmission is by direct contact, sexual and nonsexual, and by fomites. May disseminate in a line away from a central area, indicating autoinoculation by scratching.[50]

Diagnosis: Diagnosis is made by clinical examination or by expressing the core of a lesion onto a slide for visualization of basophilic, Feulgen-positive, intracytoplasmic inclusions or "molluscum bodies" or "Henderson-Paterson bodies" by histology.[50]

ⓜ Management

1. **Educate the woman** regarding her condition and its infectivity. Provide safe sex instructions. Instruct her to keep blisters dry and covered.[50]
2. **Refer** the woman to a physician for treatment.
3. **Anticipatory guidance:** A physician may perform curettage under local anesthesia, use a peeling agent, or freeze with liquid nitrogen.[20] Imiquimod (Aldara), a cream that stimulates the immune system, may be useful.[32]
4. Sexual **partners** should be treated.[20]
5. **Report** to local public health authorities.[20]

Syphilis

Syphilis is an acute and chronic disease caused by the spirochete *Treponema pallidum*. Transmission is by direct contact with body fluids or blood transfusion. Perinatal transfer may occur hematogenously through the placenta or during delivery. Infectiousness varies throughout the disease course; it is less infectious in the absence of lesions and during latency. The disease is rendered noncommunicable within 24 to 48 hours of treatment.[20] Thirty percent to 50% of those exposed develop the disease.[78]

The primary stage occurs about 3 weeks after exposure, when a painless hardened chancre appears on the finger, tongue or mouth, genitalia, anus, or cervix with a raised, defined border and scanty yellow serous drainage at the site of inoculation. Regional lymph nodes are painlessly enlarged.[78] The lesion is contagious, heals in 4 to 6 weeks if untreated, and may go unnoticed.[20]

The secondary stage occurs 6 to 8 weeks after the chancre in one third of untreated patients. A symmetrical maculopapular rash of the palms and soles, condyloma lata, alopecia and lymphadenopathy may be seen, with mild flulike symptoms. This stage lasts weeks to a year and may recur within the first 2 years of infection.[3]

Tertiary (or latent stage) syphilis is manifested by cardiac, ophthalmic, or auditory complications or "gummatous" lesions (encapsulated granuloma ≥1 mm to 1 cm in size, surrounded by inflammation and fibrosis that occur in skin, viscera, or bone) develop in 25% of untreated patients.[78] This stage lasts weeks to years.[20] The treatment goal is to prevent late manifestations.[30]

Early latent phase is defined as the first year after infection. Most patients are asymptomatic but potentially infectious during this phase.[3] Infectious lesions of skin and mucous membranes may recur.[20] Patients are categorized as being in the early latent phase only if they had a documented seroconversion during the previous year, if they had unequivocal symptoms of primary or secondary stage, or if they had a sexual partner with primary, secondary, or early latent syphilis. Otherwise, they are considered to have late latent infection and are treated accordingly.[30] **Late latent phase** is defined as 1 year or more after infection and may last for the remainder of a lifetime. Some may remain symptom free. Infection is spread only by perinatal transmission or blood transfusion. Manifestations include gummas, cardiovascular syphilis, and neurosyphilis.[3,20] **Cardiovascular syphilis** is manifested by gummas in the aorta.[20] **Neurosyphilis** is developed by 20% of untreated patients[3] and is manifested by auditory, ophthalmic, and cranial nerve symptoms or meningitis[31]—the latter potentially resulting in paralysis, seizures, cognitive and emotional deficits, ataxia, pain, and paresthesia. HIV infection increases the risk of developing neurosyphilis.[20] Neurosyphilis is not always a manifestation of tertiary syphilis.[30]

The **Jarisch-Herxheimer reaction** is an acute febrile reaction that occurs within 24 hours of therapy for syphilis. It is frequently accompanied by headache, myalgia, and other symptoms (including preterm labor or fetal distress during pregnancy). Antipyretics may be taken, and concern regarding the reaction should not prevent or delay treatment.[30]

Infection During Pregnancy: The course of syphilis is not affected by pregnancy.[3] Fetal infection may result in SAB, stillbirth, premature delivery, nonimmune hydrops, generalized congenital disease, or neonatal death. The placenta may be large and edematous and the cord may show funisitis. Congenital syphilis syndrome results in CNS deficits, with facial deformities and liver, bone, heart, lung, and kidney involvement. An infant is presumed infected if the mother had untreated syphilis at the time of delivery; was inadequately treated or followed up; was treated within 4 weeks before delivery; or if the baby has physical findings indicative of syphilis, a serum nontreponemal titer 4 times greater than the mother's, or a positive dark-field examination or fluorescent antibody test of body fluids.[78]

Laboratory Findings: Reactive tests for nontreponemal antigens (Rapid Plasma Reagin [RPR] or VDRL) are confirmed with tests for treponemal antigens (fluorescent treponemal antibody, absorbed [FTA-ABS] and *T. pallidum* particle agglutination [TP-PA]).[30] False-positive results occur with acute bacterial or viral infection, systemic lupus erythematosus, fever, vaccination, narcotic addiction, tuberculosis, and other diseases.[3] The nontreponemal antigens, reported in dilutions, rise during the primary stage, decrease during the early latent phase, and progressively decrease to a low or nonreactive titer during late latent stage. A fourfold change in titer (e.g., from 1:16 to 1:4) is required to demonstrate a clinically significant difference using the same test and the same lab. Fifteen percent to 25% revert to a negative titer 2 to 3 years after treatment, though low levels may persist for life. Most treponemal antigens are positive for life, not reflecting treatment or disease activity; most nontreponemal tests become nonreactive with time after treatment.[30]

Diagnosis: Primary and secondary syphilis are definitely diagnosed by dark-field or phase-contrast examination or by fluorescent antibody staining of exudate from lesions or lymph node aspirant. Cerebrospinal fluid (CSF) analysis determines CNS involvement in the woman with evidence of tertiary syphilis.[30]

Syphilis in the Presence of HIV: Syphilis concomitant with HIV is treated as below, with more aggressive evaluation for neurosyphilis. Penicillin is used at all stages, with desensitization if the woman is allergic.[30]

Management According to the CDC's 2002 Recommendations

1. **Educate** all women regarding safe sex, STIs, and high-risk behaviors.
2. **Screen.** During pregnancy, screen at the first prenatal visit. For high-risk women (young age, multiple or new sexual partners, lack of barrier contraception, history of STIs), screen again at 28 weeks and at delivery. Screen women who are being treated for other STIs, including HIV. Test any woman who delivers a stillborn baby after 20 weeks.
3. Evaluate for **concurrent STIs.** Offer HIV counseling and testing. If results are negative, retest in 3 months.[30]
4. Gather history of recent sexual contacts and LMP. Determine whether pregnant. If the woman is pregnant and delivery is imminent, **notify pediatric staff.**[30]
5. Perform a **pelvic examination** on all infected women before treatment to rule out internal mucosal lesions, which would affect the diagnosis of stage.[30]
6. Women with evidence of **active tertiary syphilis** such as gummas, ophthalmic or neurologic findings, treatment failure, or HIV infection with latent syphilis or syphilis of unknown duration are at risk for neurologic disease. **Refer** the woman to a physician who will consider CSF analysis.[30]
7. **Pharmacologic treatment**[30]:
   a. **Primary or secondary syphilis:**
      (1) **Nonpregnant or pregnant:** Long-acting penicillin G (benzathine penicillin) 2.4 million U IM in a single dose on the day of diagnosis of syphilis at any stage.[30] The cure rate is 98%, and it prevents congenital syphilis.[78]
      (2) **Nonpregnant penicillin-allergic:** Doxycycline 100 mg PO bid for 14 days or tetracycline 500 mg PO qid for 14 days.[30]
      (3) **Pregnant penicillin-allergic:** Confirm allergy by skin testing. After oral desensitization, treat with long-acting penicillin G (benzathine penicillin) 2.4 million U IM in a single

dose because only penicillin adequately treats the fetus.[30]
b. **Early latent syphilis** (no evidence of CNS involvement):
(1) Benzathine penicillin G 2.4 million U IM in a single dose.[30]
(2) **Nonpregnant penicillin-allergic:** Doxycycline 100 mg PO bid for 28 days or tetracycline 500 mg PO qid for 28 days.[30]
(3) **Pregnant, penicillin-allergic:** Confirm allergy by skin testing. After oral desensitization, treat with long-acting penicillin G (benzathine penicillin) 2.4 million U IM because only penicillin adequately treats the fetus.[30]

8. **Follow-up for the nonpregnant woman:**
a. **For primary or secondary syphilis:** Evaluate the woman again at 6 and 12 months. Signs or symptoms that persist, or a fourfold increase in the nontreponemal test titer sustained for 6 months, indicates a woman who has failed treatment or who is reinfected. Serologic tests may decline more slowly in the woman who has had syphilis before. Offer **HIV counseling and testing. Refer** for CSF analysis and pharmacologic treatment.[30]
b. **For latent syphilis:** Perform quantitative nontreponemal serologic testing at 6, 12, and 24 months. **Refer** to a physician if titers increase fourfold, if an initially high titer (>1:32) fails to decrease by fourfold within 12 to 24 months of treatment, or if further signs or symptoms of syphilis develop.[30]
c. **For tertiary syphilis:** Follow up according to lesions.[31]
d. **Patients who fail treatment** are at risk for CNS involvement. **Refer** them to a physician.[31]

9. **Follow-up during pregnancy:** Draw nontreponemal tests monthly throughout the pregnancy. If titer levels fail to decline fourfold within 3 to 4 months,[78] or when the nontreponemal titer increases fourfold, or when signs and symptoms recur, the patient is considered to have failed treatment or to have been reinfected. **Offer HIV counseling and testing** and **refer** to a physician. Serology is repeated at 3, 6, and 12 months after delivery.[78] The woman with latent syphilis is also tested at 24 months.[28]

10. **Outpatient instructions:** Advise outpatients to refrain from sexual intercourse until treatment is complete and until partners are treated.[20]

11. **Partner treatment:** Partners are offered counseling and testing for HIV. For **primary** syphilis, partners of the previous 3 months plus duration of symptoms are at risk. For **secondary syphilis,** partners of 6 months plus the duration of the symptoms are at risk. For purposes of partner notification only, patients with syphilis of **unknown duration** who have a titer >1:32 are assumed to have early syphilis. For **latent syphilis,** partners of the last year plus duration of symptoms are at risk. Treat all of these partners presumptively if testing is unavailable or if compliance is uncertain. For long-term partners of patients with **late syphilis,** evaluate clinically, perform serologic testing, and

treat appropriately. Refer sexual partners exposed more than 90 days prior for treatment, and treatment is given presumptively if serology testing is not immediately available or if follow-up is uncertain.[30]

12. **Report** syphilis to the local public health department.[20]

Toxic Shock Syndrome

TSS is sepsis caused by *Staphylococcus aureus* infection originating from the reproductive tract.[129] Most often arising during menses from tampon use, TSS is also associated with diaphragm and vaginal contraceptive sponge use or postpartum endometritis.[134] Symptoms include the sudden onset of fever >102° F (38.8° C), severe headache, sore throat, myalgia, nausea, vomiting, profuse watery diarrhea, sunburn-like rash (desquamation 2 to 3 weeks later) especially on palms and soles of feet, hyperemia of mucous membranes, and progressive hypotension that develops into shock. CNS symptoms, including disorientation and altered level of consciousness, may occur.[129]

Laboratory Findings: The creatine phosphokinase, serum blood urea nitrogen (BUN), creatinine, aspartate aminotransferase (AST), and alanine aminotransferase (ALT) are all greater than twice the normal level; sterile pyuria is present; platelets are <100,000/mm^3; SI units: <100 × 10^9. Blood and throat cultures and CSF are negative for the organism.[129]

Differential Diagnoses: Rocky Mountain spotted fever, leptospirosis, and measles.[129]

ⓜ Management

1. **Educate** all women regarding using low-absorbency tampons and changing them frequently; removing barrier contraception within 24 hours, learning the signs and symptoms of TSS, and, if they occur, removing any vaginal devices and seeking health care immediately. Women who have had TSS should not use barrier methods of birth control.[134]

2. The midwife **refers** the woman to a physician who will hospitalize the woman, give IV fluids, antibiotics, and manage the septic shock.[129]

• MENSTRUAL DISORDERS

The normal menstrual cycle and associated hormones are illustrated in Figure 8-3.

Amenorrhea

Primary Amenorrhea: Primary amenorrhea is defined as no menses by 16 years of age.[134] Categories include amenorrhea with normal feminization and female secondary sex characteristics, the lack of secondary sex characteristics or feminization, breast development without axillary or pubic hair, or arrested development of secondary sex characteristics.[67]

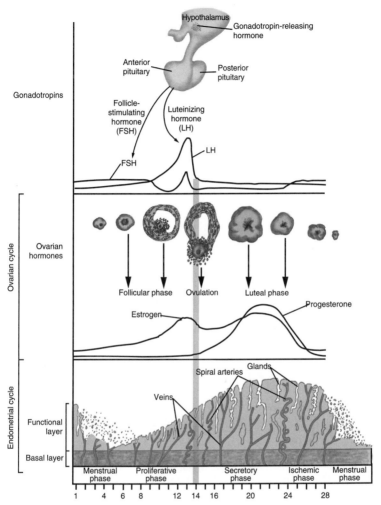

Figure 8-3 • The menstrual cycle. (From Murray SS, et al: *Foundations of maternal-newborn nursing,* 3 ed, Philadelphia, 2002, WB Saunders.)

Secondary Amenorrhea: Secondary amenorrhea is defined as 6 months without menses in the woman with the history of regular menses or 12 months in the woman with the history of oligomenorrhea or the equivalent of at least three cycle intervals.[134] Amenorrhea may be a sign of metabolic, endocrine, gynecologic, or congenital disease and is often associated with infertility, endometrial hyperplasia, or osteopenia. Incidence is higher among college students and competitive endurance athletes.[83]

ⓜ Diagnosis and Management of Primary or Secondary Amenorrhea

1. **Exclude pregnancy.**[134]
2. **Refer** the woman to a gynecologist for the remainder of the workup and treatment.

Dysfunctional Uterine Bleeding

DUB describes a variety of bleeding manifestations or anovulatory cycles in the absence of pathology or medical illness.[134] The bleeding is of endometrial origin, is painless, irregular, and may be excessive, prolonged, or unpatterned.[43] High estrogen and low progesterone levels cause the endometrium to grow rapidly. It outstrips its blood supply and sloughs, but never completely. The condition is most common in perimenarcheal and perimenopausal women and in women with polycystic ovary disease.[90]

Etiologies:

1. **Estrogen withdrawal bleeding** occurs with bilateral oophorectomy, with discontinuance of exogenous estrogen, and at midcycle with the estrogen drop before ovulation.
2. **Estrogen breakthrough bleeding** occurs when low levels of estrogen cause prolonged, light, intermittent spotting; high levels of estrogen may cause long periods of amenorrhea followed by excessive bleeding.
3. **Progesterone withdrawal bleeding** occurs when progesterone is insufficient in relation to estrogen, if estrogen has caused the endometrium to proliferate.
4. **Progesterone breakthrough bleeding** occurs when progesterone is higher than normal in relation to estrogen. Continuous progesterone administration results in breakthrough bleeding of variable duration, such as that experienced with Norplant or Depo-Provera use.[134]

ⓜ Management

1. The midwife **consults or refers** to the obstetrician/gynecologist. Advise the woman to begin a menstrual calendar noting the frequency, timing, amount, and color of bleeding.[43]
2. **Anticipatory guidance:** The diagnosis is one of exclusion after local and systemic causes have been excluded.[43] Any disruption between the hypothalamus, pituitary, ovary, and endometrium may cause vaginal bleeding. Ovulation status is determined. The bleeding is categorized as cyclic abnormal uterine bleeding (uterine abnormality or a blood dyscrasia), cyclic bleeding with superimposed abnormal bleeding (local etiology), or noncyclic bleeding (endocrine-related).[65] Pregnancy, medications, endocrine disorder, chronic medical disease, menopause, obesity, neoplasm, uterine abnormalities, adolescence, sexual practices, bleeding disorders, infection, foreign bodies, and exercise are excluded to diagnose DUB.[134,152] Treatment depends on the etiology.

Dysmenorrhea

Primary Dysmenorrhea

Primary dysmenorrhea is a diagnosis of exclusion more common before age 20 years. It may improve with pregnancy and vaginal delivery, because pregnancy decreases uterine nerve endings and may reduce pain. The tendency may be familial and is associated with early menarche increased duration of menses, nulliparity, and cigarette smoking.[139] The condition begins 6 to 12 months after the menarche with the onset of ovulation. Lower abdominal cramping (may radiate to thighs), backache, headache, fatigue, nausea, vomiting, diarrhea, and syncope are caused by prostaglandin excess. The syndrome may begin 2 days before the onset of menses and resolve in 2 to 4 days or by the end of menses.[148] Endometriosis is excluded.[134]

ⓜ Management

1. **Advise the woman** regarding lifestyle interventions:
   a. **Exercise** decreases prostaglandins, releases endorphins, and shunts blood away from the uterus.
   b. **Sexual activity** may improve symptoms by causing uterine arteriolar vasodilation.
   c. **Local heat** increases bloodflow and decreases muscle spasm.
   d. **Decrease water retention** by decreasing salt, taking in natural diuretics (including coffee).
   e. **Vitamin E** inhibits prostaglandin and reduces arteriolar spasm.[139]
2. **Pharmacologic interventions may include:**
   a. **Nonsteroidal anti-inflammatory drugs (NSAIDs)** inhibit prostaglandin synthesis and improve symptoms in 80%. Advise the woman to take at or just before the onset of pain tid on days 1 to 3. Six months may be required to establish effectiveness.[65]
   b. **OCs** suppress ovulation, diminish endometrial growth, and decrease prostaglandin levels.[134] An OC with low estrogen and high progestational activity is appropriate.[45] Three to 4 months may be necessary to establish effectiveness.[90]
   c. **Calcium antagonists**, such as verapamil and nifedipine, reduce uterine activity and contractility.[90]
3. **Transcutaneous electrical nerve stimulation** (TENS) may be used, and **surgical interruption of neural pathways** may be performed.[90]
4. **Complementary measures:**
   a. Many **homeopathy** experts recommend remedies for dysmenorrhea.[40,113,121,149]
   b. **Acupuncture** is useful in the treatment of primary dysmenorrhea.[90]
   c. Herbs: **Black cohash** is an antispasmodic that promotes healthy menstrual activity, soothing irritation and congestion of the

uterus, cervix, and vagina.* Thirty to 60 drops of tincture several times/d may be taken[153]; alternately, simmer ½ to 1 tsp dry herb in 1 cup boiling water for 10 to 15 minutes and drink tid.[71a] **Blue cohash** is an antispasmodic with a steroidal component indicated for pain due to blood stagnation or cervical spasm (pain preceding bleeding). It may be taken as a tincture or the root in a decoction.† **Chamomile** is an antispasmodic that alleviates cramping.[62,91,107,115] Take as an infusion, 1 Tblsp/cup tea or 10 drops tincture bid.[107] **Cramp bark** is indicated for dysmenorrhea.[71,91,115,149] Suggested regimens include ½ tsp tincture qh up to 6 doses or 5 to 10 mL tid, or 2 tsp dried bark simmered in 1 cup water for 10 minutes taken tid; or taking the herb in capsule form.[71a] **Ginger** is recommended for women with dysmenorrhea that is relieved by heat who have a light flow of blackish blood.[62,86,107] Dried ginger in capsule form (250 mg qid for 4 to 5 days) may be taken; chewing on a root is suggested by Parvati as an "immediate remedy."[115] **Pasque flower** may relieve menstrual cramps, especially when the woman feels irritable.[62,71,91,110] Take up to 20 gtts tincture tid or add 5 g herb to 500 mL water for tea.[110] **Wild yam** may relieve menstrual cramps.[62,71,91,117] **See information about herbs, p. 563.**

Secondary Dysmenorrhea

Secondary dysmenorrhea is associated with pelvic pathology and is more common in women older than 20 years. Possible etiologies include adenomyosis, leiomyomata, endometrial polyps, congenital malformation, cervical stenosis, endometriosis, PID, pelvic congestion syndrome, ovarian cysts/tumors, Asherman's syndrome (intrauterine adhesions), uterine prolapse, or an IUD.[45] The dull pain starts earlier and lasts longer than that of primary dysmenorrhea. It may be associated with chronic pelvic pain. It may occur with ovulation or intercourse and increases with age. There are no systemic symptoms.[139] Endometriosis, myoma, PID, and Asherman's syndrome are excluded.

ⓜ Management

1. **Rule out PID** with cervical cultures, and order an ultrasound to detect myoma.
2. Offer **comfort measures** described for primary dysmenorrhea.
3. **Refer** the woman to a physician for further evaluation.
4. **Anticipatory guidance:** Hysterosalpingogram may be performed to detect uterine abnormalities, endometrial polyps, or Asherman's syndrome; laparoscopy and hysteroscopy may detect intrauterine and other pelvic pathology.[90]

---

*References 18, 62, 71, 84, 91, 97, 107, 117, 118, 153.
†References 71a, 84, 91, 107, 110, 117.

Intermenstrual Bleeding

Intermenstrual bleeding is defined as bleeding or spotting between normal periods. It is differentiated from breakthrough bleeding due to OCs, ectopic pregnancy, endometrial or endocervical polyps, a vaginal laceration, cervicitis, cervical or endometrial cancer, and fibroids.[152]

ⓜ Management

1. **Rule out pregnancy,** including ectopic pregnancy.
2. For **breakthrough bleeding** caused by **OCs,** see p. 508.
3. Treat any identified **lesions.**
4. **If the cause of the bleeding is not identified, refer** the woman to a gynecologist for endometrial sampling or hysteroscopy.[152]

Menorrhagia (Hypermenorrhea)

Defined by Speroff et al[134] as menses occurring at regular, normal intervals with excessive flow and duration, menorrhagia is more specifically described as menstrual blood loss exceeding 80 mL/cycle or bleeding in excess of 7 days.[51] Iron-deficiency anemia indicates this diagnosis in the presence of ovulatory cycles. Regular cycles ranging from 21 to 35 days, varying only by a few days, accompanied by cramping, breast tenderness, and mood swings indicate ovulatory cycles.[152] Possible etiologies include coagulopathies, liver disease, medications, thyroid malfunction, structural lesions, pregnancy-related bleeding, or DUB,[51] although in many cases, no etiology is found.

ⓜ Management

1. Advise the woman to keep a **menstrual diary** to record the amount of bleeding for one cycle.
2. **Screen for STIs and treat** any identified infections.
3. Screen for and treat iron deficiency anemia (see p. 352).
4. If further treatment is required, **consult with or refer** the woman to a gynecologist.
5. **Anticipatory guidance:** After a thorough evaluation that may include endometrial sampling, ultrasound, hysteroscopy, and MRI,[51] the physician may offer the woman OCs, NSAIDs,[152] medroxyprogesterone (MPA) given in the luteal phase of the cycle, a progestin IUD, an antifibrinolytic agent or a derivative of vasopressin for menorrhagia related to coagulopathies, danazol or gonadotropin-releasing hormone (GnRH) agonists (both cause endometrial atrophy, but have side effects),[51] or endometrial ablation.
Endometrial ablation suppresses the menses by destroying the endometrial lining. The procedure may be done with electric cautery, laser, or thermal or electrode balloons.[51] Laparoscopy may be used to monitor this outpatient procedure performed under general anesthesia or regional block. It may cause sterility but is not guaranteed to do so.

Some women have slight cramping and fatigue for several days; others are back to full activities in 2 to 3 days. Women are asked to refrain from exercise for 3 to 4 weeks. Scant discharge is present for up to 6 weeks. Virtually all women have a reduction in menstrual flow after this procedure. The result is not known for 12 to 18 months.[76] Complications include the risks of anesthesia, the risk of injury to the uterus or pelvic organs, hemorrhage, and water intoxication from excessive absorption of the medium used to distend the uterus. The procedure may allow the woman to avoid hysterectomy. In 10% to 15%, menorrhagia returns and further treatment is required.[51] **Myomectomy** and **removal of endometrial polyps** may also be tried before resorting to hysterectomy.[152] D&C is not indicated because the blood loss is usually only reduced for one cycle after the procedure. It is used only to manage an acute bleeding episode.[51]

6. **Complementary therapies:**
   a. **Nutritional suggestions: Vitamin K** 100 μg bid and **vitamin A** 100,000 IU qd for 2 to 3 weeks, then reduced to 10,000 IU/d.[113]
   b. **Herbs: Lady's mantle** stops uterine hemorrhage[71a,91,107,110,115]: 10 drops tincture in water tid.[107] **Vitex agnus castus or chaste tree** regulates female hormones and is useful in the treatment of menstrual conditions[71,91,117,153]: 20 drops tincture 1 to 2 times daily, 3 capsules freshly powdered berries daily, or 1 cup/250 mL tea of freshly powdered berries daily.[153] The following are astringents that help stem menorrhagia when taken as tea 1 cup tid: **cranesbill**,[62,71,110,113] **raspberry leaf**,* and **periwinkle**.[71,91,110,113] **Shepherd's purse**, an astringent, is useful in the treatment of menorrhagia. The dose suggested is 1 cup tea tid before and during menses.† **See information about herbs, p. 563.**

Metrorrhagia

Metrorrhagia is defined as irregular menstrual cycles of excessive flow and duration.

Oligomenorrhea

Oligomenorrhea is defined as menstrual cycles lasting more than 35 days.

Polymenorrhea

Polymenorrhea is defined as menstrual cycles lasting less than 24 days.[134]

Premenstrual Syndrome

Seventy percent to 75% of all women have some premenstrual symptoms 1 to 2 weeks before menses. Thirty percent to 40% report symptoms

---

*References 18, 62, 97, 107, 113, 115.
†References 71a, 91, 97, 110, 113, 115, 117.

severe enough to interfere with activities of daily living; 5% report symptoms that are incapacitating.[18] Timing of premenstrual syndrome (PMS) varies from 2 to 12 days before menses, resolving within 24 hours of menses (as opposed to dysmenorrhea, which begins up to 48 hours before menses and resolves in 2 to 4 days or by the end of menses). The diagnosis of PMS requires consistent prospective ratings of signs and symptoms during the luteal phase of ovulatory menstrual cycles severe enough to interrupt daily activities, with 1 full week of the follicular phase being symptom free.[148] Speroff et al[134] describe PMS as a collection of different problems, primarily biologic but with a psychological overlay, possibly a learned response or possibly a response of certain individuals to neuroendocrine and hormonal changes involving the serotonergic system.

Classifications:

Type A: Most common, 60% to 80% of PMS patients. Anxiety, irritability, insomnia, and nervous tension result from elevated estrogen and progesterone.[97] Excessive dairy intake and magnesium deficiency contribute.[148]

Type H: Water retention, weight gain, edema, bloating, breast tenderness from aldosterone and estrogen excess and dopamine deficiency.[97] Vitamin B_6 and magnesium deficiencies may contribute.[148]

Type C: Carbohydrate and sweets cravings, headache, palpitations, dizziness, fainting, and/or fatigue. Medina[97] states that the cause is an increased binding capacity for insulin. B vitamins, zinc, magnesium, and/or vitamin C deficiencies may be involved.[148]

Type D: Least common, involving 17% to 23% of PMS patients. May occur with type A. Depression, confusion, insomnia, and suicidal tendencies. Occurs due to decreased estrogen and increased progesterone, hypothyroidism, androgen imbalance, genetic predisposition, or elevated prolactin.[97] B vitamin and magnesium deficiencies may be involved.[148]

Laboratory Studies: Glucose tolerance test (GTT), TSH, T4, serum prolactin.[148]

ⓜ Management

1. Ask the woman to keep a **diary** for at least 3 months. Assess whether symptoms are actually cyclic.[134]
2. **Advise lifestyle changes** that may relieve PMS, including:
   a. Regular **exercise.**
   b. A **low-fat, low-salt, high complex-carbohydrate diet** with at least 45 g protein daily. **Avoid alcohol, caffeine, sugar,** and **minimize dairy** products that deplete the system of needed nutrients.
   c. **Stress-reduction techniques.**
   d. Drink at least 8 glasses of **water** daily to facilitate diuresis.[148]
3. **Calcium carbonate** 1200 mg PO daily reduces mood and somatic symptoms of PMS. Women who have had kidney stones should not take calcium.[134]

4. Advise the patient to take **supplements** as indicated for each type of PMS:
   a. **Type A:** magnesium, decrease dairy intake.
   b. **Type H:** vitamin B_6 and magnesium, and vitamin E 400 IU qd to bid for breast symptoms.
   c. **Type C:** vitamins B and C, magnesium, and zinc. Vitamins A and E and evening primrose oil 1000 mg bid are suggested (the latter provides prostaglandins).
   d. **Type D:** vitamin B and magnesium. (Vitamin B_6 may cause peripheral neuropathy; low dosages are used with close monitoring. Toxicity may occur if the woman uses 50 to 100 mg bid for the entire cycle.)[148]

5. If lifestyle changes and supplements have had insufficient impact after 1 to 2 months, the following **medical interventions** may be offered to the woman:
   a. **OCs** remove endogenous steroid variability.[134] Monophasic pills are appropriate for mood disorders.[65]
   b. **Depo-Provera** helps some women.[134]
   c. Further medical interventions require physician **consultation** or management: GnRH agonists, diuretics,[134] bromocriptine, antidepressants such as selective serotonin reuptake inhibitors (SSRIs), or danazol[148] may be prescribed.

6. **Complementary measures:**
   a. **Miscellaneous: Massage,** stretching/relaxation **exercises,** and **meditation** have been linked to improvement for many women. Twenty minutes of **exposure to light** improves PMS for some women. **Avoid nicotine.**[113]
   b. **Chinese medicine: Shiatsu, acupuncture,** and **tai chi** all work to relax the reproductive organs and may be beneficial.[113] **See information regarding Chinese medicine, p. 559.**
   c. **Herbs: Chamomile** relieves cramping and other PMS symptoms[62,91,97,107,113] as an infusion, 1 Tblsp/cup tea, or 10 drops tincture bid.[107] **Chaste tree (Vitex agnus-castus)** is a regulator of the female cycle and relieves breast tenderness, bloating, irritability, mood swings, and headache[71a,91,113,117,127]: 1 tsp ripe berries steeped in 1 cup boiling water for 10 to 15 minutes tid or 1 to 2 mL tincture tid[71a,110] or 10 drops tincture taken in the morning in water for the second half of the menstrual cycle.[110] **Dandelion** is a diuretic and will relieve breast tenderness and bloating.[18,62,71,113] **Dong quai** is hormone balancing, said to stimulate the body's production of estrogen. It treats menstrual irregularity and the pain of cramping but may take several weeks to act[18,55,62,110,153]: 10 to 40 drops fresh root tincture 1 to 3 times/d, 4 to 8 oz/25 to 50 mL dried root infusion or tea daily, or a $\frac{1}{8}$ to $\frac{1}{4}$ inch (4 to 6 mm) piece of dried root chewed 2 to 3 times/d.[153] **Evening primrose oil** stimulates estrogen production, promotes

prostaglandin formation, relieves breast tenderness and bloating. 3000 mg qd is recommended* or 1 or 2 capsules tid.[117] Alternately, take 1 tsp root/cup water for decoction or chopped plant and flowers in equal parts for tea.[107] **See information about herbs, p. 563.**

• OVARIAN DISORDERS

Ovarian Cancer

Ovarian cancer is the leading cause of death from gynecologic disease. A woman's risk of developing ovarian cancer in her lifetime is 1 in 70. Most ovarian cancers arise from the epithelium of the ovary. Subclassified by cell type as serous, mucinous, endometrioid, clear cell, or undifferentiated carcinomas, there is little difference among the epithelial cell types in regard to therapy or prognosis. Other ovarian malignancies include epithelial ovarian tumors of low malignant potential, those of germ cell origin, stromal and sex chord carcinomas, mesenchymal tumors, and cancer that has metastasized to the ovary, usually from the breast or gastrointestinal (GI) tract (Krukenberg tumor).[14] Adnexal masses in younger women are usually of the low malignant or borderline type.[47]

In more than 75% of women, the disease is spread throughout the peritoneal cavity before diagnosis. Even when advanced, patients may have only nonspecific GI symptoms, such as early satiety, abdominal fullness, or gas pain.[92] Fatigue, increasing abdominal girth, urinary frequency, and shortness of breath may occur due to ascites and pleural effusion. The woman usually remains alert until major complications occur such as bowel obstruction, massive ascites, or profound edema of the lower extremities. Most women die in a matter of months from malnutrition and small bowel obstruction.[14]

On exam, the palpable postmenopausal ovary is abnormal, the normal postmenopausal ovary being <1 cm in its longest axis. A woman 12 months or more postmenopause should not have follicular or corpus luteum cysts.[92] A mass that is bilateral, irregular, solid, or fixed as well as the presence of ascites or nodularity in the cul de sac are suspicious for malignancy.[14] The differential for an adnexal mass includes physiologic or functional cysts, endometriomas, masses originating from adjacent structures, lesions of infectious origin (hydrosalpinx or TOA), and benign and malignant neoplasms.[47]

Predisposing Factors[14,35,92]:

Nulliparity and low parity	Mumps infection before
High-fat diet	menarche
Anovulation	Ovulation induction in
Perineal talc use	infertile women (controversial)

---

*References 18, 37, 62, 91, 107, 113, 117, 147.

Sedentary lifestyle   Two first-degree relatives
                                        with ovarian cancer (50% risk)

NOTE: Some families have a pattern of breast and ovarian cancer; others have ovary, breast, colon, and endometrial cancers.[14]

Ⓜ Management

1. **Refer** the woman with an ovarian mass or the woman with a family history of ovarian and breast cancer to a gynecologist.
2. **Anticipatory guidance:** Women of reproductive age may be prescribed an OC containing at least 50 μg estrogen and reevaluated again in 6 weeks or after one menses. If the mass is not diminished in size or absent, **laparoscopy**[92] or **transvaginal ultrasonography** are conducted.[14] **Suspicious related findings**, however, include ascites, abdominal masses, pleural effusion, supraclavicular or inguinal adenopathy, cachexia, and anorexia. Such findings should lead to surgical exploration, not to further imaging studies. Aggressive management of pelvic masses is required to detect ovarian cancer.[92] When cancer is diagnosed, **surgery** is performed. Removal of uterus, tubes, ovaries, omentum, lymph nodes, and all visible cancer is standard.[14] **Staging** is conducted. Aggressive **chemotherapy** is initiated. A **"second look" surgery** may be indicated to gauge the success of surgery and to determine the need for further treatment. **Palliative treatment** may include nutritional support, surgical alleviation of GI blockage, paracentesis to relieve ascites, or narcotics.[92]
3. **Women with two first-degree relatives with ovarian cancer** have a 50% chance of developing the cancer themselves and are **followed by a gynecologist.** Some experts will monitor these patients with serial ultrasound, endometrial biopsy, CA-125 measurement, and frequent pelvic exams. OCs and prophylactic oophorectomy may be offered.[14,92]

Ovarian Cysts

Benign ovarian cysts include hemorrhagic cysts, simple cysts, and endometriomas. Any cyst >4 cm is considered a possible neoplasm.[45] Assisted reproduction increases the incidence of ovarian cysts,[70] as does the use of Norplant.[134] Older, larger-dose OCs helped prevent cysts, but the newer, low-dose OCs do not.[65] Cysts decrease in volume by 50% in 21 days. A cyst that does not decrease in volume is either malignant or an endometrioma.[45] Cysts are more likely to be malignant as the size of the mass and the woman's age increase.[70]

Types of Ovarian Cysts

1. **Nonfunctional cysts: A serous inclusion cyst** forms from an invagination on the surface epithelium of the ovary, lined by epithelium, and is usually <1 cm in diameter.[45]

2. **Functional cysts:**
   a. **Simple or unilocular cysts** usually result from preovulatory follicles that contain an atretic oocyte. They may become 4 cm in size and persist into the next cycle. They may be recurrent and often occur at either end of reproductive life. Fifty percent spontaneously resolve within 60 days.[45] Pain may result from rupture, torsion, or hemorrhage.[145]
   b. **Follicular cysts** are graafian follicles undergoing atresia, lacking an ovum, that may be up to 5 cm in diameter. They usually contain clear, watery fluid and sometimes fresh or altered blood.[45] Rupture may cause acute, brief pain.[145]
   c. **Corpus luteum cysts** are the persistence of a mature corpus luteum.[45] They may delay menses, then produce menorrhagia, and are associated with intraluminal bleeding, which may cause pain. They usually resolve spontaneously in 4 to 8 weeks. They are very vascular; rupture may result in hemorrhage.[145]
   d. **Theca-lutein cysts** are caused by excessive stimulation of the theca lutein by high levels of circulating gonadotropins from an ectopic pregnancy, hydatidiform mole, exogenous hormone therapy, or choriocarcinoma.[45]
   e. **Polycystic ovary syndrome:** see p. 460.

   During Pregnancy: Adnexal pathology occurs in 1 in 600 pregnancies.[94] Most adnexal masses found on ultrasound during pregnancy are found before 16 weeks' gestation.[70] Many will resolve spontaneously.[94]

   Complications: Torsion may include the ovary, the fallopian tube, or the broad ligament of the uterus.[94] If sustained, it may lead to infarction, peritonitis, and death. Torsion is usually unilateral, associated with cysts or carcinoma, TOA, or a nonadherent mass, or it may occur in a normal ovary. It is most common among women of reproductive age. Symptoms include abrupt, severe pain in a lower abdominal quadrant, nausea, and vomiting. A tender mass is noted on the affected side. Fever and leukocytosis may be present. Laparoscopy is the treatment of choice; the adnexa are unwound ("detorsion"), viability assessed, and gangrenous adnexa are removed. Any cyst present is also removed and evaluated histologically.[145]

   Rupture of a follicular cyst causes acute, brief pain. Rupture of a corpus luteum cyst, which is highly vascular, may result in life-threatening hemorrhage. The acute pain is indistinguishable from a ruptured ectopic pregnancy, but the serum hCG is negative. Diffuse pelvic tenderness is noted on pelvic exam and is often unilateral on the affected side. A mass may be palpable. Abdominal distention and shock occur in severe hemorrhage. Ultrasound is diagnostic, showing a complex cystic adnexal mass with free fluid in the cul de sac. The presence of an intrauterine gestation is noted and decreases the likelihood of an ectopic pregnancy. Surgical removal of the cyst is required if the patient is hemodynamically unstable or if the diagnosis is uncertain. If the pregnancy is less than 12 weeks' gestation and the corpus luteum must be removed, progesterone supplementation maintains the pregnancy.[145]

ⓜ Management

1. The midwife **consults** with a gynecologist.
2. **Anticipatory guidance: Pregnancy** is ruled out by hCG. **Ultrasound** is diagnostic. Any **cyst >4 cm requires laparoscopic or surgical exploration** to exclude a neoplasm. Cysts **≤4 cm and appearing benign by ultrasound may be managed initially by a course of OCs.**[45] The woman is seen monthly to assess the size as equal or decreasing (remaining <5 cm), soft and cystic, unilateral, smooth, mobile, asymptomatic, or slightly painful. If any of these signs changes, ovarian cancer is excluded.

   During pregnancy, clear ovarian cysts <5 cm diameter are followed with anticipatory management.[70] Some experts recommend conservative management until the sixteenth week when, if they persist, they are removed to avoid the risks of torsion, infarction, hemorrhage, and obstruction of labor and to avoid delay of a diagnosis of malignancy. Masses discovered during the third trimester are observed, when possible, and removed during a cesarean delivery.[94]

Polycystic Ovary Syndrome (Stein-Leventhal Syndrome)

PCOS is the most common reason for menstrual irregularities in reproductive-age women.[45] Twenty-two percent of women have ultrasonographically identifiable cystic ovaries. The fundamental physiologic defect in PCOS is unknown.[66] The luteinizing hormone (LH) level is higher than usual in these women, stimulating the follicle without releasing the egg. The follicle undergoes luteinization, resulting in ovarian production of testosterone and indirectly changing estrogen levels. Cysts form in the ovaries because they cannot release an egg, and theca cell hyperplasia occurs. Multiple small cysts are easily seen in the ovaries on pelvic ultrasound, each generally <8 mm in diameter, with increased central stroma that causes hormonal disturbances responsible for a combination of the following symptoms: chronic anovulation, excess androgen resulting in a hirsute appearance, acne, hyperinsulinemia, hyperestrogenemia, hyperprolactinemia, weight gain, enlarged ovaries, and infertility. The disease may begin at menarche, after androgen treatment, or after prolonged periods of stress.[93]

Signs and symptoms include menstrual irregularities (amenorrhea or hypermenorrhea) usually beginning at menarche, decreased fertility, higher rate of SAB due to LH elevation, obesity, hirsute appearance and acne, abnormal insulin action, and galactorrhea.[66] PCOS increases a woman's risk for breast and ovarian cancer, triples the risk for endometrial cancer (unopposed estrogen production) and hypertension, increases by sixfold the risk of developing diabetes mellitus, and increases by sevenfold the risk of coronary heart disease (due to adverse effects on the lipid profile).[93] The differential includes hyperprolactinemia, thyroid abnormalities, nonclassic adrenal hyperplasia,[65] insulin resistance, ovarian hyperthecosis, ovarian stromal hyperplasia, ovarian and/or adrenal neoplasia, late onset adrenogenital syndrome, acromegaly, or Cushing's syndrome.[45]

Laboratory Findings: Total testosterone, dehydroepiandrosterone sulfate (DHEAS), prolactin, free testosterone, LH, and follicle-stimulating hormone (FSH) are elevated.[93]

Ⓜ Management

1. **Refer** the woman with PCOS to a gynecologist for management.
2. **Anticipatory guidance:** Ultrasound and laboratory findings are diagnostic. The **goal of management** is to alleviate symptoms and to reduce the long-term sequelae.[65] **Lifestyle recommendations** include weight loss, exercise, stress management, and dietary modification. A 5% weight loss lowers circulating androgens, decreases circulating insulin, and induces menses. Exercise decreases peripheral insulin resistance. Stress management is addressed because stress contributes to androgen excess. Physical hair removal treatment may be suggested. **Pharmacologic treatment** may include OCs or progestins to regulate menses and improve acne, OCs and/or spironolactone, GnRH agonists for hirsutism,[65,93] and/or antiandrogens to improve insulin resistance. Wedge resection or ovarian drilling is a **surgical approach** that may provide complete, temporary, or long-term relief.[89] **Conception** may occur with assisted conception techniques, but poses the risk of Ovarian Hyperstimulation Syndrome, a potentially serious condition in which too many follicles are stimulated.[65]

• UTERINE DISORDERS

Adenomyosis of the Uterus

Adenomyosis of the uterus is defined as symmetrical or localized extension of the endometrial glands and stroma into the myometrium. This condition may cause severe secondary dysmenorrhea, menorrhagia, polymenorrhea, spotting, and a tender, enlarged uterus. It may be related to endometriosis or myomas. Many patients, however, are asymptomatic. About 15% women develop some degree of adenomyosis. Endometrial biopsy, laparoscopy, laparotomy, or hysteroscopy may be used in the diagnosis and management. After excluding endometrial hyperplasia, physician management may include D&C, GnRH agonists, mifepristone, or hysterectomy.[58,129]

Anomalies of the Uterus

Figure 8-4 illustrates the most common uterine anomalies.

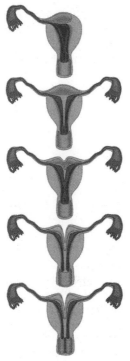

Unicornuate uterus:
Uterus having a single horn
and only one fallopian tube

Septate uterus:
Single uterus with a
midline septum

Bicornuate uterus:
Two horns
with a fundal indentation

Uterus didelphys:
Double uterus with
one vagina

Uterus didelphys and septate vagina:
Double uterus and vagina

Figure 8-4 • Anomalies of the uterus. (Modified from Murray SS, et al: *Foundations of maternal-newborn nursing*, 3 ed, Philadelphia, 2002, WB Saunders.)

Asherman's Syndrome

Asherman's syndrome is the formation of adhesions after surgical scraping of the endometrium, usually during the postpartum period. Overly vigorous scraping or the woman's idiosyncratic reaction may be causative. The condition may also result from other uterine surgeries, disseminated TB, uterine schistosomiasis, or IUD-related pelvic infections. Dysmenorrhea, hypomenorrhea,[134] amenorrhea, infertility, or SAB may result. Diagnosis is made by hysterosalpingogram and hysteroscopy. Lysis of adhesions by excision, cautery, or laser may be done through the hysteroscope, restoring menses in 90%.[83] Seventy percent to 90% of women thus treated can subsequently become pregnant, but during the pregnancy they are risk for preterm labor, placenta previa, placenta accreta, and/or postpartum hemorrhage (PPH).[134]

Myomas (Fibroids, Leiomyomata Uteri, Myomata, Fibromyoma)

These estrogen-sensitive muscle cell tumors of the uterus are usually benign. Women who are >35 years, nulliparous, and black are at greater risk.[33] Occurring in 10% of Caucasian and 30% of black women, most commonly in their 40s, the etiology of this condition is unknown. Genetic predisposition and environmental factors (such as hormonal variations) may act as triggers.[98] After menopause, they regress because of decreased estrogen stimulation.[139] Approximately 1 in 1000 cases of fibroids are leiomyosarcomas (carcinoma). This diagnosis is excluded if the fibroid is growing quickly. Otherwise, there is no link between fibroids and cancer.[98]

Fibroids are usually asymptomatic. However, the classic triad of symptoms is bleeding, pressure, and pain.[98] One third have worsening menorrhagia. A prolapsed pedunculated myoma may cause intermenstrual bleeding. One third have severe, acute episodes of pelvic pain associated with sudden degeneration or torsion. Dyspareunia, dysmenorrhea, urinary symptoms, constipation or other lower GI symptoms, increased abdominal girth without weight change, and anemia are other signs.[73] Complications may include infarction (signs include fever and elevated WBC), torsion of a pedunculated myoma, uterine inversion caused by a pedunculated myoma, anemia, infection, infertility, and sarcomatous change (0.3% to 0.7%).[41]

On exam, the fibroids may be irregular, symmetrical, or multilobular in shape. Rubbery and firm on palpation, myomas are well circumscribed, often multiple, and may be calcified.[41] The uterus is enlarged but nontender. Degenerating myomas feel softer and cyst-like. A pedunculated myoma may mimic an adnexal or ovarian mass. A retroverted uterus may mimic a posterior myoma. Myomas should regress in size in menopause.[139]

Types (Most Are Mixed):

1. **Submucosal** myomas are located just under the decidual layer of the endometrium protruding into the uterine cavity. They are problematic if they block a fallopian tube. The increased surface area of endometrium results in increased menstrual bleeding. They may cause infertility, SAB and may pedunculate.

2. **Intramural or interstitial** myomas are rounded and contained within the myometrium. They may develop a subserosal or submucosal component.

3. **Subserosal** myomas are located just under uterine serosa, bulging out through the outer uterine wall. They do not cause infertility unless they block fallopian tubes.

   a. **Pedunculated** myomas are submucus or subserosal myomas attached to the uterus by a pedicle.

4. **Parasitic** myomas extrude from the uterus with an accessory blood supply, such as one from the omentum. They may extend into the broad ligament of the uterus or may cause hydroureter.[41]

5. **Intraligamentous** myomas are located within the broad ligament.

   a. **Cervical** myomas are usually small and asymptomatic. They may become pedunculated or protrude out of the cervix and become infected.[139] They may withdraw into the uterus with pregnancy.[41]

Diagnosis: The differential includes adenomyosis, pregnancy, ectopic pregnancy, ovarian cyst or tumor, malignancy, PID, urinary tract infection (UTI), subinvolution, congenital anomaly, endometrial hyperplasia/cancer, TOA or other tubal pathology, appendicitis, bowel tumor or other pathology, endometriosis (often coexists with myoma), and ovarian and uterine cancer.[139] Presumptive diagnosis is made on the basis of the pelvic exam, confirmed by ultrasound, MRI (distinguishes adenomyoma from myoma), CT (of questionable value), hysterosalpingogram, hysterosonogram, or endoscopy. If abnormal bleeding is present or if the woman has adenomyosis, an endometrial biopsy is done to rule out endometrial hyperplasia.[98]

Myomas and Pregnancy

Although myomas may cause infertility by distortion or blockage of the fallopian tube and distortion of the uterine cavity, many women have fibroids that enlarge the uterus up to 14 to 16 weeks' gestation in size, and fertility is not affected. Submucous fibroids may cause faulty implantation and SAB. Myomectomy is not indicated until infertility is established or until habitual abortion occurs.[73]

Myomas may increase in size, regress, or stay the same during pregnancy. Large myomas tend to get smaller; small myomas tend to grow. Fifty percent do not change in size. Myomas <3 cm are generally inconsequential during pregnancy. Myomas >3 cm may cause SAB, preterm labor, pelvic pain, malpresentation, or cesarean delivery. Placental abruption, retained placenta, and PPH may occur if the placenta implants over a myoma. Pain may signal torsion or degeneration of a myoma. The uterus may measure larger than dates.[41]

Myoma and Contraception

OCs, which do not stimulate myoma growth, are used by some clinicians to concomitantly decrease bleeding and dysmenorrhea in the woman with a myoma.[6]

ⓜ *Management*

1. **Consult** with the obstetrician/gynecologist.
2. The **asymptomatic woman** requires **anticipatory management** only, with frequent examination.[98]
3. Treat **anemia.**
4. **Anticipatory guidance:** When the woman is **symptomatic, physician management** may include **pharmacologic treatment:** NSAIDs, OCs (unlikely to work), and GnRH agonists to reduce menstrual flow by reducing fibroid size by 30% to 50% in 3 to 6 months. The drugs are expensive and cause multiple side effects.[98,140]

    Surgery is indicated if there is progressive menorrhagia with anemia, pain, increasing pressure on the bladder or bowel (mild hydronephrosis is usually clinically insignificant and does not require treatment), demonstrated infertility, or for recurrent SABs.[73] The woman should be counseled that fibroids may grow back; the average time to recurrence is 7 years.[98] Surgical options include embolization (causing infarction of the fibroid, with significant but transient pain; cures 80%; effect on fertility is unknown), myomectomy (removal of fibroids, adhesions, and scarring that may predispose to infertility; may cause excessive bleeding; and may mandate cesarean delivery for future pregnancies), laparoscopy (to remove fibroids growing on the outside of the uterus[98]), hysteroscopy (to remove fibroids inside the uterus[10]), or hysterectomy.[139]

5. **Management during pregnancy:** Serial ultrasounds are considered for the pregnant woman with significant myomas. Degeneration of a myoma during pregnancy with inflammation of the surrounding peritoneum is treated with analgesia and watchful waiting. Infection is harder to eradicate with myoma involvement, short of hysterectomy. Myomectomy during pregnancy is associated with profuse blood loss, and the risk of uterine rupture in subsequent pregnancies is increased.[41]

6. **Complementary measures:**
   a. **Homeopathic** measures are suggested by some experts.[75,121] **Herbal** remedies are suggested by others.[37,91,113,153]
   b. **Nutritional suggestions:** Reduction of dietary phytoestrogens may reduce myoma growth.[140] Nutritional suggestions by Balch and Balch[18] include:
      (1) Floridix iron as directed on the label. This iron is easily assimilated.
      (2) L-Arginine 500 mg daily taken on an empty stomach with water or juice, not milk. Absorption is best when taken with vitamin B_6 50 mg and vitamin C 100 mg. The supplement enhances the immune system and anti-tumor effects.
      (3) L-Lysine 500 mg daily on an empty stomach (to balance arginine).
      (4) Multivitamin and minerals as directed on label.
      (5) Vitamin A 25,000 IU (immune system stimulant; tissue repair). Take apart from iron, which inhibits absorption.
      (6) Vitamin C 3000-10,000 mg qd in divided doses (immune; antioxidant).
      (7) Zinc 30-80 mg daily (≤100 mg total) (immune system stimulant).

   Ikenze[75] suggests avoiding red meat and high-fat foods, concentrating on eating fish, chicken, whole grains, and vegetables. Avoid caffeine. Supplement the diet with lecithin, which promotes liver function and bile flow, facilitating estrogen excretion. Dark green leafy vegetables stimulate bile flow and estrogen excretion and replace iron loss. Avoid dairy products that may contain hormones;

low or no-fat cheeses contain less of the hormones. Daily or alternate-day exercise involving pelvic motion increases bloodflow to the region. Page[113] also advocates a low-fat vegetarian diet (50% to 60% fresh foods) and achievement of an appropriate weight to promote normal estrogen levels. Caffeine, refined sugars, and fried and preserved foods are to be avoided. Increase intake of vitamin B foods; for cleansing, eat sea greens, leafy greens, diuretic foods (cucumber and watermelon), and fresh apple or carrot juice.

Uterine Polyps

A uterine polyp may actually be a myoma, carcinoma, carcinosarcoma, or polypoid endometrial hyperplasia—localized overgrowths of endometrial glands and stroma. Unopposed estrogen may be causative. Approximately 5% are malignant, most in postmenopausal women. Most are asymptomatic, though they may cause intermenstrual or postmenopausal bleeding. Diagnosis is made by hysteroscopy and is confirmed by histologic examination.[67]

ⓜ Management

1. **Perform** cultures, wet mount, CBC to evaluate bleeding, and Pap smear.[67]
2. **Refer** the woman to a gynecologist for treatment.
3. **Anticipatory guidance: D&C** is done for diagnosis and treatment.[67]

• VAGINAL AND PELVIC FLOOR DISORDERS

Dyspareunia

Dyspareunia is recurrent or persistent genital pain before, during, or after sexual intercourse.[139] The pain may be generalized (not just a specific partner and/or situation) or situational; it may be primary (with first sexual experience and more likely psychologically based) or secondary (beginning after a period of pain-free sexual functioning, more likely physically based). It involves psychological issues–anticipation of pain will decrease arousal, diminish lubrication, and worsen the problem. Interpersonal difficulties often result, with sexual avoidance and decreased sexual encounters.[81,90]

Physical etiologies may include the following[81,90,139]:

Rigid hymenal ring	Menopausal vaginal atrophy
Imperforate hymen	Vulvodynia
Hymenal strands	Vulvar vestibulitis
Coarse pubic hair	Vaginismus
Small introitus	Endometriosis
Episiotomy scar	Shortened vagina
Infection	PID
Vaginal stenosis	Pelvic adhesions

Müllerian abnormality
Bartholin's gland inflammation
Urethral conditions
Cystitis
Insufficient lubrication
Inept male technique
Varices of the broad ligament

Ovarian pathology
Bowel disease
Myoma
Adenomyosis
Diabetes (fragile mucosa)
Postoperative or
    postradiation status

Types of Dyspareunia

1. **Vulvodynia** is chronic burning, stinging, and/or pain of the vulva in the absence of abnormal clinical findings, causing distress, sexual dysfunction, limitations in other daily activities such as sitting and walking, and psychological disability in the absence of abnormal clinical findings.[119] Not a psychosomatic condition, possible etiologies of vulvodynia include cyclic vulvovaginitis, altered sensation centrally or at the nerve root, or lesions.

2. **Vulvar vestibulitis** is defined as 6 months or more of severe burning and pain on contact with localized areas of the vulvar vestibule (at the 5 and 7 o'clock positions), erythema and hyperemia of the vestibule just distal to the hymenal ring[99,128] causing difficulties with lubrication, sexual arousal, and negative emotions regarding sexual interaction with the partner.[150] Etiology is unknown.[24]

3. **Vaginismus** is an involuntary muscle spasm of the outer third of the vagina that interferes with intercourse. The muscle contraction is the physical manifestation of an emotional response to a negative initial sexual experience, sexual abuse, a painful vaginal exam, erectile problems in a partner, religious taboos, pain associated with physical problems (short vagina, imperforate hymen, tumor, recurring vulvar pain, or genital injury), or fear, such as the fear of STIs, pregnancy, sexual orientation, cancer, or HIV.[81]

Dyspareunia During Pregnancy

Pelvic congestion, weight of the growing abdomen, descent of the presenting part, or fear of damaging the pregnancy may cause discomfort.[151]

Ⓜ Management

1. In interviewing the client with sexual concerns, **guarantee privacy and confidentiality. Do not assume the nature of the patient's sexuality.** Refer to her "partner" rather than husband; ask whether the woman has relations with men, women, or both; ask the current number of sexual partners and the number in the last year.[81]

2. **Advise elimination of products** to which the woman may be **allergic.**[90] Advise discontinuance of all feminine hygiene products, cleaning instead once a day with water-moistened washcloth with one wipe from clitoris to anus.[81]

3. **Suggest counseling** and group support as part of the treatment plan from the beginning rather than as a last-ditch effort when nothing else can be done.[81]

4. Elicit a **history of sexual abuse, assault,** or an uncomfortable initial pelvic exam that may make examination difficult (see p. 376).

5. **Treat vaginal infections. Treat menopausal vaginal atrophy. Treat urinary infection.**

6. The woman with **vaginismus** may respond to **education** regarding her anatomy, relaxation techniques, behavioral deconditioning techniques, Kegel exercise to gain a sense of control, or instruction in the use of rubber dilators (or the fingers).[90]

7. **Refer** the woman with **hymenal strands and other hymenal variations** to a gynecologist. **Anticipatory guidance:** Surgery or progressive dilation may be required.[81]

8. **Refer** the woman with **vulvar vestibulitis** to a gynecologist. **Anticipatory guidance:** Interferon treatment,[24] **laser,**[90] **behavioral approaches,** a **low-oxalate diet,**[22] or **pharmacologic** interventions may be tried.[90] **Perineoplasty,** or removal of the vestibule, decreases pain significantly in 89%. Complete long-term resolution was reported by 72%.[23]

9. **Refer** the woman with **vulvodynia** to a gynecologist. **Anticipatory guidance: Candida treatment,** a **low-oxalate** diet, and oral calcium citrate to **neutralize the oxalates** in urine are prescribed; **tricyclic antidepressants** may be prescribed because of their effect on cutaneous nerves. **Other lesions** are treated according to diagnosis.[99] **Complementary measures: Acupuncture** has been used with success in women with vulvodynia.[119]

10. **Educate the pregnant woman** regarding measures to increase sexual comfort during pregnancy, including position alternatives, alternate ways of sexually satisfying the partner, reassurance regarding safety, and externally applied ice to decrease pelvic congestion.[151]

11. **Address emotional aspects:** The patient may need permission to say "no" to intercourse verbally rather than physically. The following **"PLISSIT"** model is useful for sexual counseling, with 80% to 90% of problems being resolved in the first three steps:
    Permission: validate feelings and allow discussion of sexual concerns
    Limited **I**nformation regarding sexual physiology and behavior
    Specific **S**uggestions regarding sexual practices and attitudes
    Intensive **T**herapy referral[90]

Pelvic Organ Prolapse

Prolapse describes the protrusion of pelvic organs into or out of the vaginal canal. Descent of the bladder into the anterior vaginal wall is called a cystocele; bulging of the urethra into the lower anterior vaginal wall is called urethral displacement; descent of the upper posterior vaginal wall generally contains bowel loops and is called enterocele; and bulging of the rectum forward into the lower posterior vaginal wall is called a rectocele.[67]

Signs and symptoms include stress incontinence; urinary frequency; urgency; urge incontinence; hesitancy; a weak or prolonged urinary stream; feeling incompletely emptied; manual reduction of the prolapse or positional changes to be able to begin or complete micturition; difficulty, urgency, or discomfort with defecation; incontinence of flatus or stool; digital manipulation of vagina, perineum, or anus required to complete defecation; feeling of incomplete defecation; rectal protrusion during or after defecation; dyspareunia; change in orgasmic response; incontinence during sexual activity; vaginal, perineal, low back, or abdominal pressure or pain; protrusion of tissue from the vagina; or observation or palpation of a mass.[26]

Predisposing Factors[67]:
Inherently poor connective tissue and muscle strength
Loss of connective tissue integrity during childbirth
Loss of connective tissue integrity with aging
Metabolic diseases that affect muscle strength
Failure to correct pelvic support defects in surgery
Prolonged lifting, straining, or coughing
Loss of levator function from neuromuscular damage during childbirth

Classification: ACOG's Technical Bulletin[16] on this subject gives the following classification:
Grade 0: No descent.
Grade 1: Descent between normal position and ischial spines.
Grade 2: Descent between level of the ischial spines and the hymenal ring.
Grade 3: Descent within the hymenal ring.
Grade 4: Descent through the hymen.

ⓜ Management

1. **Prevent** pelvic prolapse by treating conditions that increase intra-abdominal pressure, such as medical conditions that cause a chronic cough, constipation, or heavy lifting. Weight control, smoking cessation, and Kegel exercises are also helpful in preventing prolapse.[16]
2. **Refer** the woman with pelvic floor prolapse to a gynecologist.
3. **Anticipatory guidance: Diagnostic studies** may include PE during straining in standing or lying positions; cotton swab testing of the urethra; endoscopy; photography; imaging procedures including ultrasonography, contrast radiography, CT, and MRI; and pelvic floor testing by electromyography and pressure recordings.[26] **Treatment** is determined by the woman's age, her desire for future fertility, her desire for sexual function, the severity of the condition, and any medical conditions.[16] Vaginal pessaries are effective if the pelvic floor can hold them in place. Estrogen may preserve mucosal integrity. Surgical repair may be considered.[129]

4. **Complementary measures: Some experts suggest homeopathic** measures for prolapse.[74,121,132] **Acupuncture** may be used in the treatment of pelvic prolapse.[156]

Urinary Incontinence

There are four types of urinary incontinence: stress incontinence (the most common, leaking during exercise, sneezing, coughing, or laughing), urge incontinence (where the urge comes on so abruptly that there isn't time to get to the bathroom), mixed (stress and urge), and overflow incontinence (when the bladder cannot completely empty itself).[7] Incontinence may result in diminished ability to participate in physical activities and in diminished self-esteem.[123]

Thirty percent to 60% of all women have incontinence during pregnancy.[100] The rate of incontinence among older women living at home has been estimated at 17% to 55%; among perimenopausal women, 31%; and among younger and middle-aged nonpregnant women, 12% to 42%.[123,124] After spontaneous vaginal birth, 21% of women have urinary incontinence. After instrumental vaginal delivery, 34% women have urinary incontinence.[100] Twenty percent of women report incontinence after hysterectomy.[124]

Extraurethral support and intraurethral support and innervation maintain urinary continence.[122] Thirty percent of urinary incontinence is temporary, caused by infection, extended bed rest, diuretics, or other medical problems. Advanced cancer of the pelvis, fistulas between the urinary tract and the vagina, side effects of some medications,[7] atrophic vaginitis/urethritis, urinary retention, constipation, irritable bowel, UTI, hematuria, the use of anticholinergics that decrease urethral tone, or neurologic deficits such as MS, cerebrovascular accident (CVA), or spinal cord injury may cause incontinence.[122]

ⓜ Management

1. **Screen:** Questions regarding incontinence should be a part of the routine written history given to each woman at her GYN visit.[122]
2. **Exclude causes** of incontinence such as medication and infection.
3. **Refer** women who have medical complications.
4. The first line of treatment for other women reporting urinary incontinence is **behavioral intervention;** the success rate is significant and there is no harm.[122]
   a. Advise patient to **avoid caffeine.**[7]
   b. Suggest **"double-voiding"**: the woman empties the bladder, rests a moment, then attempts to empty her bladder a second time.[7]
   c. To increase cortical control over micturition as well as building pelvic floor strength, women with urge, stress, and mixed incontinence benefit from both **bladder and pelvic floor training.** This training improves the frequency of incontinence, the amount of urine lost, and the limitation of activities from this condition[124]:

(1) Teach the woman that the **bladder** first gives the **signal to void** when it is about half full.[122]

(2) **Pelvic floor exercise** (Kegel): Teach the woman that the Kegel exercise is the tightening of the pelvic muscles as though she is holding back the unwanted passage of intestinal gas or as though she is clasping the penis during intercourse; moving the clitoris back toward the vagina and the rectum forward toward the vagina. The thigh and the gluteal muscle are relaxed. Thirty contractions/d are advised, of moderate to near maximum intensity, lasting 3 seconds each, relaxing slowly, with at least 10 seconds' relaxation between. Several weeks are required to see results.[125]

(3) Have the woman keep a **2-day diary of voiding and incontinent episodes.** Calculate the shortest interval and suggest that she void at that interval while awake, with or without the urge (a 5- to 10-minute grace period is suggested.) Mental distraction or two or three 10-sec Kegel exercises will usually quiet the urge signal. The schedule is increased in 15- to 30-minute increments every week, with a goal of every 3 to 4 hr, although some women are more comfortable at every 2 to 2.5 hours.[122]

(4) Teach the woman to perform Kegel exercises when she anticipates a **sneeze or heavy lifting** in the case of stress incontinence or when she initially feels the urge to void.[122]

5. **Complementary measures: Biofeedback** may improve incontinence.[113] **Homeopathic** remedies are suggested by some experts,[121,132] whereas **herbal** remedies are suggested by others.[71,97,110,153] **Acupuncture** may control incontinence symptoms.[113]

Fecal Incontinence

Although usually unreported, recent studies have found a 5.6% to 15.9% incidence of fecal incontinence in the general female population. Risk factors for incontinence in the general population include female sex, poor general health, and physical impairment.[109] A 4% to 25% incidence in fecal incontinence is reported after vaginal delivery.[57,100] Studies have focused on the effect of vaginal delivery on the integrity of the rectal sphincter. Damage to the sphincter occurs by two mechanisms during vaginal birth: by pudendal neuropathy that occurs due to stretch or compression with descent of the vertex, by third-degree laceration, or by a combination of these mechanisms. Risk factors for third-degree lacerations include forceps use (vacuum extraction is not implicated), primiparous delivery, macrosomia, a long second stage, and the occiput posterior fetal position. Epidural anesthesia may increase the risk of anal injury by prolonging the second stage. Neurologic damage occurs cumulatively and is associated with multiparity as well as high birthweight and instrumental delivery. The role of episiotomy is unclear, although midline episiotomy is associated with a higher rate of anal sphincter mechanical injuries than is mediolateral episiotomy. Cesarean section performed late in labor does not necessarily prevent neurologic damage. Neurologic injury may recover with time; mechanical disruption will not. Continence may be regained after some months postpartum.[57,109]

Endoanal ultrasound is the tool for evaluating the integrity of the internal and external anal sphincters. Endoanal ultrasound has identified occult sphincter defects in up to 35% of asymptomatic women in whom no sphincter damage was suspected after one vaginal delivery. After multiparous deliveries, 40% had occult disruption of internal and/or external sphincters in one study.[143] In another study among women who sustained occult injuries in their first delivery, 42% experienced fecal incontinence after a second delivery.[57] Among women who sustained a recognized sphincter injury and had a third- or fourth-degree repair, more than 66% had a full-thickness defect after a seemingly satisfactory repair, with 50% of these women reporting incontinence after 3 months and 30% having permanent incontinence. Management of subsequent deliveries is controversial. Fecal incontinence is a serious social handicap. Twenty-one percent of women who had sustained third- and fourth-degree lacerations in their first delivery stated in one study that they would prefer an elective cesarean section to a vaginal delivery for subsequent pregnancies.[53] An alternative to elective cesarean would be expectant management, with cesarean delivery if risk factors occur during labor.

ⓜ Management

1. **Educate** women regarding the frequency with which women experience fecal incontinence to reduce the associated stigma and encourage reporting of symptoms. At the postpartum visit and at routine gynecology visits, **all women should be asked whether they experience fecal incontinence.**

2. Some clinicians suggest **consideration of routine postpartum endoanal endoscopy.** This intervention would evaluate those women who are symptomatic and would detect occult injuries that put a woman at risk for incontinence after subsequent deliveries.

3. After approximately 6 months, allowing for spontaneous recovery of continence, women who report symptoms should be **referred** for an evaluation, which would include endoanal endoscopy.

4. Women who have **pudendal neuropathy** are referred for augmented **biofeedback** therapy.[57]

5. Some clinicians suggest that women who sustain an occult anal sphincter injury after one delivery be given **informed consent** regarding the risk for deterioration of sphincter function after subsequent vaginal delivery and be offered an elective cesarean section **for further deliveries.** Because waiting until the woman has finished her childbearing does not seem reasonable, repair of the sphincter followed by elective cesarean delivery may be considered for the woman who is symptomatic.[57]

Vaginitis

General Principles

1. R/O secondary infections.
2. If the disease is sexually transmitted, treat partner.
3. Treat any infection and have the woman return in 2 months for a Pap smear. If compliance is in doubt, gently remove purulent matter from the cervix with a moistened cotton swab and obtain a Pap smear.[31]
4. Infection may flare with menses.
5. For recurrent infections, consider pockets such as Skene's and Bartholin's glands, urethra, bladder, or rectum.
6. An ectropion may cause excess secretions.
7. Normal vaginal pH is 3.8 to 4.2.[52]
8. Consider advising prophylactic antifungal treatment with antibiotics.
9. Chemical causes of vaginitis include bubble baths, deodorant soaps and sprays, home remedies, hot tub water, laundry soap (especially cold water enzyme activated), OTC drugs, perfume, perfumed toilet paper, spermicide, and swimming pool water.
10. Mechanical causes of vaginitis include condoms, diaphragms, dildos, bicycle riding, masturbation, horseback riding, nonporous panties, foreign bodies, tampons, and vibrators.

Instructions for Women With Vaginitis

1. Wipe the perineal area from front to back.
2. Wear underwear and pantyhose with cotton crotches.
3. Do not use feminine hygiene sprays, bath oils, strong soaps, or anything deodorized.
4. Do not douche unless it is curative.
5. Cut down on simple sugars and increase intake of yogurt, acidophilus milk, protein, and acid-forming grains and beans.
6. Rest, exercise, and decrease stress.
7. Increase pelvic bloodflow by relaxation or sitz baths.
8. Acidify the system to discourage infection: drink cranberry juice or a mixture of 1 tsp vinegar, 1 tsp lemon juice, and 1 tsp honey in hot water, or take vitamin C.
9. Take the complete course of any medication ordered.
10. Abstain from intercourse or use a condom until the course of treatment is complete.
11. Refrain from tampon use during treatment.
12. Avoid reinfection by not reusing towels, washcloths, clothes, douching tips, and diaphragms or having sex with an untreated partner.
13. **Complementary measures:**
    a. **Homeopathic** measures are suggested by some experts.[40,121,149]
    b. **Nutritional suggestions: Plain yogurt** may be used internally or externally. **Garlic** is antiviral and antibacterial when taken in the diet.[62,71]

c. **Herbs: Goldenseal, contraindicated in pregnancy,** is indicated for vaginal infections.[18,97,107] Take 30 to 120 drops of tincture a day PO or diluted in water for a douche.[107] **See information about herbs, p. 563.**

d. **Reflexology:** Massage along the Achilles tendon in increase blood-flow to the pelvic region. See information about reflexology, p. 567.

14. **For specific treatment, see monilia (p. 476), trichomonas (p. 480), bacterial vaginosis (below), or atrophic vaginitis (p. 544).**

Bacterial Vaginosis (Previously Haemophilus or Gardnerella)

BV is the alteration of vaginal flora with a decrease in the normally dominant lactobacilli, resulting in the dominance of anaerobic organisms.[3] Fifty percent of women are asymptomatic. If symptoms are present, it is usually a gray, foul or fishy-smelling, profuse, homogenous, thin or thick vaginal discharge that may or may not be irritating. The odor may be more noticeable after intercourse or during menses. Although the discharge may be adherent, the vaginal wall and cervix do not appear inflamed on examination.[39] The vaginal pH is >4.5. A wet mount shows "clue cells," which are epithelial cells so covered with bacteria that they appear stippled and have serrated edges. When 10% potassium hydroxide (KOH) is added, a fishy odor is noted. A decrease in lactobacilli and the presence of Mobiluncus (small bacteria that move in a rapid, corkscrew manner) may be noted. Culture is not suggested (many false-positive results),[3] but Gram stain identification of bacteria is acceptable for diagnosis. The Pap smear has low sensitivity.[30]

Predisposing Factors[39]:

Vaginal douching	Presence of an IUD
Spermicide use	Antibiotic use
Cigarette smoking	Multiple and/or uncircumcised
Increased parity	partners
Sexual intercourse	Presence of trichomonas
Lower socioeconomic status	Pregnancy

Transmission: The infection may be sexually transmitted according to many authorities. BV is associated with multiple sexual partners and concomitant STIs. Treatment of male partners does not improve cure rates, but women who are not sexually active rarely have BV.[30]

Complications: Women with BV are at increased risk for UTIs,[68] PID, postoperative vaginal cuff cellulitis, and cervical intraepithelial neoplasia. An association exists between the presence of BV and HIV seropositivity.[39] Increased rates of infection occur in the presence of BV after endometrial biopsy, hysterectomy, hysterosalpingography, IUD placement, cesarean section, and uterine curettage, and some clinicians screen and treat BV before these procedures.[30]

Complications During Pregnancy: SAB in the first and second trimesters,[120] preterm labor and birth,[54] UTI,[114] chorioamnionitis, PPROM, and puerperal endometritis have been reported.[78]

m *Management of the Nonpregnant Woman According to the CDC's 2002 Recommendations*

1. Treat all women who are symptomatic.[30]
2. **Pharmacologic treatment:**
   a. Metronidazole 500 mg PO bid for 7 days is the drug of choice for nonpregnant women (cures 78% to 84%) *or*
   b. Metronidazole gel 0.75%, one full applicator (5 g) PV qd for 5 days (cures 75%) *or*
   c. Clindamycin cream 2%, one full applicator (5 g) PV at hs for 7 days (cures 82%); less efficacious than metronidazole preparations[30]
3. **Alternate regimens[30]:**
   Metronidazole 2 g PO in a single dose *or*
   Clindamycin 300 mg PO bid for 7 days *or*
   Clindamycin ovules 100 g PV at hs for 3 days
   NOTE: Both metronidazole regimens are equally efficacious. Some women may tolerate the vaginal preparation better than the oral preparation.[30] Alcohol and vinegar must be avoided by women for 24 hours after taking metronidazole. The intravaginal route may produce less GI side effects. Clindamycin cream is oil-based and may weaken latex condoms and diaphragms.[30]
4. Treatment of the **partner** is not suggested routinely. Consider if infection is recurrent.[30,114]
5. **Follow-up:** Instruct the woman to return if symptoms recur. If this occurs, order a different recommended treatment regimen. Prophylactic, long-term therapy is not recommended.[30]
6. **HIV-positive women** are treated with the same regimens.[30]

m *Management During Pregnancy According to the CDC's 2002 Recommendations*

1. Some specialist physicians recommend **screening** those **pregnant women at high risk for preterm delivery** at the fist prenatal visit; treatment of these women decreased preterm delivery in 3 out of 4 clinical trials. Screening and treatment of **pregnant women at low risk for preterm delivery** has been studied and found in one study to reduce spontaneous preterm delivery and in another to reduce postpartum infections. All **symptomatic pregnant women** should be screened and treated.[30]
2. **Pharmacologic treatment of pregnant women:**
   a. Metronidazole 250 mg PO tid for 7 days[30] *or*
   b. Clindamycin 300 mg PO bid for 7 days[30]
   NOTE: Some experts suggest systemic therapy for low-risk pregnant women to treat subclinical upper genital tract infections. Clindamycin cream has shown adverse effects (prematurity and neonatal infection) and is no longer recommended. Metronidazole use during pregnancy has not been associated with teratogenic or mutagenic effects in newborns.[30]

3. **Test of cure is necessary** after 1 month for the pregnant woman at high risk for a preterm birth.[30]

Chemical Vaginitis (Contact Dermatitis or Reactive Vulvitis)

Chemical vaginitis is irritation of vaginal tissue from an irritant, possibly aggravated by perspiration, heat, friction, or pressure or initiated by bicycle riding, horseback riding, coitus, saliva, spermicides, laundry detergent, fabric dyes, perfumes, soap, or ingredients in swimming pools. Symptoms may include itching, burning, irritation, tenderness, and urinary retention in severe cases. Erythematous, edematous, exudative, weeping papulovesicular lesions or bullae may be present; thickening; scaling; or wheals may occur, especially in skin folds.[139]

m Management

1. **Exclude infectious vaginitis.**[139]
2. **Identify and remove irritant.**[139]
3. **Teach the woman comfort measures,** including avoidance of intercourse until healed, use of a hair dryer to keep the perineum dry, using only cornstarch to powder perineum, avoiding tampon use, wearing loose clothes and underwear with cotton crotches, external application of Burrow's solution for comfort by cool baths, or wet dressings. Avoid topical anesthetics.[139]
4. Prescribe low-potency **corticosteroid cream** for local use (oil-based is more effective for scaly areas; cream for other areas).[139]
5. In **severe cases,** systemic antihistamines and corticosteroids may be needed and physician **consultation** is indicated.[139]

Monilial Vaginitis (Vulvovaginal Candidiasis)

Monilial vaginitis is a fungal infection caused by *Candida albicans* or other candida species.[30] These organisms are present in the vaginas of approximately 20% women without causing symptoms. *C. albicans* causes 80% to 90% of cases. Other species (*C. parapsilosis, C. tropicalis, C. kefyr, C. krusei,* and *C. glabrata*) are involved less frequently but are more refractory to treatment. Clinical presentation of all species is the same.[52] Transmission is by contact with secretions from the mouth, skin, vagina, or feces of infected individuals. A fetus may be infected vertically through hematogenous spread or from the mother's birth canal. Although usually not sexually transmitted, candida may infect the glans and prepuce of males or the area under the foreskin.[20]

Signs and symptoms include vulvar pruritus or burning, external dysuria, soreness, dyspareunia,[30] vulvar and vaginal erythema, fissures, curd-like vaginal discharge, or no discharge.[52] The vaginal pH is normal (<4.5).[30] Discrete pustulopapular peripheral lesions may be present.[52]

Predisposing Factors[20,49,52,59,135]:

OCs (cause 11% to 12% of recurrent cases)
Tight clothes
Summer weather
Pregnancy
Atrophic vaginitis
Menses
General debilitation`
Hematologic malignancies
Diabetes mellitus
Obesity
Psychogenic factors
Supraphysiologic doses of adrenal corticosteroids
Therapy with broad-spectrum antibiotics
Douching
Condom or spermicide use
Luteal phase of the menstrual cycle
Young age
Sexual intercourse more than 4 times a month
Sanitary pad use
Rectal intercourse
Receptive oral intercourse
Presence of STIs
Black or minority race
History of vulvovaginal candidiasis (VVC) in the previous year
Immunosuppression (including HIV, local allergic, or hypersensitivity reactions)

Classifications:

1. **Uncomplicated VVC** is infection with *C. albicans* mild to moderate in severity, sporadic, and nonrecurring in a normal host responding to medical therapy.[30]

2. **Complicated VVC** is severe local or recurrent VVC in an abnormal host (e.g., the woman with uncontrolled diabetes) or infection caused by a less susceptible fungal pathogen (e.g., *Candida glabrata*) that requires a longer duration of therapy (10 to 14 days) with topical or oral azoles.[30]

3. **Recurrent VVC** (RVVC) is defined as 4 or more episodes of symptomatic VVC in 1 year confirmed microscopically or by culture. Etiology is unknown. Predisposing factors include diabetes, immunosuppression, corticosteroid use,[31] use of commercial perineal hygiene or vaginal douche products, and a greater number of lifetime sexual partners. Whether OCs contribute is controversial.[135]

Laboratory Findings: Wet mount with KOH shows pseudohyphae and yeast cells in 50% of the patients who have a positive culture for *C. albicans*. Gram stain of vaginal discharge shows pseudohyphae or yeasts.[30] Some yeast infections cannot be detected by microscope, either because there are few organisms or because they are not albicans specimens without pseudohyphae.[39] Microscopic examination of non–*C. albicans* shows budding yeast or blastospores without pseudomycelia or hyphae.[133]

ⓜ Management According to the CDC's 2002 Recommendations

1. Treatment is not indicated for the **asymptomatic woman.**[30]

2. For the woman who is symptomatic with negative wet mount findings, send a **culture for *C. albicans*.**[49]
3. **Recurrent VVC** requires a screen for underlying medical conditions.[31]
4. **Pharmacologic treatment:**
   a. **Uncomplicated VVC**
      (1) **Topical preparations** (treatment with azoles is more effective than nystatin):
         (a) Butoconazole 2% cream, 5 g PV for 3 days* *or*
         (b) Butoconazole 2% cream 5 g (Butoconazole 1—sustained release), single intravaginal application,* *or*
         (c) Clotrimazole 1% cream*:
            (i) 5 g PV for 7 to 14 days *or*
            (ii) 100 mg vaginal tablet two PV for 3 days *or*
            (iii) 100 mg vaginal tablet one PV for 7 days *or*
            (iv) 500 mg vaginal tablet one PV in a single application *or*
         (d) Miconazole 2% cream (Monistat)*:
            (i) 5 g at hs for 7 days PV *or*
            (ii) 200 mg suppository one PV at hs for 3 days *or*
            (iii) 100 mg suppository one PV at hs for 7 days *or*
         (e) Nystatin (Nilstat or Mycostatin): one 100,000 U vaginal tablet PV for 14 days *or*
         (f) Tioconazole* 6.5% ointment 5 g PV at bedtime in a single application *or*
         (g) Terconazole*
            (i) 0.4% cream 5 g PV for 7 days *or*
            (ii) 0.8% cream 5 g PV at hs for 3 days *or*
            (iii) 80 mg suppository one PV at hs for 3 days[30]
      (2) **Oral preparation:** Fluconazole (Diflucan) 150 mg PO in a single dose.[30]
   b. **Complicated VVC** (note definition on p. 477):
      (1) Obtain a vaginal culture to confirm the diagnosis and to identify the non-albicans species.
      (2) Topical therapy is prescribed for 7 to 14 days; or fluconazole 150 mg PO is repeated in 3 days before prescribing a maintenance antifungal regimen.
      (3) Maintenance antifungal regimen—continue for 6 months[30]:
         (a) Clotrimazole 500 mg vaginal suppository once weekly *or*
         (b) Ketoconazole 100 mg once daily (monitor woman for hepatotoxicity) *or*
         (c) Fluconazole 100 to 150 mg once weekly *or*

---

*These medications are available OTC and may be used by a woman who has been examined by a health care provider and diagnosed with VVC once and is having a **recurrence** of the same symptoms. The woman whose symptoms persist or return within 2 months of self-treatment should see a health care provider.[30]

(d) Itraconazole 400 mg once monthly or 100 mg once daily

c. **Severe VVC** (extensive erythema, edema, excoriation, and fissure formation)[30]:

(a) Prescribe 7 to 14 days of topical azole *or*

(b) Fluconazole 150 mg PO; repeat dose in 72 hours

d. NOTES:

(1) The creams and suppositories are **oil-based and may weaken latex condoms or diaphragms.**[30]

(2) **Choice of anti-fungal:** The initial therapy for a non-albicans VVC in a non-fluconazole azole drug for 7 to 14 days.[30] Tioconazole acts against *C. albicans, C. glabrata, C. tropicalis, C. krusei, C. kefyr,* and *C. parapsilosis.* Clotrimazole, miconazole, and butoconazole are less effective against *C. glabrata* or *C. tropicalis.* Ketoconazole is less effective against *C. glabrata.* Fluconazole is less effective against *C. glabrata* and *C. krusei.* Use of the broadest spectrum antifungal should result in the highest cure rates and in less promotion of resistant yeasts. Oral antifungals achieve therapeutic levels at the site but cannot provide the rapid local relief of topical medications.[52] If recurrence occurs, boric acid 600 mg in a gelatin capsule PV qd for 2 weeks is recommended. For further recurrence, refer to specialist physician.[30]

(3) **Side effects** seen most often include headache (0.2%), abdominal cramps (0.2%), and local burning, itching, or discomfort (0.9% to 6%). With oral therapy, GI symptoms occur in 5% to 12.5%, and rarely hives and anaphylaxis or hepatotoxicity. Frequent doses of oral fluconazole during pregnancy are teratogenic.[52]

(4) **Drug interactions:** Oral anti-fungals should not be taken concurrently with astemizole, calcium channel antagonists, cisapride, warfarin, cyclosporin A, oral hypoglycemic agents, phenytoin, protease inhibitors, tacrolimus, terfenadine, theophylline, trimetrexate, and rifampin.[30]

5. **Treatment of the pregnant woman:** Prescribe a topical azole therapy for 7 days.[30]

6. Advise the woman to **abstain from sexual intercourse** until treatment is complete for best results.[20]

7. **Comfort suggestions:** Baking powder, baking soda, or plain yogurt applied externally may be comforting. Mycolog cream can be applied externally to excoriated skin.[107] A 50% solution of vinegar and water applied externally is comforting.[149]

8. **Partner treatment:** Consider treating the partner of the woman with recurrent infections.[30]

9. **Patient education:** Advise the woman to discontinue use of commercial douches or perineal hygiene products. Advise her, if applicable, that the OCs may be predisposing her to the infection.[136]

10. **Follow-up** is necessary only if symptoms persist or recur within 2 months.[30]
11. **Complementary measures:**
    a. Some experts suggest **homeopathy** remedies for vaginal yeast infection.[40,132]
    b. **Nutritional suggestions:** Balch and Balch[18] suggest that **garlic** is safer and as effective in neutralizing fungi as antifungal medications. They suggest taking 2 capsules tid with meals. **Vitamin B complex** 50 mg tid with pantothenic acid (vitamin B_5) 50 mg tid, **vitamin C with flavonoids** 5000 to 20,000 mg daily in divided doses, **vitamin E** 400 to 800 IU daily, and **zinc** 50 mg qd support the body's immune function. **Acidophilus or L bifidus** replacement is also suggested. The eating of raw foods and avoidance of sugar, meat, dairy, grains, and processed and greasy foods is helpful.[18]
    c. **Herbs: Calendula, contraindicated in pregnancy,** is an antifungal, astringent, anti-inflammatory, and immune system restorative that promotes the growth of new tissue, promoting wound healing. Diluted tincture of calendula as a rinse to the external vulva will ease itching.[62,107,138] The tea may be used as a douche or cream; or infused oil may be applied externally.[110] **Goldenseal, also contraindicated in pregnancy,** acts as an antibiotic as well as an immune system stimulant.[62] As a rinse to the external vulva, goldenseal eases itching[107]; as a douche it treats candida vaginitis.[91] Place one peeled (not nicked) clove of **garlic** in the vagina, wrapped in a small piece of gauze, morning and night.[62,91,107,110,138] **Pau d'arco** is an antifungal. Three cups of pau d'arco tea may be taken daily.[18,62,97] Medina[97] warns never to use the bark directly on the skin, but douche with a one quarter strength infusion. **See information about herbs, p. 563.**

Trichomonas

Trichomonas vaginalis is a unicellular, flagellate parasitic protozoan infection of the genitourinary tract.[3] Nearly half of infected women are asymptomatic.[39] For those who are symptomatic, a thin, profuse, foamy gray or yellow-green discharge with foul odor is present. Itching, pain, and erythema of vulva,[3] abdominal pain, fullness, dyspareunia, dysuria, cystitis, urinary frequency, spotting, and inflamed Bartholin's cysts and urethra may be present.[78] On exam, the cervix is edematous and friable.[3] "Strawberry cervix" is seen in <25%.[39] The organism promotes an anaerobic environment, causing a pH between 5 and 8 and supporting the growth of BV.[78]

Sexually transmitted to 70% of exposed partners, trichomonas is infectious as long as the organism is present.[20] It is infrequently transmitted by warm, wet fomites[107] but requires intravaginal or intraurethral inoculation, and the incubation period is up to 21 days.[39]

Predisposing Factors:

Young age[78]

Poor education[78]

History of gonorrhea[78]

Multiple sexual partners[78]

Tobacco use[78]

Nonbarrier contraception[39]

Single marital status[78]

Black race[3]

Complications During Pregnancy: Preterm birth, PPROM, and intrauterine growth restriction (IUGR) have been reported as associated with trichomonas[30]; however, these may actually be related to the BV that so often coexists with trichomonas.[78] When trichomonas coexists with BV, the risk for preterm delivery is higher than the risk with BV alone. This synergistic effect may actually reflect the high-risk behaviors behind acquisition of these infections or a racial bias for preterm births, because black women are at significantly higher risk to have both trichomonas and preterm labor. Trichomonas may cause transient vaginitis or cystitis in newborns 4 to 6 weeks after delivery.[54]

Laboratory Findings: A wet mount with normal saline identifies the organism in 60% to 70% of cases.[30] Culture is the most sensitive way to identify the organism.[20,78] Pap smears are nonspecific and infection should be confirmed before treatment.[3]

Ⓜ *Management According to the CDC's 2002 Recommendations*

1. **Educate** all women regarding safe sex, STIs, and high-risk behaviors.
2. Perform **wet mount and/or culture** for trichomonas.
3. **Exclude concurrent STIs.** Offer HIV counseling and testing.
4. **Pharmacologic treatment** (including for the HIV-positive woman):
   a. **Nonpregnant woman:** Metronidazole (Flagyl or Protostat) 2 g PO in a single dose or 500 mg PO bid for 7 days.[30]
   b. **Pregnant woman:** Metronidazole (Flagyl or Protostat) 2 g PO in a single dose.[30] Although trichomonas is associated with adverse outcomes in pregnancy, treatment has not been shown to improve these outcomes. Treat only the woman who is symptomatic.[30]
   c. **NOTE:** The single-dose regimen is recommended for **pregnant** women. Because the drug is excreted in breastmilk, for the **lactating** woman prescribe the single dose and advise discontinuance of breastfeeding for 12 to 24 hours to clear the dose, instructing the woman to pump and discard her milk.[28] The use of alcohol and vinegar products are contraindicated during metronidazole administration and for 24 hours afterward.[3]
   d. **Metronidazole-allergic patients:** No alternative medical therapy exists. Desensitization followed by treatment with metronidazole is suggested.[30]
5. **Follow-up:** Test of cure is not necessary if the woman is asymptomatic and does not suspect reinfection.[30]
6. **Recurrences:** Although some strains are developing resistance to metronidazole, most will respond to higher doses. After either

of the above regimens fail, give metronidazole 500 mg PO bid for 7 days. If this fails, give metronidazole 2 g PO qd for 3 to 5 days.[30]

7. **Refer** the partner for treatment.[30]

8. **Advise abstinence** until both partners have been treated and are asymptomatic.[30]

9. **Complementary measures:**

   a. Some experts recommend **homeopathic** remedies for a trichomonas infection.[132]

   b. **Nutritional suggestions: Garlic** is believed to be effective against trichomonas.[91,107]

   c. **Herbs: Goldenseal** in a douche, **contraindicated in pregnancy,** acts as an antibiotic and stimulates the immune system and is effective against trichomonas.[62,91,97] **See information about herbs, p. 563.**

• OTHER GYNECOLOGIC DISORDERS

Diethylstilbestrol Exposure

Diethylstilbestrol (DES) is a nonsteroidal estrogen that was prescribed for pregnant women between 1940 and 1971 for threatened abortion, preeclampsia and other hypertensive disorders, diabetes, and preterm labor.[41] The timing and the dosage of the drug affected its manifestation in the offspring.[67] A list of medications containing DES may be accessed online at http://www.desaction.org/deswhat.html.

Women who were prescribed DES during pregnancy appear to have an increased risk for breast cancer. Men who were exposed to DES in utero (DES sons) have an increased risk for epididymal cysts and other genitourinary abnormalities.[143a]

DES daughters may have vaginal changes that include adenocarcinoma, clear cell carcinoma, adenosis, or columnar epithelium in the vaginal wall.[41] Clear cell adenocarcinoma increases in the 40 to 46 year age group.[4] Adenosis usually resolves spontaneously with squamous maturation.[67] Cervical changes may include ectropion or eversion; cervical ridges, collar, hood, or hypoplasia[41]; cervical cockscomb[67]; pseudopolyps; fusion of the cervix to the vagina; and an abnormal or absent fornix.[151] Uterine changes may include hypoplasia, a T-shaped endometrial canal, constricting bands in the endometrium, and transverse septa. Ovaries may show shortening, narrowing, and the absence of fimbriae. Infertility, SAB, and ectopic pregnancy occur with more frequency among these women.[41] DES exposure increases the risk of preterm labor by 1.6 to 5.4 times.[69]

The children of DES daughters may also be at increased risk for reproductive cancers and abnormalities known as a "third generation effect."[4]

ⓜ *Management*

1. In 2000, these women were between ages 29 and 52 years. **Examination, Pap smear, and colposcopy** should have been done at menarche or when they became sexually active. Clear cell carcinoma usually occurs before the age of 30 years. Some clinicians take smears circumferentially for the **Pap smear** from the upper two thirds of the vagina as well as the cervical smear.[17] **Follow annually** if findings are normal or for simple adenosis.
2. For other symptoms, **refer** to a gynecologist who will see the woman every 6 months.
3. **Anticipatory guidance:** For infertility, **surgical correction of structural abnormalities** of cervix and vagina may result in pregnancy. Zygote transferring techniques are also used with success. **Clear cell carcinoma,** if identified, is treated by irradiation or by surgical excision.[41]
4. Resources for providers and patients are available at http://www.cdc.gov/DES or by phone (888-232-6789).

ⓜ *Management During Pregnancy*

1. The midwife **co-manages or refers** this woman to an obstetrician.[41]
2. **Anticipatory guidance: Ectopic gestation** is excluded with an early ultrasound.[41] The woman is followed for **cervical competence**[41] and **preterm labor.**[58]

Endometriosis

Endometriosis is the presence of estrogen-sensitive tissue outside the uterus that has the histologic structure and function of the uterine mucosa.[90] This tissue is most commonly found on the ovaries, posterior and uterosacral ligaments, and anterior and posterior cul de sacs.[82] The fallopian tubes, posterior broad ligament, bowel, and extraperitoneal sites such as the lungs may also be affected. Cyclic hormonal changes stimulate this tissue, which responds with proliferation, secretion, necrosis and sloughing, causing peritoneal inflammation. Prostaglandins, cytokines, and complement are produced and contribute to the severe cramping. Adhesions form throughout the pelvis, cause further pain, and may distort genital structures.[34]

The woman usually has a history of chronic pain and dysmenorrhea. She may have acute exacerbations. Lesions may also be present without pain. The etiology is unknown. One theory postulates "retrograde menstruation" with an abnormal immunologic response.[65] Retrograde menstruation actually occurs in 90% of all women, but in women who develop endometriosis, apparently due to an autoimmune disease or environmental differences, the tissue successfully implants, proliferates, develops its own blood supply and becomes an independent growing mass. A piece of the tissue can break off, migrate by the lymph, and implant elsewhere.[34]

Signs and symptoms include short cycles with prolonged and heavy menstrual flow,[82] dysmenorrhea, dyspareunia, rectal bleeding, pain with bowel movements during menses, colonic obstruction, diarrhea, urethral obstruction, dysuria, hematuria, postcoital bleeding, cyclic sciatica, cyclic hemoptysis,[139] chronic pelvic pain, and low back pain.[34] Intensity may range from nonexistent to incapacitating.[34] On exam, retroversion of the uterus; limited mobility; an irregular, tender adnexal mass; adherent, enlarged nodular tube and ovary; nodular thickening of uterosacral ligaments; and diffuse pelvic tenderness may be found.[82] These findings are more pronounced premenstrually.[34]

Predisposing Factors[34]:

Early menarche
Short menstrual cycles
Long duration of flow
Dysmenorrhea
Asian race
First-degree relative with endometriosis (increases risk sevenfold)

Uterine abnormalities that obstruct outflow
IUD use
Having sexual intercourse during menses

Risk-Reducing Factors: Frequent pregnancies, cigarette smoking (decreases estrogen), intense physical training, breastfeeding and, of course, menopause reduce the risk.[34]

Complications: Infertility, possibly SAB, and rarely endometriomas that have become neoplastic have been reported.[139]

Differential Diagnoses: PID, myoma, ovarian cysts, appendicitis, bowel disease, urinary tract disease, neoplasm, and ectopic pregnancy.[139]

ⓜ Management

1. The midwife **gathers information** that would identify the woman with endometriosis at any gynecology visit. The information is useful as a baseline in the asymptomatic woman. **Listen to the woman's concerns**, **provide information** about endometriosis, and give **referrals for support groups** to help the woman with the emotional burden of the disease.[34]

2. When the midwife suspects endometriosis, she **refers** the woman to a gynecologist.

3. **Anticipatory guidance:** Definitive diagnosis is made by laparoscopy or laparotomy, during which visible lesions are ablated with laser or electrocauterized and biopsies are taken.[65] Goals of therapy include halting the destruction of the pelvic organs by halting the progression of present lesions and preventing development of new ones, relieving pain and other symptoms, maintaining fertility, and validating symptoms.[34]

4. **Complementary measures:**
   a. All **stress-reduction** therapies such as massage and acupuncture are helpful.[113] Several herbalists suggest **herbal** remedies for endometriosis.[18,107,113,153]

b. **Reflexology:** Press both sides of the foot just below the ankle bone for 10 seconds bid (uterine and ovary areas).[113] **See charts and information about reflexology, p. 567.**

c. **Nutritional suggestions:**
   (1) **Vitamin A** 400 IU qd aids hormonal balance.[18]
   (2) **Vitamin K** 200 µg qd for blood clotting.[18]
   (3) **Essential fatty acids** 1500 mg qd.[18] **Omega fish oil** or **primrose oil** will help properly metabolize estrogen.[113]
   (4) **Iron** if iron deficiency anemia is present (ferrous fumarate the best form according to Balch & Balch).[18]
   (5) **Vitamin B complex** for cell productivity and hormone balance taken as directed on the label plus vitamin B_5 100 mg tid for stress and vitamin B_6 50 mg tid for diuresis.[18]
   (6) **Vitamin C with bioflavonoids** 2000 mg tid (buffered form) for healing.[18]
   (7) **Zinc 50 mg** qd (not to exceed 100 mg daily total) for tissue repair and immune function.[18,107]
   (8) Supplement manganese, copper, and magnesium.[107]
   (9) Fifty percent of the diet should be raw fruits and vegetables. Use whole grain products, nuts, and seeds rather than refined flours.[18]
   (10) Avoid alcohol, caffeine, animal fats, dairy products, fried foods, additives, red meat, poultry (except organic skinless), salt, shellfish, and sugar.[18,113]
   (11) Fast for 3 days each month at the end of the menstrual cycle, drinking steam-distilled water and fresh juices.[18,113]
   (12) **Garlic** decreases cholesterol and may affect estrogen levels.[18,62]

Pelvic Mass Differential

Box 8-2 lists diagnoses to be considered when a pelvic mass is noted.

Sheehan's Syndrome

The woman who experiences severe PPH and hypovolemic shock may undergo infarction and necrosis of the pituitary.[134] Her prolactin level is lower than normal (<5 ng/mL) and she fails to lactate postpartum.[67] Severity is determined by the degree of necrosis and the subsequent failure to secrete one or more of the anterior pituitary hormones—growth hormone, gonadotropins, or adrenocorticotropic hormone (ACTH). Least often, TSH deficiencies may be seen. Loss of pubic and axillary hair,[134] breast atrophy, superinvolution of the uterus, sterility, signs of hypothyroidism, and adrenocortical insufficiency may be observed.[154] Diagnosis is delayed an average of 7 years from onset of symptoms. Some patients are misdiagnosed with postpartum depression when the woman is actually hypothyroid. Failure of the menses to return after 6 months postpartum in a nonlactating woman is cause to investigate.

• Box 8-2 / Pelvic Masses—Differential •

Vaginal

Developmental anomalies
- Imperforate hymen
- Vaginal septum

Relaxation
- Cystocele
- Rectocele
- Enterocele

Foreign body

Bartholin's/Gartner's duct cyst

Neoplasm

Cervical

Nabothian cyst

Fibroid

Ectopic pregnancy

Carcinoma

Uterine

Pregnancy
- Cornual
- Cervical

Displacement
- Retro
- Lateral

Fibroids

Adenomyosis

Round ligament tumors

Malignancies

Rare tumors

Congenital anomalies

Hematometra/pyometra
- Transverse vaginal septum
- Vaginal atresia
- Cervical stenosis
- Cervical cancer

Tubal

Mesonephric duct remnants

Ectopic pregnancy

Acute salpingitis
- Pyosalpinx
- TOA

Chronic salpingitis
- Hydrosalpinx

Tuberculosis

Ovarian

Epithelial stroma tumors

Germ cell tumors

Sex-cord stromal tumors

Lipid (lipoid) cell tumors

Gonadoblastoma

Soft tissue tumors

Unclassified tumors

Secondary (metastatic) tumors

Tumor-like conditions
- Pregnancy luteoma

Extragenital

Endometriosis

Inflammatory
- Appendicitis
- Diverticulitis
- Perirectal abscess

Hematocele

Ascites

Urologic
- Bladder
- Urachal cysts
- Pelvic kidney
- Transplant
- Tumor

GI
- Inflammatory
- Tumor
- Stool/gas

- Hyperplasia of
  ovarian stroma,
  hyperthecosis
- Massive edema
- Follicle cyst
- Corpus luteum cyst
- Polycystic ovaries
- Luteinized follicle
  cysts and/or
  corpora lutea
- Endometriosis
- Surface-epithelial
  inclusion cysts
- Simple cysts
- Paraovarian cysts
- Inflammatory
  lesions

Retroperitoneal
- Teratoma
- Meningomyelocele
- Presacral chordoma
- Lymphocyst
- Lymphoma
- Sarcoma group

Abdominal wall lesions
- Hematoma
- Muscle tumor
- Abscess
- Lipoma
- Scar implants
- Foreign body

Modified from Star WL et al: Women's primary health care: protocols for practice, Washington, DC, 1995, American Nurses Association.

The preexisting vascular changes of diabetes predispose the diabetic woman to Sheehan's syndrome.[116]

ⓜ Management

1. The midwife who suspects Sheehan's syndrome may **order relevant laboratory tests** (levels of ACTH, TSH, T4, FSH, LH, estradiol, prolactin, electrolytes, BUN, and creatinine) and then **refer** the woman to a physician.[116]

2. **Anticipatory guidance:** Other testing may be performed to evaluate the degree to which the pituitary has been injured and to exclude other pathology.[116] Replacement of thyroid and adrenocorticosteroid hormones is the treatment.[129] Future reproduction is accomplished with careful medical induction of ovulation.[116]

Vaginal Bleeding: Abnormal, Differential

See p. 66 for a decision tree regarding the diagnosis and management of vaginal bleeding during pregnancy.

Possible Causes of Vaginal Bleeding During the Childbearing Years: Not Related to Pregnancy:

Anovulation

Vaginitis

Psychogenic factors

Ovarian cysts

OCs

IUD

Cervical erosion

Foreign bodies

Endometritis (PID)

Vaginal or cervical lacerations or other trauma

Stein-Leventhal cervical polyps (after age 25 years)

Uterine myoma (after age 25 years)

Endometriosis and adenomyosis (after age 35 years)

Anorexia nervosa or obesity

Endometrial hyperplasia (after age 35 years)

Medications (phenothiazines, hypothalamic depressants, anticoagulants, anticholinergics, thiazide diuretics)

Systemic disease, such as a blood dyscrasia, hypothyroidism, leukemia, or TB

Possible Causes of Vaginal Bleeding During the Postmenopausal Years:

Carcinoma

Polyps

Coital injuries due to atrophy, estrogen therapy, myoma, atrophic vaginitis, or endometrial hyperplasia (see dysfunctional uterine bleeding, p. 450)

• REFERENCES

1. Aboulghar MA, Mansour RT, Serour GI: Controversies in the modern management of hydrosalpinx, *Hum Reprod Update* 4:882-890, 1998.

2. Al-Tawfiq JA et al: Experimental infection of human volunteers with *Haemophilus ducreyi* does not confer protection against subsequent challenge, *J Infect Dis* 179: 1283-1287, 1999.

3. Ament LA, Whalen E: Sexually transmitted diseases in pregnancy: diagnosis, impact, and intervention, *J Obstet Gynecol Neonatal Nurs* 25:657-666, 1996.

4. American College of Nurse-Midwives (ACNM): DES: a problem we cannot forget, *Quickening* 32:9, 2001.

5. ACNM: Position statement: adolescent health care, *Quickening* 8:8, 2000.

6. American College of Obstetricians and Gynecologists (ACOG): *The use of hormonal contraception in women with coexisting medical conditions*, Practice Bulletin No. 18, Washington, DC, 2000, ACOG.

7. ACOG: *Breaking the silence on a common problem*, Washington, DC, 1999, ACOG. Available at: *http://www.acog.com/from_home/publications/womans_health/wh11-24-7.htm*.

8. ACOG: *Deciphering the news about breast cancer risks*, Washington, DC, 1999, ACOG. Available at: *http://www.acog.com/from_home/publications/womans_health/wh10-6-7.htm*.

9. ACOG: *Federal study shows conventional Pap test remains most effective way to diagnose cervical cancer*, Washington, DC, 1999, ACOG. Available at: *http://www.acog.com/search97 cgi/s97_cgi.exe*.

10. ACOG: *Getting the facts on fibroids*, Washington, DC, 1999, ACOG. Available at: *http://www.acog.com/from_home/publications/womans_health/wh9-22-7.htm*.

11. ACOG: *Management of herpes in pregnancy*, Practice Bulletin No. 8, Washington, DC, 1999, ACOG.

12. Reference deleted in galleys.

13. ACOG: *Confidentiality in adolescent health care*, Educational Bulletin No. 249, Washington, DC, 1998, ACOG.

14. ACOG: *Ovarian cancer*, Educational Bulletin No. 250, Washington, DC, 1998, ACOG.

15. ACOG: *Now is the time to help adolescent girls avoid lifelong health problems, report ob/gyns*, news release, Washington, DC, 1997, ACOG. Available at: *http://www.acog.com/from_home/publications/press_releases/nr12-9-97.htm*.

16. ACOG: *Pelvic organ prolapse*, Technical Bulletin No. 214, Washington, DC, 1995, ACOG.

17. ACOG: *Cervical cytology: evaluation and management of abnormalities*, Technical Bulletin No. 183, Washington, DC, 1993, ACOG.

18. Balch JF, Balch PA: *Prescription for nutritional healing*, ed 2, Garden City Park, NY, 1997, Avery.

19. Bedinghaus JM: Care of the breast and support of breastfeeding, *Women's Health* 24: 147-160, 1997.

20. Benenson AS, editor: *Control of communicable diseases manual*, ed 16, Washington, DC, 1995, American Public Health Association.

21. Bergeron C et al: Human papillomavirus testing in women with mild cytologic atypia, *Obstet Gynecol* 95:821-827, 2000.

22. Bornstein J et al: Persistent vulvar vestibulitis: the continuing challenge, *Obstet Gynecol Rev* 54:S212-S217, 1999.

23. Bornstein J et al: Vulvar vestibulitis: physical or psychosexual problem? *Obstet Gynecol* 93:876-880, 1999.

24. Bornstein J et al: Polymerase chain reaction for viral etiology of vulvar vestibulitis syndrome, *Am J Obstet Gynecol* 175:139-144, 1996.

25. Boronow RC: Death of the Papanicolaou smear? *Am J Obstet Gynecol* 179:391-396, 1998.

26. Bump RC et al: The standardization of terminology of female pelvic organ prolapse and pelvic floor dysfunction, *Am J Obstet Gynecol* 175:10-17, 1996.

27. Burman ML et al: Effect of false-positive mammograms on interval breast cancer screening in a health maintenance organization, *Ann Intern Med* 131:1-6, 1999.

28. Burst HV: Sexually transmitted diseases and reproductive health in women, *J Nurse Midwifery* 43:431-444, 1998.

29. Carter JE: Surgical treatment for chronic pelvic pain, *J Soc Laparendoscopic Surg* 2: 129-139, 1998.

30. Centers for Disease Control and Prevention (CDC): Sexually Transmitted Diseases Treatment Guidelines—2002, *MMWR* 51(RR06):1-80, 2002. Available at: http://www.phppo.cdc.gov/cdcrecommends/showarticle.asp?a_artid+1653++++&TopNum=50& CallPG=Adv.

31. CDC: Guidelines for treatment of sexually transmitted diseases, *MMWR* 47:1-116, 1998.
32. Conant MA: Immunomodulatory therapy in the management of viral infections in patients with HIV infection, *J Am Acad Dermatol* 43:S27-S30, 2000.
33. Coronado GD, Marshall LM, Schwartz SM: Complications in pregnancy, labor, and delivery with uterine leiomyomas: a population-based study, *Obstet Gynecol* 95:764-769, 2000.
34. Corwin EJ: Endometriosis: pathophysiology, diagnosis, and treatment, *Nurse Practitioner* 22:35-55, 1997.
35. Cottreau CM, Ness RB, Kriska AM: Physical activity and reduced risk of ovarian cancer, *Obstet Gynecol* 96:609-614, 2000.
36. Crane-Okada R: Early stage breast cancer: hope for the future, *Nurseweek* 4:16-17, 1999.
37. Crawford AM: *Herbal remedies for women*, Rocklin, Calif, 1997, Prima.
38. Creasy RK, Resnick R: *Maternal fetal medicine*, ed 3, Philadelphia, 1994, WB Saunders.
39. Cullins Ve et al: Treating vaginitis, *Nurse Practitioner* 24:46-63, 1999.
40. Cummings S, Ullman D: *Everybody's guide to homeopathic medicines*, New York, 1997, Putnam.
41. Cunningham FG et al: *Williams obstetrics*, ed 20, Stamford, Conn, 1997, Appleton & Lange.
42. Daly SF et al: Can the number of cigarettes smoked predict high-grade cervical intraepithelial neoplasia among women with mildly abnormal cervical smears? *Am J Obstet Gynecol* 179:399-402, 1998.
43. Dealy MF: Dysfunctional uterine bleeding in adolescents, *Nurse Practitioner* 23:12-23, 1998.
44. Desforges WL: Evaluation of a palpable breast mass, *N Engl J Med* 327:937-942, 1992.
45. Dickey RP: *Managing contraceptive pill patients*, ed 10, Dallas, 2000, EMIS Medical Publishers.
46. Dillon SM et al: Prospective analysis of genital ulcer disease in Brooklyn, New York, *Clin Infect Dis* 24:945-950, 1997.
47. Drake J: Diagnosis and management of the adnexal mass, *Am Fam Physician* 57:2471-2477, 1998.
48. Early Breast Cancer Trialists' Collaborative Group: Favourable and unfavourable effects on long-term survival of radiotherapy for early breast cancer: an overview of the randomised trials, *Lancet* 355:1739-1740, 2000.
49. Eckert LO et al: Vulvovaginal candidiasis: clinical manifestations, risk factors, management algorithm, *Obstet Gynecol* 92:757-765, 1998.
50. Emmons L et al: Primary care management of common dermatologic disorders in women, *J Nurse Midwifery* 42:228-253, 1997.
51. Engstrom JL et al: Midwifery care of the woman with menorrhagia, *J Nurse Midwifery* 44:89-105, 1999.
52. Faro S et al: Treatment considerations in vulvovaginal candidiasis, *Female Patient* 22:21-38, 1997.
53. Fitzpatrick MB et al: A randomized clinical trial comparing primary overlap with reapproximation repair of third-degree obstetric tears, *Am J Obstet Gynecol* 183:1220-1224, 2000.
54. Franklin TL, Monif GRG: *Trichomonas vaginalis* and bacterial vaginosis: coexistence in vaginal wet mount preparation from pregnant women, *J Reprod Med* 45:131-134, 2000.
55. Freeman SB: Menopause without HRT: complementary therapies, *Contemp Nurse Practitioner* 1:40-49, 1995.
56. Fremgen AM et al: Clinical highlights from the National Cancer Data Base, 1999, *CA Cancer J Clin* 49:145-158, 1999.
57. Fynes M et al: Effect of second vaginal delivery on anorectal physiology and faecal incontinence: a prospective study, *Lancet* 354:983-986, 1999.
58. Gabbe SG, Niebyl JR, Simpson JL: *Obstetrics: normal & problem pregnancies*, ed 3, New York, 1996, Churchill Livingstone.
59. Geiger AM, Foxman B: Risk factors for vulvovaginal candidiasis: a case-control study among university students, *Epidemiology* 7:182-187, 1996.

60. Gordon JD et al: *Obstetrics gynecology & infertility,* Glen Cove, NY, 1998, Scrub Hill Press.
61. Grabrick DM et al: Risk of breast cancer with oral contraceptive use in women with a family history of breast cancer, *JAMA* 284:1791-1798, 2000.
62. Griffith HW: *Healing herbs: the essential guide,* Tucson, Ariz, 2000, Fisher Books.
63. Grimes DA, editor: Patient Update: Facts about breast cancer and hormones, *Contracept Rep* 11, 2000.
64. Grimes DA, editor: Hormonal contraception and sexually transmitted disease, *Contracept Rep* 10:11-14, 1999.
65. Grimes DA, editor: Using oral contraceptives to treat medical conditions, *Contracept Rep* 10:4-10, 1999.
66. Guzick D: Polycystic ovary syndrome: symptomatology, pathophysiology, and epidemiology, *Am J Obstet Gynecol* 179:S89-S93, 1998.
67. Hacker NF, Moore JG: *Essentials of obstetrics and gynecology,* ed 3, Philadelphia, 1998, WB Saunders.
68. Harmanli OH et al: Urinary tract infections in women with bacterial vaginosis, *Obstet Gynecol* 95:710-712, 2000.
69. Heffner LJ et al: Clinical and environmental predictors of preterm labor, *Obstet Gynecol* 81:750-757, 1993.
70. Hill LM et al: The role of ultrasonography in the detection and management of adnexal masses during the second and third trimesters of pregnancy, *Am J Obstet Gynecol* 179:703-707, 1998.
71. Hoffmann D: *The complete illustrated holistic herbal,* Boston, 1996, Element Books.
71a. Hoffmann D: *The holistic herbal,* Findhorn, Scotland, 1985, Findhorn Press.
72. Hunter DJ et al: Cohort studies of fat intake and the risk of breast cancer: a pooled analysis, *N Engl J Med* 334:356-361, 1996.
73. Hutchins FL: Uterine fibroids: diagnosis and indications for treatment, *Obstet Gynecol Clin North Am* 22(4):659-665, 1995.
74. Idarius B: *The homeopathic childbirth manual,* ed 2, Talmage, Calif, 1999, Idarius Press.
75. Ikenze I: *Menopause and homeopathy,* Berkeley, Calif, 1998, North Atlantic Books.
76. Internet Health Resources: *Endometrial ablation,* 1995. Available at: http://www.ihr.com/bafertil/articles/formendo.html.
77. Ivey JB: The adolescent with pelvic inflammatory disease: assessment and management, *Nurse Practitioner* 22:78-91, 1997.
78. Jackson SL, Soper DE: Sexually transmitted diseases in pregnancy, *Obstet Gynecol Clin North Am* 24(3):631-644, 1997.
79. Jacobs AJ, Gast MJ: *Practical gynecology,* Norwalk, Conn, 1994, Appleton & Lange.
80. Jancin B: Try intravaginal boric acid for candida glabrata, *OBGYN News* 36:18, 2001.
81. Jones KD, Hewell SW: Dyspareunia: three case reports, *J Obstet Gynecol Neonatal Nurs* 26:19-23, 1997.
82. Kennedy HP, Griffin M, Frishman G: Enabling conception and pregnancy: midwifery care of women experiencing infertility, *J Nurse Midwifery* 43:190-207, 1998.
83. Kiningham RB, Apgar BS, Schwenk TL: Evaluation of amenorrhea, *Am Fam Physician* 53:1185-1194, 1996.
84. Kloss J: *Back to Eden,* New York, 1981, Benedict Lust.
85. Koehler N: *Artemis speaks: V.B.A.C. stories & natural childbirth information,* Occidental, Calif, 1985, Jerald R. Brown.
86. Kolasa KM, Weismiller DG: Nutrition during pregnancy, *Am Fam Physician* 56:205-212, 1995.
87. Koutsky LA et al: A controlled trial of a human papillomavirus type 16 vaccine, *N Engl J Med* 347(21):1645-1651, 2002.
88. Lee KR et al: Comparison of conventional Papanicolaou smears and a fluid-based, thin-layer system for cervical cancer screening, *Obstet Gynecol* 90:278-284, 1997.
89. Legor RS: Polycystic ovary syndrome: current and future treatment paradigms, *Am J Obstet Gynecol* 179:S101-S108, 1998.
90. Leppert PC, Howard FM: *Primary care for women,* Philadelphia, 1997, Lippincott-Raven.

91. Mabey R et al, editors: *The new age herbalist*, New York, 1988, Collier Books.
92. Mann WJ: Diagnosis and management of epithelial cancer of the ovary, *Am Fam Physician* 49:613-618, 1994.
93. Marantides D: Management of polycystic ovary syndrome, *Nurse Practitioner* 22:34-41, 1997.
94. Mayer IE, Hussain H: Pregnancy and gastrointestinal disorders, *Gastroenterol Clin* 27:1-36, 1998.
95. McCance KL, Jorde LB: Evaluating the genetic risk of breast cancer, *Nurse Practitioner* 23:14-29, 1998.
96. McCool WF, Stone-Condry M, Bradford HM: Breast health care: a review, *J Nurse Midwifery* 43:406-430, 1998.
97. Medina IM: *Issues in women's health care: nutrition and herbs from menarche to menopause*, course syllabus 3/28-29/98, State University of New York Health Science Center at Brooklyn College of Health Related Professions Midwifery Education Program.
98. Meisler J: Toward optimal health: the experts respond to fibroids, *Womens Health & Gender-based Med* 8:879-883, 1999.
99. Metts JF: Vulvodynia and vulvar vestibulitis: challenges in diagnosis and management, *Am Fam Physician* 59:1547-1556, 1999.
100. Meyer S et al: *The effects of birth on urinary continence mechanisms and other pelvic-floor characteristics*, *Obstet Gynecol* 92:613-618, 1998.
101. Mitchell MF et al: A randomized clinical trial of cryotherapy, laser vaporization, and loop electrosurgical intraepithelial lesions of the cervix, *Obstet Gynecol* 92:737-744, 1998.
102. Molander P et al: Laparoscopic management of suspected acute pelvic inflammatory disease, *J Am Assoc Gynecol Laparosc* 7:107-110, 2000.
103. Morris VM, Rorie JL: Nutritional concerns in women's primary care, *J Nurse Midwifery* 42:509-520, 1997.
104. National Cancer Institute (NCI): Human papillomaviruses and cancer, 1998. Available at: *http://cis.nci.nih.gov/fact/3_20.htm*.
105. Nettina SM: *The Lippincott manual of nursing practice*, Philadelphia, 1996, Lippincott.
106. Newcomb PA et al: Lactation and a reduced risk of premenopausal breast cancer, *N Engl J Med* 330:81-87, 1994.
107. Nissim R: *Natural healing in gynaecology: a manual for women*, San Francisco, 1996, HarperCollins.
108. Nyirjesy I, Billingsley FS, Forman MR: Evaluation of atypical and low-grade cervical cytology in private practice, *Obstet Gynecol* 92:601-607, 1998.
109. O'Boyle AL, Davis GD, Calhoun BC: Informed consent and birth: protecting the pelvic floor and ourselves, *Am J Obstet Gynecol* 187:981-983, 2002.
110. Ody P: *The complete medicinal herbal*, New York, 1993, Dorling Kindersley.
111. Olivotto IA et al: Adjuvant systemic therapy and survival after breast cancer, *N Engl J Med* 330:805-810, 1994.
112. Paavonen J: Pelvic inflammatory disease: from diagnosis to prevention, *Dermatol Clin* 16:747-756, 1998.
113. Page L: *Healthy healing*, ed 11, Carmel Valley, Calif, 2000, Healthy Healing Publications.
114. Paige DM et al: Bacterial vaginosis and preterm birth: a comprehensive review of the literature, *J Nurse Midwifery* 43:83-89, 1998.
115. Parvati J: *Hygieia: a woman's herbal*, Berkeley, Calif, 1985, Bookpeople.
116. Payton RG, Gardner R, Reynolds D: Pharmacologic considerations and management of common endocrine disorders in women, *J Nurse Midwifery* 42:186-206, 1997.
117. *Physician's desk reference (PDR) for herbal medicines*, Montvale, NJ, 1998, Thomas Medical Economics.
118. Polone K: Nature in your birth bag, *Midwifery Today* 26:34, 1993.
119. Powell J, Wojnarowska F: Acupuncture for vulvodynia, *J Soc Med* 92:579-581, 1999.
120. Ralph SG, Rutherford AJ, Wilson JD: Influence of bacterial vaginosis on conception and miscarriage in the first trimester: cohort study, *BMJ* 319:220-223, 1999.
121. Rose B, Scott-Moncrieff C: *Homeopathy for women*, London, 1998, Collins & Brown.

122. Sampselle CM: Behavioral intervention for urinary incontinence in women: evidence for practice, *J Midwifery Womens Health* 43:94-103, 2000.

123. Sampselle CM et al: Continence for women: a test of AWHONN's evidence-based protocol in clinical practice, *J Obstet Gynecol Neonatal Nurs* 29:18-26, 2000.

124. Sampselle CM et al: Continence for women: evaluation of AWHONN's third research utilization project, *J Obstet Gynecol Neonatal Nurs* 29:9-17, 2000.

125. Sampselle CM et al: Continence for women: evidence-based practice, *J Obstet Gynecol Neonatal Nurs* 26:375-385, 1997.

126. Sawaya GF, Grimes DA: New technologies in cervical cytology screening: a word of caution, *Obstet Gynecol* 94:307-310, 1999.

127. Schellenberg R: Treatment for the premenstrual syndrome with agnus castus fruit extract: prospective, randomised, placebo-controlled study, *BMJ* 322:134-137, 2001.

128. Schultz W et al: Behavioral approach with or without surgical intervention to the vulvar vestibulitis syndrome: a prospective randomized and non-randomized study, *J Psychom Obstet Gynecol* 17:143-148, 1996.

129. Scott JR et al: *Danforth's handbook of obstetrics and gynecology*, Philadelphia, 1996, Lippincott-Raven.

130. Singingtree D: Herbal helps, *Midwifery Today* 26:16, 1993.

131. Slap GB et al: Recognition of tubo-ovarian abscess in adolescents with pelvic inflammatory disease, *J Adolesc Health* 18:397-403, 1996.

132. Smith T: *Homeopathy for pregnancy and nursing mothers*, Worthing, England, 1993, Insight Editions.

133. Soper DE, Chez RA: Treating vaginitis: beyond the basics, *OBG Manage* 12:36-40, 45, 2000.

134. Speroff L, Glass RH, Kase NG: *Clinical gynecologic endocrinology and infertility*, Philadelphia, 1999, Lippincott Williams & Wilkins.

135. Spinillo A et al: The impact of oral contraception on vulvovaginal candidiasis, *Contraception* 51:293-297, 1995.

136. Spinillo A et al: Epidemiologic characteristics of women with idiopathic recurrent vulvovaginal candidiasis, *Obstet Gynecol* 81:721-727, 1993.

137. Spitzer M: Cervical screening adjuncts: recent advances, *Am J Obstet Gynecol* 179:544-556, 1998.

138. Stapleton H, Tiran D: Herbal medicine. In Tiran D, Mack S, editors: *Complementary therapies for pregnancy and childbirth*, ed 2, Edinburgh, 2000, Baillière Tindall.

139. Star, WL, Lommel LL, Shannon MT: *Women's primary health care: protocols for practice*, Washington, DC, 1995: American Nurses' Association.

140. Stewart EA, Nowak RAL: Clinical commentary: new concepts in the treatment of uterine leiomyomas, *Obstet Gynecol* 92:624-627, 1998.

141. Stowe A: Continuing education forum: diagnostic workup of breast cancer in females, *J Am Acad Nurse Practitioners* 11:71-79, 1999.

142. Strandell A, Thorburn J, Hamberger L: Risk factors for ectopic pregnancy in assisted reproduction, *Fertil Steril* 71:282-286, 1999.

143. Sultan AH et al: Anal-sphincter disruption during vaginal deliver, *N Engl J Med* 329:1905-1911, 1993.

143a. Summers L: CDC DES update provides resources for health care providers, consumers, *Quickening* 33:18-19, 2003.

144. Tenti P et al: Perinatal transmission of human papillomavirus from gravidas with latent infections, *Obstet Gynecol* 93:475-479, 1999.

145. Terraza HM, Moore RD: Gynecologic causes of the acute abdomen and the acute abdomen in pregnancy, *Surg Clin North Am* 77:1371-1394, 1997.

146. Thune I et al: Physical activity and the risk of breast cancer, *N Engl J Med* 336:1269-1275, 1997.

147. Tuso P: The herbal medicine pharmacy: what Kaiser Permanente providers need to know, *The Permanente J* 3:33-37, 1999.

148. Ugarriza DN, Klingner S, O'Brien S: Premenstrual syndrome: diagnosis and intervention, *Nurse Practitioner* 23:40-58, 1998.

149. Ullman R, Reichenberg-Ullman J: *Homeopathic self-care*, Rocklin, Calif, 1997, Prima.
150. Van Lankveld JJDM, Weijenborg PTM, Kuile MMT: Psychologic profiles of and sexual function in women with vulvar vestibulitis and their partners, *Obstet Gynecol* 88:65-70, 1996.
151. Varney H: *Varney's midwifery*, ed 3, Sudbury, Mass, 1997, Jones and Bartlett.
152. Wathen PI, Henderson MC, Witz CA: Abnormal uterine bleeding, *Med Clin North Am* 79(2):329-344, 1995.
153. Weed S: *Menopausal years: the wise woman way*, Woodstock, NY, 1992, Ash Tree Publishing.
154. Willis CE, Livingstone V: Infant insufficient milk syndrome associated with maternal postpartum hemorrhage, *J Hum Lac* 11:123-126, 1995.
155. Wright TC et al: HPV DNA testing of self-collected vaginal samples compared with cytologic screening to detect cervical cancer, *JAMA* 283:81-86, 2000.
156. Yelland S: *Acupuncture in midwifery*, Cheshire, England, 1996, Books for Midwives Press.

Chapter 9

Contraception

• CONTRACEPTION VISIT FORMAT

Initiation

1. Conduct a gynecologic (GYN) visit (see p. 403).
2. Assess sexual history (number of partners, frequency, expected cooperation of partners in chosen method), contraceptive history, absolute and relative contraindications, ability to use method, likelihood of compliance, conception plans and fertility history, and need for barrier contraception for sexually transmitted infection (STI) protection.
3. Discuss risks and benefits of contraceptive methods, method of action, side effects, absolute and relative contraindications, required follow-up, and cost.
4. Prescribe the client's choice of method and teach the method, danger S/S, side effects, and STIs.
5. Arrange for follow-up and document.

Revisit

1. Update the menstrual, gynecologic, and medical histories: last menstrual period (LMP), nature of menses, general health changes, medications, tobacco use history, and STI risk.
2. Obtain the current contraceptive history, including satisfaction with method and side effects. Review and exclude danger signs and verify correct usage of method. With an intrauterine device (IUD), inquire regarding signs of infection; with a diaphragm, check for fit, comfort, urinary tract infection (UTI), signs and symptoms. Answer the woman's questions, if any.
3. Perform a physical examination (PE) annually. Perform Pap, BP, weight, hematocrit and hemoglobin (H&H) as indicated. For the woman taking oral contraceptives (OCs), check liver.
4. Prescribe client's choice of method; teach use of the method, danger S/S, and side effects. Discuss the protection from STIs offered by the method and the precautions that are still required to ensure protection.
5. Arrange follow-up visit and document.

• CONTRACEPTIVE METHODS

Natural Methods

Coitus Interruptus

Method of Action: Withdrawal of the erect penis out of the vagina before ejaculation to prevent deposit of sperm into vagina. Requires foreknowledge of orgasm and self-control by the male partner.

Advantages: Absence of drugs and devices, convenience, and no cost.

Disadvantages: Lack of STI protection and a high pregnancy rate (sperm may be present in the pre-ejaculate fluid).

Effectiveness Rate: It has been hypothesized that with perfect execution the pregnancy rate might be 4%; with typical use, 19%.[7]

Natural Family Planning (Abstinence and Fertility Awareness)

Method of Action: Abstinence from sexual intercourse during times that the woman is likely to be fertile. Methods include the calendar, symptothermal, ovulation, and postovulation methods.[7] The methods are based on the following assumptions: The woman's fertile period lasts approximately 5-13 days of the menstrual cycle. Physiologic events such as cervical mucus, cervical changes, and body temperature indicate fertility. The ovum is viable for about 24 hours. If a second ovum is released, it is released within 24 hours of the first ovum. Sperm are viable for approximately 72 hours.[56]

Advantages: Increased self-reliance; partner involvement; absence of side effects[7]; "marriage-enhancing" according to proponents; natural, safe, consistent with the Catholic faith, inexpensive; and increased familiarity with the body.[56]

Disadvantages: Lack of STI protection, need for partner cooperation, and periods of abstinence when initiating the method and during each fertile period. The woman who wants to have intercourse during the ovulatory period can use a barrier method at those times,[7] but this is discouraged because contraceptive jelly obscures cervical mucus signs.[56] Abstinence is required during the periods of the month when the woman's testosterone is the highest and her libido is peaking. The methods are ineffective during lactation, when secretions and the cycle are altered.

Effectiveness Rate: When used perfectly, the calendar method has the lowest effectiveness rate of 91%; the postovulation method has a 99% effectiveness rate. The ovulation method's first-year effectiveness rate is 97%. The symptothermal method's effectiveness rate is 98%. Typical use failure rates for all methods combined is 20%.[7]

Initiating the Method: Most natural family planning teachers suggest abstaining from intercourse for a full cycle or until postovulation infertility to learn to observe the cyclic changes. Abstinence is usually suggested during menses because menses could hide changes in the cervical mucus, or be confused with ovulatory spotting. Each method has its own guidelines for determining the fertile time.[56]

METHODS
OVULATION MODEL. The ovulation method is also known as the basal body temperature method (BBT). Ovulation may be preceded by a small decrease in the BBT, followed by a sustained rise in BBT (about 0.4° F).[8] By using the beginning of the fertile time according to the cervical mucus, the fertile time ends 2 to 4 days after the peak day and when the BBT has been elevated for 3 days, or whichever is later. Factors that affect the temperature include electric blanket use, environmental temperature, illness, medications, intercourse, alcohol, immunizations, time of day, oral intake, inadequate sleep, and early morning activities. Other symptoms, such as cervical mucus, are used to confirm the BBT findings.[56]

SYMPTOTHERMAL METHOD. This method combines the BBT, the mucus, and the symptom methods.[8] The follicular phase is considered to be "relatively infertile," and the luteal phase "infertile." The following factors are noted to determine fertility: days of the cycle and month, coitus, cervical mucus, BBT, peak day, cervical condition, any miscellaneous symptoms or routine changes, "fullness," or mittelschmerz.[56] Used properly, this method is 98% effective.[8]

Cervical Mucus Changes: In the perimenopausal woman or the lactating woman (when ovulation may not be occurring regularly) cervical mucus is the first sign of impending ovulation.[56] After approximately 5 days of menses, 3 to 4 "dry days" follow. The next 3 days viscous, sticky, tacky, cloudy/white/yellow mucus—called non-peak mucus—is present, and this begins the fertile time. Estrogen rises and the fertile ovulatory mucus becomes copious, clear, slippery like raw egg-white, and can be stretched between the fingers (a feature called spinnbarkeit). This mucus ferns microscopically as it dries and is favorable to sperm penetration.[8] The last day of fertile mucus occurs near ovulation and is called the peak day, when the possibility of conception is greatest (66.7%). As the quality of the mucus declines thereafter, so does the possibility of conception. Three days later the possibility has decreased to 8.9%. Note that ovulatory mucus may be blood-tinged and confused with menses. The fertile mucus of the woman with short cycles may be hidden in menstrual blood. Cervical mucus is not a reliable indicator of ovulation for several cycles after discontinuing OCs.[56]

Cervical Changes: Around the time of ovulation, the cervix softens and rises slightly as the os dilates to allow sperm to enter more easily. After ovulation, the cervix lowers and becomes more firm as the os closes. The cervix should be checked with clean fingers 2 to 3 times a day.[56]

Biochemical and Mechanical Aids:
1. Dipstick kits detect the luteinizing hormone (LH) surge.
2. Volumetric vaginal aspirators test the volume of vaginal fluids.

3. Personal computer-assisted fertility indicators predict the fertile period.

4. Ovarian monitor (which measures urinary estrogens and urinary pregnanediol) predicts ovulation in 99%, shortening the period of abstinence.[8]

Barrier Contraceptive Methods

Cervical Cap

Method of Action: The cap is a barrier that is individually fitted and then covers the cervix to prevent entry of sperm and pregnancy.

Advantages: Control of the method by woman, STI protection, no systemic side effects, and effective episodic birth control for the woman who has sex irregularly.

Disadvantages: Lack of participation by partner, need for fitting by a health care provider, increased incidence of UTI or toxic shock syndrome (see p. 448), modesty issues (requires touching genitals),[7] odor depending on length of time left in place (especially after intercourse), and lowered effectiveness for multiparous women.

Effectiveness Rate: Eighty percent to 91% with perfect use and 64% to 82% with typical use.[7] The cap is more effective for nulliparous women in the first year of use. Twenty-six percent of parous women using the cap perfectly will conceive within the first year.[57]

Prescription and Fitting: After a routine initial GYN visit, specially trained providers fit the cap. Six percent to 40% of women are "unfittable" because of the shape or size of their cervix.[57]

Contraindications:

1. Inability to be fitted (e.g., cervical lacerations and diethylstilbestrol [DES] malformations of the cervix).
2. Inability to understand instructions or to place cap.
3. History of toxic shock syndrome.
4. Abnormal Pap smear or suspected cervical or uterine cancer.
5. Vaginitis or cervicitis.
6. Use during menses, postpartum, or after cervical procedures until healing and refitting occur.
7. Allergy to rubber or spermicide.

Client Instructions:

1. Fill the cap one third full with spermicide. Keep the rim dry to facilitate suction.
2. Insert the cap at least 30 minutes and up to several hours before intercourse. Empty the bladder, compress the cap for insertion into the vagina, then release or place onto the cervix.
3. Leave the cap in place 8 to 48 hours after intercourse. After 24 hours, an odor may develop. Remove the cap by pushing or pulling the rim to break the suction. Bear down to facilitate reaching the cap.
4. For multiple acts of intercourse, check placement of the cap. No jelly addition is required.

5. The cap is refitted after pregnancy, abortion, or any cervical procedure.
6. Have a Pap smear after 3 months of use and again at 12 months. Annual Pap smears are indicated thereafter.
7. Care of the cap: Wash the cap in mild soap and water, fill with water and look for leaks, dust with cornstarch, and store away from sunlight or heat. If it develops an odor, soak the cap in 1 qt water with 1 tsp apple cider vinegar; this may change the color of the cap.
8. Do not use the cap with petroleum products.
9. Be aware of the S/S of UTI and toxic shock syndrome (see p. 448) and report promptly.[57]

Condom (Male)

Method of Action: A condom is a polyurethane, latex, or membranous sheath that covers the erect penis, providing a barrier and acting as a receptacle for semen.

Advantages: Male participation, simplicity of use, over-the-counter (OTC) accessibility, portability.[7] The latex condom offers protection from those STIs transmitted by fluids from mucosal surfaces.[9]

Disadvantages: Interruption of foreplay for application, contraindicated with latex allergy, and decreased sensation.[7] Nonoxynol-9–coated condoms have been associated with UTIs in women.[9] Condoms are less effective in preventing transmission of those STIs transmitted skin to skin, such as herpes, HPV, syphilis, and chancroid.[9]

Effectiveness Rate: The condom is 88% to 97% effective when used alone and 99.9% effective when used with spermicide.[7] The first-year failure rate is 14% among typical users.[31] Two in 100 condoms break.[9] Non-latex condoms have higher slippage and breakage rates.[9]

Client Instructions:

1. Place the condom before each act of entry, handling carefully to avoid puncture. Apply the condom after the penis is erect and before any genital contact with partner. When placing the condom, a small "nipple" of space, but no air, is left at the tip.
2. Ensure adequate lubrication during intercourse. Only water-based lubricants can be safely used with latex products, such as K-Y jelly, Astroglide, Aqualube, coconut oil, and glycerin. Oil-based lubricants such as petroleum jelly, shortening, mineral oil, massage oils, body lotions, and cooking oil can weaken the condom.[9] Polyurethane is less susceptible to this deterioration than latex; latex is superior to the membranous sheath.[7]
3. After securing the base of the condom, the man withdraws from the vagina while the penis is erect to avoid leakage. Before discarding, examine the condom for holes. If there was breakage, the woman should immediately use spermicidal foam.
4. The condom is a single use form of contraception and STI protection.
5. Store condoms in a clean, dry place for up to 1 year. Condoms lubricated with nonoxynol-9 expire sooner.[9]

Condom (Female)

Method of Action: A female condom is a single-use, one-size pre-lubricated polyurethane sheath, one end of which is placed into the vagina like a diaphragm while the other end, which is attached to a larger ring, opens outside the introitus, where it lays against the labia and provides barrier protection from sperm and STIs.

Advantages: Control of method by woman, OTC accessibility, potential for use during menses, no need for concomitant spermicide, and STI protection, including HIV.[9]

Disadvantages: Unfavorable appearance and necessary skill to apply the condom. Penile or vaginal irritation occasionally occurs.[7]

Effectiveness Rate: Similar to male condom and diaphragm.[7] Average pregnancy rate in the first year of use is 21% and 5% with perfect use.[13]

Contraceptive Sponge

Method of Action: The sponge is a donut-shaped device permeated with the spermicide nonoxynol-9. It is placed over the cervix like the diaphragm and acts as a barrier contraceptive.[28]

Advantages: Rare side effects, easy availability, and relative ease of use.[28] The sponge protects against cervical gonorrhea and chlamydia, but whether it prevents HIV transmission is unknown.[9]

Disadvantages: The sponge rarely causes toxic shock syndrome.[41]

Effectiveness Rate: Typical user failure rate is 20% in nulliparous women and higher in multiparous women.[28]

Client Instructions:
1. Insert up to 24 hours before intercourse.[28]
2. Do not use during menses or when passing lochia after delivery.
3. Remove the sponge after 24 hours.[41]

Teach the woman to report symptoms of toxic shock syndrome (see p. 448).

Diaphragm

Method of Action: The diaphragm is a barrier method of latex or rubber stretched over a flexible ring. It is placed over the cervix and mechanically prevents sperm from entering the cervical os.

Advantages: Control of method by woman, STI protection, no systemic side effects, and effective episodic birth control for the woman who has sex irregularly. The diaphragm may protect against cervical gonorrhea, chlamydia, and trichomoniasis.[9]

Disadvantages: Lack of participation by partner, need for fitting by a health care provider, modesty issues (requires touching genitals), and increased risk for UTI[9] and toxic shock syndrome.[7] The diaphragm must be placed before every act of intercourse and the contraceptive cream is messy. Use requires motor skills and awareness of time intervals and may be difficult for some women. The diaphragm should not be assumed to be protective against HIV.[9]

Effectiveness Rate: Used with spermicide, the diaphragm is 94% effective with perfect use and 82% effective with typical use.[7] Grimes[27] cites 14% typical user failure rate during the first 12 months of use.

Types of Diaphragms:

1. The flat spring rim is appropriate for the woman with good muscle tone and a shallow pubic arch. Prescribe the Ortho-White diaphragm sizes 55 to 95.
2. The coil spring rim is appropriate for the woman with average muscle tone and pubic arch. This diaphragm folds flat and can be placed with an inserter, which may be easier for some women. Prescribe the Koromex diaphragm sizes 50 to 105 or the Ortho diaphragm sizes 50 to 105.
3. The arcing-spring rim diaphragm may be easier to insert and is appropriate for the woman who has more lax muscle tone, cystocele, or rectocele. Prescribe the Koroflex diaphragm sizes 60 to 95, Allflex diaphragm (an Ortho product) sizes 55 to 95, or Ramses Bendex diaphragm sizes 65 to 95.

Client Instructions:

1. Use for every act of intercourse.
2. Place 1 tsp contraceptive jelly in the well, spreading a small amount of cream around the rim.
3. Insert the diaphragm; the cervix should be felt behind the diaphragm to confirm correct placement. (Demonstrate insertion and removal and have the woman give a return demonstration.)
4. The diaphragm may be placed up to 6 hours before the act of intercourse and should remain in place for 8 to 24 hours after intercourse. The diaphragm can be worn during activities of daily living.
5. For a second act of intercourse, add 1 full applicator of contraceptive jelly into the vagina without moving the diaphragm. Leave the diaphragm in place for 8 hours after the second act of intercourse.
6. Do not douche with the diaphragm in place.
7. Bring the diaphragm to the annual Pap exam so that the fit can be reassessed.
8. Have the diaphragm refit yearly, after pelvic surgery, after pregnancy, after weaning, when the frequency of intercourse has increased, with any 10 lb weight change, or with recurrent UTIs.
9. Wash the diaphragm with a mild soap and water and observe for tears or leaks. After drying thoroughly, dust the diaphragm with cornstarch and store in a cool dry place. Do not use petroleum products or perfumes with the diaphragm.
10. Use a backup contraceptive method until a follow-up visit in 2 weeks, when placement of the diaphragm and satisfaction with the method are assessed.
11. The woman should be aware of the S/S of UTI and toxic shock syndrome (see p. 448) and should know to contact her care provider promptly if she develops them.[7]

Spermicide

Method of Action: A foam, gel, cream, or suppository that contains surfactants that destroy sperm membrane integrity. The active agent is usually nonoxynol-9 or octoxynol.[7]

Advantages: Control of the method by the woman, OTC accessibility, and increased vaginal lubrication.[7]

Disadvantages: Skin irritation, an unpleasant taste, incomplete melting of suppositories, and interruption of foreplay for application.[7] Nonoxynol-9 has been shown to increase heterosexual transmission of HIV by increasing the incidence of genital lesions. Other products (including C31G and polystyrene sulfate) with bactericidal and virucidal properties are being developed.[6,9] Nonoxynol-9 is also ineffective against gonorrhea and chlamydia.[9]

Effectiveness Rate: Spermicide is 80% to 94% effective with perfect use and 99.9% effective when used in conjunction with a condom.[7]

Client Instructions for Use of Spermicidal Foam:

1. Shake 20 times before using.
2. Apply the cream far back into the vagina after lying down for the final time before intercourse.
3. Reapply if standing before intercourse.
4. Lie flat for 30 minutes after the act of intercourse so the foam does not slip away from the os.
5. Do not douche after intercourse.
6. Wash the applicator with soap and water.
7. Always have a spare container of foam on hand.
8. Reinsert another dose of foam for a second act of intercourse.
9. Dosage: Emko and Dalkon: 1 full applicator (10 to 17 mL); Delfen and Koromex: 2 full applicators (5 mL)

Client Instructions for Use of Spermicidal Suppositories: Use in the same way as contraceptive foam, with the following additions:

1. Allow 10 to 30 minutes to dissolve. If vaginal lubrication is decreased, effectiveness of the method is decreased. If the suppository is undissolved, the partner may perceive "grittiness" and it may cause burning of the penis or the vagina.
2. Use one suppository per act of intercourse.
3. May cause a discharge after intercourse.
4. Keep in the refrigerator during hot weather.

Hormonal Contraceptive Methods

Combination Contraceptive Injection (Medroxyprogesterone [MPA]/estradiol cypionate [E_{2C}]) (Lunelle)

Method of Action: This first once-a-month IM combination contraceptive option for women was approved by the FDA in October 2000. It inhibits ovulation, decreases and thickens cervical mucus, and thins the endometrium. The estrogen promotes a monthly cycle.[38]

Advantages: No daily pill-taking, privacy, regular menses with decreased flow, and improved dysmenorrhea. The manufacturer expects a protective effect against pelvic infections, ectopic pregnancy, functional ovarian cysts, and endometrial and ovarian cancers, as seen with the combination oral OC.[44] Return of ovulation occurs within approximately 60 to 90 days, depending on body weight and injection site.[38]

Disadvantages: Requires a prescription and a monthly visit to the provider. As with other hormonal contraceptives, there is no protection from STIs.[44]

Effectiveness Rate: More than 99.0% effective when administered as directed in testing by the manufacturer.[44]

Method: Single monthly IM injection.[44]

Dosage: 0.5 mL IM (in arm, thigh, or buttock) equaling 5 mg E_{2C} and 25 mg MPA (regardless of body weight) administered every 28 to 30 days, not to exceed 33 days; within 10 days of a first trimester abortion or between 4 and 6 weeks postpartum. If necessary, reinjection can be given as early as 23 days.[44]

Adverse Effects: Most common (57% in first 3 months) are menstrual irregularities (irregular, frequent, and/or prolonged bleeding), improving at 3 months and more after the first year (30% of users will still have irregularities). Headache, breast tenderness, acne, and mood changes subside after the first 3 months, as with oral OCs. Weight gain (average 4 lb in the first year) is the most common reason for discontinuance.[38]

Safety: The lipid profile is statistically more favorable than that seen with OCs, showing a greater reduction in triglycerides and total cholesterol, apparently because of lower androgenic activity. There are fewer effects on clotting factors than OCs (no thromboembolic events among 17,000 women). It may be an acceptable method for diabetic women because there is no effect on carbohydrate metabolism.[44]

Cost: About $30 per month, equal to that of OCs.[38]

Contraindications and Relative Contraindications: The same as those of the combination OC.[44] (See p. 515.)

Client Instructions:
1. Timely administration of the drug is required; expect menses within 2-3 weeks after the first injection and thereafter on the twenty-second day after the injection. Flow is lighter starting the second cycle.
2. Side effects, as with the OCs, often improve spontaneously after 3 months.
3. Danger signs are the same as OCs.
4. If an injection is missed, backup contraception is used; emergency contraception can be considered if there has been unprotected intercourse.
5. Condom use is still recommended to protect against STIs unless the woman is in a mutually monogamous relationship.[44]

Depo Provera (depot medroxyprogesterone)

Method of Action: Progestin crystals in suspension, insoluble in water or lipids, are deposited in the tissue by injection and slowly absorbed. The progestin suppresses the LH surge, inhibits ovulation, makes cervical mucus inhospitable to sperm,[10] and causes the endometrium to atrophy and be unreceptive to a blastocyst.[33]

Advantages: Best suited for the woman who needs contraception for several months to years. It may be useful for noncompliant women and can be used during lactation and when estrogen is contraindicated. Decreases menstrual flow (improving anemia) and decreases the risk of pelvic inflammatory disease (PID) and endometrial cancer. Women with epilepsy have fewer seizures while using depot medroxyprogesterone (DMPA).[50]

Disadvantages: Patients must use condoms for STI protection.[29] Approximately one third of DMPA users discontinue the method after 1 year, and one half discontinue by the end of the second year. Menstrual irregularities, especially amenorrhea, are often cited as the reason.[33] After receiving DMPA, an average of 5 to 8 months is required to clear the body of the hormone and resume normal fertility.[10]

Effectiveness Rate: 99.7% per year.[50]

Side Effects and Their Management:

- **Irregular bleeding** (irregular in 30%; amenorrhea in 50% at 1 year and 80% at 3 years[50]: prescribe ibuprofen 800 mg q8h for 1 week; conjugated estrogens 1.25 mg or estradiol 2 mg PO for 7 days; or MPA 2.5 mg PO qd for 30 days.
- **Weight gain** (average weight gain at 1 year, 5.4 lb; at 2 years, 8.1 lb.; at 6 years, 16.5 lb[10]): advise lifestyle and nutrition changes.
- **Depression** (whether caused by DMPA is controversial[33]): advise counseling or recommend another contraceptive method.
- **Bone loss** may occur after 5 years or more, completely reversing after discontinuance.[50] In adolescents, DMPA may adversely affect bone mineralization during a critical growth period; whether these changes are reversible is unknown.[33]: Give with caution to adolescents, women at risk for osteoporosis, and perimenopausal women.[3] Recommend calcium supplementation, especially for amenorrheic women.
- **Alopecia:** Recommend avoiding harsh chemicals on hair. Reassure that alopecia is transient. Hair loss may be a postpartum change.[5]
- **Other side effects include** headache, gastrointestinal (GI) upset, dizziness,[50] loss of libido, nervousness, fatigue,[33] acne, abdominal bloating, and breast tenderness.[5] Causes mild deterioration in glucose metabolism: 25% decrease in triglyceride, high-density lipoprotein (HDL), and total cholesterol levels,[10] although dyslipidemia may be transient.[50] Small increased risk of breast cancer after long-term use; possible decreased risk of endometrial cancer.[10]

Contraindications to DMPA Use: Liver disease, breast cancer, clotting dyscrasias, or cerebrovascular disease.[50] According to ACOG,[3] the package labeling is incorrect when it states that DMPA is unsafe for the woman with a history of venous thromboembolic disease, and DMPA does NOT increase the risk of venous thrombosis.

Discontinue DMPA: Sudden partial or complete loss of vision, diplopia, proptosis (eyes forced downward), migraine, or for any thrombolic disorder.[10]

Give DMPA with Caution: In the presence of any condition that might be affected by fluid retention such as epilepsy, asthma, cardiac or renal disorders, or depression.[10]

DMPA and Epilepsy: Circulating contraceptive steroid levels are lowered by many anti-convulsant drugs, causing breakthrough bleeding and concerns regarding the efficacy of contraceptive effects. DMPA, however, has an intrinsic anticonvulsant effect and may be suggested in combination with condom use.[3]

DMPA and Sickle Cell Disease: DMPA reduces the frequency of sickle cell crises and may be a particularly appropriate contraceptive choice for these women.[3]

Dosage: DMPA 150 mg IM q3mo, ideally within the first 5 days of the cycle.[3] The manufacturer suggests beginning 6 weeks after delivery in the breastfeeding mother and within 5 days of delivery in the bottle-feeding mother.[10] ACOG[3] states that the 6-week start suggested on the packaging may be overridden by an informed breastfeeding mother who wishes to start birth control earlier because lactation and infant development are not affected. DMPA is detectable in breastmilk but does not affect composition or quantity. No developmental or behavioral effects have been detected in exposed children.[10]

If amenorrhea is present at the time for the next injection, 10 to 14 days abstinence followed by a negative pregnancy test are required before the next dose. A barrier contraception method is suggested for the first 2 weeks after the injection.[5]

Norplant (Levonorgestrel Implants)

Method of Action: Six implants, each containing 36 mg of levonorgestrel in a Silastic capsule, are implanted through a trocar into the inner aspect of the upper arm.[10] Cervical mucus is rendered inhospitable to sperm, ovulation is inhibited, and oocyte maturation is impaired by blocking the LH surge and by luteal insufficiency.[50]

Advantages: Long-term contraception, no action required at time of intercourse, and the method is controlled by the woman. The return to fertility occurs immediately on removal of the device. Lipid and glucose metabolism is unaffected.[50]

Disadvantages: No partner involvement, lessened effectiveness for heavier women, and no STI protection.[29] Removal may be difficult due to fibrotic changes,[50] and serious side effects and complications during insertion and removal have been alleged in many lawsuits.[33]

Effectiveness Rate: Implants are 99.2% effective averaged over a 5-year period and 98% in the sixth year.[50] In women who weigh 70 kg or more, the pregnancy rate was 5.1 per 100 women in the third year of use and 8.5 per 100 women after 5 years.[10]

Contraindications: Not for use in lactating women.[10] ACOG[3] suggests that implants might be placed 6 weeks postpartum or earlier at the discretion of the informed client. If pregnancy occurs, it should be removed immediately because of potential masculinizing effects on the fetus. Other contraindications are the same as for OCs (see p. 515).[10]

Side Effects: Variable bleeding (5% to 10% amenorrheic), headache, mood changes, local dermatitis, acne, mastalgia, hair changes, functional ovarian cysts, weight gain or loss, nausea, and depression. Expulsion of capsule at the insertion site occurs in 0.7%; infection at the site occurs in 0.7%.[33]

Dosage: The 6 rods release 30 μg progestin into the bloodstream daily.[33] The rods are replaced every 5 years, except in women who weigh more than 70 kg (154 lb), in whom replacement should occur every 2 years.[10]

Placement: Ideally, within 7 days of onset of menstruation, the capsules are placed into the subcutaneous tissue in the upper arm under local anesthesia by a trained clinician. Insertion may occur immediately after abortion or after delivery in the bottlefeeding woman. Backup contraception should be used for 72 hours after insertion.[10]

Removal: Half of removals take less than 30 minutes, but 19% last for more than 1 hour. Rarely, the woman has to return for a second procedure. Twenty-five percent report substantial pain.[33]

Oral Contraceptives (OCs)

COMBINATION PREPARATIONS

Method of Action: Combination OCs contain synthetic estrogens and progestins that suppress hypothalamic and pituitary secretions, prevent ovulation, and render cervical mucus hostile to sperm penetration. The endometrium is rendered inhospitable for implantation. Two synthetic estrogens and 12 synthetic progestins are available in various combinations. Table 9-1 lists the biologic activity of these synthetic drugs. Many combination OCs supply a constant dose of estrogen and progesterone for 21 days, with an inert or ferrous fumarate tablets for 7 more days in some preparations. In triphasic, or low-dose OCs, the estrogen or progestin dose varies throughout the cycle to duplicate the normal fluctuation of the ovulatory cycle.[10]

Advantages: Action is taken apart from the sexual act; menses are regular; the woman is in control of the method; and there is decreased menstrual flow, anemia, dysmenorrhea, and mittelschmertz.[30] OCs are protective against ectopic pregnancy,[10] endometrial cancer,[15,39] ovarian cancer,[15,37] and possibly osteoporosis and colon cancer.[18] Acne and benign cystic changes of the breast may improve, and ovarian cysts are

Table 9-1 / Biologic Activity of Oral Contraceptive Components

Class Compound	Progestational Activity[a]	Estrogenic Activity[b]	Androgenic Activity[c]	Endometrial Activity[d]	Andro: Prog Ratio[e]
Progestins[f]					
19 Nor-Testosterone Progestins Estrane					
Norethindrone	1.0	1.0	1.0	1.0	1.0
Norethindrone acetate	1.2	1.5	1.6	0.4	1.3
Ethynodiol diacetate	1.4	3.4	0.6	0.4	0.4
5(10) Estrane					
Norethynodrel	0.3	8.3	0	0	0
Gonane					
Norgestimate	1.3	0	1.9	1.2	1.5
dl-Norgestrel	2.6	0	4.2	2.6	1.6
Levonorgestrel	5.3	0	8.3	5.1	1.6
Desogestrel	9.0	0	3.4	8.7	0.4
Gestodene	12.6	0	8.6	12.6	0.7
Pregnane Progestins					
Medroxyprogesterone acetate	0.3	0	0	NA	0
Other					
Drospirenone	0.5	0	0	NA	0
Estrogens[g]					
Ethinyl estradiol	0	100	0	0	0
Mestranol	0	67	0	0	0

From Dickey RP: Managing contraceptive pill patients, ed 11, Dallas, 2002, EMIS Medical Publishers.
[a]Based on amount required to induce vacuoles in human endometrium. Desogestrel, gestodene, levonorgestrel, and norgestimate based on oral stimulation of endometrium in immature estrogen-primed rabbits relative to levonorgestrel = 5.3.
[b]Comparative potency based on oral rat vaginal epithelium assay. Norethindrone = 1.0 when methyl-testosterone = 50.
[c]Comparative potency (oral) based on rat ventral prostate assay. Norethindrone = 1.0 when methyltestosterone = 50. Levonorgestrel and desogestrel relative to norethindrone = 1.0. Norgestimate, relative to levonorgestrel = 8.3. Gestodene relative to levonorgestrel = 8.3.
[d]Based on estimation of amount required to suppress bleeding for 20 days in 50% of women.
[e]Androgenic + progestational activity, based on oral animal assays. Actual activity in women may be different and will be modified by the dose of estrogen.
[f]Calculated on the basis of norethindrone = 1.0 in activity.
[g]Calculated on the basis of ethinyl estradiol = 100 in activity.

decreased with larger dose OCs.[10] The risk of acquiring PID for which hospitalization is required is reduced. The combination OC may be a useful intervention in the treatment of dysfunctional uterine bleeding, bleeding disorders, polycystic ovary syndrome, acne, hirsutism, endometriosis, and perimenopausal symptoms.[30]

Disadvantages: Hypercoagulability increases the risk of thrombophlebitis and pulmonary embolus. The OC does not protect against STIs or HIV. Side effects may be troublesome. OCs are costly, ongoing health care is required, and a pill must be remembered each day.[7] Combination OCs reduce the quality and quantity of breastmilk and reduce the duration of lactation. Detectable in the milk, its effect on the infant is unknown.[10]

Effectiveness Rate of Combination OCs: Effectiveness rate with perfect use is 99.5% to 99.9% and 97% with typical use.[7]

Combination OC Suppression of Menses: Seasonale: As of 2003, the FDA is considering approval of Seasonale, a monophasic OC designed to be taken for up to 84 days, or 12 weeks, continuously. The pill contains 30 μg ethinyl estradiol and 150 μg of levonorgestrel. The 7-day hormone-free interval with withdrawal bleeding is reduced to a frequency of as few as 4 times annually. Researchers plan to study shortening the hormone-free period to fewer than 7 days, potentially further reducing the symptomatology of menses. Indications for prescription include menstrual disorders (particularly endometriosis and dysmenorrhea) and other conditions that worsen cyclically (such as headaches, epilepsy, and arthritis), as well as convenience. Disadvantages include breakthrough bleeding at 6 to 7 weeks, increased cost, and the lack of a monthly menses in the woman who prefers the 28-day cycle. Contraindications, complications, and effectiveness rates are equivalent to other OCs. The studies have followed women on this regimen for 7 years; long-term safety is unknown.[6,54a,55a]

Side Effects of Combination OCs and Their Management: The first step in managing any side effect is to decide whether the side effect is the sign of a serious complication, in which case the OC is discontinued immediately. Determine the cause of the symptom. Determine what would happen if the OC was continued (some side effects resolve with continued use). Change to another OC with a smaller or larger dose of the hormonal component responsible for the side effect.[10]

1. **Amenorrhea:** The woman who misses 2 consecutive periods should discontinue the OC until pregnancy has been excluded. If not pregnant, she may continue the OC and remain amenorrheic. If she desires menstruation, prescribe an OC with the same estrogen and a progestin with greater endometrial activity, an OC with the same progestin in a lower dose, or a multiphasic OC. If these are ineffective, she can remain on the same OC and take supplemental estrogen or take an OC with a higher estrogen content for 1 to 2 cycles before returning to the lower dose OC. Only if this fails should the woman remain on the higher estrogen OC.[10]

2. **Heavy menses:** Exclude neoplasm of uterus, myoma, adenomyosis, abnormal pregnancy, or endometrial polyps when this less common side effect occurs. Prescribe an OC with greater progestational and androgenic effects and/or a lower estrogen dose.[10]

3. **Breakthrough bleeding (BTB):** Experienced by 32% of users, BTB is the most common reason for discontinuing OCs. Occurs 30% more often among smokers. Decreases after the second to fourth cycle. BTB may indicate incomplete efficacy of the OC, and additional contraception should be used as long as the bleeding continues. Exclude spontaneous abortion (SAB), ectopic pregnancy, PID, and endometriosis before altering the OC preparation. If BTB occurs in the first half of the cycle, increase the estrogen compo-

nent. If BTB occurs in the latter half of the cycle, increase the progesterone component. Alternately, prescribe an OC with higher androgenic activity, which usually decreases bleeding at any time in the cycle. If this does not stop BTB, investigate other causes of vaginal bleeding.[10]

4. **Depression:** Fourteen percent of OC users experience mood swings, fatigue, sleepiness, nervousness, or irritability. Hypoglycemia may be causative. Vitamin B_6 deficiency may cause depression; suggest supplementing vitamin B_6 10 mg qd. Decreasing the progesterone component may help. If irritability is accompanied by edema, decrease the estrogenic component of the pill. Monophasic pills may help the woman who has mood swings. Closely monitor the woman with a history of depression while taking OCs for a return of symptoms.[10]

5. **Weight gain:** Fourteen percent of users gain weight, although as many or more lose weight. Overweight women tend to gain less than underweight women.[10] If the weight gain is associated with increased hunger and hypoglycemia, decrease the progesterone component. If the weight gain is cyclic (i.e., fluid retention) and has to do with fat deposition mainly in breasts, hips, and thighs, advise diet and exercise and decrease the estrogen in the OC. This side effect is reduced in the newer progestins.[50]

6. **Nausea and vomiting with OC ingestion** occurs in 19% of OC users.[10] Advise taking the OC at bedtime, with meals, or try decreasing the estrogen component of the pill.

7. **Libido changes:** Decreased libido occurs most often with high estrogen/high progestin preparations. To increase libido, decrease both components while increasing androgenic activity.[10]

8. **Hypertension (HTN):** Five percent of women who take OCs for 5 years develop HTN. HTN may occur at any time, is usually mild to moderate, reverses 1 to 3 months after discontinuance, and rarely progresses to malignant HTN. The risk increases with age, a family history of HTN or preeclampsia, and duration of use. The HTN appears to be caused by the progestin component, which may be decreased. If BP does not normalize in 3 months, discontinue OCs. Combining antihypertensive medication with OCs is undesirable.[10]

9. **Acne:** Prescribe a less androgenic progesterone component.[10]

10. **Breast tenderness:** Experienced by 11% of OC users, breast tenderness occurs less with low-dose formulations. When swelling is generalized and there is no palpable mass, instruct the woman to reduce caffeine intake. Lower either the estrogen or progesterone components to relieve this symptom. Some providers may suggest giving diuretics and lowering sodium intake as well.[10]

11. **Dizziness** may be caused by fluid excess, anemia, hypoglycemia, or hypotension. The symptom should improve after the first 3 months, but if not, try decreasing the estrogen component of the OC. If it does not improve, pursue other causes.[10]

12. **Headaches** are experienced by 11% of OC users. R/O HTN. Tension headaches are unrelated to OC use. Fluid retention headaches may be related to the OC, may be associated with other fluid retention symptoms, and may improve with an OC with a lower estrogen component. If headaches persist, discontinue OCs.[10] See headache discussion on p. 380.

13. **Mild bilateral tingling and numbness** of the extremities may be caused by fluid retention. An OC with lower estrogenic activity may be tried, but if it does not improve, discontinue OCs.[10]

14. **Predisposition to moniliasis** or other vaginal infections may occur, sometimes doubling the frequency of infection. Decrease progesterone or increase estrogen in the OC.[10]

15. **Chloasma:** Exclude other causes of hyperpigmentation such as Addison's disease. Changing to a lower progestational and estrogenic activity OC may decrease the pigmentation, although it may never disappear completely.[10]

16. **Hirsutism** may be caused by an androgenic progestin and should occur less with the newer progestins.[50] However, it is more likely caused by low estrogenic activity more than increased androgenic activity.[10]

17. **Mucorrhea** or **leukorrhea** is caused by estrogen excess.[10]

18. **Insufficient lubrication** may be caused by excessive progestin and/or deficient estrogen.[10]

19. **Lipid changes:** Newer progestins have less of an adverse affect on the lipids than did older progestin preparations.[50]

20. **Dysmenorrhea** may be experienced by women who were anovulatory before OC use. Exclude adenomyosis and endometriosis, uterine prolapse, and pelvic infection. If no pathology is found, prescribe an OC higher in progestational and androgenic activity and lower in estrogenic activity.[10]

21. New-onset **impaired glucose tolerance** may be improved by supplementing vitamin B_6 10 mg qd.[10] Newer progestins are not associated with the insulin resistance noted in the original preparations.[50]

22. **Cervical hypertrophy or ectopy:** The estrogen predisposes the woman to endocervicitis and PID. Prescribe an OC with less estrogenic activity. For recurrent cervicitis, prescribe an OC with lower progestational and androgenic properties.[10]

23. The following **visual changes** may be caused by cerebral vascular spasm and may precede cerebrovascular accident (CVA): scintillating scotoma (a luminous patch in the visual field with an irregular outline), proptosis (downward displacement of the eyeball), sudden diminished vision, or temporary cessation of vision. Discontinue the OC immediately and the woman should call her medical provider to arrange a workup. Women with retraction difficulties benefit from an OC with less estrogenic activity.[10]

24. **Respiratory infections** appear to be increased in OC users and may be caused by the immunosuppressive effects of progestin or the increased nasal congestion effect of estrogen. Prescribe an OC lower in estrogen and progesterone and discontinue if infections recur.[10]

25. For **increased cystitis episodes** or if the woman is symptomatic but the urine is sterile, prescribe an OC with lower estrogenic activity. If **urinary incontinence** develops or new **pelvic floor prolapse** is noted, prescribe an OC with a higher estrogenic component.[10]

26. **Uterine fibroid changes:** Fibroids may increase or decrease in size and number with OC use. Estrogen stimulates endometrial growth while progesterone antagonizes this effect. When growth is noted, prescribe an OC with lower estrogenic activity. If myoma do not regress in size, exclude pregnancy or uterine or ovarian neoplasm.[10]

PROGESTIN-ONLY PREPARATIONS

Method of Action: Progestin OCs inhibit ovulation, render cervical mucus impenetrable, and thin and atrophy the endometrium, rendering it inhospitable to implantation. Premature luteolysis is induced,[7] and cilia transport of the ovum in the fallopian tubes is slowed.[32]

Advantages: Progestin OCs do not contain estrogen and do not enhance coagulability, as do combination OCs. Menstrual bleeding and thus anemia are decreased. Dysmenorrhea is diminished, and mittelschmerz is eliminated. They offer a protective effect against endometrial and ovarian cancer, PID, and ectopic pregnancy. The woman controls the method. Use during lactation does not diminish the milk supply. Detected in the milk, its effect on the infant is unknown.[10]

Disadvantages: The need to remember and take the pill at the same hour every day, irregular menstrual bleeding or amenorrhea, no protection from STIs or HIV, no partner involvement, cost, and the need for continued contact with a health care provider are disadvantages. Ovarian cysts and ectopic pregnancy occur more frequently compared with combination OCs. A transient decrease in bone mass from low estrogen levels appears to be remineralized on discontinuance. Anticonvulsants decrease the efficacy of the progestin.[7]

Effectiveness Rate: Taken perfectly progestin-only OCs are 95.5% effective; with typical use, they are 86.8% to 98.9% effective.[7]

Side Effects: Menstrual cycle disruption (intermenstrual bleeding, amenorrhea, shortened cycles) is the most common side effect. Others include breast tenderness, headache, nausea, and dizziness.[32]

COMBINATION AND PROGESTIN-ONLY ORAL CONTRACEPTIVES

Pregnancy During OC Use: Studies have not confirmed the increased incidence of birth defects in fetuses when the mother takes OCs during pregnancy. An increased rate of SAB is seen. Some contraceptive failures result in ectopic pregnancies.[10]

Pregnancy After OC Use: Menses may be delayed after OC discontinuance. The woman who had regular menses before taking OCs will probably resume menses in an average of 5 weeks. The woman who had oligomenorrhea or irregular menses may wait as long as 3 months for menses. The average delay before pregnancy is 2 months. Most women are able to conceive within 24 months. A 3-month window after discontinuance of OCs and before conception is advised. No increased frequency in SABs has been noted.[10]

SERIOUS COMPLICATIONS WITH ORAL CONTRACEPTIVES

Venous Thromboembolism: All combination and multiphasic OCs have a procoagulation effect caused by an increase in hepatic production of clotting factors. The risk increases with the dose of ethinyl estradiol. The risk is less than that of pregnancy, and although the relative risk is increased, the absolute risk remains very low. For non-OC users, the absolute risk is 0.4 per 10,000 woman-years; for women taking low-dose OCs it is 1.0 to 1.5 per 10,000 woman-years; and for pregnant women it is 6.0 per 10,000 woman-years.[50]

Stroke: The risk of stroke among women aged 20 to 44 years who are taking regular- to high-OC is 0.5 per 10,000. There is no increased risk among women using low-dose OCs.[51]

Myocardial Infarction (MI): Although the older, high-dose OCs were associated with an increased risk for MI, OCs containing <50 µg ethinyl estradiol do not increase the risk of MI in nonsmoking women. Whether there is an increased risk of MI among hypertensive women who take OCs is controversial. Synergistic interaction of the vascular changes of smoking and the procoagulation effect of OCs cause a marked increase in the risk of MI for the woman who smokes, and a nonhormonal means of birth control is recommended for her.[51] Progestin-only pills do not appear to increase the risk for cardiovascular disease and may be an appropriate contraceptive choice for the woman who smokes cigarette or who is hypertensive at risk for thrombosis, or older than 35 years.[32]

Breast Cancer: A 1996 study of 53,297 women who had breast cancer and 100,239 women who did not have breast cancer revealed that the incidence of breast cancer is slightly increased with OC use, although the risk decreases with increased duration of use. The OC users who developed breast cancer had less advanced disease than did other women.[51] Some experts understand this risk as that of being diagnosed with breast cancer rather than that of developing breast cancer.[34] Women who have a first-degree relative with breast cancer more than triple their risk of developing breast cancer if they take higher-dose OCs (risk ratio, 3.3). It is unknown whether low-dose OCs pose the same risk.[12] All women, especially those with additional risk factors for breast cancer, should do monthly breast exams, receive annual provider examinations, receive mammograms as recommended, and do monthly breast exams and report breast changes to their provider immediately.[10] The effect of progestin-only pills on the risk of breast cancer is unknown.[32]

Cervical Cancer: A small increased incidence of cervical cancer occurs among women taking OCs, possibly because of increased susceptibility to HPV (increased ectropion).[10]

Ectopic Pregnancy and the Progestin-Only Pill: Among the contraceptive failures that result in pregnancies, a higher proportion of the pregnancies will be ectopic pregnancies. The overall risk for ectopic pregnancy, however, is 0.7%—3 times lower than the general population.[32]

Diabetes Mellitus and the Progestin-Only Pill: The progestin-only OC triples the risk for developing diabetes mellitus type 2, the risk increasing with duration of use.[32]

INITIATION. See the contraceptive initiation visit, p. 495.

Physical Assessment Specific to OCs: BP, weight, thyroid, heart, lungs, breasts, abdomen (liver), pelvic exam (pap), skin condition, and presence of peripheral vascular disease.

Lab Work: CBC, urinalysis (UA), Pap, gonococcus, serology. For women ≥40 years with a family history of heart disease, add cholesterol, including HDL and low-density lipoprotein (LDL). For women with a family history of diabetes, add a fasting insulin and blood sugar. For women with a personal or family history of venous thromboembolism of unknown etiology, add Leiden factor V.

The visit should include elements described on p. 495 and, for OCs, include a description of common side effects (as well as the likelihood of many resolving spontaneously by 3 months) and the desirability of waiting until 3 months to switch types as long as the side effect is not a danger sign or too annoying. The danger signs should be reviewed with instructions regarding whom to call if they should occur.[10]

Considerations in Timing Initiation of OCs (Rationale: to Ensure the Woman is Not Pregnant and to Begin before Ovulation):
1. Start the pill on days 1 through 5 of the menstrual cycle.[10]
2. **Day of week:** Some pills suggest a Sunday start as a memory tool and to time the menses mid-week. The patient is instructed to begin the pill on Sunday if she begins her menses on Sunday, or on the first Sunday after the menses begins if it begins on any other day.[10]
3. **Postpartum:** The risk of thromboembolism is increased for 3 to 4 weeks postpartum. Ovulation before 3 to 4 weeks postpartum is rare. At 3 to 4 weeks, the woman who is not breastfeeding may begin combination or multiphasic OCs without waiting for a menstrual cycle.[3,10,31]

The woman who is breastfeeding may begin progestin-only OCs 6 weeks postpartum.[31] Because steroid components of the OC can be detected in the breastmilk, and because combination OCs may inhibit lactation, many providers do not prescribe OCs to lactating women until after their babies are weaned.[10] The American Academy of Pediatrics (AAP) states that use of the combination OCs is acceptable after lactation is well established.[31]

4. **After abortion:** After a first-trimester SAB or therapeutic abortion (TAB), the pill can be started immediately or within 7 days. After a second-trimester abortion, begin as after a term pregnancy.[10]

5. **Irregular cycles:** Women with irregular cycles may begin OCs at any time, after ascertaining that they are not pregnant, but they should use backup contraception for the first cycle.[10]

Client Instructions:

1. **Initiate** the pills as described above. Use a **backup** contraceptive method for the first month on OCs. Be familiar with a backup contraceptive method and keep it on hand.[31]

2. Take **one pill a day.** If prescribed a 21-day pack, take a week off between packs.

3. Take the pill **at the same time** every day (especially important when using progestin-only or combination low-dose OCs). Identify a daily activity to associate with pill-taking as a memory assist.[10] If the pill is taken 3 hours or more after the appointed time, it is considered late. Backup contraception must be used for at least 48 hours; some advocate using it for 7 days.[31]

4. **If pills are missed:**
   a. If one pill is missed, take it as soon as noticed and take the next pill at the regular time. Use backup contraception for 2 to 7 days.[31]
   b. If 2 pills are missed in the first 2 weeks of the cycle, take 2 pills daily for 2 days then resume the regular schedule. Use backup contraception for the remainder of the cycle.
   c. If 2 pills are missed in the third week of the cycle, take 2 pills daily until all the active pills have been taken, restarting with 1 pill on the twenty-eighth day. Use backup contraception until the next cycle is begun and for the first 7 days of the next cycle.
   d. If 3 or more pills are missed at any time during the cycle, stop the OCs. Restart within 7 days with 1 pill a day. Use a backup method for the first 7 days of the next cycle.[10]

5. **If you have missed two periods,** even if you have not missed a pill, use a backup contraceptive method and see a health care provider to exclude pregnancy.

6. There is a slightly increased risk of congenital defects **if you take OCs while you are pregnant.**

7. If you have **vaginal spotting** for more than 2 months, call your health care provider.

8. When seeing any **health care provider** for any problem, mention that you are taking OCs.

9. If **pregnancy is desired,** discontinue the pill for 3 months before the time that you intend to start trying to conceive and use a non-hormonal backup contraceptive method for those 3 months to allow your cycles to return to normal.

10. Notify the surgeon that you take OCs if **surgery** is planned. Discontinue combination OCs (not progestin-only pills) at least 4 weeks before inpatient surgery or immobilization of an extremity (twofold to sixfold increased risk of thromboembolism).[10]

11. Notify your health care provider immediately if you have the following danger signs:

    Signs of Life Threatening Complications = ACHES
    A   severe Abdominal pain
    C   severe Chest pain or shortness of breath
    H   severe Headache
    E   Eye problems: spots, burning, blindness
    S   Severe leg pain

12. Call your provider immediately if you develop **symptoms of thrombophlebitis:** swelling, redness, heat, and pain in a leg.[26]

13. **Emergency contraception** is available if unprotected intercourse occurs.[31]

14. **Barrier contraception** must be used for protection against STIs.[9]

ABSOLUTE CONTRAINDICATIONS FOR COMBINATION OR PROGESTERONE-ONLY ORAL CONTRACEPTIVES

1. **Thromboembolic disease.** The risk of venous thromboembolic disease (VTE) is quadrupled due to the estrogen component of the combination OC.[10] A personal history of a VTE precludes the use of combination OCs. Make a risk/benefit judgment for the patient with a strong family history of VTE.[3] The progestins desogestrel or gestodene cause a slightly higher risk of VTE than do levonorgestrel or norgestimate.[58] ACOG[3] states that package labeling, which states that certain brands of progestin-only OCs are contraindicated for use in the patient with a history of VTE, is incorrect.

2. **Cerebrovascular disease** is a contraindication because of the increased risk for VTE, lipid metabolism changes, and HTN. OC users with HTN have a tenfold risk of stroke, and those who smoke increase the risk by 50%.[10]

3. **Cardiovascular disease.** Women who smoke and are older than 35 years should use another method of birth control because of the risk for coronary disease.[3] The progestin-only pill seems to have little effect on cardiovascular disease and may be a good contraceptive choice for the woman with risk factors.[32]

4. **Liver disease.** Impaired liver function, hepatic adenoma, carcinoma, or benign liver tumors preclude OC use.[10] There is no increased risk of liver cancer with OCs.[17]

5. **Malignancy** of the breast or reproductive tract is a contraindication.[10] Benign breast disease, a history of fibroadenoma, or a family history of breast cancer in a first-degree relative are not contraindications to OCs.[3]

6. Undiagnosed abnormal **genital bleeding.**[10]

7. **Pregnancy.**[10]

8. Type II **hyperlipidemia** (hypercholesterolemia) or hypertriglyceridemia. An alternative contraceptive choice is chosen for the woman with an LDL >160 mg/dL; or for multiple risk factors for coronary artery disease (family history, smoking, diabetes, obesity, HTN, HDL <35 mg/dL, or triglyceride level >250 mg/dL).[3]

9. **Factor V Leiden mutation**. Use of OCs in the woman with this coagulation disorder increases the woman's risk for VTE by 30 times.[10] A polymerase chain reaction test identifies factor V Leiden mutation.[3]

RELATIVE CONTRAINDICATIONS FOR ORAL CONTRACEPTIVES

1. **Diabetes,** history of gestational diabetes mellitus (GDM), or impaired glucose tolerance.[10] ACOG[3] specifies diabetes with vascular disease in the woman older than 35 years and specifies that combination OCs can be used in women with diabetes who are otherwise healthy, nonsmoking, and younger than 35 years. These women are followed closely, monitoring BP, weight, and lipid profile. Screen women with the following risk factors every 3 years: GDM, a family history of diabetes, obesity, HTN, or race (Hispanic, African American, and Native American are high risk).[3] Newer progestins are not associated with insulin resistance, as were original preparations.[50]

2. **Hepatitis** or acute **mononucleosis** within the last year.[10]

3. **Headaches.** Distinguish the type of headache that the woman is experiencing.
   a. OCs have variable effects on headache frequency.[19]
   b. OCs do not increase the CVA risk of the woman with migraines without aura.[19]
   c. Women with classic migraine with aura have a fourfold increase in the risk for CVA. The World Health Organization (WHO) and ACOG[3] recommend that women who have migraines with aura not use OCs.
   d. Tension headache is not a contraindication for the OC.[19]
   e. If headaches worsen in severity, persistence, or intensity; change qualitatively; are associated with new neurologic signs; or if new-onset headaches occur, OCs should be discontinued at least temporarily while an evaluation is made. A month or two of nonhormonal birth control will determine the role of OCs. A different pill formulation, including progestin-only preparations, may be useful.[19]

f. The risk of CVA is increased when the woman has unilateral numbness, tingling, or paralysis before a migraine. Such symptoms mandate OC discontinuance.[10]

4. **Cholestatic jaundice** during pregnancy.[10] OCs slightly increase the risk of gallbladder disease.[16]

5. The incidence of **hypertension** is slightly increased by both low- and high-dose OCs. Preparations containing 30 μg of estrogen increase the ambulatory systolic pressure by 7 to 8 mm Hg. The relative risk of vascular events is increased for hypertensive women taking the pill, but the absolute risk remains low. Consider the risk inherent in the woman's HTN, her age (increased risk >35 years), the risk to her health that pregnancy would pose, and her ability to implement alternative methods of birth control.[3] Cigarette smoking adds a substantial risk for cardiovascular disease and should be avoided. Younger hypertensive patients whose BP can be controlled with medication can use low-dose OCs with close monitoring. Women who are older or who have poorly controlled HTN should probably use progestin formulations or another method.[55] Dickey[10] states that combining antihypertensives and OCs is undesirable. Limited experience suggests that women with a history of eclampsia or preeclampsia can safely use OCs. Progestin-only methods may be superior for women with a history of thrombophilia.[59]

6. **Sickle cell anemia or sickle cell-hemoglobin C disease.** The first choice of contraception for this patient is DMPA because it actually decreases the number of sickle cell crises.[10] The combination OC is now thought to be the second best choice for this patient. The sludging of sickled cells in sickle cell anemia does not act synergistically with the OC-induced clotting changes to increase the risk for VTE. Furthermore, the risks inherent in pregnancy are high for these women.[20]

7. **Heart or renal disease.**[10]

8. **Depression.**[10]

9. **Age >35 if a smoker.** Some providers consider this an absolute contraindication.[3]

10. First-order family history of **nonrheumatic cardiovascular disease before age 50.**[10]

11. **Ulcerative colitis.**[10]

12. **Varicose veins.**[10]

13. Use of **drugs that interact** with OCs.[10]

14. Status less than 2 weeks **postpartum.** See p. 513.

15. **Systemic lupus erythematosus** (SLE) with vascular disease, nephritis, or antiphospholipid antibodies (increased risk for VTE). Combination OCs may be associated with SLE flare-ups; progestin-only OCs are not. Avoid combination OC use, but progestin-only

OCs are acceptable.[3] See p. 370 regarding SLE and p. 371 regarding antiphospholipid syndrome.

16. **Worsening of any chronic disease during pregnancy.**[10]

ORAL CONTRACEPTIVES AND THE WOMAN WHO IS IMMOBILIZED AFTER TRAUMA. VTE with pulmonary embolism is a leading cause of death after surgery. Women taking OCs have twice the risk of postoperative VTE. Six weeks or more are required to normalize clotting factors after discontinuing OCs with 30 μg estrogen. The risk of unintended pregnancy is weighed. Heparin prophylaxis may be considered. Brief surgical procedures have a very low risk of VTE, and OCs do not need to be discontinued.[3]

ORAL CONTRACEPTIVES AND INTERACTIONS WITH OTHER MEDICATIONS. OCs interact with other medications. The activity of the OC and that of the other drug may increase or decrease. Consider such interactions when prescribing OCs to a woman taking any other medications. See Dickey[10] for specific information.

ORAL CONTRACEPTIVES AND INTERACTIONS WITH LABORATORY STUDIES. Many laboratory tests are affected by OCs. Specific data may be found in Dickey.[10]

Transdermal Hormonal Preparation (Ortho-Evra)

Method of Action: Ortho-Evra is a combination hormonal preparation. It delivers estrogen and progestin transdermally through a beige skin patch the size of a matchbook and lasts 7 days.[45]

Advantages: Weekly rather than daily tasking, as with OCs.[45] Delivers progestin and estrogen continuously, directly into the circulation, bypassing interference from GI disturbances and avoiding the daily peaks and troughs of OCs. The hormonal patch is associated with a higher level of compliance than OCs[53] and has the same benefits.[45]

Disadvantages: Requires medical contact and a prescription. Not as effective for women weighing ≥198 lb. The cost is the same as OCs, approximately $40 per month; risks are the same as OCs.[45]

Effectiveness Rate: The patch is 99% effective in clinical trials but less effective in women ≥198 lb.[45]

Side Effects: Side effects are those typical of hormonal contraception, usually mild to moderate in severity. The incidence of breakthrough bleeding is low. Reasons for discontinuance in one study were local reactions at application site (1.9%), nausea (1.8%), emotional lability (1.5%), headache (1.1%), and breast discomfort (1%). Breast discomfort improves after the first 3 cycles.[53]

Client Instructions:
1. Replace the patch q7d and use for 3 weeks out of 4.[45]

2. Apply new patches to buttocks, upper outer arm, lower abdomen, or upper torso, excluding the breast and excluding the site just used.
3. Do not use oils, creams, and cosmetics around the site.
4. If the patch accidentally becomes detached, apply a replacement patch immediately and wear it for the rest of the week.
5. The patch continues to release progestin and estrogen for a full 9 days and does not have to be changed at the same hour each week.[53]
6. Instructions regarding side effects, danger signs, and notification of other health care providers are the same as those for OCs.

Vaginal Ring (NuvaRing)

Method of Action: A transparent, flexible ring, 2 inches in diameter, is inserted into the vagina. It releases Etonogestrel 0.12 mg and ethinyl estradiol 0.015 mg daily for a 3-week period,[40] achieving serum levels equivalent to OCs and preventing conception primarily by suppressing ovulation, as do OCs.[1]

Advantages: Task is required only once a month.[1]

Disadvantages: Requires medical contact and prescription. Risks and side effects are similar to those of OCs (see below). Some women may have local irritation, discharge, or infection. Does not offer protection from STIs.[1]

Effectiveness Rate: The ring is 99% effective in clinical trials.[1]

Method: The ring is inserted once a month, then discarded and replaced on or before the fifth day of the cycle.[1]

Intrauterine Device

Method of Action: The IUD is a small device placed into the endometrial cavity.[7] The copper-impregnated IUD alters endometrial and tubal fluids, inhibits egg transport, fertilization, sperm motility, and integrity. A local foreign body inflammatory reaction disturbs the endometrium and the myometrium, eventually affecting the oviduct and the cervix as well.[23,46] The progesterone-impregnated IUD renders the endometrium unfavorable for implantation, thickens the cervical mucus, and may inhibit ovulation.[36]

Advantages: Reliable, low maintenance, viable during lactation, lack of action required during the sexual encounter, length of effectiveness (some effective for up to 10 years). Progesterone-releasing IUDs may decrease menstrual bleeding and dysmenorrhea.[7] The levonorgestrel IUD may have a protective effect against PID.[36]

Disadvantages: Higher incidence of PID and HIV after insertion; and spontaneous expulsion (2% to 10% within the first year). Half the pregnancies that occur with an IUD in place end in SAB, and cycle length increases as does menstrual bleeding with the Cu-T380A IUD.[7]

Effectiveness Rates: IUDs are effective in 98.5% to 99.9% with perfect use and 98% to 99% with typical use.[7]

Devices Available in the United States:

1. **Cu-T380A:** Annual pregnancy rate of <1/100 users for the 10-year lifespan. First year continuation rate is 77% to 86%. Expulsion rate is 5% to 6% in the first year and 1% to 2% thereafter. Twelve percent are removed for pain and bleeding in the first year and 3% in subsequent years. Perforation rate is 0.6 per 1000 insertions.[47]

2. **Progesterone T:** Releases 65 µg progesterone daily. Approved to be used for 1 year.[22] Expulsion rate is 2.7%; perforation rate is 1.1 per 1000 insertions.[47] Incidence of ectopic pregnancy is greater than other IUDs or OCs. There is less menstrual bleeding and cramping and increased intermenstrual spotting.[10]

3. **Mirena levonorgestrel-releasing intrauterine system:** A T-shaped device that releases approximately 20 µg levonorgestrel daily for 5 years. May protect against PID. It is 99.9% effective in the first year and has a 99.3% cumulative rate in 5 years of use. Side effects are the same as the other IUDs, abdominal cramping being the most common but subsiding after 3 months.[22] The woman may have side effects related to progesterone such as acne, mood changes, and nausea. After increased spotting initially, the woman with menorrhagia experiences an 86% to 94% reduction in flow during the first 3 months and 97% at 12 months. May decrease endometrial hyperplasia, endometrial cancer, and adenomyosis and may be used to supply the progesterone component of hormone replacement therapy.[22]

Absolute Contraindications:

1. Pregnancy.[21]
2. PID, acute or within 3 months.
3. Cervical, ovarian, or uterine carcinoma or malignant trophoblastic disease.
4. Severely distorted uterine cavity that precludes safe insertion.
5. Undiagnosed abnormal vaginal bleeding.
6. Pelvic tuberculosis.
7. Postpartum endometritis or septic abortion.[21]
8. Wilson's disease (a copper-accumulating disease) or copper allergy contraindicate the copper IUD.
9. Increased susceptibility to infection (HIV-positive or IV drug-abusing women).[47]

Relative Contraindications: The midwife consults with a gynecologist before placing an IUD in women with the following:

1. Previous ectopic pregnancy, especially if future pregnancies are desired.
2. History of anemia.
3. History of difficulty with an IUD.
4. Corticosteroid use (may mask infection).
5. Multiple sexual partners or a partner with multiple partners.
6. Emergency treatment difficult to obtain.

7. Endometrial polyps, fibroids, cervical stenosis, bicornuate uterus, or any uterine abnormality.
8. Valvular heart disease (increases risk for development of SBE).
9. History of a vasovagal response to past IUD insertion.[41]

Other Considerations in Choosing This Contraceptive Method:

1. Often causes dysmenorrhea (progesterone IUD may improve).[10]
2. Often causes menorrhagia (progesterone IUD may improve, copper IUD may worsen).[21]
3. History of metrorrhagia (progesterone IUD may improve).[10]
4. Whether the woman can check the string and note the danger signs.
5. The nulliparous woman concerned with fertility may want to choose another method.[40]
6. Marked anteflexion or retroflexion may make placement difficult or dangerous.[35]
7. More nulliparous women expel the IUD.[21]
8. HIV-positive women: Increased blood loss with copper IUDs may increase female-to-male transmission, and the woman's suppressed immunologic response to pelvic infection may be dangerous.[21]
9. A woman at risk for STIs should not use an IUD (increased PID risk).[21]
10. Progesterone IUD may cause oligomenorrhea or amenorrhea.[50]
11. Progestasert increases the risk of ectopic pregnancy.[10]

Insertion of the IUD:

1. **Data collection before insertion:** During the PE, carefully assess the heart for signs of valvular disease. During the pelvic examination, note the size, shape, position, and normalcy of the uterus. A wet mount excludes the presence of bacterial vaginosis.[9] Note laboratory studies, including hemoglobin (Hb), hematocrit (Hct), Pap smear, and gonococcus and chlamydia cultures. Exclude pregnancy, PID, and contraindications.
2. **Timing of insertion:** Insertion is safe at any point during the menstrual cycle as long as the woman is not pregnant. Mid-cycle insertions result in fewer expelled IUDs (a 3% rate). Expulsion occurs more frequently with postpartum placement (10.5%), so this technique is generally only used in circumstances in which the patient is unlikely to return for postpartum care. Insertions between 48 hours and 6 weeks postpartum result in more perforations, however, although the "postplacental" insertion is not associated with an increased risk for perforation. Breastfeeding is safe with the IUD and probably does not increase the risk of perforation. Insertion is safe after a SAB or TAB unless there has been infection, excessive bleeding, genital tract injury, or anemia. Insertion after a late abortion (>16 weeks) requires special training. Otherwise, the IUD may be inserted at the 6-week visit.[24]

3. **Procedure:**
   a. Place speculum. Wash the cervix with a Betadine-saturated sponge 3 times. Place a tenaculum at the 10 and 2 o'clock positions, closing notch by notch.
   b. Pull on the tenaculum to straighten the uterine canal; sound the uterus, noting the direction of the canal and the lack of obstruction and marking the depth with a cotton-tipped swab.
   c. Load IUD according to directions.
   d. Insert IUD according to directions for that IUD.
   e. Cut string to 5 cm and give the tail to the client to familiarize her with the type of string.
   f. Remove the tenaculum and watch the sites for bleeding.
   g. Have client feel the string in place.

Removal of the IUD:
1. Use a tenaculum (as described above) to straighten the uterine canal.
2. Grasp the string with a hemostat and pull the IUD out.

Side Effects of the IUD:
1. Spotting, bleeding, hemorrhage, and anemia (worsened with the Cu IUD, reduced with the progesterone IUD). Improves after 3 months. Follow the woman whose bleeding is heavy with annual Hct measurement, and suggest iron supplementation. Speroff et al[54] suggest the use of prostaglandin synthetase inhibitors during menses to decrease the bleeding caused by IUDs.
2. Dysmenorrhea improves after 3 months. R/O ectopic pregnancy, PID, SAB, incorrectly unfolded IUD, and partial expulsion of the IUD.
3. IUD expulsion. Symptoms are bleeding, pain, or dyspareunia for the woman or her partner.
4. Lost IUD string.
5. Partner irritated by string.
6. Difficult removal.
7. Contraceptive failure resulting in septic abortion indicated by flu-like symptoms.
8. The perforation rate is 1 in 1000 woman-years. Symptoms include pain, bleeding, absence of the string, pregnancy, or no symptoms. Perforations are a function of clinician skill and uterine configuration.[47]
9. PID: Remove IUD if PID is suspected. A woman's risk of PID is primarily related to her exposure to STIs. Women at low risk for STIs have little long-term risk of PID from an IUD.[23]
10. When compared with women who don't use contraception, ectopic pregnancy rates are elevated slightly with the Progestasert (absolute numbers very low) and are decreased with the levonorgestrel-containing IUD.[10] With the copper IUD, the number of ectopic pregnancies is halved.[47]
11. The IUD may actually have a protective effect against endometrial cancer.[47]

12. The levonorgestrel-progesterone IUD may cause oligomenorrhea or amenorrhea.[10]

Returning IUD User History:

1. LMP?
2. Satisfaction with the method?
3. Presence of any life-threatening complications?
4. Signs or symptoms of pregnancy?
5. Effect of IUD on menses?
6. Has she seen another health care provider for a problem since IUD placement?
7. Signs or symptoms of infection?
8. Does she check for strings?
9. Lab work: Hb and Hct.
10. On pelvic examination, note the presence of the string, vaginal discharge, tenderness, uterine enlargement, or signs of pregnancy.

IUD and Pregnancy: Easy IUD removal or expulsion during the first trimester of pregnancy is not associated with an increase in SAB. If the string is visible, the IUD must be removed. At approximately 12 weeks, the string may be drawn into the uterus. When this occurs, removal is more difficult and is more likely to result in SAB. Continuing a pregnancy with the IUD in situ is associated with a 40% to 50% risk of SAB and a fourfold increase in the incidence of preterm labor and delivery. The incidence of congenital anomalies is not increased.[47]

Locating a Lost IUD:

1. Measure serum human chorionic gonadotropin (hCG) to exclude pregnancy.
2. Use an alligator clamp to attempt to grasp the IUD string or the IUD itself in the cervical canal.
3. Use the IUD retriever to sound the uterus.
4. Consult. X-ray with a sound or marker IUD in place to indicate the endocervical canal, sonogram, or hysteroscopy may be used to locate the IUD.

Client Instructions:

1. After menses and after abnormal cramping, check for the presence of the string. If the string is gone or if the hub can be felt, call the health care provider and use another birth control method. Observe tampons and sanitary napkins for the IUD.
2. Expect side effects (increased flow, cramping, spotting). These ease after 3 months.
3. If the menses is missed, see the midwife immediately.
4. If pregnancy is suspected, see the midwife immediately. The IUD is removed, and the risk of SAB and infection is increased.
5. The IUD must be replaced (at the appropriate time).
6. Make a follow-up visit 6 weeks after insertion; thereafter return annually.
7. Refrain from intercourse for 24 hours after placement.

8. Do not remove the IUD.
9. Danger signs with the IUD: "PAINS"
   Period late/no period
   Abdominal pain
   Increased temperature with chills
   Noticeable foul discharge
   Spotting, bleeding, heavy menses

Surgical Sterilization

Tubal Ligation

Method of Action: Surgical ligation of the fallopian tubes, preventing fertilization.

Advantages: Long-term contraception with no further action required. The risk of ovarian cancer is reduced. Sterilization is protective against PID, although not absolute.[4]

Disadvantages: Initial cost, lack of STI protection, increased risk of ectopic pregnancy with procedure failure, permanence, and the need for certainty about future child-bearing plans.[7] Some women have menstrual changes, but most do not.[54] Women who undergo sterilization before age 30 years are more likely to undergo hysterectomy than women who undergo sterilization after age 30 years. Physician and patient bias for surgery in the woman who is beyond her child-bearing years is thought to bias these findings.[4]

Effectiveness Rate: The effectiveness rate for tubal ligation is 99.6% to 99.9%.[7] When failures occur, they are likely to be ectopic pregnancies.[4]

Complications: The most common complications are anesthesia-related. Sepsis from thermal bowel injury (seen most with unipolar electrocoagulation, described below) or bleeding (major vessel lacerations upon entry to abdomen for laparoscopic sterilization procedures) may occur.[4]

Timing and Technique: The procedure may be performed during a cesarean section, after a vaginal delivery through a 2- to 5-cm mini-laparotomy incision, after an abortion by laparoscope or a suprapubic mini-laparotomy incision, or during the follicular phase with the patient's confirmation of strict adherence to a contraceptive method, verified by a sensitive pregnancy test.[4]

Counseling:
1. All operative sterilization procedures are intended to be permanent. Approximately 6% of women request information about reversal of sterility. The strongest indicator of future regret after sterilization is young age. Marital instability is the second greatest indicator. Success rate in reversal procedures depends on the type of sterilization, interval between sterilization and reversal, age, and length of tube remaining.[4] Many women (40% in one report) are turned down as poor candidates for reanastomosis. Those who do have the surgery

are at risk for tubal pregnancy. One author reported a 60% pregnancy rate among women who did undergo the surgery.[52]

2. Suggest alternate methods of birth control.
3. Discuss the procedure used, anesthesia, risks, and benefits.
4. Discuss the possibility of procedure failure, including ectopic pregnancy.
5. Discuss the need to use barrier contraception for STI protection.[9]
6. Discuss postprocedure changes in physiology, including possible changes in menstruation.
7. Provide answers to any questions.
8. Have the woman sign the consent.

Essure: Nonincisional Permanent Birth Control for Women

FDA-approved in late 2002, Essure is a small metal implant that is placed into each fallopian tube. Scar tissue builds around the device, obliterating the tube. The woman who desires placement of the device has a Pap smear and is tested for the presence of pelvic infection. The devices are placed hysteroscopically by a gynecologist during a 35-minute office visit. Local anesthetic and IV sedation are used for comfort during the procedure. The woman rests for 45 minutes and is discharged home. She is instructed to report fever, unusual pain, or bleeding. She may experience some lightheadedness, nausea, or vomiting during the procedure and may experience light vaginal discharge and cramping afterward. She can resume normal activities in 1 to 2 days. For 3 months after placement of the devices, another birth control method (other than an IUD) is continued. The woman returns for a hysterosalpingogram (HSG). If correct placement of the devices and complete obstruction of the tubes is demonstrated, no further birth control is required.

Advantages: Advantages include permanent birth control that does not require an incision or general or regional anesthetic, with an effectiveness rate of 99.8% at 1 and 2 years (data not available after 2 years).

Disadvantages: Disadvantages include unsuccessful implantation of the devices, which occurs in approximately 14% of women. Some of these women return for a successful second placement. An attempt to reverse infertility after the insertion of Essure would involve major surgery with a poor chance for success. Essure is new, so safety and effectiveness data are available for only 2 years. No data are available regarding the safety of pregnancy for the mother or infant in the presence of Essure.

Risks: Risks include the possibility of pregnancy several years after the procedure (no long-term studies have been conducted to date) and the increased risk of ectopic pregnancy if pregnancy does occur. Three percent of women do not form scar tissue at the 3-month HSG sufficient enough to be able to rely on this method for birth control. Infection or expulsion, perforation, migration, or breakage of the device may occur (the latter during placement; not associated with problems in studies).

The risks inherent in hysteroscopy, HSG, and anesthesia apply. Undiagnosed pregnancy at the time of the procedure is associated with complications. Some women report temporary menstrual changes that include menorrhagia and intermenstrual bleeding and spotting. Permanent changes are rare. Pelvic, back, or abdominal pain episodes are reported by some women, but persistent pain is rare. There is a risk that subsequent pelvic procedures may interfere with the performance of the device or that the presence of the device may preclude a procedure (such as hysteroscopy, uterine ablation, or D&C). The device is safe during MRI, although it may obscure visualization in the vicinity.

Contraindications

1. Uncertainty about the desire for permanent infertility.
2. Current pregnancy.
3. Status less than 6 weeks postpartum (abortion or term delivery).
4. Active or recent pelvic infection.
5. Unusual uterine shape.
6. Sensitivity to dye (contrast media for HSG) or nickel (confirmed by skin test).
7. History of a tubal ligation.
8. Unwillingness to use alternate birth control for 3 months after placement or to undergo HSG at that time.

Relative Contraindications:

1. Immunosuppressive therapy, which may suppress the body's tendency to create scar tissue in the tube.
2. History of pelvic surgery.[9a]

Vasectomy

Method of Action: Ligation of the vas deferens preventing transmission of sperm into seminal fluid.[25]

Advantages: Compared with female sterilization, vasectomy is less expensive, safer, and equally effective.[4] It provides long-term contraception with no further action required.[7]

Disadvantages: Vasectomy is a surgical procedure. Permanent contraception results, and 5% to 10% have postprocedure regret.[7] Alleged associations with atherosclerosis,[4] MI, CVA,[43] testicular cancer, and prostate cancer have not been confirmed in studies.[25] Complications occur in <3%.[4] Pain and swelling may be present for a week. Scrotal hematoma may require ligation, scrotal abscess and sperm granuloma may require operative excision, and epididymitis may occur.[25] Less than 1% of procedures fail.[4]

Effectiveness Rate: The effectiveness rate for vasectomy is 99.6% to 99.9%.[7]

Counseling/Education (Midwife Would Not Be Consenting Client):

1. Should be considered permanent. Five percent to 10% have postprocedure regret,[7] and 1% to 2% seek information about reversal.[4]

Success of reversal procedures depend on type of procedure done, interval between the procedure and reversal, age, and length of tube remaining.[4] Reversal is more effective if done within 10 years.[25]

2. Procedure itself.
3. Risks and benefits.
4. Need for barrier contraception as STI protection.[9]
5. Client's questions.

Procedure: Under local anesthesia, two small incisions are made in the scrotum to reach the vas deferens. Alternatively, the "no-scalpel" vasectomy is made through one puncture with a special instrument. Vasectomy is ineffective until all the sperm in the system are ejaculated, which takes about 20 ejaculations or 12 weeks.[4] The procedure is simple, lasts 10 to 15 minutes, and is done on an outpatient basis.

Emergency Contraception ("Morning-After" Contraception)

Prevention of conception after unprotected intercourse may be appropriate as an intervention after rape, condom breakage, inadvertent displacement of a barrier device, or failure to use birth control when pregnancy is not desired.

Method of Action: Mechanism of action is unclear. May make endometrium inhospitable for implantation, prevent or delay ovulation,[50] interfere with fertilization, disrupt the luteal phase of the menstrual cycle, change the cervical mucus, or alter tubal transport.[1a]

Effectiveness Rate: Emergency contraception (EC) effectiveness ranges from 55.3% to 94.2% depending on the method and where the woman was in her cycle.[7]

Absolute Contraindication: Known **pregnancy**.[50] Once implantation has occurred, EC has no effect on the pregnancy.[1a] EC is not abortifacient and pregnancies carried to term have not shown adverse effects. The woman with a current, active **migraine** headache with neurologic complications should avoid taking EC because of an increased risk of cardiovascular events during the headache.[42]

Side Effects: Nausea, vomiting, headache, breast tenderness, dizziness, abdominal cramping, fatigue, early or late menses.[10] VTE has not been identified as a complication of EC.[3]

Contraindications: Because of its short duration of action, EC has not been shown to have adverse effects for women with contraindications to the routine use of OCs.[42]

Self-Administration: The midwife may choose to offer an advance prescription for a woman to have EC available.[1b] A study conducted in 1998 found that women who had EC on hand did not show an increase in high-risk sexual behaviors.[11]

Methods:

Diethylstilbestrol: Approved by the FDA for emergencies only. Probably interferes with implantation; is 75% effective. The woman is advised that if the method fails, there is an increased risk of congenital abnormalities. Requires a history and physical, including breast exam.[2] Side effects include nausea, headache, vomiting, menstrual irregularities, and breast tenderness. No long-term side effects are proven.[7]

- Dose is 25 mg qd for 5 days begun within 72 hours of intercourse.[7]

Progestins: Progestins have a high success rate. They contain less hormone than DES and are theoretically safer.

- Dose is 2 tablets PO within 24 hours of coitus, repeat in 12 hours[7] or **levonorgestrel** 0.75 mg (20 Ovrette mini-pills) given twice, 12 hours apart, within 48 hours of intercourse (nearly 2 boxes of pills).[50]

IUD: IUDs have a toxic effect on sperm as well as impair implantation by changes in the endometrium. The IUD can be used for women who are not at risk for STI if the woman does not have another contraindication.[50] To be effective, before ovulation, the IUD must be inserted within 5 to 7 days of intercourse; after ovulation it must be inserted within 5 days of intercourse. Failure rate is ≤0.1%. Thereafter, it provides ongoing contraception.[14]

Oral Contraceptives: Side effects are nausea and vomiting.[50]

- Dose is two doses of 100 μg ethinyl estradiol and 0.5 mg levonorgestrel 12 hours apart within 72 hours of unprotected intercourse.[50] The following are dosages of different brands of OCs that contain the prescribed amount: Ovral, 2 white; LoOvral, 4 white; Nordette, 4 orange; Levlen, 4 orange; Levora, 4 white; Trilevlen, 4 yellow, Triphasil, 4 yellow, Trivora, 4 pink, Alesse, 5 pink, and Levlite, 5 pink.[42]

Mifepristone (RU486): An antiprogesterone agent that inhibits ovulation and causes corpus luteum regression in 50% of women. A prescription for RU486 requires three office visits and a signed consent. The effectiveness rate is 85% to 100%. Side effects include nausea and vomiting, headache, breast tenderness, and delayed menses. Contraindications include possible ectopic pregnancy or adnexal mass, IUD in place, chronic adrenal failure, corticosteroid use, allergy to any prostaglandin, coagulopathy or anticoagulation, inherited porphyria, and no access to emergency care.

- Dose is 600 mg taken within 120 hours of unprotected intercourse. (Lower doses have been used with equal success.)[35]

Preven Emergency Contraception Kit: This kit contains an early pregnancy test to exclude prior pregnancy and two doses of 2 pills, each containing levonorgestrel 0.25 mg and ethinyl estradiol 0.05 mg. The first dose is taken within 72 hours of unprotected sex, and the second is taken 12 hours later.[50] Side effects are nausea and vomiting.[42]

• REFERENCES

1. American College of Nurse-Midwives (ACNM): FDA approves new birth control option, *Quickening* 32:30, 25, 2001.
1a. American College of Nurse-Midwives (ACNM): Position statement: emergency contraception: expanding education and access, *Quickening* 32:20, 2001.

1b. New ACOG recommendations on emergency contraception, *Quickening* 32:9, 2001.

2. American College of Obstetrics and Gynecology (ACOG): Public uninformed about, and physicians underutilizing, emergency oral contraception, Washington, DC, May 31, 1997, http://www.acog.com/from_home/publications/press_releases/oral-contra.htm, News release; retrieved May 31, 1997.

3. ACOG: The use of hormonal contraception in women with coexisting medical conditions, July 2000, Practice bulletin No 18.

4. ACOG: Sterilization, April 1996, Technical bulletin No 222.

5. Archer B et al: Depot medroxyprogesterone: management of side-effects commonly associated with its contraceptive use, *J Nurse-Midwifery* 42:104-111, 1997.

6. Archer D: New contraceptive options: contraception for the 21st century, *Clin Obstet Gynecol* 44:122-126, 2001.

7. Branden PS: Contraceptive choice and patient compliance: The health care provider's challenge, *J Nurse-Midwifery* 43:471-482, 1998.

8. Cavero C: Using an ovarian monitor as an adjunct to natural family planning, *J Nurse-Midwifery* 40:269-276, 1995.

9. Centers for Disease Control and Prevention (CDC): Sexually transmitted diseases treatment guidelines, *MMWR* 51(RR 06):1-80, 2002.

9a. Conceptus, Inc: A non-incisional approach to permanent birth control: patient information booklet. San Carlos, CA, 2002, Conceptus. Available at: http://www.essure.com/Patient_Information_Booklet.pdf.

10. Dickey RP: *Managing contraceptive pill patients*, 10 ed, Dallas, 2000, EMIS Medical Publishers.

11. Glasier A et al: The effects of self-administering emergency contraception, *N Engl J Med* 339:1-4, 1998.

12. Grabrick DM et al: Risk of breast cancer with oral contraceptive use in women with a family history of breast cancer, *JAMA* 284:1791-1798, 2000.

13. Grimes DA, editor: Patient Update: Latex allergy and contraception, *The Contraceptive Report* 8(1), 1997.

14. Grimes DA, editor: Emergency contraception options, *The Contraceptive Report* 8(2):11-14, 16, 1997.

15. Grimes DA, editor: Health benefits of oral contraceptives, *The Contraceptive Report* 8(2):4-10, 16, 1997.

16. Grimes DA, editor: Benign gallbladder disease: newer data suggest little or no excess risk with oral contraceptive use, *The Contraceptive Report* 8(5):9-11, 1997.

17. Grimes DA, editor: Oral contraceptives and liver cancer, *The Contraceptive Report* 8(5):4-8, 1997.

18. Grimes DA, editor: Patient Update: Health benefits of oral contraceptives, *The Contraceptive Report* 8(5), 1997.

19. Grimes DA, editor: Headache, migraine, and oral contraceptives, *The Contraceptive Report* 8(6):12-14, 16, 1998.

20. Grimes DA, editor: Oral contraceptives and sickle cell disease, *The Contraceptive Report* 8(6):9-11, 1998.

21. Grimes DA, editor: Modern IUDs Part I: Increasing access to IUDs, *The Contraceptive Report* 9(4):9-11, 1998.

22. Grimes DA, editor: Modern IUDs Part I: Worldwide perspective on IUD use, *The Contraceptive Report* 9(4):4-8, 16, 1998.

23. Grimes DA, editor: Modern IUDs Part II: IUDs: understanding their mechanisms of action, *The Contraceptive Report* 9(5):4-5, 16, 1998.

24. Grimes DA, editor: Modern IUDs Part II: Timing of IUD insertions, *The Contraceptive Report* 9(5):6-8, 1998.

25. Grimes DA, editor: Patient Update: Questions and answers about vasectomy, *The Contraceptive Report* 9(6):1999.

26. Grimes DA, editor: Desogestrel- and gestodene-containing combination OCs and venous thromboembolism: where are we now? *The Contraceptive Report* 10(1):4-8, 1999.

27. Grimes DA, editor: New estimates of contraceptive failure rates, *The Contraceptive Report* 10(2):10-11, 14, 1999.

28. Grimes DA, editor: Return of the contraceptive sponge expected, *The Contraceptive Report* 10(2):9, 1999.
29. Grimes DA, editor: Hormonal contraception and sexually transmitted disease, *The Contraceptive Report* 10(3):11-14, 16, 1999.
30. Grimes DA, editor: Using oral contraceptives to treat medical conditions, *The Contraceptive Report* 10(3):4-10, 1999.
31. Grimes DA, editor: Counseling suggestions for successful OC use, *The Contraceptive Report* 10(4):12-14, 1999.
32. Grimes DA, editor: Progestin-only oral contraceptives: an update, *The Contraceptive Report* 10(4):4-7, 11, 1999.
33. Grimes DA, editor: Contraceptive implants and injectables: recent developments, *The Contraceptive Report* 10(6):26-30, 2000.
34. Grimes DA, editor: Patient Update: facts about breast cancer and hormones, *The Contraceptive Report* 11(2), 2000.
35. Grimes DA, editor: FDA approval of mifepristone: an overview, *The Contraceptive Report* 11(4):4-12, 2000.
36. Grimes DA, editor: FDA approves levonorgestrel-releasing intrauterine system, *The Contraceptive Report* 12(2):9-14, 2001.
37. Grimes DA, editor: Low-dose OCs protect against ovarian cancer, *The Contraceptive Report* 12(2):4-8, 14, 2001.
38. Grimes DA, editor: FDA approves combined monthly injectable contraceptive, *The Contraceptive Report* 12(3):8-11, 2001.
39. Grimes DA, editor: Health benefits of oral contraceptives: update on endometrial cancer protection, *The Contraceptive Report* 12(3):4-7, 2001.
40. Grimes DA, editor: Current design of the etonogestrel/ethinyl estradiol contraceptive vaginal ring, *The Contraceptive Report* 12(5):7, 2001.
41. Hatcher RA et al: *Contraceptive technology* 16 ed, New York, 1994, Irvington Publishers.
42. Judge DE: Emergency contraception: it's not too late, *Journal Watch Women's Health* 4: 23-24, 1999.
43. Manson JE et al: Vasectomy and subsequent cardiovascular disease in US physicians. *Contraception* 59:181-186, 1999.
44. National Association of Nurse Practitioners in Women's Health (NPWH): New option in hormonal contraception, Dayton, NJ, 2001, NP Communications.
45. Neegaard L: FDA approves world's first contraceptive skin patch, *The Press Democrat* p A8, November 21, 2001.
46. Ortiz ME, Croxatto HB, Bardin CW: Mechanisms of action of intrauterine devices, *Obstet Gynecol Surv* 51:S42-S51, 1996.
47. Pasquale S. Clinical experience with today's IUDs, *Obstet Gynecol Surv* 51:S25-S29, 1996.
48. Reference deleted in galleys.
49. Reference deleted in galleys.
50. Qureshi M, Attaran M: Review of newer contraceptive agents, *Cleveland Clinic J Med* 66:358-366, 1999.
51. Shulman LP: Oral contraception: safety issues re-examined, *Int J Fertil* 44:78-82, 1999.
52. Siegler AM, Hulka J, Peretz A: Reversibility of female sterilization, *Fertil Steril* 43: 499-510, 1985.
53. Smallwood GH et al: Efficacy and safety of a transdermal contraceptive system, *J Obstet Gynecol* 98:799-805, 2001.
54. Speroff L, Glass RH, Kase NG: *Clinical gynecologic endocrinology and infertility,* Philadelphia, 1999, Lippincott Williams & Wilkins.
54a. Sulak PJ et al: Acceptance of altering the standard 21-day/7-day oral contraceptive regimen to delay menses and reduce hormone withdrawal symptoms, *Am J Obstet Gynecol* 186:1142-1149, 2002.
55. Sullivan JM, Lobos RA: Considerations for contraception in women with cardiovascular disorders, *Am J Obstet Gynecol* 168:2006-2011, 1993.

55a. Thomas SL, Ellertson C: Nuisance on natural and healthy: should monthly menstruation be optional for women? *Lancet* 355:922-924, 2000.

56. Trent AJ, Clark K: What nurses should know about natural family planning, *J Obstet Gynecol Neonatal Nurs* 26:643-648, 1997.

57. Varney H: *Varney's midwifery*, 3 ed, Sudbury, Mass, 1997, Jones and Bartlett.

58. Winkler UH: Effects on hemostatic variables of desogestrel- and gestodene-containing oral contraceptives in comparison with levonorgestrel-containing oral contraceptives: a review, *Am J Obstet Gynecol* 179:S51-S60, 1998.

59. Witlin AG: Counseling for women with preeclampsia or eclampsia, SeminPerinatol 23:91-98, 1999.

Chapter 10

Menopause

• DEFINITIONS

Menopause: When the ovaries cease functioning; the permanent cessation of menses for 1 year.
Perimenopause: The period leading up to menopause, generally lasting 3 to 5 years.
Postmenopause: Begins 1 year after the last menses.[3]

• PHYSIOLOGY OF MENOPAUSE

Each woman is born with a finite number of follicles that are eliminated by ovulation and atresia. As they diminish, less estrogen and progesterone are produced by the ovaries in response to follicle-stimulating hormone (FSH) from the pituitary, until there fails to be a luteinizing hormone (LH) surge. During the following anovulatory cycles, the pituitary increases FSH production in an effort to increase estrogen production. The LH level rises as well. Cycles may lengthen and periods may become lighter. Cycles become increasingly anovulatory and irregular, with vaginal bleeding occurring at the end of an inadequate luteal phase or after an estradiol peak without ovulation or corpus luteum development. Surges of estrogen may cause heavier menses and enlargement of uterine fibroids. The hormones continue to fluctuate in this way for months to years. After approximately 400 ovulations, the capacity for reproduction is exhausted, and menopause occurs.[69]

The ovaries continue to produce small amounts of estrogen. The precursor hormone androstenedione is converted to estrone, a form of estrogen, in fat cells. Estrone (E1) is the predominant postmenopausal estrogen. Estriol (E3) is a biologically weak estrogen created by the metabolism of estrone. The ovaries continue to produce testosterone in amounts only slightly less than those produced during the reproductive years, now proportionately excessive in most postmenopausal women.[69]

About 75% of women experience menopausal symptoms. Twenty-five to thirty percent of women consult their health care providers regarding these symptoms. LH and FSH levels are used clinically to confirm the onset of menopause. Maximum levels occur 1 to 2 years after natural menopause and remain elevated for 10 to 15 years. Surgical menopause occurs when the ovaries are removed or when ovarian failure occurs after hysterectomy as a result of compromised ovarian blood flow. After surgical menopause, FSH and LH levels rise within 20 to 30 days.[75]

As estrogen diminishes, blood flow to the reproductive and urinary tracts diminishes. Mitotic activity of the epithelium decreases, and in the vaginal walls, the production of superficial epithelial vaginal cells is gradually reduced, resulting in shortened, narrow, friable walls. The pH increases, the number of lactobacilli diminishes, and resistance to vaginitis is decreased. Bladder and urethral tissue atrophy, resulting in increased proximity of the urine to the sensory nerves. Increased frequency, dysuria, nocturia, and urge incontinence may result. The urethral and vaginal openings move closer together and, with the more basic pH, the risk for urinary tract infection (UTI) is increased. Collagen synthesis, also stimulated by estrogen, is decreased. Stress incontinence and prolapse of pelvic organs may result.[56]

• TIMING OF MENOPAUSE

The average age at the onset of menopause is 51 to 52 years. Thin women, nulliparous women, and women who smoke experience menopause earlier. Exposure to toxic chemicals (such as chemotherapy) usually causes menopause to occur earlier. Familial tendency, the woman's age at menarche, her height, race, parity, marital status, and geographical location are unrelated to the age at menopause.[69] Menopause before the age of 40 is termed *premature ovarian failure*. The average length of perimenopause is approximately 4 years.[44] The expected life span for women is 79.2 years, so most women can expect to live about 3 decades after menopause.

• OBESITY AND MENOPAUSE

The obese woman, because of her larger fat stores, produces more estrone. She tends to have higher estrogen levels. Although she is at less risk for osteoporosis, she is at higher risk for complications that arise from unopposed estrogen-endometrial hyperplasia and cancer. She is also at increased risk for cardiovascular disease.[69]

• PERIMENOPAUSE/MENOPAUSE-RELATED SYMPTOMS AND THEIR TREATMENT

Affective Symptoms

During perimenopause, a loss of concentration, insomnia, memory lapses, mood changes, and depression may be experienced. Estrogen increases cerebral perfusion, and estrogen receptors have been localized in many neuronal tissues.[6] Research has demonstrated that estrogen serves many functions in the nervous system and that its withdrawal may have a pervasive effect. By affecting the neurochemistry, architecture, stress response, and nerve-communication pathways of the brain, estrogen has an impact on memory, learning, the ability to pay attention, moods and emotions, and the ability of the brain and the individual as a whole to withstand stress.[77] Symptoms of psychologic distress correlate with the history of psychological distress and with socioeconomic factors. Preexisting depression or panic disorder may be exacerbated by menopause.[69]

m Management

1. The use of **estrogen replacement therapy (ERT)** for these symptoms alone **is not justified.**[44]
2. Supplementation with **vitamin B** complex, **calcium,** and **zinc** is suggested for depression.[43]
3. **Alcohol, caffeine, and sugar** may intensify mood swings, fatigue, and depression and should be **avoided or used in moderation.**[7]
4. **Complementary measures:**
   a. **Homeopathy** experts recommend their remedies for affective symptoms of menopause.[20,32,60]
   b. **Herbs: Ginkgo biloba,** rich in bioflavonoids that improve circulation to the brain, is suggested for depression or fatigue, memory loss, loss of concentration, and emotional fatigue.[7,24,41,47,71] It takes 2 weeks to see results[7]: dose is 60 to 80 mg of dried extract tid.[71] **Ginseng *(Panax ginseng)*** stimulates the brain and reduces stress and fatigue; it may increase stamina, improve short-term memory, and act as an aphrodisiac.* **Siberian ginseng is contraindicated with hypoglycemia, heart disease, or hypertension.**[30] **Oat straw** is said to "nourish" the nervous system, soothe nerves, and lend energy.† Medina[47] suggests drinking no more than 2 cups/d. **Skullcap** may be taken for anxiety, fatigue, stress, or nervous disorders.‡ **St Johns' wort** is useful in the treatment of mild to moderate but not severe depression, especially that of menopause, because it normalizes female hormone levels. It may take several weeks before an effect is noted.§ Twenty-five drops of tincture may be taken qd to tid for several months.[78] It should not be used for more than 6 months.[2] **See information on herbs p. 563.**

---

*References 7, 14, 24, 30, 41, 46, 47, 52, 58, 71, 78.
†References 7, 36, 41, 47, 52, 78.
‡References 7, 30, 36, 38, 41, 46.
§References 2, 7, 24, 30, 36, 46, 47, 58, 71.

Cardiovascular Disease

The number one killer of Americans, including women,[69] cardiovascular disease is the major cause of death and disability among older women.[22] Total serum cholesterol levels are lower before menopause and increase after menopause. Triglyceride levels rise, the body mass index (BMI) increases, the waist-to-hip ratio increases, and insulin levels rise.[44] Major risk factors for heart disease include smoking, dyslipidemia, diabetes mellitus, age >60 years, postmenopausal status, and a family history of heart disease in a woman <65 years.[70] Box 10-1

• *Box 10-1 /* Lipids •

The four principal circulating lipids are triglycerides, free cholesterol, cholesterol esters, and phospholipids. They are transported in macromolecules called *lipoproteins* that carry cholesterol, triglycerides, and proteins as very low density lipoproteins (VLDLs); intermediate density lipoproteins; low density lipoproteins (LDLs); and high density lipoproteins (HDLs).[62]

VLDLs: Main transporters of triglycerides. Indicated by fasting triglyceride level.[27]

LDL: A high LDL level is atherogenic.[13] Increases if VLDLs increase. 60% to 70% of cholesterol is carried on LDL, and a fasting cholesterol determination indicates the LDL level.[27]
- Normal: 60 to 130 mg/dL (conversion factor 0.0259;1.6-3.4 mmol/L)[66]
- High risk: ≥160 mg/dL
- Moderate risk: 130 to 159 mg/dL[13]

HDL: Removes cholesterol from circulation by transporting it to the liver. High levels decrease the risk of coronary artery disease. Levels increase with the endogenous or exogenous estrogen level, exercise, weight loss, alcohol use, and age and decrease with progesterone administration (especially androgenic), obesity, and smoking.[27]
- (Normal: 30 to 70 mg/dL (conversion factor 0.0259; 0.8-1.8 mmol/L)[66]; ≥35 mg/dL is a desirable level.[13]

Cholesterol: Dietary cholesterol, dietary saturated fats, lack of insulin or thyroid hormone increase serum cholesterol.[27] Plays a part in assembly of cell membranes, production of bile salts, and steroid hormones.[62]
- Desirable: <200 mg/dL (conversion factor 0.0259; <5.2 mmol/L), with HDL exceeding LDL.
- High: >240 mg/dL.

Triglycerides: Normal: 40 to 250 mg/dL (0.5-2.8 mmol/L).[66]

Variables:
- Timing of testing—Defer with acute illness, after trauma, surgery, or weight loss.[13]
- Estrogen—Increases HDL, increases biliary cholesterol, decreases bile acid concentration, thereby increasing gallstone formation.[13]
- Effect of oral contraceptives—See p. 510.

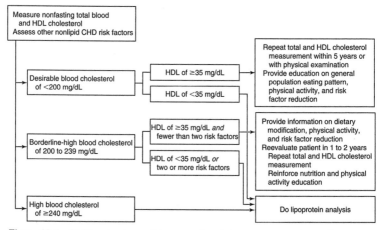

Figure 10-1 • Lipid evaluation and treatment in relation to coronary heart disease. (From the National Cholesterol Education Program Report of the Second Expert Panel on Detection, Evaluation and Treatment of High Cholesterol in Adults: adult treatment panel II, *Circulation* 89:1357, 1994.)

reviews the lipids that circulate in the body, and Figure 10-1 outlines the evaluation and treatment of lipids in relation to coronary heart disease.

m Management

1. A **fiber-rich, low-fat diet, treatment of hypertension,** maintenance of **normal blood glucose levels** in diabetic women, **weight control,** and possibly **low-dose aspirin** and **antioxidant vitamin supplementation** may reduce the risk of cardiovascular disease.[43]

2. All **hormone replacement therapy (HRT)** regimens increase high-density lipoprotein (HDL) levels, decrease mean low-density lipoprotein (LDL) levels, and increase triglyceride levels.[83,84] The American Heart Association has concluded that primary prevention of coronary heart disease is not an indication for initiation of HRT.[50] The Women's Health Initiative[84] demonstrated an increase of 7 more coronary heart disease events per 10,000 healthy woman-years.

3. **The woman who has a history of heart disease has an increased risk for myocardial infarction (MI) during the first year of ERT**, and so prescription for this client must be done with careful discussion of risks and benefits.[31] The American Heart Association has concluded that HRT should not be prescribed for the secondary prevention of coronary heart disease, and whether it is prescribed at all for women with coronary heart disease is based on an analysis of noncoronary and coronary risks and benefits and the woman's preference.[50]

4. **Selective estrogen receptor modulators** (SERMs) (tamoxifen, raloxifene, and droloxifene) bind to estrogen receptors, mimicking the

action of estrogen in some tissues, while acting as estrogen antagonists in others.[22] They may prescribed for their effect on the lipid profile.

5. **Complementary measures:**
   a. **Nutritional suggestions:** Long-term intake of **soy and isoflavones** may improve lipoprotein profiles but is contraindicated in women with estrogen-dependent cancer.[2] **Phytoestrogens** are chemicals with estrogenic properties that are found in a number of foods (e.g., soy products, potatoes, yams, apples, carrots, coffee, bean sprouts, rye, wheat, sesame seeds, flaxseed, and some alcoholic beverages). Phytoestrogens, found in higher levels in vegetarian women, appear to reduce the risk of cardiovascular disease.[43,55] **Bioflavonoids**, chemicals found in certain foods, have a mild estrogenic effect, as well as an estrogen receptor–blocking effect. They decrease the risk of cerebrovascular accident (CVA) and MI[7,78] but are contraindicated in women with estrogen-dependent cancer.

   b. **Herbs: Evening primrose oil** guards against coronary artery disease, reduces BP, slows blood clotting, and apparently reduces weight. It stimulates estrogen production, lowering cholesterol levels, which makes it beneficial for women with heart disease.[7,14,41] Results show in 3 to 6 weeks. The dose is 8 to 10 500-mg capsules/d.[14] It may be taken as a decoction (1 tsp root/cup water); or as a tea made with equal parts chopped plant and flowers.[52] **Garlic** reduces the risk of heart disease by reducing cholesterol levels and BP* and by slowing blood clotting.[7,46,58,71] Two to four grams of dried bulb may be taken tid.[71] Odorless supplements are available. **Hawthorn** is known as a nourisher of the circulatory system. It increases the blood flow to the heart and dilates the coronary blood vessels; it may decrease cholesterol levels and may reduce elevated BP. It is suggested for hypertension, "weakness of the heart," and for palpitations.[14,24,30,46] **See information on herbs, p. 563.**

Headaches

Individuals with migraines may find that headaches occur less frequently with menopause; or they may experience worsening.[69] See p. 380 regarding the evaluation of headaches.

ⓜ Management

1. The woman taking HRT may benefit from **continuous HRT** rather than cyclic HRT to prevent headaches that are related to cyclic hormonal changes.[69]
2. **Complementary measures:** Several experts recommend **herbal** remedies for headaches.[30,46,57,78] See p. 33 for other measures.

---

*References 14, 24, 30, 41, 46, 58.

Insomnia

Poor sleep may be a sign of a chronic disease, depression, or a sleep or breathing disorder; or it may be caused by night sweats interrupting sleep.[69]

ⓜ Management

1. **Refer** the woman to a physician if a medical illness is suspected. See p. 533 regarding **affective symptoms** of perimenopause. Refer the woman for significant depression. Address **night hot flashes.** See p. 546.
2. **Make the following lifestyle suggestions: Exercise** during the day to enhance sleep. **Avoid caffeine, alcohol, cigarettes,** and **spicy foods**—all of which may cause insomnia. **Winding-down activities** should precede bedtime. Take a **warm bath** or shower, and drink **warm milk** at bedtime. Sleep in a **cool room and dress in light,** natural fabrics. **Go to bed and rise at regular times.**[47,80]
3. **Complementary measures:**
   a. **Homeopathy** experts suggest their remedies for insomnia.*
   b. **Chinese medicine: Acupuncture** may be used in the treatment of insomnia,[12] as may **shiatsu.**[34] **Acupressure** points for insomnia are on the back of the head, at the hairline on either side of the spine (Bladder 10).[55] Alternately, someone can apply 10 to 15 lb of pressure with the heel of one hand to the sacrum for 2 to 3 minutes at bedtime to bring on relaxation and sleep (Bladder 31 and 32).[68] **See charts and information on Chinese medicine, p. 559.**
   c. **Nutritional suggestions: Calcium and magnesium,** taken in combination at bedtime, may improve sleep.[47] Alternately, **magnesium** (a 500-mg supplement), taken between meals, will deepen sleep.[78] Balch and Balch[7] suggest that **vitamin B** deficiencies can cause insomnia. Consumption of oats may help sleep.[14,24,55]
   d. **Aromatherapy: Lavender** can be delivered on a hanky, in a small pillow, or in the bath to induce sleep.[78] **See information on aromatherapy, p. 559.**
   e. **Herbs: Chamomile** provides tryptophan, aiding sleep.† It may be taken as an infusion (1 Tblsp/cup tea) or as tincture 10 drops bid.[52] **Hops** may be used as a sedative and sleep inducer. Hops may be taken as a tea at bedtime, or a pillow may be filled with hops.‡ Three cups of tea/d (made with 30 g of cones per liter) or tincture 20 to 80 drops per day.[52] Sleep may be improved with an **oat straw** infusion, which eases night sweats, anxiety, depression, and headaches. Fresh, green, flowering organic oat straw should be used. Drinking a cup of oat straw infusion at bedtime with milk

---

*References 15,16, 20, 28, 32, 47, 55, 60, 65, 72.
†References 7, 30, 46, 47, 55, 73.
‡References 7, 30, 38, 39, 41, 46, 47, 52, 54, 58, 67, 72.

and one at breakfast or sleep on an oat hull pillow will deliver these effects.* Chamomile can be added for taste. Tincture has a more sedative effect.[47] **Passion flower** improves sleep by increasing serotonin levels.† The dose of passion flower tincture is 15 to 60 drops before bed.[78] **Skullcap** tea may relieve insomnia.[14,39,55,67,72] **Valerian** acts as sedative and is indicated for insomnia and anxiety.‡ Dosage is 10 to 25 drops of tincture, bid to tid[52] or 1 cup of tea 1 hour before bed (made with 1 tsp herb to 150 mL water).[58] Prolonged use and large doses can be addictive and are to be avoided.[30,52] Catnip tea is also suggested.[24,39,68] **See information on herbs, p. 563.**

Loss of Libido

There is no evidence that menopause itself is associated with a loss of libido. Many older women do not have sexual partners because of divorce or death. Arousal time is increased for both men and women with aging. Symptoms of menopause including urogenital discomfort, fatigue, insomnia, and depression may secondarily affect libido.[69]

ⓜ *Management*

1. **Address primary physical problems.**
2. Make the following **lifestyle suggestions:** Consider **counseling** if needed. **Limit alcohol** intake.[80]
3. **Androgen/estrogen combination therapy** is controversial. Libido is multifactorial and difficult to quantify. Androgen improves mood and one's sense of well-being and is sometimes prescribed for loss of libido postmenopause. Risks and side effects must be carefully considered.[6,44]
4. **Complementary measures: Herbs: Damiana** has been used over time as an aphrodisiac[7,24,29,46] and may have testosterone-like actions, but it is a nerve tonic that treats depression and fatigue.[30,46] **See information on herbs, p. 563.**

Menstrual Irregularities

Menstrual irregularities may continue for months to years, as discussed on p. 532.[69]

ⓜ *Management*

1. See the discussions regarding premenstrual syndrome (p. 454) and dysmenorrhea (p. 451) for descriptions of management of these disorders. Intermenstrual bleeding (see p. 453) or heavy bleeding (see p. 453) should be investigated for pathologic causes.

---

*References 7, 24, 47, 52, 55, 78.
†References 7, 14, 24, 30, 41, 46, 47, 54, 55, 72.
‡References 7, 30, 41, 46, 47, 52, 58.

2. **Educate** the woman about menopause.
3. **Complementary measures** (See also information on menorrhagia, p. 454).
   a. **Homeopathic** measures are recommended by some experts.[60,78]
   b. **Nutritional measures:** The woman with heavy menses should have adequate **iron intake.** See p. 355. According to Weed,[78] menstrual irregularities are reduced if dietary intake of **animal fats** is reduced because animal fats are converted to estrogen in the body. Fresh wheat germ oil also helps to **regulate menses.**
   c. **Herbs:** *Vitex agnus-castus,* or chaste tree, regulates female hormones and is used to treat the menstrual irregularities associated with menopause.[14,30,41,46] *Vitex* berries in tincture, 25 drops several times daily for several months, will decrease heavy bleeding, although the effect is slow to appear.[78] For other menstrual irregularities, see the specific disorder in the gynecology chapter with its complementary measures. **See information on herbs, p. 563.**

Osteoporosis

Bone loss occurs at a rate of approximately 3% during the first 5 years after the onset of menopause and at a rate of 1% thereafter. Osteoporosis is diagnosed when bone mineral density decreases to <2.5 standard deviations below the young adult peak value.[6] About 40% of postmenopausal women will have a fracture due to osteoporosis.[9] Hip fractures frequently occur 15 to 25 years after menopause, and a 30% mortality rate accompanies such a fracture within the first year.[6] See Box 10-2 for the factors that predispose women to osteoporosis. Factors protective against osteoporosis include increased parity, android body fat distribution (higher waist-to-hip ratio), lactation,[44] and large, dense bones in early adult life.[7]

ⓜ *Management*

1. **Dietary suggestions:**
   a. A **high calcium intake** throughout the life cycle is recommended. See Box 10-3 for suggested calcium intake.
   b. **Limit protein** (6 oz/d), **phosphorous,** and **sodium** (found, for example, in soft drinks and processed foods)—all of which decrease calcium in the system. **Caffeine and sugar** cause the blood to become more acidic, which causes calcium to be released from the bones to act as a buffer. **Salt** increases the urinary excretion of calcium. Foods containing **oxalic acid,** which inhibits calcium absorption, should be consumed in moderation and include spinach, rhubarb, almonds, asparagus, beet greens, cashews, and chard. **Citrus fruits and tomatoes** may inhibit calcium absorption.[7] **Alcohol** reduces the body's ability to use calcium, alters the retention of calcium in the kidneys, and thus contributes to osteoporosis.[41]

• *Box 10-2* / **Predisposing Factors for Osteoporosis** •

- Northern European and Asian ancestry
- Family history
- Thin body habitus
- Early menopause
- Impaired ovarian function
- Early pregnancy
- Medical illnesses including cancer
- Smoking
- Sedentary lifestyle
- Alcohol and caffeine intake
- Inadequate calcium intake
- High dietary salt, sugar, phosphorus
- Medications including antineoplastic agents, anticonvulsants, steroids, heparin, drugs used for endometriosis, long-term levothyroxine sodium replacement, and the use of depot medroxyprogesterone acetate (DMPA)

Data from Balch JF, Balch PA: *Prescription for nutritional healing*, ed 2 Garden City Park, New York, 1997, Avery; and Lichtman R: Perimenopausal and postmenopausal hormone replacement therapy. Part 2. Hormonal regimens and complementary and alternative therapies, *J Nurse Midwifery* 41:195-210, 1996.

• *Box 10-3* / **Suggested Daily Calcium Intake** •

- Young adult women: 1000 mg qd
- Females 11 to 24 years: 1200 to 1500 mg qd
- Postmenopausal females not taking estrogen: 1200 to 1500 mg qd
- Postmenopausal females taking HRT: 1000 mg qd[5]
- Maximum daily dose: 2500 mg qd[49]

---

   c. **Phytoestrogens** are chemicals with estrogenic properties found in a number of foods including apples, potatoes, yams, soy products, bean sprouts, red clover sprouts, sunflower seeds, rye, wheat, sesame seeds, flaxseed, and some alcoholic beverages that may have a favorable effect on bone mass.[43,80] ACOG[6] states that relatively high doses of these substances would have to be consumed to equal the effect of HRT.

   d. Long-term intake of **soy and isoflavones** may protect against osteoporosis, but they are contraindicated in the woman with estrogen-dependent cancer.[2]

2. **Calcium supplementation:** When choosing a **calcium supplement,** note the amount of elemental calcium in the tablet. Calcium carbonate

contains the highest percentage of elemental calcium.[7] **Vitamin D,** 400 IU/d (obtained by being in the sun for 15 minutes 3 times/wk), facilitates absorption of calcium and should be supplemented after menopause to prevent osteoporosis if the woman is not exposed to the sun for adequate periods.[47] Calcium must be balanced with **magnesium** and **phosphorus.** The calcium dose should be double the magnesium dose and should be 66% to 100% of the phosphorus dose.[14,47] The woman who takes a **diuretic** should consult with her physician before supplementing calcium because different diuretics affect calcium needs. The woman replacing **thyroid hormone** should increase her calcium replacement by 25% to 50%.[7] **Iron, zinc, and vitamins A and C** assist the body in utilizing calcium and must be obtained in the diet or by supplementation.[20]

3. Provide the following **lifestyle suggestions:**

   a. **Exercise** increases bone mass. It potentiates the increase in bone mass that ERT provides. Weight-bearing exercise is the most beneficial, and benefits have been seen with a twice-a-week regimen. For cardiovascular benefits, the exercise should be continuous for at least 20 minutes and should increase the heart rate to 60% to 80% of the age-predicted maximum.[7,43]

   b. **Smoking** tobacco, which interferes with the body's ability to use calcium, should be discontinued.[20]

4. **Pharmacologic interventions:** Prevention of osteoporotic fractures has been considered the most widely accepted indication for **ERT.**[9] Estrogen protects against postmenopausal bone loss. Estrogen plus calcium is the most protective combination. Estrogen must be continued indefinitely to maintain its protective effects.[44,81] The 2002 Women's Health Initiative[84] found that **HRT** prevented five hip fractures (a reduction of one third compared with a placebo group) per 10,000 woman-years. However, the risk of heart disease was increased by seven events; the risk of breast cancer, by eight more invasive cases; and the risk of pulmonary embolism by eight more cases per 10,000 woman-years. They concluded that the substantial cardiovascular and breast cancer risks must be weighed against the prevention of fractures.[84] Calcitonin, biphosphonates, alendronate, tibolone, selective estrogen receptor modulators, and sodium flouride are other medications prescribed to increase and preserve bone mass.

5. **Complementary measures:**

   a. Some experts suggest **homeopathic** remedies for osteoporosis.[60]

   b. **Herbs:** Herbal remedies suggested are those herbs known to be rich in calcium. **Horsetail** increases calcium absorption; strengthens bones, nails, hair, and teeth; and promotes healthy skin and healing of bones and cartilage.[7,14,20,41,78] Weed[78] suggests drinking 1 cup tea tid (1 tsp/1 cup water steeped 5 minutes). **Nettle** is high in calcium[7,14,78]: one cup of infusion may be consumed tid.[78] **Oat straw** is also calcium-rich.[14,20,41,78] **See information on herbs p. 563.**

Skin Changes

Estrogen receptors are present in the epidermis and dermis. Dryness, increased tendency to bruise, slower healing, decreased melanocytic activity, and sometimes acne are seen in the perimenopausal woman. Skin tags (fibroepitheliomas), seborrheic keratoses (sharply defined, flat, brown papules), De Morgan's spots (cherry angiomas—red, dome-shaped papules), and acne rosacea (inflammatory condition of the sebaceous glands) occur with increasing frequency.[73] Smoking and stress exacerbate these symptoms.[44]

During perimenopause, some women experience odd skin sensations such as "creepy crawly" feelings. Other women experience dryness of the oral mucosa.

ⓜ Management

1. Provide **lifestyle suggestions** for dry skin. Educate the woman to **drink 8 glasses of water** every day and **avoid caffeine.** Advise her to control **environmental humidity.** Large house plants or open containers of water in each room maintain humidity. Use of **mild soaps, such as moisturizing castile soap,** and **emollients** with 10% to 20% urea or lactic acid may reduce drying. **Regular exercise and deep breathing** open the small skin capillaries and keep them vital. Advise the woman to use a **sunscreen** when in the sun. **Smoking cigarettes** has an antiestrogenic effect, causes premature aging of the skin, and should be **discontinued.**[32]
2. **For dry mouth, review medications** being taken to determine whether dry mouth is a side effect.[78] **Lifestyle suggestions** include **consumption of raw foods** for maintaining blood flow to the gums. Good **oral hygiene** is important to maintain oral and dental health. **Acidic and sugar-containing drinks should be avoided.**[32]
3. **Medical intervention: Estrogen** appears to reduce the skin changes associated with menopause, including dry oral membranes, and although this alone does not justify prescribing ERT, the benefit may assist the woman in making her treatment decision.[44,69]
4. **Complementary measures:**
   a. Some experts suggest **herbal remedies** for dry skin and for "crawling" skin sensations.[14,78]
   b. **Homeopathic remedies** are suggested for oral dryness.[32]
   c. **Nutritional measures:** For moisturizing the skin, take 2 tsp of uncooked flaxseed oil daily (e.g., in salad dressing).[14,20] **Dry mouth** can be relieved by drinking **barley or rice water.** Boil a handful of grain in 4 cups of water for 1 hour.[78]

Urinary Symptoms

Urinary tract changes are discussed on p. 533. Incontinence has been reported in 15% to 60% of postmenopausal women, though many studies have been conducted in women >60 years of age.[44,69] Urinary symptoms may be related to chronic constipation or sexual activity.[32]

m Management

1. **Exclude UTI** (see p. 389) and **associated factors** (sexual activity or chronic constipation) as causative.[32]
2. See p. 470 regarding urinary incontinence.
3. **Medical intervention:** Systemic and intravaginal **estriol** prevents recurrent UTI in postmenopausal women. The efficacy of estrogen on urinary incontinence is unclear, though it appears to be useful, particularly for urge incontinence.[6,44]
4. **Complementary measures:**
   a. **Homeopathic remedies** are suggested for urinary symptoms of menopause by Ikenze.[32]
   b. **Acupuncture** has helped some women with chronic bladder problems.[78]
   c. **Aromatherapy:** Freeman[20] suggests that the essential oil of **fennel** may be placed directly on the skin, used as a bath oil, or inhaled as treatment for cystitis. **See p. 559 for information on aromatherapy.**
   d. **Nutritional measures: Bioflavonoids**, chemicals found in certain foods, have a mild estrogenic effect, as well as an estrogen receptor–blocking effect, strengthening the bladder. **Bladder irritants** include coffee, alcohol, black tea, sodas, chocolate, citrus juices, cayenne, and hot peppers. **Bladder infections** will be reduced with the elimination of all forms of sugar (even fruit) for a month.[78]

Vaginal Changes

Vaginal changes of menopause are discussed on p. 533.

m Management

1. Consider elimination of any **medication** that causes drying of the mucous membranes, such as antihistamines, which may also cause vaginal dryness.[20]
2. **Lifestyle suggestions: Continuation of sexual activity** is recommended to maintain vaginal lubrication and suppleness.[43,56] Increased foreplay assists in lubrication. A coital position in which the woman can control thrusting may relieve dyspareunia.[20,56] Many older adults remain sexually active into the ninth decade, although they may feel embarrassed to discuss it. If widowed, they may feel guilt or performance anxiety about relating to a new partner. Frank discussion, new positions, or the use of vibrators, creams, or oils may help the woman more fully enjoy sexual activity.[59]

   The **Kegel exercise** helps to maintain vaginal muscle tone and increase blood supply to the perineal area and may be beneficial to the sexual response.[56] The home may be **humidified,** and women should **drink** 8 glasses of water each day to maximize hydration. *Replens,* a nonhormonal vaginal moisturizer, compares favorably with Premarin in vaginal lubrication. Intravaginal use is recommended every 2 to 3 days.[43] Other **water-soluble lubricants** may be used[20]; almond or coconut **oil** may be applied to the vagina for relief of dryness. Vitamin E alone[56] or mixed with a water-soluble lubricant may be used. However, many water-soluble lubricants contain glycerin, to which some women are allergic.[32] **Vitamin E** cream (without fragrance) or the oil from a vitamin E capsule applied locally stops vaginal itching and treats dryness.[55] Remind clients that vitamin E preparations, because they are oil-based, *cannot* be used with latex condoms.

Oral **zinc** supplementation (15 mg daily) is suggested for **vaginal lubrication.**[14,20] Crawford[14] suggests that **vitamin E,** 400 to 600 IU/d PO, increases vaginal lubrication for many women. It may be better absorbed, she states, if taken with vitamin C 1000 to 3000 mg. Supplementation of more than 100 IU of vitamin E may be contraindicated in women with diabetes, hypertension, or rheumatic heart conditions and in women receiving digitalis or anticoagulants.[75]

3. **Medical intervention: Intravaginal ERT** increases vaginal lactobacilli, vaginal acidity, and the vaginal epithelium maturation index after 2 weeks of daily treatment.[44] Unfortunately, maturation is reversed when the dose is reduced for a maintenance schedule, and compliance with use of vaginal cream is often poor because it is messy.[56]

4. **Complementary measures:**
   a. Some experts recommend **homeopathic remedies** for vaginal atrophy.[32,78]
   b. **Nutritional measures: Bioflavonoids**, chemicals found in certain foods, have a mild estrogenic effect, as well as an estrogen receptor–blocking effect, and increase vaginal lubrication.[78] Increasing **phytoestrogen** intake may be beneficial,[41,80] although one study could not demonstrate improvement in vaginal maturation indices in a supplemented group.[1] **Women who have any of the contraindications for estrogen replacement should avoid bioflavonoids and phytoestrogens, because the estrogenic properties of these herbs and foods may cause the same complications as estrogen therapy.**
   c. **Herbs: Chickweed,** used regularly, reduces vaginal dryness and may reduce itching. The dose is 25 to 40 drops of tincture, taken qd to bid.[24,47,78] **Dong quai** contains phytoestrogens and relieves vaginal dryness.* Dong quai is an estrogen precursor and should

---

*References 7, 20, 41, 47, 75, 78.

be **avoided if estrogen is contraindicated.** The dose is 10 to 40 drops fresh root tincture qd to tid; 4 to 8 oz of dried root in 25 to 50 mL of infusion or tea may be consumed qd; or a piece of dried root (1/8 to 1/4 inch [4 to 6 mm]) may be chewed bid to tid.[78] Consumption of dong quai in the form of a tea or a few drops in tincture form placed under the tongue stimulates the body's production of estrogen but may take several weeks to have any affect.[20] **See information on herbs, p. 563.**

Vasomotor Symptoms

Vasomotor symptoms, called *hot flushes* or *flashes* and *night sweats*, were reported by 72% of menopausal American women in one study.[44] In 57% of women, hot flashes persist for more than 5 years; 10% will experience the flashes for more than 15 years, and some, for 30 years.[75] The flashes are described as a feeling of intense heat rising from the upper chest or neck to the face and head. Vasodilation occurs in the skin, moving from one part of the body to another, and may be accompanied by palpitations, vertigo, weakness, perspiration, and anxiety.[44] Frequency ranges from rare to every 10 to 30 minutes.[75] Hot flashes occur in both surgical and naturally occurring menopause but are more intense and frequent during the first 6 months after surgical menopause.[44] The exact cause of hot flashes is not understood, but it is thought that the hypothalamic neurotransmitters are altered because of the loss of negative feedback from estrogen. The increased norepinephrine level stimulates the thermoregulatory center in the hypothalamus.[75]

ⓜ *Management*

1. Begin by **identifying the triggers** for hot flashes.[20] Common triggers are listed in Box 10-4. **Record-keeping** may help to sort out causative events and agents.[75] Then identify **lifestyle change solutions.** For example, dressing in light layers will ease coping with the hot flashes, allowing layers to be taken off and replaced. Freeman[20] suggests regular exercise, wearing natural fibers, and keeping water and a fan nearby when the environment cannot be controlled. Exercise, biofeedback, yoga, meditation, prayer, relaxation,[43] slow deep-breathing exercises, and guided imagery have been shown to be effective.[75]

2. **Dietary interventions:** Problematic foods may be avoided or combined with other foods. Alcohol should be used in moderation and is less irritating if taken with food. Smaller, more frequent meals will decrease the dilation of blood vessels and may reduce the frequency of hot flashes.[20]

    Phytoestrogens, partial estrogen agonists and antagonists, are nonsteroidal plant compounds that have been suggested for the relief of vasomotor symptoms. However, in one study, postmenopausal women were given 60 g of soy powder daily for 3 months and no

> ### • *Box 10-4 /* Common Triggers for Hot Flashes •
>
> - Chocolate
> - Fats
> - Hot and humid weather
> - Hot tubs, saunas
> - Clothing made of synthetic fibers
> - Tobacco
> - A warm bed
> - Intense exercise, including sexual activity
> - Stress and anxiety
> - Anger, especially unexpressed
> - Alcohol
> - Marijuana
> - Spicy foods
> - Hot drinks and soups
> - Dairy products
> - Acidic foods such as pickles, citrus, or tomatoes
> - Caffeine
> - White sugar
>
> ---
>
> Data from Balch JF, Balch PA: *Prescription for nutritional healing*, ed 2, Garden City Park, New York, 1997, Avery; Freeman SB: Menopause with HRT: complementary therapies, *Contemp Nurse Pract* 1:40-49, 1995; and Weed S: *Menopausal years: the wise woman way*, Woodstock, NY, 1992, Ash Tree.

reduction in vasomotor symptoms was noted.[1] Other researchers have found that a diet supplemented with soy products increased HDL cholesterol levels by 5.5% and reduced LDL levels by 9%. Levels of osteocalcin, a marker of bone formation, increased by 13%, whereas the number of osteoclasts, cells that cause bone loss, decreased by 14.5%. Genistein, one of the soy isoflavones, is said to inhibit metastatic uterine cancer and a type of endometrial cancer.[53]

Vitamin E is thought to decrease FSH and LH production, and some believe it provides relief from hot flashes.[7,75] Supplementation has been advocated in doses of 200 to 600 IU daily, but supplements >100 IU/d are contraindicated for women with diabetes, high BP, or rheumatic heart conditions and women receiving digitalis or anticoagulants.[43] Freeman[20] suggests a maximum dose of 400 IU/d for the latter chronically ill women and doses of up to 800 IU/d for healthy women, warning that this fat-soluble vitamin may cause side effects including nausea and blurred vision. It should be taken after a meal or with lecithin.[43]

Foods high in **vitamin C** such as citrus fruits, rose hips jam, and fresh broccoli will relieve hot flashes.[14] Balch and Balch[7] also suggest vitamin C for hot flashes at a dose of 3000 to 10,000 mg qd. **Vitamin B complex** is also said to help with hot flashes.[75] Vitamins B_2, B_6, and B_{12} are helpful for hot flashes.[78] Balch and Balch[7] state that the entire vitamin B complex is useful in supporting cellular function; vitamin B_5 100 mg tid, supports adrenal function; and vitamin B_6, 50 mg tid, eases vasomotor symptoms and minimizes water retention. **Magnesium,** 500 mg, taken between meals will prevent **palpitations.**[78] Magnesium is found in whole grains and vegetables and may be depleted by diarrhea, excess alcohol intake, diuretic therapy, and stress, as well as by the intake of processed foods from which magnesium has been removed.[47]

3. **Pharmacologic interventions: ERT** may be prescribed on a short-term basis for vasomotor symptoms.[44] Palpitations, also a vasomotor response, respond to ERT.[69] **HRT** increases the risk for cardiovascular and thromboembolic events (although not the risk for breast cancer) when used on a short-term basis, and prescribing the smallest dose for the shortest period is recommended.[84] Clonidine hydrochloride, danazol, Bellergal (a combination of belladonna, ergotamine tartrate, and phenobarbital),[6,75] progesterone products,[42] and tranquilizers or sedatives[41] may also be prescribed for the vasomotor symptoms of menopause. **Fluoxetine** (Prozac, a selective serotonin reuptake inhibitor [SSRI]) (20 mg qd) was shown to reduce hot flashes by 50% compared with placebo in one study.[45]

4. **Complementary measures:**
   a. **Homeopathy** experts recommend their remedies for hot flashes.[32,55,60,78] Some recommend **homeopathic** measures specifically for palpitations.[60] **Acupuncture** may reduce the frequency and intensity of hot flashes.[43,75]
   b. **Herbs: Black cohosh, dong quai, and ginseng contain phytoestrogens and are contraindicated in the patient for whom estrogen supplementation is contraindicated. Black cohosh** is effective for relief of vasomotor symptoms. It may relieve palpitations as well.* ACOG[6] states that black cohosh may be helpful in the short term (≤6 months) for relief of hot flashes. For profound hot flashes, usually experienced after surgical menopause, black cohosh root tincture, 30 to 60 drops, may be taken up to qid.[78] **Dong quai** *(Angelica sinensis)* may reduce hot flashes and palpitations.† Ten to 40 drops of fresh root tincture may be taken qd to tid; 4 to 8 oz of dried root in 25 to 50 mL of water for infusion or tea may be consumed daily; or a piece of dried root ($\frac{1}{8}$ to $\frac{1}{4}$ inch [4 to 6 mm]) may be chewed bid to tid.[78] It may take several weeks to have any effect.[20,75] **Ginseng** may reduce stress that may be triggering hot flashes; may increase the pain threshold and reduce depression, increasing feelings of well-being; and may reduce fatigue and improve stamina.[14,24,75,78] Results are seen in 2 to 3 weeks.

   For palpitations related to hot flashes, motherwort combines a cardiovascular tonic with a relaxant and a hormonal

---

*References 14, 24, 41, 47, 71.
†References 7, 20, 24, 41, 47, 75, 78.

tonic.[14] Described as "soothing the heart," it is helpful for palpitations and anxiety and has a sedative effect.[30,46,47,58] Weed[78] suggests a dose of 10 to 20 drops of tincture with meals and at bedtime or 25 to 50 drops of tincture when palpitations are experienced. **Hawthorn,** a "nourisher of the circulatory system," increases blood flow to the heart, dilates the coronary blood vessels, and may decrease cholesterol levels and lower elevated BP. It is suggested for hypertension, "weakness of the heart," and palpitations.[14,24,30,46]

Garden sage reduces or eliminates night sweats.[24,46,52,78] Infusion (1 to 4 Tblsp/20 to 60 mL) may be taken in a cup of hot or cold water. Results are usually prompt and last up to 2 days. Alternately, 1 to 2 spoonfuls of dried leaf tea can be consumed 1 to 8 times/d; or 5 to 40 drops of fresh leaf tincture may be taken 1 to 3 times/wk.[78] **Valerian** acts as a sedative and is indicated for insomnia and hot flashes.[7,30,46,52,58] A water-soluble extract is the best form.[7] Dosage is 10 to 25 drops of tincture, bid to tid.[52] **Avoid prolonged use and large doses of valerian because it is addictive. See information on herbs, p. 563.**

• HORMONE REPLACEMENT THERAPY

In 1992, 39 million prescriptions were written for estrogen replacement, up from 16 million in 1982. Fifteen to twenty-five percent of all eligible women took the preparations[3] before the Women's Health Initiative Study was published. Administration of estrogen only is referred to as *ERT*; administration of estrogen in combination with progesterone is referred to as *HRT* or *combination therapy*. The hormonal preparation, dosage, and duration are determined by the indications for use.[43] Box 10-5 lists factors the woman and her provider should consider when determining whether she should use hormone replacement. Box 10-6 lists contraindications to various hormone replacements.

Risks of Hormone Replacement Therapy

Unopposed ERT is associated with a 2.3 to 4.0 increased relative risk of **endometrial cancer** as compared with no therapy; the risk continues for 5 years after cessation of use.[82] Concomitant administration of progestins is protective against endometrial cancer, although whether the effect is complete is controversial.[10]

A year 2000 multicenter study of more than 46,000 postmenopausal women demonstrated that the relative risk of receiving a diagnosis of **breast cancer** for lean women (BMI ≤24.4) who had taken ERT within 4 years was 1.2, increasing annually by 0.01. The relative risk for women taking HRT within the last 4 years was 1.4, increasing annually by 0.08. No increased risk was found for heavy women.[63] A sec-

• *Box 10-5* / Factors To Consider: Whether To Use Hormone Replacement •

- Desire for symptom relief
- Degree of disability caused by a symptom
- One's own philosophy and belief symptoms regarding exogenous hormones
- Individual risk factors for osteoporosis, cardiovascular disease, colon cancer, and breast cancer
- Previous experience with daily medication compliance
- Interest in and experience with alternative treatments
- Willingness to alter lifestyle
- Concerns about the affects of aging
- Fear of various diseases
- Economic considerations

Data from Lichtman R: Perimenopausal and postmenopausal hormone replacement therapy. Part 2. Hormonal regimens and complementary and alternative therapies, *J Nurse Midwifery* 41:195-210, 1996; and Writing Group for the Women's Health Initiative Investigators: Risks and benefits of estrogen plus progestin in healthy postmenopausal women: principal results from the Women's Health Initiative Randomized Controlled Trial, *JAMA* 288:321-333, 2002.

• *Box 10-6* / Contraindications to Hormone Replacement Therapy •

Absolute Contraindications to HRT	Relative Contraindications to HRT	Absolute Contraindications to Unopposed ERT
Breast or endometrial cancer	History of breast or uterine cancer	Contraindicated for the woman with her uterus because of risk of endometrial hyperplasia[82]
Other estrogen-dependent tumors	Large fibroids	
Acute liver disease	Chronic liver disease	
Acute thrombophlebitis	Endometriosis	
Thromboembolic disorder	Hyperlipidemia	
Undiagnosed vaginal bleeding	Gallbladder disease	
Pregnancy	Fibrocystic breast disease	
	History of thromboembolic events, including CVA, MI	
	Hypertriglyceridemia	
	Hypertension aggravated by estrogen	
	Migraine headaches	
	Hepatic porphyria	
	Possibly seizure disorders	
	Possibly bronchial asthma	

Data from Waldman TN: Menopause: when hormone replacement therapy is not an option. Part I. *J Womens Health* 7: 559-565, 1998.

ond year 2000 study demonstrated an increased risk for breast cancer only after 15 years of ERT use, especially in thin women, with a relative risk of 1.24. Most of these cancers were in situ when they were diagnosed. The risk of breast cancer increased 10% for every 5 years of HRT use, and the cancer identified was comparable for all stages. Authors suggested that adding progestin to decrease the risk of endometrial cancer might be reconsidered in light of the increased risk for breast cancer.[61] Kuller[40] concluded that "there is little question" that both ERT and HRT are "associated with an increased risk for breast cancer, especially with long-term use." The Women's Health Initiative of 2002[84] measured the outcomes after administration of HRT and found an increase of 8 invasive breast cancer cases/10,000 woman-years, exceeding, along with increased cardiovascular risks, the benefits of that therapy.

For the **woman with a history of breast cancer,** HRT does not cause a tumor to occur; rather, existing tumor cells may be stimulated to grow more quickly. Therefore HRT should be prescribed only after careful consideration in consultation with the woman's oncologist.[6]

The risk of **gallbladder disease** is doubled with estrogen replacement.[64]

The risk of **venous thromboembolism** is increased by 2 to 3.5 times with HRT, though the absolute risk remains small and the risk is greater for women with other risk factors.[17,33] Women currently receiving ERT and HRT are at increased risk for **pulmonary embolism,**[17,33] at an absolute risk rate of 5/100,000 person-years of use by women 50 to 59 years of age.[26] The Women's Health Initiative of 2002[84] documented an increase of 8 more pulmonary embolisms per 10,000 woman-years among women taking HRT.[84]

HDL levels increase with ERT; estrogen with cyclic progesterone replacement showed the next highest increase, and estrogen with continuous progesterone therapy showed some increase, whereas placebo showed a decrease in HDL levels. All of the hormonal regimens showed **decreased mean LDL levels and increased triglyceride levels** when compared with placebo, and the placebo group alone experienced a rise in fibrinogen levels.[83] The American Heart Association concluded that the evidence does not support initiation of HRT for the purpose of primary prevention of **coronary heart disease.** Rather, noncoronary benefits and risks should be considered in making the decision.[50] In fact, the Women's Health Initiative of 2002 documented an increase of 7 coronary heart events among healthy women per 10,000 woman-years among women receiving HRT.[84]

The 1998 Heart and Estrogen/Progestin Replacement Study (HERS) indicated that the woman with a history of cardiovascular disease receiving estrogen with progestins actually has an increased risk of fatal and nonfatal coronary heart disease in the first year of HRT therapy. The authors conclude that **HRT is not useful in the secondary prevention**

of coronary heart disease.[31] The woman who develops cardiac disease while taking HRT should be evaluated, and discontinuance should be considered.[50]

Some researchers report that **BP** appears not to be affected by ERT or HRT.[83] Others report idiosyncratic increases in BP. Transdermal estrogen causes no such idiosyncratic increase and may be preferable for women with hypertension.[69]

Estradiol does not reduce mortality or the risk of having a stroke among women who are prescribed estradiol after a CVA or transient ischemic attack (TIA), and it is not indicated for **secondary prevention of cerebrovascular disease.**[74] The Women's Health Initiative of 2002 documented an increase of 8 more CVAs per 10,000 woman-years among women taking HRT.[84]

Exacerbation of **endometriosis** may occur. Recurrence of endometriosis should be treated by discontinuing the ERT, and possibly by initiating progestin-only replacement therapy.[6] **Fibroids** may enlarge with estrogen stimulation. If metromenorrhagia or vaginal discomfort occurs, ERT may need to be discontinued.[41]

Estrogen has been causally related to adult-onset **asthma.**[64]

Estrogen

Action: Stimulation of estrogen receptors in body tissues.

Benefits of ERT: Perimenopausal symptoms are reduced by ERT, which is generally given for this indication for about 5 years. **Bone mineral density** (BMD) is improved,[81] although replacement must be continued for life to maintain the benefit. Miscellaneous benefits of ERT include significant reduction of the risk of fatal **colon cancer**, improving with longer duration of use and remaining even in former users.[25] The effect of estrogen on **osteoarthritis** has been beneficial according to some studies,[51] but results are not definitive.[21]

Side Effects of Oral Estrogen: Side effects may include breast tenderness, nausea, weight gain, and headaches; and irritability similar to that associated with premenstrual syndrome (PMS) may be experienced.

Estrogen Preparations: Estrogen may be administered orally; transdermally; in the form of vaginal cream or vaginal rings; or as a subcutaneous implant. Unopposed estrogen may be taken cyclically—3 weeks on, 1 weeks off—or continuously. Alcohol abuse, cigarette smoking, surgically induced menopause, and the use of psychotropic medications increase the required dose. The woman who desires monthly withdrawal bleeding may require a higher dose. The woman who takes ERT for relief of menopausal symptoms may require up to twice this dose, to be tapered later. Side effects may be minimized by switching compounds.

Three classes of exogenous estrogens are available for postmenopausal hormone replacement:

1. Endogenous estrogens including estradiol, estriol, and estrone
2. Conjugated equine estrogens (Premarin) extracted from the urine of pregnant mares, composed of estrone (50%), and estrogens not found in humans
3. Synthetic estrogens (more potent than the estrogens used in hormone replacement, used primarily for contraception)[44]

Progestin

Actions: Progesterone opposes estrogen's effect on the **endometrium,** decreasing the risk of endometrial adenocarcinoma.[41] Progesterone alone **reduces the incidence of hot flashes** by 60% to 80%. Progestin therapy may be especially effective when a woman is having hot flashes while continuing to menstruate regularly with high endogenous estrogen levels. However, the PEPI study showed that hot flashes were not affected by the addition of progestin to ERT.[23] Progestin may also be useful when a woman has a contraindication to ERT. Progestin is thought by some to **increase bone mass.**[41,42]

Side Effects: Side effects are dose-related and may include depression and anxiety, breakthrough bleeding, weight gain, headaches, bloating, breast tenderness, abdominal cramping, fatigue, skin disorders, and malaise.[23,43]

Progestin Preparations: Progestins are available in the following forms: oral capsules, transdermal patches, vaginal creams, subcutaneous implants, intramuscular injections, percutaneous gels, vaginal rings, and facial creams.

Natural progesterones are biologically unavailable when taken orally because they are rendered ineffective by the gastric secretions and by absorption into and metabolism by the liver. Synthetic progesterones have androgenic properties, which probably cause the side effects including dysphoria, depression, headaches, bloating, and weight gain. Four are used for HRT: depot medroxyprogesterone, medroxyprogesterone acetate, norethindrone acetate, and micronized progesterone. Progesterone cream, extracted from Mexican yams, provides precursors of progesterone. Proponents state that this cream is identical to the natural progesterone of the human ovaries or placenta, increases bone density, and increases feelings of well-being; and that compliance with use is excellent because of a lack of side effects.[79] However, in a 1999 study no protective benefit in bone density was demonstrated after one year of use, although 83% of subjects noted a reduction in vasomotor symptoms.[42] Some creams marketed as progesterone creams actually contain the herbal precursors sarsasapogenin and diosgenin, from which the body cannot make progesterone—no active drug is present in the creams.[79]

Oral Contraceptives

Low-dose oral contraceptives (OCs) replace the ovarian estrogen, progesterone, and androgen needed for HRT. If serum lipid levels are normal and the patient does not smoke cigarettes, the healthy perimenopausal woman ≤50 years old may use OCs for HRT during perimenopause. OCs suppress vasomotor symptoms, regulate menses, provide birth control, and protect bone mass.[69] The protective effect against ovarian and endometrial cancers is beneficial. However, the dose of estrogen, even in low-dose OCs, is 4 times the dose needed for postmenopausal hormone replacement, and switching to HRT is suggested after menopause.[18] Women who have been taking OCs in their forties can be tested yearly after age 50 for their FSH levels on day 6 or 7 of the non-hormone week. They may begin taking HRT when the FSH level exceeds 30 mIU/mL.[43]

Testosterone

Testosterone may be added to ERT or HRT to increase libido or to relieve vasomotor symptoms that estrogen has not helped. Although it is controversial, this treatment may be especially beneficial for the woman who has experienced surgical menopause. Androgens will increase total cholesterol levels (both HDL and LDL), may interact with other medications, and are associated with many side effects.[6,43]

• REFERENCES

1. Albertazzi P et al: Dietary soy supplementation and phytoestrogen levels, *Obstet Gynecol* 94:229-231, 1999.
2. American College of Obstetricians and Gynecologists (ACOG): *Use of botanicals for management of menopausal symptoms*, Practice Bulletin No. 28, Washington, DC, June 2001, ACOG.
3. ACOG: *September is National Menopause Awareness Month* [news release], Washington, DC, 1999, ACOG. Available at: http://www.acog.com/from_home/publications/press_releases/898mam.htm; downloaded January 31, 1999.
4. Reference deleted in galleys.
5. ACOG: *Women are never too young to protect against bone loss* [Woman's Health Column], Washington, DC, 1999, ACOG. Available at: http://http:www.acog/com/from_home/publications/womans_health/wh5-12-7.htm; downloaded January 31, 1999.
6. ACOG: *Hormone replacement therapy*, Educational Bulletin No. 247, Washington, DC, May 1998, ACOG.
7. Balch JF, Balch PA: *Prescription for nutritional healing*, ed 2, Garden City Park, New York, 1997, Avery.
8. Reference deleted in galleys.
9. Barrett-Connor E et al: Hormone and nonhormone therapy for the maintenance of postmenopausal health: the need for randomized controlled trials of estrogen and raloxifene, *J Womens Health* 7:839-847, 1998.
10. Beresford SA et al: Risk of endometrial cancer in relation to use of oestrogen in combination with cyclic progestagen therapy in postmenopausal women, *Lancet* 349:458-461, 1997.
11. Reference deleted in galleys.
12. Budd S: Acupuncture. In Tiran D, Mack S, editors: *Complementary therapies for pregnancy and childbirth*, Philadelphia, 2000, Baillière Tindall.
13. Campbell C: Primary care for women: comprehensive cardiovascular assessment, *J Nurse Midwifery* 40:137-149, 1995.
14. Crawford AM: *Herbal remedies for women*, Rocklin, Calif, 1997, Prima.

15. Cummings B, Tiran D: Homeopathy for pregnancy and childbirth. In Tiran D, Mack S, editors: *Complementary therapies for pregnancy and childbirth*, Philadelphia, 2000, Baillière Tindall.

16. Cummings S, Ullman D: *Everybody's guide to homeopathic medicines*, New York, 1997, Jeremy P. Tarcher/Putnam.

17. Daly E et al: Risk of venous thromboembolism in users of hormone replacement therapy, *Lancet* 348:977-980, 1996.

18. Dickey RP: *Managing contraceptive pill patients*, ed 10, Dallas, Tex, 2000, EMIS Medical.

19. Reference deleted in galleys.

20. Freeman SB: Menopause with HRT: complementary therapies, *Contemp Nurse Pract* 1:40-49, 1995.

21. Gharib SD: Osteoarthritis prevention: another role for estrogen? *Journal Watch: Women's Health* 1(9):67-68, 1996.

22. Goldstein SR: Selective estrogen receptor modulators: a new category of therapeutic agents for extending the health of postmenopausal women, *Am J Obstet Gynecol* 179:1479-1484, 1998.

23. Greendale GA et al: Symptom relief and side effects of postmenopausal hormones: results from the Postmenopausal Estrogen/Progestin Interventions Trial, *Obstet Gynecol* 92:982-988, 1998.

24. Griffith HW: *Healing herbs: the essential guide*, Tucson, 2000, Fisher Books.

25. Grimes DA, editor: Weighing the risks and benefits of hormone replacement therapy after menopause, *The Contraception Report* 6(4):4-11,16, 1995.

26. Grodstein F et al: Prospective study of exogenous hormones and risk of pulmonary embolism in women, *Lancet* 348:983-987, 1996.

27. Guyton AC: *Textbook of medical physiology*, ed 8, Philadelphia, 1991, WB Saunders.

28. Hanafin MJ: *An introduction to homeopathy* [lecture handout and notes], American College of Nurse-Midwives Annual Convention, San Francisco, May 1998.

29. Hoffmann D: *The complete illustrated holistic herbal*, Boston, 1996, Element Books.

30. Hoffmann D: *The holistic herbal*, Findhorn, Scotland, 1985, The Findhorn Press.

31. Hulley S et al: Randomized trial of estrogen plus progestin for secondary prevention of coronary heart disease in postmenopausal women. Heart and Estrogen/progestin Replacement Study (HERS) Research Group, *JAMA* 280:605-613, 1998.

32. Ikenze I: *Menopause and homeopathy*, Berkeley, Calif, 1998, North Atlantic Books.

33. Jick H et al: Risk of hospital admission for idiopathic venous thromboembolism among users of postmenopausal oestrogens, *Lancet* 348:981-983, 1996.

34. Johnson E: Shiatsu. In Tiran D, Mack S, editors: *Complementary therapies for pregnancy and childbirth*, Philadelphia, 2000, Baillière Tindall.

35. Reference deleted in galleys.

36. Johnson LC: Menopausal choices. Part I. *Northern California Woman*, pp 11-13, Feb 1996.

37. Reference deleted in galleys.

38. Kloss J: *Back to Eden*, New York, 1981, Benedict Lust Publications.

39. Koehler N: *Artemis speaks: V.B.A.C. stories & natural childbirth information*, Occidental, Calif, 1985, Jerald R. Brown.

40. Kuller LH: Re: Effect of hormone replacement on breast cancer risk: estrogen versus estrogen plus progestin, *J Natl Cancer Inst* 92:1100-1101, 2000 (letter).

41. Lark SM: *The estrogen decision*, Berkeley, Calif, 1995, Celestial Arts.

42. Leonetti HB, Longo S, Anasti JN: Transdermal progesterone cream for vasomotor symptoms and postmenopausal bone loss, *Obstet Gynecol* 94:225-228, 1999.

43. Lichtman R: Perimenopausal and postmenopausal hormone replacement therapy. Part 2. Hormonal regimens and complementary and alternative therapies, *J Nurse Midwifery* 41:195-210, 1996.

44. Lichtman R: Perimenopausal and postmenopausal hormone replacement therapy. Part 1. An update of the literature on benefits and risks, *J Nurse Midwifery* 41:3-28, 1996.

45. Loprinzi CL et al: Phase III evaluation of fluoxetine for treatment of hot flashes, *J Clin Oncol* 20:1578-1583, 2002.

46. Mabey R et al, editors: *The new age herbalist*, New York, 1988, Collier Books.
47. Medina IM: *Issues in women's health care: nutrition and herbs from menarche to menopause 3/28-29/98* [course syllabus], Brooklyn, NY, State University of New York Health Science Center at Brooklyn College of Health Related Professions Midwifery Education Program, 1998.
48. Reference deleted in galleys.
49. Morris VM, Rorie JL: Nutritional concerns in women's primary care, *J Nurse Midwifery* 42:509-520, 1997.
50. Mosca L et al: Hormone replacement therapy and cardiovascular disease: a statement for healthcare professionals from the American Heart Association, *Circulation* 104:499-503, 2001.
51. Nevitt MC, et al: Association of estrogen replacement therapy with the risk of osteoarthritis of the hip in elderly white women, *Arch Intern Med* 156:2073-2080, 1996.
52. Nissim R: *Natural healing in gynecology*, San Francisco, 1996, Pandora (HarperCollinsPublishers).
53. Northrup C: Answers to your most frequently asked questions about soy, *Health Wisdom for Women* 6:4-5, 1999.
54. Ody P: *The complete medicinal herbal*, New York, 1993, Dorling Kindersley.
55. Page L: *Healthy healing*, ed 11, Carmel Valley, Calif, 2000, Healthy Healing Publications.
56. Papera S: Urogenital atrophy, *Quickening* 28:9,14, 1997.
57. Parvati J: *Hygieia: a woman's herbal*, Berkeley, Calif, 1985, Bookpeople.
58. *Physician's desk reference for herbal medicines*, Montvale, NJ, 1998, Medical Economics.
59. Read J: Sexual problems associated with infertility, pregnancy, and ageing, *BMJ* 318: 587-589, 1999.
60. Rose B, Scott-Moncrieff C: *Homeopathy for women*, London, 1998, Collins & Brown.
61. Ross RK et al: Effect of hormone replacement therapy on breast cancer risk: estrogen versus estrogen plus progestin, *J Natl Cancer Inst* 92:328-332, 2000.
62. Sacher RA, McPherson RA: *Widmann's clinical interpretation of laboratory tests*, ed 10, Philadelphia, 1991, FA Davis.
63. Schairer C et al: Menopausal estrogen and estrogen-progestin replacement therapy and breast cancer risk, *JAMA* 283:485-491, 2000.
64. Scharbo-Dehaan M: Hormone replacement therapy, *Nurse Pract* 21:1-13, 14-15, 1996.
65. Smith T: *Homeopathy for pregnancy and nursing mothers*, Worthing, England, 1993, Insight Editions.
66. Speroff L, Glass RH, Kase NG: *Clinical gynecologic endocrinology and infertility*, Philadelphia, 1999, Lippincott Williams & Wilkins.
67. Stapleton H, Tiran D: Herbal medicine. In Tiran D, Mack S, editors: *Complementary therapies for pregnancy and childbirth*, Philadelphia, 2000, Baillière Tindall.
68. Tarr K: *Herbs, helps, and pressure points for pregnancy and childbirth*, ed 3, Provo, Utah, 1984, Sunbeam.
69. Thacker H: Menopause, *Prim Care* 24:205-221, 1997.
70. Tobin LJ: Evaluating mild to moderate hypertension, *Nurse Pract* 24:22-43, 1999.
71. Tuso P: The herbal medicine pharmacy: what Kaiser Permanente providers need to know, *The Permanente Journal* 3:33-37, 1999.
72. Ullman R, Reichenberg-Ullman J: *Homeopathic self-care*, Rocklin, Calif, 1997, Prima.
73. Varney H: *Varney's midwifery*, ed 3, Sudbury, Mass, 1997, Jones and Bartlett.
74. Viscoli CM et al: A clinical trial of estrogen-replacement therapy after ischemic stroke, *N Engl J Med* 345:1243-1249, 2001.
75. Waldman TN: Menopause: when hormone replacement is not an option. Part II. *J Womens Health* 7:673-683, 1998.
76. Reference deleted in galleys.
77. Warga C: *Menopause and the mind*, New York, 1999, Simon and Schuster.
78. Weed S: *Menopausal years: the wise woman way*, Woodstock, NY, 1992, Ash Tree.
79. Wetzel W: Micronized progesterone: a new option for women's health care, *Nurse Pract* 24:62-76, 1999.

80. Whitlock EP: Managing menopause: alternatives to HRT, *Journal Watch: Women's Health* 3(3): 23-24, 1998.
81. The Writing Group for the PEPI Trial: Effects of hormone therapy on bone mineral density. Results from the Postmenopausal Estrogen/Progestin Interventions (PEPI) Trial, *JAMA* 276:1389-1396, 1996.
82. The Writing Group for the PEPI Trial: Effects of hormone replacement therapy on endometrial histology in postmenopausal women. The Postmenopausal Estrogen/Progestin Interventions (PEPI) Trial, *JAMA* 275:370-375, 1996.
83. The Writing Group for the PEPI Trial: Effects of estrogen or estrogen/progestin regimens on heart disease risk factors in postmenopausal women. The Postmenopausal Estrogen/Progestin Interventions (PEPI) Trial, *JAMA* 273:199-208, 1995.
84. Writing Group for the Women's Health Initiative Investigators: Risks and benefits of estrogen plus progestin in healthy postmenopausal women: principal results from the Women's Health Initiative Randomized Controlled Trial, *JAMA* 288:321-333, 2002.

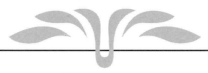

Chapter 11

Complementary Measures

Recent surveys show that more than 80% of Americans use complementary and alternative therapies, although many do not report this fact to their Western medical care providers.[26] People seek out alternatives to Western medicine because they are dissatisfied with conventional medicine, because they want greater control over their health, because the alternatives are philosophically and spiritually attractive, and because they cost less.[14,41]

Many of these therapies have come into use traditionally and have not been studied extensively in the Western scientific manner. In 1992, the U.S. Congress created the Office of Alternative Medicine within the National Institutes of Health to promote research and evaluation and to establish an information clearinghouse for these therapies.[26] Western health care providers express concern that consumers may attempt to self-treat with alternative approaches, delaying—possibly too long—definitive Western medical care. They also may use a product without sufficient information and suffer serious side effects or drug interactions.[14] Historic use of substances does not guarantee their safety, critics state, offering as evidence that tobacco's capacity to cause lung cancer was unknown for so long. Single and occasional use of a substance may not result in side effects as would the chronic use of some drugs.[12] Furthermore, calling many of these mass-produced and packaged preparations "natural" is considered ludicrous by some.[9]

This chapter offers a brief overview of the theory and practices of only some of these alternatives; approximately 350 techniques and treatments are available.[1] Further study is urged for midwives who are interested in integrating these measures into their practice. Although some of the remedies may be harmless, others have side effects, drug interactions, toxicities, and quality, standardization, and contamination problems. Others are powerful interventions that must be respected and used with caution, especially during pregnancy. Before incorporating alternative therapies into practice, midwives should study the area of interest to develop a knowledge base, determine what they consider to be safe and acceptable ethical practice, and give their clients informed consent.

• AROMATHERAPY

The ancient practice of aromatherapy involves administration of highly concentrated oils or essences distilled from plants to utilize a therapeutic property of that plant.[34] Nerve fibers in the nose carry the sensory input through the olfactory bulb directly to the limbic system of the brain—the evolutionarily ancient center where instincts, memories, and vital functions are formed and regulated. All other sensory information is perceived first by more sophisticated portions of the brain and then sent to the limbic system. Thus the sense of smell is primal and compelling. Smells are also absorbed through the alveoli and the skin and are excreted by urine, feces, sweat, and exhalation. Essential oils are used to relieve stress and are suggested for a variety of medical conditions.[37] Some oils are contraindicated throughout pregnancy. Others are suggested only after the fifth month and then only in small, dilute amounts. Many oils are contraindicated for children. Toxic effects of oils may include skin irritation, liver toxicity, cardiac failure, hypertension or hypotension, potentiation of alcohol, or photosensitivity.

• CHINESE MEDICINE

Traditional Chinese medicine visualizes the human being as the integrated "bodymindspirit." The life force is called Ch'i (or Qi), which, in good health, flows like water in streams and rivers in a balanced, harmonious fashion. Ch'i flows along energy paths in the body known as the meridians. The 12 meridians correspond to the 12 "main functions" of the body.[5,29] Chinese medicine is ideally used to maintain good health rather than to be consulted only for symptoms of disease.[27] According to Chinese medicine, symptoms are signals that there is a disruption in the flow of energy—clues to an underlying imbalance and not something in themselves to be suppressed.[5,23]

The human body is regarded as a microcosm of the universe, also containing all the elements and being governed by the forces of yin and yang.[27] The "organs" in Chinese medicine refer to concepts developed in ancient times, and the functions assigned to them are not always the same as the literal organ functions known by Western scientists. Each organ is associated with an element (fire, wood, metal, earth, or water), an emotion, a taste, a color, a time of day, a season, an odor, a sound, a sense organ, a body orifice, a direction, a flavor, a body fluid, and a pathway (meridian) where Ch'i energy flows.[5]

Acupuncture involves the placement of needles at points along the meridians. Some practitioners see a pattern of all the body's meridians

> • **Box 11-1** / Acupoints to Be Avoided During Pregnancy
> (May Be Useful at the End of Pregnancy): •
>
> • BL-60, BL-67, LI-4, and SP-6[2,6]
> • Points on the lower abdomen[2,6]
> • Points on the lower back[2,6,19]
> • Points on the lower inner leg[19]
> • Points on the sacrum[19]

in the ear and treat only the ear points.[39] Acupuncture should be avoided during pregnancy, and the use of a number of points is forbidden to minimize the risk of miscarriage or preterm labor (Box 11-1). Only an experienced acupuncturist should treat a condition during pregnancy.[10]

Acupressure

Pressure may be used to stimulate acupoints in a treatment, or a small bean or seed can be positioned to stimulate a point over a period of time.[4] To perform acupressure, identify the desired point on a chart and then on the body (Figure 11-1). Points are the size of a pinhead and are quite tender. The tip of the index and/or middle fingers, the edge of a fingernail, or the blunt end of a pair of tweezers is used. "Digging stimulation" provides deep massage to the point.[29] Pressure is applied for 30 seconds, then let go for 10 seconds, and repeated 3 to 5 times.[6] This treatment may be repeated on the opposite side or may be performed bilaterally and simultaneously for the most effect.[29]

Shiatsu (meaning "finger pressure") is a form of acupressure that is combined with massage, integrating knowledge of the meridians and involving the holding of acupoints.[19,27] Moxibustion involves the application of heat to these points. Transcutaneous electrical nerve stimulation (TENS) is a technique in which electrical stimulation is applied to electrodes attached to the skin at acupoints.

Point locations (described in terms of "divisions," the measurement of the patient's thumb between the proximal and distal phalanges) relevant for the midwife include:

Bladder 10: Located on the neck, 1.3 divisions lateral to the median line, at the base of the occipital bone and on the trapezius muscle.[38]

Bladder 23: Located on the back, between the second and third lumbar vertebrae, just behind the navel, 2.5 divisions lateral to the median line.[27,38]

Bladder 31 and Bladder 32: Located on the sacrum, under the first and second sacral vertebrae in the upper foramen and second foramen.[6,38]

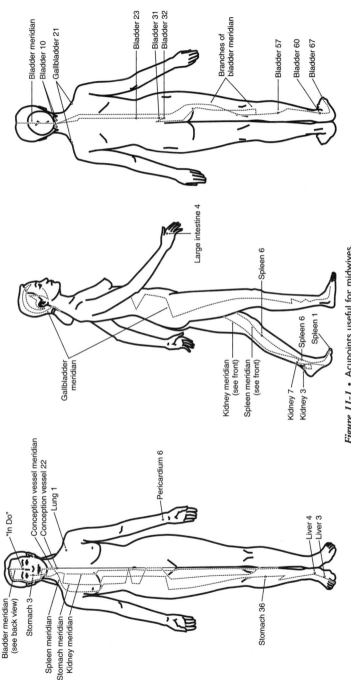

Figure 11-1 • Acupoints useful for midwives.

Bladder 57: Located on back of the thigh, in the depression between the lateral and medial heads of the gastrocnemius muscle.[38]

Bladder 60: Located on the outer aspect of the leg near the ankle, one half division posterior to the prominence of the lateral malleolus, halfway between this prominence and the Achilles tendon.[6,38]

Bladder 67: Located on the little toe, one eighth inch proximal to the lateral base of the fifth toenail.[6,38,39]

Conception Vessel 22: Located on the neck, on the median line just below the cricoid cartilage.[38]

Gallbladder 21: Located on the upper back above the scapula, at the juncture of two imaginary lines: one from the seventh cervical to the acromion, and one from the nipple to the highest point on the shoulder. Locate using the thumb and middle finger to grasp the muscle and using the index finger to press down on the middle of the muscle until you feel the muscle divide in half. The acupoint is between the two halves.[6]

Kidney 3: Located on the inside of the thigh, located 1 division above the prominence of the medial malleolus over the posterior tibial artery.[38]

Kidney 7: Located at the inner ankle, 3 divisions above the prominence of the medial malleolus behind the flexor digitorum longus.[38]

Large Intestine 4: Located on the top of the hand, along the lateral edge of the second metacarpal, just distal to its junction with the first metacarpal.[6,39]

Liver 3: Located on the top of the foot, in a depression on the pulse distal to the junction of the bases of the first and second metatarsals.[6,38]

Liver 4: Located on the top of the foot, in a straight imaginary line from between the great and second toes, at the flexure of the ankle.[38]

Lung 1: Located on the upper chest wall, 1.6 divisions below the inferior border of the clavicle, between ribs 1 and 2.[38]

Pericardium 6: Located on the inside of either wrist between the two tendons, 3 fingerbreadths above the wrist fold.[2,39]

Spleen 1: Located on the great toe, on the medial side at the base of the nail.[38]

Spleen 6: Located on the inner aspect of the leg above the ankle, 3 divisions superior to the prominence of the medial malleolus and just posterior to the medial edge of the tibia. Look for the most sensitive area because the point may vary by up to three fourths of a division.[6,38,39]

Spleen 9: Located on the inner aspect of the leg, on the medial ridge of the tibia is a depression between the posterior border of the tibia and the gastrocnemius muscle. Find it by sliding the finger up the inner aspect of the tibia, to the place the finger stops, noting its tenderness.[6]

Stomach 3: Located on the face, directly under the center of the orbit, at the level of the nares.[38]

Stomach 36: Located on the lower leg, 1 division below the tibial tuberosity and 3 inches below the lower border of the patella in a depression between the edge of the tibia and the tibialis anticus muscle.[38]

In Do: A point not related to a meridian; located on the face between the eyebrows.[38]

• HERBAL REMEDIES

Herbalism may be defined as the use of crude plant-based products to treat, prevent, or cure a disease.[14] Proponents characterize herbal medicine as health oriented rather than illness oriented and offer herbs they consider more in harmony with the natural rhythms of the body. The whole plant is used rather than isolating active constituents, reducing side effects and potency and allowing the various ingredients of a given plant to work together synergistically. Herbalists set aside concerns regarding standardization, noting that individuals even respond differently to standardized drugs such as insulin or digoxin.[31] Concerns of Western medical caretakers regarding herbal remedies include:

1. **Have all the components of the herb been researched?**
2. How are the **raw materials** chosen? (Soil, temperature, season, maturity, and location affect composition.)[8]
3. How are the herbs **processed:** extraction, drying process, and storage?[15]
4. Is the drug **standardized?**
5. Are there any **potentially harmful additives?**
6. Are there **warnings,** cautions, an **ingredient list**, and an **expiration date** on the container?[8]
7. Are there data regarding **interactions with other drugs?**
8. Is the herb **being used properly** by the consumer?

Glisson et al[14] suggest the following guides when prescribing natural products:

• Recommend only pure, standardized products.
• Develop experience with one or two specific herbal product lines and educate clients regarding the quality variations in herbal products.
• Develop a relationship with a knowledgeable pharmacist in your area who is willing to consult regarding herbal products.
• Educate the client regarding the proper use, length of use, side effects, food and drug interactions, and possible side effects.
• Educate the client regarding lifestyle and medical interventions that remain essential while the herb is being used.
• Include questions regarding alternative health care in ongoing care.

Throughout this text, herbal remedies are noted as complementary measures under management. This author is not an herbalist and has concerns about the use of herbs, especially during pregnancy. However, the first step in integrating herbal remedies into practice would be to identify those herbs suggested by many herbalists, eliminating those that are suggested by one practitioner who may have had anecdotal experience with an herb and inferred a causal relationship. The remedies given in this text are herbs suggested by 3 or more herbalists. Report suspected side effects of herbs and drug interactions with herbs to the Food and Drug Association Medwatch at 1-800-FDA-1088.

• *Box 11-2* / Herbs Contraindicated During Pregnancy*† •

- Aloe leaf; Mediterranean, Curacao, or Barbados aloe; Aloe vera, barbadensis, or officinalis[11,25,29]
- Angelica[11,15,29] (European or garden or Angelica archangelica
- Anise or Pimpinella anisum[15]
- Arborvitae[31]
- Arnica[25]
- Autumn crocus[11,16]
- Barberry (European) or Berberis vulgaris[11,15,21,25,29,31]
- Beth root, birthroot, or Trillium erectum or pendulum[25]
- Bittermelon[25]
- Black cohash, black snake root, rattle root, squaw root, or Cimicifuga racemosa (safe only in the last 4 weeks' gestation)[11,25,29,31]
- Bladderwrack or Fucus vesiculosus[25]
- Blood root[21,25]
- Blue cohash, papoose root, squaw root, or Caulophyllum thalictroides[13,22,25,31]
- Blue flag[25]
- Broom[25]
- Buchu (honey or short-leaf mountain) or Barosma betulina[15,25,29]
- Buckthorn or Rhamnus cathartica[15,29]
- Burdock (great or edible), lappa or Arctium lappa[15]
- Calamus root; rat, sweet, or flagroot; acore; sweet flag; sweet myrtle; sweet cane or sweet sedge; calamus or Acorus calamus[15,21]
- Calendula, pot marigold, or Calendula officinalis[25]
- Cascara sagrada (buckthorn) or Rhamnus purshiana[15,21,25,29]
- Cat's claw, una de gato, or Uncaria tomentosa[15]
- Cayenne, red or red-hot; Spanish, Africa, chili, or American pepper; capsaicin or Capsicum frutescens or annuum[21]
- Celandine[21]
- Celery seed[11,15]
- Chamomile, Anthemis nobilis or flores[15]
- Chaparral[25]
- Cinchona[31]
- Cinnamon, camphor, or Cinnamonum camphora (medicinal)[11,15,25]
- Coltsfoot, coughwort, horse-hoof, or Tussilago farfara[25]
- Comfrey, knitbone, or Symphytum officinale[15,29]
- Cotton root[25,31]
- Couch grass, dog grass, triticum, or Agropyrum repens[15]
- Cranesbill, crowfoot, or Geranium maculatum[25]
- Damiana or Turnera diffusa[15,25]
- Devil's claw[11]
- Dogwood (American), American boxwood, or Cornus florida[15]
- Dong quai, Chinese angelica, dang gui, tank kwei, or Angelica sinensis[25]
- Echinacea, purple coneflower, or Echinacea augustifolia or pallida[28]
- Elecampane[25]
- Eleutherococcus[25]
- Ephedra[21,25,29]

---

*NOTE: This list is not exhaustive but contains more commonly used herbs. Note that the variation among authors is significant.
†Reference citations correspond with reference list at the end of this chapter.

• *Box 11-2 /* Herbs Contraindicated During Pregnancy*†—cont'd •

- Eucalyptus[25]
- Fennel, finocchio, or foeniculum[15,21]
- Feverfew, altamisa, bachelor's buttons, or Tanacetum parthenium[15,25,35]
- Flaxseed, linseed, or Linum usitatissimum[15,21]
- Gentian, yellow gentian, or Gentiana lutea[25]
- Gingko (biloba) or ginkgoaceae[25,28]
- Ginseng (Asian, panax, American, Korean, or Chinese)[23,25]
- Goldenseal or Hydrastis canadensis[11,13,15,16,21,22,24,25,29,31]
- Greater celandine[31]
- Guaiacum[25]
- Hops[25]
- Horsetails, bottle brush, shave grass, or Equisetum arvense[15]
- Hyssop or Hyssopus officinales[11,15,25]
- Inmortal[25]
- Ipecac[25]
- Juniper or Juniperus communis[11,15,16,21,25,29,31]
- Lavender (medicinal use)[21,25]
- Licorice (common), Spanish or Glycyrrhiza blabra[15,21,25]
- Liferoot, ground groundsel, squaw weed, Senecio vulgaris or aureus[15]
- Lobelia, Indian tobacco, asthma weed, or Lobelia inflata[15,25]
- Lovage[29]
- Male fern, aspidium, or Dryopteris filix-mas[11,15,16,21,29]
- Mandrake, love apple, Satan's apple, or Mandragora officinarum[11,15,16,25,29]
- Marjoram[31]
- Mayapple, American mandrake, podophyllum, or Podophyllum peltatum[21]
- Meadow saffron[31]
- Milkwort, Polygala vulgaris, senega[15]
- Mistletoe, Phoradendron serotinum, or Viscum album[13,15,21,22,25,29]
- Mitchella[25]
- Motherwort[25,31]
- Mugwort[25,29,31]
- Mulberry or Morus rubra[15]
- Myrrh or Commiphora molmol[25]
- Ocotillo[25]
- Oregon grape root[25]
- Osha[13,22,25]
- Parsley or Petroselinum crispum (medicinal use)[11,15,25]
- Passion flower, maypop, or Passiflora incarnata[15,21]
- Pennyroyal, Mentha pulegium, or Hedeoma pulegioides[11,13,15,21,22,25,29,31]
- Periwinkle (cape), Madagascar, old maid, Catharanthus roseus, or Vinca rosea[15,21]
- Pleurisy root, butterfly weed, or Asclepias tuberosa[15,25]
- Poke, pokeweed, stoke, or Phytolacca americana[11,15,21,25,31]
- Pulsatilla, May flower, or pasque flower[15,25]
- Rhubarb (not the fruit)[15,21,29]
- Rosemary or Rosmarinus officinalis[11]
- Rue (garden, German, or Rue graveolens)[11,15,22,25,29,31]
- Saffron (saffron crocus or Crocus sativus)[15]
- Saw palmetto[25]
- Sage[11,16,25,31] (avoid while attempting conception)[21]

Continued

- Sarsaparilla[25]
- Sassafras or Sassafras albidum[15,25]
- Senna[25,29]
- Shepherd's purse[29]
- Slippery elm, red elm, Ulmus rubra or fulva[15]
- Snakeroot (Virginia), serpentaria, or Aristolochia serpentaria[15]
- Snakeplant or Rivea corymbosa[15]
- Snakeweed, bistort, or Polygonum bistorta[15]
- Southernwood[11,16]
- Squaw vine, partridgeberry, or Mitchella repens[15,31]
- St. John's wort, klamath weed, or Hypericum perforatum[28]
- Tansy or Tanacetum vulgare[11,13,15,16,21,22,25,29,31]
- Thorn apple, jimson weed, sacred datura, stramonium, or Datura stramonium[15]
- Thuja[11,16,25]
- Thyme (common) or Thymus vulgaris[21]
- Uva ursi (controversial)[25]
- Vervain (European), Verbena, or Verbena officinalis[25]
- Vitex agnus-castus, or chaste tree[16,24,30]
- Western red cedar[13]
- Wild carrot[25]
- Wild cherry[21,25]
- Wild ginger[15,29]
- Wild indigo or Baptista tinctoria[15,25]
- Wild yam root, rheumatism root, or Dioscorea villosa[15,25]
- Witch hazel or Hamamelis virginiana[15,25]
- Wormseed, pigsweed, or Chenopodium ambrosioides[15,25]
- Wormwood, absinthium, or Artemisia absinthium[11,16,21,25,29,31]
- Yarrow or Achillea millefolium (contains thujone)[11,21,22,25,29]
- Yellow dock or Rumex crispus[15,25]
- Yucca[25]

*NOTE: This list is not exhaustive but contains more commonly used herbs. Note that the variation among authors is significant.
†Reference citations correspond with reference list at the end of this chapter.

Herbs to Avoid During Pregnancy

Routine use of herbs is not advocated during pregnancy, while breastfeeding, or for children less than 2 years of age.[15,31] Box 11-2 lists herbs that were noted by one or more authors to be contraindicated during pregnancy.

• HOMEOPATHIC MEDICINE

Homeopathy, first described by Hippocrates, is practiced around the world, especially in Asia, Europe, and Latin America. In 1990, it was estimated that 1% of the U.S. population uses homeopathy.[18] Homeopathy proponents believe that the vital force is the body's healing, balancing energy, and that illness reflects an imbalance in this energy. Symptoms represent the body's effort to heal itself. A homeopathic remedy is chosen to address the mental, spiritual, emotional, and physical dimensions of the individual.[17] Homeopathic remedies are actually energetic treatments.[7] The doses are so small that they are typically safe for use in pregnancy or with infants.[36] The basis of homeopathy is called the "law of similars," which states that a substance that causes symptoms like that of a particular disease in a healthy individual can be used to treat that disease.[29] The remedies stimulate the body's own healing abilities.[36] Because choosing a remedy involves a lengthy, holistic assessment, specific remedies could not be included in this text. Rather, the reader is referred to homeopathy authors who suggest remedies for the problem being discussed.

• REFLEXOLOGY

Developed in ancient Egypt, reflexology is based on the theory that each body part is connected through the nervous system to representative areas of the hands and feet, where a "map" of the body's zones may be visualized. Reflexologists believe that stress accounts for 80% of illness. Reflexology reduces stress and improves the flow of energy, thereby improving lymphatic drainage and stimulating a better blood supply. The therapist does not treat illness but stimulates the body to do so. Illness, tension, or injury in a body part result in tenderness in a corresponding foot zone. Pressure to a reflex point for a specific organ within that foot zone improves function in that organ.[29,33] See Figure 11-2 for a reflexology map. The right foot relates to the right part of the body, whereas the left foot relates to the left side of the body. The exception is in the brain and nervous system because the nervous system crosses (the left brain controlling the right side of the body). The top of the foot represents the front of the body, including muscles, and the sole of the foot represents the back of the body and the internal organs.[33]

Technique

Light or deep pressure is applied in the desired zone, concentrating on tender spots. A rounded tool may also be used. Pressure is applied to the reflex point (using about 15 lb of pressure) 3 times for 10 seconds over a 20- to 30-minute period twice a week.[29,33]

The heel represents the pelvic area, and vigorous massage of this area is avoided during pregnancy to prevent affecting the uterus. Reflexology and reflex zone therapy are contraindicated during pregnancy only when there is a risk of fetal loss, placental pathology, ectopic pregnancy, or any instability.[33]

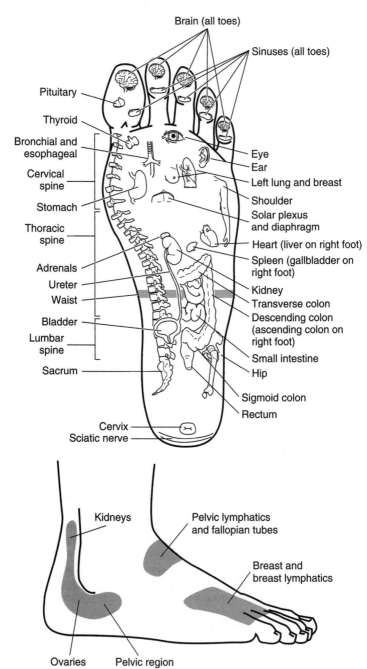

Figure 11-2 • Reflexology points on the foot.

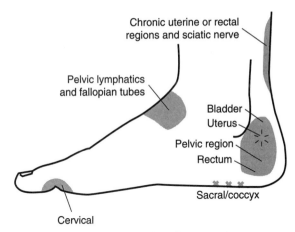

Chronic uterine or rectal regions and sciatic nerve

Pelvic lymphatics and fallopian tubes

Bladder
Uterus
Pelvic region
Rectum

Sacral/coccyx

Cervical

Figure 11-2 • cont'd. For legend, see opposite page.

• REFERENCES

1. American College of Obstetricians and Gynecologists (ACOG): Complementary and alternative medicine: ACOG committee opinion No. 227, Nov 1999.
2. Beal M: Acupuncture and related treatment modalities. Part II: Applications to antepartal and intrapartal care, *J Nurse-Midwifery* 37:260-268, 1992.
3. Reference deleted in galleys.
4. Budd S: Acupuncture. In Tiran D, Mack S, editors. *Complementary therapies for pregnancy and childbirth*. Philadelphia, 2000, Baillière Tindall.
5. Connelly DM: *Traditional acupuncture: the law of the five elements*, Columbia, Md, 1979, The Centre for Traditional Acupuncture.
6. Cook A, Wilcox G: Pressuring pain: alternatives for labor pain management, *Lifelines* April: 36-41, 1997.
7. Cummings B, Tiran D: Homeopathy for pregnancy and childbirth. In Tiran D, Mack S, editors: *Complementary therapies for pregnancy and childbirth*, Philadelphia, 2000, Baillière Tindall.
8. D'Epiro NW: The analytical study of herbs: as yet, a fledgling science, *Patient Care for the Nurse Practitioner* 3:12-18, 2000.
9. Dubick MA: Historical perspectives on the use of herbal preparations to promote health, *J Nutr* 116:1348-1354, 1986.
10. Flaws B: *The path of pregnancy*, Brookline, Mass, 1983, Paradigm Publications.
11. GardenGuides: *Herbs and Pregnancy*, 2000,http://www.gardenguides.com/herbs/preg.htm.
12. Gardiner P, Kemper KJ: Herbs in pediatric and adolescent medicine, *Pediatr Rev* 21: 44-57, 2000.
13. Gardner J: *Healing yourself*, ed 7, Trumansburg, NY, 1982, The Crossing Press.
14. Glisson J, Crawford R, Street S: Review, critique, and guidelines for the use of herbs and homeopathy, *Nurse Practitioner* 24:44-69, 1999.
15. Griffith HW: *Healing herbs*, Tucson, Ariz, 2000, Fisher Books.
16. Hoffmann D: *The complete illustrated holistic herbal*, Boston, Mass, 1996, Element Books.
17. Ikenze I: *Menopause & homeopathy*, Berkeley, Calif, 1998, North Atlantic Books.
18. Jacobs J et al: Treatment of acute childhood diarrhea with homeopathic medicine: a randomized clinical trial in Nicaragua, *Pediatrics* 93:719-725, 1994.

19. Johnson E: Shiatsu. In Tiran D, Mack S, editors: *Complementary therapies for pregnancy and childbirth*, Philadelphia, 2000, Baillière Tindall.
20. Reference deleted in galleys.
21. Kennedy HP, Griffin M, Frishman G: Enabling conception and pregnancy: midwifery care of women experiencing infertility, *J Nurse-Midwifery* 43:190-207, 1998.
22. Koehler N: *Artemis speaks: V.B.A.C. stories & natural childbirth information*, Occidental, Calif, 1985, Jerald R. Brown.
23. Koren G, Pastuszak A, Ito S: Drugs in pregnancy, *N Engl J Med* 338:1128-1137, 1998.
24. Mabey R et al, eds: *The new age herbalist*, New York, 1988, Collier Books.
25. Medina IM: *Issues in women's health care: nutrition and herbs from menarche to menopause*, course syllabus 3/28-29/98, State University of New York Health Science Center at Brooklyn College of Health Related Professions Midwifery Education Program.
26. Murphy PA, Kronenberg F, Wade C: Complementary and alternative medicine in women's health, *J Nurse-Midwifery* 44:192-204, 1999.
27. Ohashi W: *Do-it-yourself shiatsu*, New York, 1976, Dutton.
28. Ondrizek RR et al: An alternative medicine study of herbal effects on the penetration of zona-free hamster oocytes and the integrity of sperm deoxyribonucleic acid, *Fertil Steril* 71:517-522, 1999.
29. Page L: *Healthy living*, 11 ed, Carmel Valley, Calif, 2000, Healthy Healing Publications.
30. *Physician's desk reference for herbal medicines*, Montvale, NJ, 1998, Medical Economics.
31. Stapleton H, Tiran D: Herbal medicine: In Tiran D, Mack S, editors: *Complementary therapies for pregnancy and childbirth,* Philadelphia, 2000, Baillière Tindall.
32. Reference deleted in galleys.
33. Tiran D: Reflexology in midwifery practice. In Tiran D, Mack S, editors: *Complementary therapies for pregnancy and childbirth*, Philadelphia, 2000, Baillière Tindall.
34. Tiran D: Massage and aromatherapy. In Tiran D, Mack S, editors: *Complementary therapies for pregnancy and childbirth,* Philadelphia, 2000, Baillière Tindall.
35. Tuso PJ: The herbal medicine pharmacy: what Kaiser Permanente Providers need to know, *The Permanente Journal* 3:33-37, 1999.
36. Ullman R, Reichenberg-Ullman J: *The patient's guide to homeopathic medicine*, Edmonds, Wash, 1995, Picnic Point Press.
37. Walters C: *Aromatherapy: a basic guide*. New York, 1998, Barnes and Noble.
38. Worsley JR: *The traditional Chinese acupuncture, vol 1: meridians and points*, Longmead Shaftesbury, Dorset, England, 1982, Element Books.
39. Yelland S: *Acupuncture in midwifery*, Cheshire, England, 1996, Books for Midwives Press.
40. Reference deleted in galleys.
41. Ziment I: Eastern "alternative" medicine: what you need to know, *J Respir Dis* 19: 630-644, 1998.

Appendix A

Conversion Tables

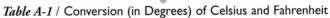

Table A-1 / Conversion (in Degrees) of Celsius and Fahrenheit

Celsius	Fahrenheit	Celsius	Fahrenheit
34.0	93.2	38.6	101.4
34.2	93.6	38.8	101.8
34.4	93.9	39.0	102.2
34.6	94.3	39.2	102.5
34.8	94.6	39.4	102.9
35.0	95.0	39.6	103.2
35.2	95.4	39.8	103.6
35.4	95.7	40.0	104.0
35.6	96.1	40.2	104.3
35.8	96.4	40.4	104.7
36.0	96.8	40.6	105.1
36.2	97.1	40.8	105.4
36.4	97.5	41.0	105.8
36.6	97.8	41.2	106.1
36.8	98.2	41.4	106.5
37.0	98.6	41.6	106.8
37.2	98.9	41.8	107.2
37.4	99.3	42.0	107.6
37.6	99.6	42.2	108.0
37.8	100.0	42.4	108.3
38.0	100.4	42.6	108.7
38.2	100.7	42.8	109.0
38.4	101.1	43.0	109.4

Table A-2 / Conversion of Centimeters and Inches

Centimeters	30	40	50	60
0	11¾ inches	15¾ inches	19¾ inches	23½ inches
1	12¼	16¼	20	24
2	12½	16½	20½	24½
3	13	17	21	24¾
4	13½	17¼	21¼	25¼
5	13¾	17¾	21¾	25½
6	14¼	18	22	26
7	14½	18½	22½	26½
8	15	19	22¾	26¾
9	15¼	19¼	23¼	27¼

Table A-3 / Conversion of Pounds and Ounces to Grams

Pounds \ Ounces	0	1	2	3	4	5	6	7	8	9	10	11	12	13	14	15
0	—	28	57	85	113	142	170	198	227	255	283	312	340	369	397	425
1	454	482	510	539	567	595	624	652	680	709	737	765	794	822	850	879
2	907	936	964	992	1021	1049	1077	1106	1134	1162	1191	1219	1247	1276	1304	1332
3	1361	1389	1417	1446	1474	1503	1531	1559	1588	1616	1644	1673	1701	1729	1758	1786
4	1814	1843	1871	1899	1928	1956	1984	2013	2041	2070	2098	2126	2155	2183	2211	2240
5	2268	2296	2325	2353	2381	2410	2438	2466	2495	2523	2551	2580	2608	2637	2665	2693
6	2722	2750	2778	2807	2835	2863	2892	2920	2948	2977	3005	3033	3062	3090	3118	3147
7	3175	3203	3232	3260	3289	3317	3345	3374	3402	3430	3459	3487	3515	3544	3572	3600
8	3629	3657	3685	3714	3742	3770	3799	3827	3856	3884	3912	3941	3969	3997	4026	4054
9	4082	4111	4139	4167	4196	4224	4252	4281	4309	4337	4366	4394	4423	4451	4479	4508
10	4536	4564	4593	4621	4649	4678	4706	4734	4763	4791	4819	4848	4876	4904	4933	4961
11	4990	5018	5046	5075	5103	5131	5160	5188	5216	5245	5273	5301	5330	5358	5386	5415
12	5443	5471	5500	5528	5557	5585	5613	5642	5670	5698	5727	5755	5783	5812	5840	5868
13	5897	5925	5953	5982	6010	6038	6067	6095	6123	6152	6180	6209	6237	6265	6294	6322
14	6350	6379	6407	6435	6464	6492	6520	6549	6577	6605	6634	6662	6690	6719	6747	6776
15	6804	6832	6860	6889	6917	6945	6973	7002	7030	7059	7087	7115	7144	7172	7201	7228

Appendix B

Body Mass Index

Body mass index (BMI) identifies the degree of adiposity according to the relationship of height to weight and is used to determine the appropriateness of a woman's weight. The following equations may be used to calculate BMI:

$$BMI = [weight\ (kg)/height\ (m^2)] \times 100$$
OR
$$BMI = [weight\ (lb)/height\ (in^2)] \times 705$$

Table B-1 / Evaluation of BMI in Women

BMI	Status
<18.5	Underweight
18.5-24.9	Normal for most women
25-29.9	Overweight
30.0-34.9	Obesity I
35-39.9	Obesity II
≥40	Extreme obesity

From National Heart, Lung, and Blood Institute: *Clinical guidelines on the identification, evaluation, and treatment of overweight and obesity in adults,* Washington, DC, 1998, National Institutes of Health.

Table B-2 / Body Mass Index

Weight (lb)	4'10"	4'11"	5'0"	5'1"	5'2"	5'3"	5'4"	5'5"	5'6"	5'7"	5'8"	5'9"	5'10"	5'11"	6'0"	6'1"	6'2"
							Height (ft, in)										
125	26	25	24	24	23	22	22	21	20	20	19	18	18	17	17	17	16
130	27	26	25	25	24	23	22	22	21	20	20	19	19	18	18	17	17
135	28	27	26	26	25	24	23	23	22	21	21	20	19	19	18	18	17
140	29	28	27	27	26	25	24	23	23	22	21	21	20	20	19	19	18
145	30	29	28	27	27	26	25	24	23	23	22	21	21	20	20	19	19
150	31	30	29	28	27	27	26	25	24	23	23	22	21	21	20	20	19
155	32	31	30	29	28	28	27	26	25	24	24	23	22	22	21	20	20
160	34	32	31	30	29	28	28	27	26	25	24	24	23	22	22	21	21
165	35	33	32	31	30	29	28	28	27	26	25	24	24	23	22	22	21
170	36	34	33	32	31	30	29	28	28	27	26	25	24	24	23	22	22
175	37	35	34	33	32	31	30	29	28	27	27	26	25	24	24	23	23
180	38	36	35	34	33	32	31	30	29	28	27	27	26	25	24	24	23
185	39	37	36	35	34	33	32	31	30	29	28	27	27	26	25	24	24
190	40	38	37	36	35	34	33	32	31	30	29	28	27	27	26	25	24
195	41	39	38	37	36	35	34	33	32	31	30	29	28	27	27	26	25
200	42	40	39	38	37	36	34	33	32	31	30	30	29	28	27	26	26
205	43	41	40	39	38	36	35	34	33	32	31	30	29	29	28	27	26
210	44	43	41	40	38	37	36	35	34	33	32	31	30	29	28	28	27
215	45	44	42	41	39	38	37	36	35	34	33	32	31	30	29	28	28
220	46	45	44	42	40	39	38	37	36	35	34	33	32	31	30	29	28
225	47	46	44	43	41	40	39	38	36	35	34	33	32	31	31	30	29
230	48	47	45	44	42	41	40	38	37	36	35	34	33	32	31	30	30
235	49	48	46	44	43	42	40	39	38	37	36	35	34	33	32	31	30
240	50	49	47	45	44	43	41	40	39	38	37	36	35	34	33	32	31

Continued

Table B-2 / Body Mass Index—cont'd

Weight (lb)	4'10"	4'11"	5'0"	5'1"	5'2"	5'3"	5'4"	5'5"	5'6"	5'7"	5'8"	5'9"	5'10"	5'11"	6'0"	6'1"	6'2"
245	51	50	48	46	45	43	42	41	40	38	37	36	35	34	33	32	32
250	52	51	49	47	46	44	43	42	40	39	38	37	36	35	34	33	32
255	53	52	50	48	47	45	44	43	41	40	39	38	37	36	35	34	33
260	54	53	51	49	48	46	45	43	42	41	40	38	37	36	35	34	33
265	56	54	52	50	49	47	46	44	43	42	40	39	38	37	36	35	34
270	57	55	53	51	49	48	46	45	44	42	41	40	39	38	37	36	35
275	58	56	54	52	50	49	47	46	44	43	42	41	40	38	37	36	35
280	59	57	55	53	51	50	48	47	45	44	43	41	40	39	38	37	36
285	60	58	56	54	52	51	49	48	46	45	43	42	41	40	39	38	37
290	61	59	57	55	53	51	50	48	47	46	44	43	42	41	39	38	37
295	62	60	58	56	54	52	51	49	48	47	45	44	42	41	40	39	38
300	63	61	59	57	55	53	52	50	48	47	46	44	43	42	41	40	39
305	64	62	60	58	56	54	52	51	49	48	46	45	44	43	41	40	39
310	65	63	61	59	57	55	53	52	50	49	47	46	45	43	42	41	40
315	66	64	62	60	58	56	54	53	51	49	48	47	45	44	43	42	41
320	67	65	63	61	59	57	55	54	52	50	49	47	46	45	43	42	41
325	68	66	64	62	60	58	56	54	53	51	50	48	47	45	44	43	42

Appendix C

Clinical Procedures

• AMNIOINFUSION

Indications

1. To thin meconium-stained amniotic fluid and decrease the incidence of meconium aspiration syndrome.[9]
2. To prevent cord compression and fetal heart rate variables[19] (improvement of neonatal outcome and lowering of cesarean rates have not been consistently demonstrated).
3. In the presence of oligohydramnios to prevent cord compression and fetal heart rate variables, theoretically decreasing cesarean section rate. No study has shown improved Apgar scores or cord gas results.[9]
4. Rarely, for irrigation/diluent/delivery of prophylactic antibiotics for postpartum endometritis; although studies have shown that the maternal temperature drops but the incidence of postpartum endometritis does not decrease.[14]
5. Transabdominal amnioinfusion has been used to prevent pulmonary hypoplasia in midtrimester PPROM, but its success is unclear.[9]

Complications[19]

Uterine hypertonus or overdistention
Increased incidence of cord prolapse
Maternal respiratory or cardiac compromise and death
Fetal bradycardia (caused by rapid infusion of cool fluid or secondary to maternal compromise)

Contraindications

Placenta previa
Multiple gestation
Known uterine anomalies
History of a vertical uterine incision
When amniotomy is undesirable, such as in a preterm pregnancy
Vaginal bleeding, especially if placental abruption is suspected
Late decelerations, absent short-term variability, or signs of fetal metabolic acidosis: do not delay delivery

Known fetal anomaly incompatible with life
Uterine hypertonus
Nonvertex presentation
Polyhydramnios

Procedure

1. Rupture membranes if intact.
2. Using the introducer, place the fluid-filled IUPC through the cervix into the uterus to the depth indicated by a mark on the catheter.
3. Transfuse a 250- to 800-mL bolus of NS or LR and follow with a maintenance drip (100 to 200 mL/h). Other protocols suggest 10 to 20 mL/min for 1 hour followed by a maintenance drip of 3 mL/min or until the amniotic fluid index is >5 or >8. Warming the fluid is unnecessary.[9]
4. While administering the amnioinfusion, assess the maternal comfort level, take vital signs hourly, and take the temperature every 2 hours. Record uterine activity, resting tone, and uterine intake and output. The FHR tracing is continually recorded and observed.
5. Discontinue amnioinfusion if the uterine resting tone exceeds 25 mm Hg; continue when it returns to this level.[13]

• STERILE SPECULUM EXAMINATION

A **sterile speculum examination** is indicated to determine whether the amniotic membranes are ruptured or intact. Other functions of the examination include obtaining cultures; observing the cervix for cervicitis, prolapse of umbilical cord, or fetal part; and estimating cervical dilation or effacement.[12] A vaginal examination with a sterile speculum and sterile gloves is performed in case the membranes are ruptured to avoid moving organisms toward the fetus in the intrauterine environment. Lubricant is not used because it may alter findings. The following factors indicate ruptured membranes:

- Trickling of amniotic fluid through the cervix
- Pooling of fluid in the vaginal vault
- Nitrazine paper demonstrating an alkaline reaction to the vaginal fluid (turning blue, approximate pH 7.15)
- Ferning of the vaginal fluid when dried on a microscope slide and examined microscopically

Various substances and conditions in the vagina may alter the accuracy of this examination:

- A **false-negative result of all measures** may occur if the membranes have been ruptured and leaking for a prolonged period, or if the membranes are leaking from a site above the presenting part and minimal fluid is present in the vagina at the time of examination.[5,12,17]
- A **false-positive Nitrazine** result may occur when the paper is contaminated with blood, semen, cervical mucus, urine, bath water, alkaline antiseptics, or water-soluble lubricant.[5,12,17]

• A **false-positive ferning** result will occur if cervical mucus or blood contaminates the slide specimen. Cervical mucus ferning appears "more floral," and ferning of blood is "more skeletal" in appearance than the ferning of amniotic fluid. Meconium, vaginal pH, and blood in the amniotic fluid (up to 20%) will not alter ferning.[1,5]

• THE WET MOUNT

During a speculum examination of the vagina, a wet mount may be prepared of the vaginal secretions by placing a small amount on a slide with a drop of normal saline, then placing a cover slip. Clue cells, bacteria (see p. 474), red blood cells, trichomonas (see p. 480), and sperm may be seen. Another slide is made with 10% potassium hydroxide (KOH) solution. An amine odor after applying the KOH suggests bacterial vaginosis (the "whiff test") (see p. 474). Yeast or pseudohyphae of candida are more easily seen with KOH (see p. 476).[4]

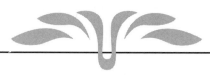

Appendix D

Food and Drug Administration Categories for Safety of Drugs During Pregnancy

The Food and Drug Administration has established the following categories for drugs and medications during pregnancy:

Category A: Controlled studies in women fail to demonstrate a risk to the fetus in the first trimester (and there is no evidence of a risk in later trimesters), and the possibility of fetal harm appears remote.

Category B: Animal studies indicate no fetal risks, but no controlled human studies have been performed. Or, adverse effects have been demonstrated in animals (other than a decrease in fertility) that have not been confirmed in controlled studies in women in the first trimester (and there is no evidence of a risk in later trimesters).

Category C: Adverse effects (teratogenic, embryocidal, or other) have been demonstrated in animal studies, and there have been no controlled studies in women. Drugs should be given only if the potential benefit justifies the potential risk to the fetus.

Category D: There is evidence of fetal risk, but benefits may outweigh the risks.

Category E: Animal studies have proven fetal risks, or there is evidence of fetal risk based on human experience, or both, and the risk clearly outweighs any benefit. The drug is contraindicated in any woman who is pregnant or may become pregnant.

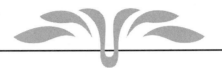

Appendix E

Fetal Skull Landmarks

Determination of Fetal Position by Vaginal Examination

The abdomen is assessed by Leopold's maneuvers (p. 5) and fetal position is determined. The position is confirmed and further defined by vaginal examination and palpation of fetal scalp landmarks.

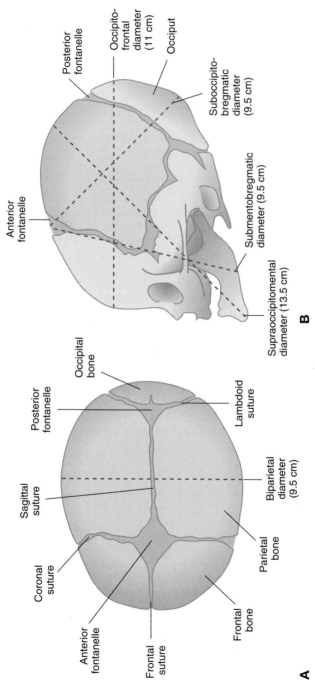

Figure E-1 • The fetal skull and its landmarks. **A,** Lateral view. **B,** Superior view. (From Matteson PS: *Women's health during the childbearing years: a community-based approach*, St Louis, 2001, Mosby.)

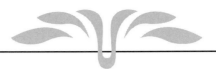

Appendix F

Nutrition Information

In September 2002, the Institute of Medicine's Food and Nutrition Board released a report that analyzed biochemical measurements of energy intake and expenditure for healthy adults. Reference Daily Intakes (RDIs) replaced the decade-old U.S. Recommended Daily Allowance (RDA). An RDA is the average daily intake of a certain nutrient. Daily Reference Values (DRVs) describe nutrients that are not covered by RDIs. These numbers are intended as guidelines and are to be altered for the individual based on total calorie intake and activity.

Table F-1 / Dietary Guidelines for Women

Nutrient	Life Stage	RDA/AI	UL
Calcium	14-18 yr	1300 mg/d*	2500
	19-50 yr	1000 mg/d*	2500
	>50 yr	1200 mg/d*	2500
	Pregnancy		
	≤18 yr	1300 mg/d*	2500
	19-50 yr	1000 mg/d*	2500
	Lactation		
	≤18 yr	1300 mg/d*	2500
	19-50 yr	1000 mg/d*	2500
Iron	14-18 yr	15 mg/d	45
	19-50 yr	18 mg/d	45
	>50 yr	8 mg/d	45
	Pregnancy		
	All ages	27 mg/d	45
	Lactation		
	≤18 yr	10 mg/d	45
	19-50 yr	9 mg/d	45
Magnesium	14-18 yr	360 mg/d	350
	19-30 yr	310 mg/d	350
	≥31 yr	320 mg/d	350
	Pregnancy		
	≤18 yr	400 mg/d	350
	19-30 yr	350 mg/d	350
	31-50 yr	360 mg/d	350

From Institute of Medicine's Food and Nutrition Board: Dietary Reference Intakes of Elements and Vitamins, 2000.
*Adequate intakes.
ND, Not determined; *RDA*, Recommended Daily Allowance; *UL*, tolerable upper intake levels.

Continued

Nutrient	Life Stage	RDA/AI	UL
	Lactation		
	≤18 yr	360 mg/d	350
	19-30 yr	310 mg/d	350
	31-50 yr	320 mg/d	350
Phosphorus	14-18 yr	1250 mg/d	4000
	19-70 yr	700 mg/d	4000
	>70 yr	700 mg/d	3000
	Pregnancy		
	≤18 yr	1250 mg/d	3500
	19-50 yr	700 mg/d	3500
	Lactation		
	≤18 yr	1250 mg/d	4000
	19-50 yr	700 mg/d	4000
Zinc	14-18 yr	9 mg/d	34
	≥19 yr	8 mg/d	40
	Pregnancy		
	≤18 yr	12 mg/d	34
	19-50 yr	11 mg/d	40
	Lactation		
	≤18 yr	13 mg/d	34
	19-50 yr	12 mg/d	40
Folate	14-18 yr	400 g/d	800
	≥19 yr	400 g/d	1000
	Pregnancy		
	≤18 yr	600 g/d	800
	19-50 yr	600 g/d	1000
	Lactation		
	≤18 yr	500 g/d	800
	19-50 yr	500 g/d	1000
Niacin	14-18 yr	14 mg/d	30
	≥19 yr	14 mg/d	35
	Pregnancy		
	≤18 yr	18 mg/d	30
	19-50 yr	18 mg/d	35
	Lactation		
	≤18 yr	17 mg/d	30
	19-50 yr	17 mg/d	35
Riboflavin (B_2)	14-18 yr	1.0 mg/d	ND
	≥19 yr	1.1 mg/d	ND
	Pregnancy		
	All ages	1.4 mg/d	ND
	Lactation		
	All ages	1.6 mg/d	ND
Thiamin (B_1)	14-18 yr	1.0 mg/d	ND
	≥19 yr	1.1 mg/d	ND
	Pregnancy		
	All ages	1.4 mg/d	ND
	Lactation		
	All ages	1.4 mg/d	ND
Vitamin A	14-18 yr	700 g/d	2800
	≥19 yr	700 g/d	3000
	Pregnancy		
	≤18 yr	750 g/d	2800
	19-50 yr	770 g/d	3000

From Institute of Medicine's Food and Nutrition Board: Dietary Reference Intakes of Elements and Vitamins, 2000.
*Adequate intakes.
ND, Not determined; *RDA*, Recommended Daily Allowance; *UL*, tolerable upper intake levels.

Nutrient	Life Stage	RDA/AI	UL
	Lactation		
	≤18 yr	1200 g/d	2800
	19-50 yr	1300 g/d	3000
Vitamin B$_6$	14-18 yr	1.2 mg/d	80
	19-50 yr	1.3 mg/d	100
	>50 yr	1.5 mg/d	100
	Pregnancy		
	≤18 yr	1.9 mg/d	80
	19-50 yr	1.9 mg/d	100
	Lactation		
	≤18 yr	2.0 mg/d	80
	19-50 yr	2.0 mg/d	100
Vitamin B$_{12}$	≥14 yr	2.4 g/d	ND
	Pregnancy		
	All ages	2.6 g/d	ND
	Lactation		
	All ages	2.8 g/d	ND
Vitamin C	14-18 yr	65 mg/d	1800
	≥19 yr	75 mg/d	2000
	Pregnancy		
	≤18 yr	80 mg/d	1800
	19-50 yr	85 mg/d	2000
	Lactation		
	≤18 yr	115 mg/d	1800
	19-50 yr	120 mg/d	2000
Vitamin E	14-18 yr	15 mg/d	800
	≥19 yr	15 mg/d	1000
	Pregnancy		
	≤18 yr	15 mg/d	800
	19-50 yr	15 mg/d	1000
	Lactation		
	≤18 yr	19 mg/d	800
	19-50 yr	19 mg/d	1000
Iodine	14-18 yr	150 µg/d	900
	≥19 yr	150 µg/d	1100
	Pregnancy		
	≤18 yr	220 µg/d	900
	19-50 yr	220 µg/d	1100
	Lactation		
	≤18 yr	290 µg/d	900
	19-50 yr	290 µg/d	1100
Vitamin D (in absence of sunlight)	14-50 yr	5 µg*	50
	50-70 yr	10 µg*	50
	>70 yr	15 µg*	50
	Pregnancy		
	All ages	5 µg*	50
	Lactation		
	All ages	5 µg*	50
Vitamin K	14-18 yr	75 g/d*	ND
	≥19 yr	90 g/d*	ND
	Pregnancy		
	≤18 yr	75 g/d*	ND
	19-50 yr	90 g/d*	ND
	Lactation		
	≤18 yr	75 g/d*	ND
	19-50 yr	90 g/d*	ND
Biotin	14-18 yr	25 g/d*	ND
	≥19 yr	30 g/d*	ND
	Pregnancy		
	All ages	30 g/d*	ND
	Lactation		
	All ages	35 g/d*	ND

Table F-2 / Daily Servings Recommended for the Pregnant Woman[8]

	Dairy Products or Other Calcium-Rich Foods	Fruits (Including One Vitamin C Source)	Grain Products	Protein Foods	Vegetables (Including One Vitamin A Source)
Age 11-24 yr, nonpregnant	2-3	2-4	6-11	2-3	3-5
Age ≥25 yr, pregnant or lactating	3	2-4	6-11	2-3	3-5
Examples of serving size	1 cup milk	6 oz juice	1 slice bread	2-3 oz cooked lean meat, poultry, or fish	½ cup cooked or 1 cup raw spinach
	1 cup yogurt	1 medium orange	1 oz dry cereal	1 egg	6 oz juice
	2 oz processed cheese	½ grapefruit	½ cup cooked cereal, rice, or pasta	2 Tbsp peanut butter	½ cup cooked greens
	3 oz tofu	¼ cantaloupe	½ bagel or roll	½ cup beans	½ cup vegetable
		¼ mango			

From Hally SS: Nutrition in reproductive health. J Nurse-Midwifery 43:459-470, 1998.

Nutrition of the Vegetarian Pregnant Woman

The vegetarian woman who excludes meat but allows fish and/or poultry in her diet will probably receive ample essential amino acids.[20] The source of dietary protein does not appear to affect birth weight as long as the woman supplements with prenatal vitamins, calcium, and iron and applies protein-matching principles.[3]

The strict vegan (no consumption of any food of animal origin, which includes women on macrobiotic diets) will need vitamin B_{12} supplementation because of the elimination of meat—its main source. The high fiber and phytate consumption of the vegetarian diet also binds calcium and reduces its availability. Calcium-fortified soy milk, vitamin B_{12}–fortified soy products, nutritional yeasts, or vitamin-mineral supplements may be taken as sources of these nutrients.[20] Magnesium and zinc may need to be supplemented.[10] Vitamins A and D are usually obtained in animal milks, so other sources must be used.[15]

A daily servings plan for the lacto-ovo vegetarian during pregnancy has been proposed by Medina[11]: milk or milk substitute, 4 servings; protein combo, 6 servings; dark greens, 2 servings; whole grains, 5 servings; vitamin C fruits, 3 servings; fats and oils, 5 servings; vitamin A source, 2 servings; and calcium supplementation as needed.

Appendix G

Laboratory Values

Hematocrit (Hct) (percent of blood that is matter)

- 35% to 47% nonpregnant[6]
- Cutoffs for diagnosis of anemia during pregnancy according to CDC (1998):
  First trimester: <33.0%
  Second trimester: <32.0%
  Third trimester: <33.0%
  - Add 1.0% to 1.5% for smoking ½ pack to 2 packs per day.
  - Add 0.5% for 3000 ft, 1.5% for 5000 ft, and 4.0% for 8000 ft elevation.

Hemoglobin (Hb) (oxygen-carrying pigment in RBCs)

- 11.7 to 15.7 g/dL nonpregnant[6]
- Cutoffs for diagnosis of anemia during pregnancy according to CDC (1998):
  First trimester: <11.0 g/dL
  Second trimester: <10.5 g/dL
  Third trimester: <11.0 g/dL
  - Add 0.3 to 0.7 g/dL for smoking ½ pack to 2 packs per day.
  - Add 0.2 g/dL for 3000 ft, 0.5 g/dL for 5000 ft, and 1.3 g/dL for 8000 ft elevation.

RBC Count

- 3.8 to 5.2 × 10 μ/mL

RBC Indices

Mean Corpuscular Volume (MCV) (average RBC volume)

- 82 to 98 fL

Mean Corpuscular Hemoglobin (MCH) (Hb/L divided by the number of RBCs/L)

- 27 to 34 pg

Mean Corpuscular Hemoglobin Concentration (MCHC) (Hb divided by Hct)

- 32 to 36 g/dL

RBC Distribution Width (RDW) (Elevation indicates variable cell size or anisocytosis)

- 11.5% to 14.6%[6]

Reticulocyte Count (Immature RBCs)

- >2.5% indicates hemolysis; <0.5% indicates marrow failure[2]
- Rises 2% to 5% during pregnancy

Erythrocyte Sedimentation Rate (ESR) (Ability of RBCs to aggregate)

- If the globulin/albumin ratio increases, or the fibrinogen is high (body's response to injury, inflammation, neoplasm, or pregnancy), the ESR rises[16]
- 15 mm/hr[16]

Serum Ferritin

- Best indicator of iron stores[16]
    Female (18 to 50 yr of age): 6 to 81 µg
    Female >50 yr of age: 14 to 186 µg
    Early pregnancy: Wide variations adequate, ranging 20 to 50 µg[7]

Serum Iron

- Drawn in morning after 12-hr fast and no iron supplementation for 12 to 24 hr
- Falls slightly during pregnancy[16]
- 37 to 170 µg/dL[6]

Serum Folate

- During pregnancy, concentration in serum drops; RBC concentration remains constant[16]
- >2.0 ng/mL[2]

Total Iron Binding Capacity (TIBC)

- Increased in iron deficiency anemia and during pregnancy[16]
- 250% to 450%[16]

Transferrin

- Iron transport protein; increases during pregnancy[2]
- 230 to 430 mg/dL[6]

Haptoglobin

- Binds free Hb, decreases when Hb is escaping from cells (e.g., in hemolysis)[16]
- 50 to 320 mg/dL[6]

• PERIPHERAL BLOOD SMEAR TERMINOLOGY AND INTERPRETATION

- **Normocytosis:** Normal, consistent shape, staining, and size of the RBCs
- **Hypochromia:** Diminished RBC color, indicating Hb concentration
- **Microcytosis or macrocytosis:** Small cell size caused by iron deficiency or large cell size caused by megaloblastic anemia, liver disease, or hypothyroidism
- **Anisocytosis:** Variation in RBC size; seen in reticulocytosis
- **Polychromatophilia:** RBCs not fully hemoglobinized; seen in reticulocytosis
- **Leptocytosis:** Hypochromic cells with small central zone of Hb, also called *target cells*; seen in thalassemias and obstructive jaundice
- **Poikilocytosis:** Variations in cell shape, seen in sickle cell disease, leukemia, hemolysis
- **Spherocytosis:** RBCs that are not biconcave in shape; hereditary
- **Schistocytosis:** RBC fragments in circulation due to hemolysis
- **Acanthocytosis:** Irregularly arranged dart-like projections on RBCs caused by membrane lipid content in liver disease; irreversible
- **Echinocytosis:** Regularly arranged dart-like projections on RBCs that represent reversible membrane lipid abnormalities due to lipid, bile acid, or drug content of blood
- **Stomatocytosis:** Elongated slit-like area in center of RBC caused by hereditary membrane sodium-transport defect
- **Elliptocytosis:** Oval RBCs, an inherited—usually harmless—variation
- **Basophilic stippling:** RNA in immature red cells may be seen as stippling
- **Howell-Jolly bodies:** Nuclear DNA fragments in the RBC; present after splenectomy or with intense reticulocytosis in the presence of hemolysis or ineffective erythropoiesis
- **Siderotic granules:** Iron-containing granules in RBCs; seen after splenectomy or with iron overload. Called *Pappenheimer bodies* on Wright-Giemsa–stained smears

- **Heinz bodies:** Masses of denatured hemoglobin; seen with severe oxidative stress, such as G6PD deficiency or thalassemias or seen after splenectomy

• WHITE BLOOD CELL COUNT AND DIFFERENTIAL

During pregnancy, **white blood cell count (WBC)** (leukocytes or neutrophils) should be between 4.0 and 11.0 K/μL.[6] Leukocytosis but not lymphocytosis is normal during pregnancy.[16] The "shift to the left" seen with infection indicates an increase in the less mature polymorphonuclear leukocytes (PMNs), revealing the body's response to infection. Hematologic lab findings may be noted as follows[6,16]:

$$\text{WBC} \xleftrightarrow{\begin{array}{c}\text{Hemoglobin}\\\\\text{Hematocrit}\end{array}} \text{Platelet count}$$

Granulocytes make up ≥50% of the WBCs and include neutrophils, eosinophils, and basophils:
- **PMNs:** 42.7% to 73.3%.[6] Mature white cells.[16]
- **Bands:** 0.0% to 11.0%.[6] Less mature than PMNs, with a band-shaped nucleus.[16]
- **Eosonophils:** 0.0% to 7.5%.[6] Contain histaminase and participate in immunologically mediated inflammation.[16]
- **Basophils:** 0.0% to 2.0%.[6] Function in serum is unknown; in tissue they are called mast cells. They contain histamine and cause allergic tissue reactions.[16]

Monocytes: 2.0% to 11.0%.[6] Begin as stem cells, then differentiate into macrophages (phagocytes) and circulate in small numbers.[16]

Lymphocytes: 12.5% to 40.0%.[6] The second most common WBC; interact with antigens and mount a humoral, a cytotoxic, or a cell-mediated defense.[16]

Laboratory Testing of Renal and Liver Function

Blood urea nitrogen (BUN): 5 to 25 mg/dL.[6] Urea from the metabolism of protein, cleared by the kidneys; levels are elevated in renal failure.[16]

Serum creatinine: 0.5 to 1.4 mg/dL.[6] End product of creatine metabolism, produced by muscles as they use energy. Levels decrease in pregnancy.[16]

Magnesium: 1.5 to 2.0 mEq/L.[6] Levels usually parallel calcium levels.[16]

Uric acid: 2.5 to 7.5 mg/dL.[6] End product of purine metabolism, which occurs with RNA and DNA synthesis. Synthesized mostly in the liver and secreted by the kidneys.[16]

Total protein: 26.3 to 8.2 g/dL.[6]

Albumin: 3.9 to 5.0 g/dL.[6] Creates the oncotic pressure of the serum. Synthesized in the liver; levels are decreased in liver disease, renal disease with proteinuria, inadequate dietary intake, and other conditions.[16] Levels decrease 20% to 50% during pregnancy.[2]

Aspartate transaminase (AST; formerly called SGOT): 8 to 39 IU/L.[6] Widely distributed in the body but especially abundant in the liver.[16] Levels undergo no significant change during pregnancy.[2]

Alanine aminotransferase (ALT; formerly called SGPT): 9 to 52 IU/L.[6] Widely distributed in the body but especially abundant in the liver because hepatocytes are the only cells with high levels.[16] Levels undergo no significant change during pregnancy.[2]

Gamma glutamyl transferase (GGT): 8 to 78 IU/L.[6] Present in large amounts in renal tubular epithelium and in the liver.[16]

Creatinine clearance (24-hour collection): Analyzes serum creatinine and creatinine excreted in 24 hr. Levels fluctuate little except in the case of a large crushing injury or degenerative disease because tubular secretion compensates for alterations in blood flow. It may be used, therefore, to judge the accuracy of subsequent 24-hr urine collections for other measures. Variation in the value is a good test of renal function because the serum quantity is so uniform. Reported as milliliters per minute per 1.73 square meters body surface area. Formula[16]:

$$\text{Creatinine clearance} = \frac{98-16([age-20]/20)}{\text{Plasma creatinine}} = \underline{\hspace{1cm}} \text{ mL/min}$$

OR

$$\frac{140-age \times 0.85}{\text{Serum creatinine}} = \underline{\hspace{1cm}} \text{ mL/min}$$

Normal range for women is 75 to 115 mL/min.[6]

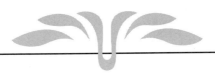

Appendix References

1. American College of Obstetrics and Gynecology (ACOG): Premature rupture of membranes, *Int J Gynecol Obstet* 63:75-84, 1998.
2. Burrow GN, Ferris TF: *Medical complications during pregnancy*, Philadelphia, 1995, WB Saunders.
3. Carter JP, Furman T, Hutcheson HR: Preeclampsia and reproductive performance in a community of vegans, *South Med J* 80:692-697, 1987.
4. Centers for Disease Control and Prevention: Recommendations to prevent and control iron deficiency in the United States, *MMWR* 47:1-29, 1998.
5. Gabbe SG, Niebyl JR, Simpson JL, editors: *Obstetrics: normal & problem pregnancies*, 3 ed, New York, 1996, Churchill Livingstone.
6. Gordon JD et al: *Obstetrics gynecology & infertility*, Glen Cove, NY, 1998, Scrub Hill Press.
7. Graves BW, Barker MK: A "conservative" approach to iron supplementation during pregnancy, *J Midwifery Womens Health* 46:156-166, 2001.
8. Hally SS: Nutrition in reproductive health, *J Nurse Midwifery* 43:459-470, 1998.
9. Kilpatrick SJ: Therapeutic interventions for oligohydramnios: amnioinfusion and maternal hydration, *Clin Obstet Gynecol* 40:328-336, June 1997.
10. Kolasa KM, Weismiller DG: Nutrition during pregnancy, *Am Fam Physician* 56:1205-1212, 1995.
11. Medina IM: *Issues in women's health care: nutrition and herbs from menarche to menopause*, course syllabus 3/28-29/98, State University of New York Health Science Center at Brooklyn College of Health Related Professions Midwifery Education Program.
12. Mercer BM: Management of preterm premature rupture of the membranes, *Clin Obstet Gynecol* 41:870-882, 1998.
13. Murray M: *Antepartal and intrapartal fetal monitoring*, 2 ed, Albuquerque, NM, 1997, Learning Resources International.
14. Parilla BV, McDermott TM: Prophylactic amnioinfusion in pregnancies complicated by chorioamnionitis: a prospective randomized trial, *Am J Perinatol* 15:649-652, 1998.
15. Reifsnider E, Gill SL: Nutrition for the childbearing year, *J Obstet Gynecol Neonatal Nurs* 29:43-55, 2000.
16. Sacher RA, McPherson RA: Widmann's clinical interpretation of laboratory tests, 10 ed, Philadelphia, 1991, FA Davis.
17. Steer P, Flint C: Preterm labour and premature rupture of the membranes, *BMJ* 318:1059-1062, 1999.
18. Weismiller DG: Transcervical amnioinfusion, *Am Fam Physician* 57:504-510, 1998.
19. Wenstrom K, Andrews WW, Maher JE: Amnioinfusion survey: prevalence, protocols, and complications, *Obstet Gynecol* 86:572-576, 1995.
20. Worthington-Roberts BS, Williams SR: *Nutrition and lactation*, 6 ed, Madison, Wis, 1997, Brown & Benchmark.

Index

Page numbers followed by f indicate
figures; t, tables; b, boxes.

595

KEEP UP-TO-DATE WITH THE AUTHORITATIVE RESOURCE FOR YOUR PROFESSION:

JOURNAL OF MIDWIFERY & WOMEN'S HEALTH
The Official Journal of the American College of Nurse-Midwives

Journal of Midwifery & Women's Health (JMWH) publishes peer-reviewed, clinically oriented, original articles pertinent to women's health in a variety of practice settings. The journal's focus is on current research and new knowledge in maternal-child health, well-woman gynecology, primary health care, family planning, and health care policy. **JMWH** provides a forum for interdisciplinary exchange across a broad range of women's health issues.

RESERVE YOUR FREE TRIAL ISSUE TODAY! TRY IT FREE FOR 30 DAYS WITH OUR MONEY BACK GUARANTEE. SEE ORDER FORM FOR DETAILS…

If you decide to subscribe to **JMWH**, you will also receive **JMWH ONLINE** at no additional cost.

Visit www.jmwh.org.

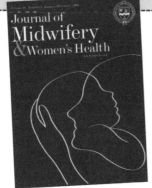

☑**YES!** Please send me my FREE trial issue of **Journal of Midwifery & Women's Health (JMWH)**, Volume 48.

After I receive my first issue, I will receive an invoice. If I choose to subscribe, I will return the invoice with a payment of $123.00 (US individuals) to continue my bimonthly subscription for a full year, including full-text online access. If not, I will write "cancel" on the invoice, return it, and owe nothing. The first issue is mine to keep.

Method of Payment
☐ Check enclosed
☐ Credit Card
☐ Bill Me

Credit card # _____

Exp. date _____

Signature _____

NAME _____

ADDRESS _____

CITY _____

STATE/ZIP _____

PHONE _____

E-MAIL _____

© 2003 Elsevier. Printed in USA. Offer valid in USA only. Prices subject to change without notice. **MO7087 DD8287**

JOURNAL OF MIDWIFERY & WOMEN'S HEALTH

The Official Journal of the American College of Nurse-Midwives

JMWH Online includes the text, photographs, illustrations, and tables from each article, with high-resolution detail in formats that download rapidly. Click on a reference and you will go to that reference. Click again and link to MEDLINE to view the abstract of that reference.

Visit www.jmwh.org.

NO POSTAGE
NECESSARY
IF MAILED
IN THE
UNITED STATES

BUSINESS REPLY MAIL

FIRST-CLASS MAIL   PERMIT NO. 7135   ORLANDO FL

POSTAGE WILL BE PAID BY ADDRESSEE

PERIODICALS ORDER FULFILLMENT DEPT
ELSEVIER SCIENCE
6277 SEA HARBOR DR
ORLANDO, FL 32821-9802